GASTRIC CARCINOMA - MOLECULAR ASPECTS AND CURRENT ADVANCES

Edited by **Mahmoud Lotfy**

Gastric Carcinoma - Molecular Aspects and Current Advances
Edited by Mahmoud Lotfy

Published by InTech

Janeza Trdine 9, 51000 Rijeka, Croatia

Publishing Process Manager Davor Vidic

Technical Editor Teodora Smiljanic

Cover Designer InTech Design Team

Additional hard copies can be obtained from orders@intechopen.com

Gastric Carcinoma - Molecular Aspects and Current Advances, Edited by Mahmoud Lotfy
p. cm.
ISBN 978-953-307-412-2

For EU product safety concerns:
IN TECH d.o.o., Prolaz Marije Krucifikse Kozulić 3, 51000 Rijeka, Croatia,
info@intechopen.com or visit our website at intechopen.com.

Meet the editor

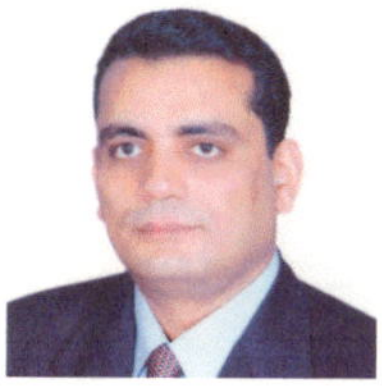

Dr. Mahmoud Lotfy began his career in a center of excellence in Egypt. It is the gastroenterology center, Mansoura University, Mansoura, Egypt. Here, Dr. Lotfy has learned the research methodologies and curricula in the Biotechnology Research Laboratories under supervision of Prof. Dr. Abdel-Fattah Attallah. Currently, Dr. Lotfy is an associate professor of molecular cell biology and immunology, molecular and cellular biology department, genetic engineering and biotechnology research institute (GEBRI) at Minufiya University, Sadat City, Minufiya, Egypt and department of applied medical sciences at Jouf University, Saudi Arabia. The research interests of Dr. Lotfy are concerned mainly with the molecular, cellular and immunologic backgrounds of the GIT diseases such as cancers, viral hepatitis and schistosomiasis. He completed and published many relevant studies. Dr. Lotfy is a reviewer in many international journals with high impact factor and his biography is included in who is who in medicine and healthcare.

Contents

Preface

Gastric cancer is one of the most common tumors worldwide. It has a heterogeneous milieu with alteration of many genes, gene products, along with gene polymorphisms. Further, the tumor immunology, oxidative stress, and microbial infections such as Helicobacter pylori and Epstein-Barr hold a vital link to gastric tumorigenesis. These diverse factors are playing a key role and have a direct impact on the prognosis of the gastric cancer and the survival of gastric cancer patients. In spite of the great advances of science, medicine and modern technology, the trend of gastric cancer in the last decades is directed toward the stability for many areas and decreasing in some other parts of world. The thankful enterprise to open more novel windows for the development of innovative therapeutic strategies against gastric cancer is greatly appreciated for scientists all over the world. This book is appropriate for scientists and students in the field of oncology, gastroenterology, molecular biology, immunology, cell biology, biology, biochemistry, pathology, and many other fields - this authoritative text carefully explains the fundamentals, providing a general overview of the principles followed by more detailed explanations of these recent topics efficiently. With its easy-to-read writing style, this book introduces in-depth coverage on such hot topics as signaling pathways, H. pylori, epigenetic and oncogenic background of gastric cancer, and recent treatment modalities. The authors are a sincere and diverse team of scientists who firmly contributed in that field. The topics presented herein contain the most recent knowledge in gastric cancer concerning the oncogenic signaling, genetic instability, the epigenetic aspect, molecular features and their clinical implications, miRNAs, integrin and E-cadherin, carbohydrate-associated-transferases, free radicals, immune cell responses, mucins, Helicobacter-pylori, neoadjuvant and adjuvant therapy, prophylactic strategy for peritoneal recurrence, and hepatic metastasis.

Our authentic gratitude is due to our brilliant authors, co-authors, reviewers, secretaries, and the publisher with his sincere team, especially Mr. Vidic. Finally, I would like to convey my faithful appreciation for the families of this wonderful team for their patient, support and encouragement. This book is dedicated faithfully to the devoted families of the authors and the amazing family of the editor, the wife, the kids (Nada, Nadeem and Nour) who all ultimately made this book possible.

Mahmoud Lotfy
Associate Professor of Molecular Cell Biology & Immunology,
Molecular and Cellular Biology Department,
Genetic Engineering and Biotechnology Research Institute,
Minufiya University, Sadat City, Minufiya, Egypt
& Department of Applied Medical Sciences,
Jouf University,
Saudi Arabia

Part 1

Molecular and Cellular Biology

1

Oncogenic Signaling in Gastric Cancer

Natália R. Costa, Andreia Sousa, Cristina Teixeira, Joana Castro, Nuno Guimarães and Filipe Santos-Silva
IPATIMUP and Faculdade de Medicina da Universidade do Porto Portugal

1. Introduction

Gastric cancer is one of the most common and life-threatening cancers worldwide (for review see Power et al., 2010). The late diagnosis and high mortality of this disease reflects the reduced understanding of its etiological factors and pathogenesis model and the lack of effective treatments. This disease results from the complex interplay between genetic and environmental factors at the gastric mucosa level that deregulates cell potentially oncogenic signaling pathways, leading to gastric cancer development. It is known that more than 80% of gastric cancer cases can be attributed to deregulation of signaling pathways caused by *Helicobacter pylori* infection (Houghton & Wang, 2005). Some of these signaling pathways are important during gastric embryogenesis and during the normal lifetime of a gastric cell, but can be tumorigenic if deregulated and therefore their better understanding is crucial for the development of new therapeutic drugs. In this review we will summarize the most important intracellular signaling pathways that have been found to be deregulated in gastric carcinoma and we will include new data recently obtained in our laboratory, focused on MUC1 mucin-mediated signaling pathways.This new information is a relevant contribution for the understanding of the gastric oncogenic signaling scenario and opens new perspectives for the development of innovative therapeutic strategies against the disease.

2. Signaling pathways involved in gastric carcinogenesis

2.1 EGFR and the extracellular signal-regulated MAPK pathway

The mitogen-activated protein kinases (MAPKs) pathway is activated either by extracellular ligand binding or intracellular stimuli, and regulates a series of cell activities such as proliferation, differentiation and cell death. The extracellular signal-regulated kinase (ERK) MAPK pathway has been often found to be deregulated in cancers and consists of several kinases (Ras, Raf, MEK) that are activated by phosphorylation upon ligand binding to a membrane receptor, ending up in the activation of several proteins involved in processes of cell invasion, apoptosis, transcription, survival and drug resistance (for review see Kim EK & Choi E, 2010). Members of this cascade have been found to be deregulated in gastric cancers, such as RAS family members (Adjei, 2001; Velho et al., 2010). Ras/MAPK activation was found to be associated with cell proliferation in gastric carcinomas (Regalo et al., 2010). ERK1/2, the final effectors of this pathway, were also found to be activated in gastric cancers (Liang et al., 2005) and in *Helicobacter pylori* related gastric cancers (Hatakeyama ,

2006; Chen et al., 2006). In contrast, ERK2 activity was found to be reduced by nonsteroidal anti-inflammatory drugs NSAIDS, therefore inhibiting the proliferation of gastric carcinoma cells (Husain et al., 2001). All of these events were found in cell lines, but when examining human gastric carcinoma specimens, a decrease in the activation of ERK1/2 was found (Wu et al., 2008). One possible explanation for this fact is that gastric cells start expressing molecules that attenuate ERK-mediated signaling upon its activation, or on the other hand, the cells act by activating negative feedback mechanisms.

The epidermal growth factor receptor (EGFR) is a member of the growth factor family HER and works as a cell surface receptor of extracellular ligands. Ligand binding to EGFR extracellular domain leads to its activation, with subsequent homodimerization, leading to the phosphorylation of its intracellular tyrosine kinase domain. This will initiate a series of intracellular signals, including activation of the central Ras/Raf/mitogen activated protein kinase (MAPK) signaling pathway (Figure 1). This molecule modulates processes of cell , migration, adhesion and proliferation and it is known to provide tumor cells with growth and survival advantages (for review see Nicholson et al., 2001). EGFR expression was found to be deregulated in several types of cancers, including gastric cancer. High EGFR levels in gastric carcinoma have been associated with the disease prognosis (Kim et al., 2008) and presence of lymph node metastasis (Choi et al., 2009). Therapies against EGFR have been developed and are active in gastric cancer treatments (Pinto et al., 2007; Liu et al., 2011), although not completely effective. The EGFR/MAPK pathway has also been shown to be activated in gastric carcinomas with microsatellite instability (Corso et al., 2011).

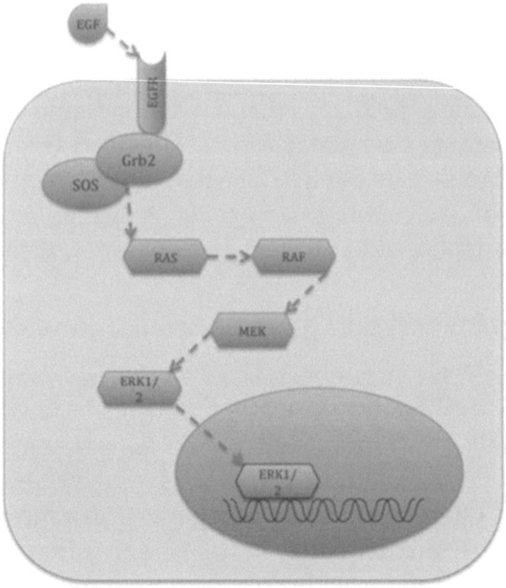

Fig. 1. EGFR/MAPK signaling pathway.

2.2 E-cadherin and Wnt/beta-catenin pathway

E-cadherin is a calcium-dependent cell-cell adhesion molecule that is essential for the maintenance of the normal epithelium architecture (for review see Van Roy & Berx , 2008). Loss of expression of this molecule has been found in gastric cancers, relating with tumor dedifferentiation, invasiveness, metastasis and prognosis (Shino et al.,1995; Gabbert et al., 1996). Mutations of this molecule have been often found in familial gastric cancers (for review see Oliveira et al., 2006). The cytoplasmic domain of this molecule interacts with the molecule beta-catenin, forming strong cohesive nets between the actin cytoskeleton (Leckband & Sivasankar, 2000), essential for processes of cell-cell adhesion and cell shape, polarity, migration and invasion.

EGFR and E-cadherin were found to interact through the respectives extracellular domains and signaling mediated by EGFR was found to be inhibited by E-cadherin (Qian et al., 2004). EGFR was found to be hyper-activated in cells where the extracellular domain of E-cadherin is not present (Bremm et al., 2008). Therefore, it may be of therapeutic value to use EGFR inhibitors in the treatment of gastric cancers in which there is a deregulation of E-cadherin.

Beta-catenin is important in mediating the E-cadherin related cell adhesion and also by participating in Wnt signaling pathways. The Wnt signaling pathway regulates several processes during development, such as determination of cell fate, morphology, polarity, adhesion and growth. Wnt signaling can be divided into canonical and non-canonical pathways. In the canonical one, wnt signals (extracellular ligands, such as wnt-1) stabilize beta catenin, therefore activating gene transcription by interaction of beta-catenin with transcriptional factors (Figure 2).

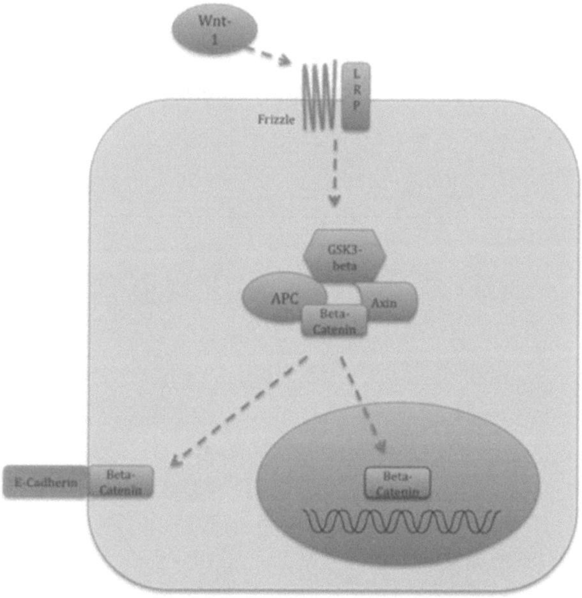

Fig. 2. Wnt signaling pathway (canonical).

This pathway was found to be deregulated in several cancers (for review see Polakis, 2007), including gastric carcinoma (Katoh et al., 2001; Clements et al., 2002; Nabais et al., 2003). The non canonical pathway is not related to beta-catenin and is involved in embryonic development and cell polarity and has also been linked to the development of gastric cancers (Kurayoshi et al., 2006; Gencer et al., 2010). This pathway seems to be repressed by Notch1 receptor in keratinocytes (Nicolas et al., 2003). Beta catenin was found to be activated by the bacterium *Helicobacter pylori* in gastric cancers (Franco et al., 2005).

In gastric cancer tissues, the expression of Wnt-1, beta-catenin and E-cadherin was found to be increased when compared to normal gastric tissue, as well as tumor size, tumor invasive depth, lymph node metastasis, pTNM stage, differentiation and five-year survival rate (Zhang & Xue , 2008). Therefore, these molecules are promising therapeutic targets for gastric carcinoma.

2.3 Hedgehog pathway

Hedgehog (Hh) signaling plays an important role during embryonic development and differentiation, proliferation and maintenance of adult tissues through the maintenance of stem cells population. Until now, three different members of the Hh family have been identified: Sonic Hedgehog (Shh), Indian Hedgehog (Ihh) and Desert Hedgehog (Dhh). All of them are secreted-type glycoproteins with a N-terminal signal peptide, a Hedgehog signaling domain and a Hint domain that signals through ligation to the hedgehog receptor Patched (Ptch), which usually acts by inhibiting the seven-span transmembrane receptor Smoothened (Smo) (Katoh and Katoh, 2005).

Of all Hh members, Shh is the most studied signaling pathway in vertebrates and plays a crucial role in stomach development. Shh protein expression is increased in parietal cells of the normal adult, gastric corpus and antrum (Saqui-Salces and Merchant, 2010). It is believed that Shh is important for regulation of gastric epithelial differentiation and its silencing causes gastric atrophy and subsequent disruption of glandular differentiation (Van den Brink, 2007). Recently, with the development of a mouse model expressing a parietal cell-specific Shh deletion, the function of this protein in adult stomach has been better clarified (Xiao et al., 2010).

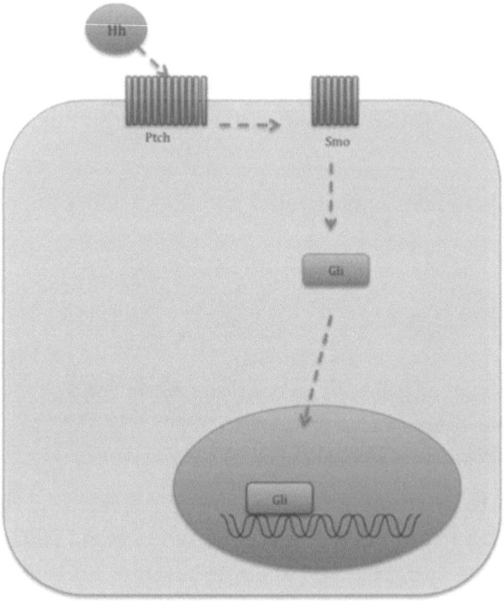

Fig. 3. Human Hedgehog signaling pathway.

Shh ligand is expressed as a 45-kDa precursor that is cleaved autocatalytically to yield a 19kDa amino terminal fragment, that contains all the signaling functions and a 26-kDa carboxy-terminal fragment (ShhC), that acts as a cholesterol transferase (Goetz et al., 2006; Zavros et al., 2007). This activation process depends on the acid-activated protease pepsin A. Gastrin increases acid secretion in parietal cells leading to conversion of pepsinogen A to pepsin A, mediating Shh processing (Zavros et al., 2007). In the stomach, Shh binds directly to Ptch receptor but not to Smo being the activity of Smo controlled indirectly by Ptch (Figure 3). In Shh absence Ptch supresses Smo activity. The binding of Shh to Ptch results in loss of Ptc activity and consequently Smo activation. Smo activation triggers Hh signal into the cytoplasm by triggering activation of Glioblastoma family transcription factors (Gli1, Gli2 and Gli3) that induce transcription of signaling targets like Wnt and the zinc finger transcription factor, Snail (Martin et al., 2010). Gli 1 induces the transcription of Snail that inhibits E-cadherin transcription. The inhibition of E-cadherin, a protein that plays an important role in cell adhesion, is associated with an increase in nuclear beta-catenin, triggering the activation of Wnt pathway targets like CD44, c-Myc and cyclin D1 (Li et al., 2006; Medici et al., 2008; Tanaka et al., 2002).

Alterations in Hh signaling pathway activation are related to different types of cancer such as gastric cancer, breast cancer, small-cell lung cancer, skin and pancreatic cancer (Kubo et al., 2004; Thayer et al., 2003; Watkins et al., 2003; Yang et al., 2010). The expression of Hh ligands, Ptch1, Smo and the three Gli transcription factors (Gli1, Gli2 and Gli3) has been related with more than two-thirds of primary gastric cancers and correlated with poorly differentiated and more aggressive tumors (Fukaya et al., 2006; Lee et al., 2007). Hh signaling activation is triggered by expression of hedgehog ligands like Shh and Ihh or an increased Ptch receptor expression (Wu et al., 2010; Zavros, 2008). Inhibition of Shh signaling pathway using Smo or antagonists like cyclopamine or Hedgehog neutralizing antibody 5E1 causes growth inhibition and regression of xenograft tumors in vivo (Berman et al., 2003). However, in the presence of precancerous lesions such as gastric atrophy (loss of parietal cells) or intestinal metaplasia, Shh protein expression is reduced or totally lost (Shiotani et al., 2005; Suzuki et al., 2005; van den Brink et al., 2001). This observation is associated with *Helicobacter pylori* infection, which is directly linked to the development of gastric cancer (Correa et al., 1975; Uemura et al., 2001). Taken together, these evidences may indicate that the inactivation of Hh signaling mediates in part the precancerous tissue alterations induced by *Helicobacter pylori* infection while its re-activation confers survival advantages in later stages of gastric carcinogenesis.

2.4 Notch pathway

Notch signaling pathway is evolutionary conserved and plays a role in many important and fundamental processes in cell and tissues such as proliferation, differentiation, apoptosis, cell fate determination, and maintenance of stem cells (Koch and Radtke, 2007; Leong and Karsan, 2006; Radtke and Raj, 2003). Notch signaling is activated during cell-to-cell contact through four receptors (Notch1-4) that can interact with ligands of the Delta (Dll-1, Dll-3, Dll-4) and Jagged (Jagged-1 and Jagged-2) family (Bray, 2006). Notch-ligand binding induces the cleavage of Notch receptor through a cascade of proteolytic cleavages by the metalloprotease tumor necrosis factor-α-converting enzyme (TACE) and γ-secretase, releasing the intracellular domain of Notch (NICD) (Katoh, 2007a; Wang et al., 2009). The NICD is translocated into the nucleus to associate with CSL transcription factor triggering the activation of Notch target genes (Androutsellis-Theotokis et al., 2006; Miele, 2006). Until now, few Notch target genes have been identified in different cellular and developmental contexts (Borggrefe and Oswald, 2009), such as Hes-1 (Hairy enhance of split-1), Cyclin D1, Nuclear factor-κB (NF-κB) and c-myc (Miele, 2006) (Figure 4).

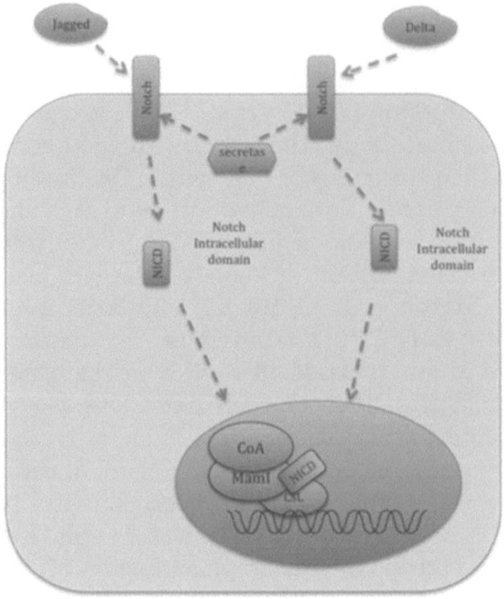

Fig. 4. Notch signaling pathway.

Recently, it has been described an association between Notch signaling and progression of gastric cancer. Three Notch receptors (Notch1-Notch3) and Notch ligand Jagged1 are expressed in human gastric cancer (Katoh, 2006; Sander and Powell, 2004; Sekine et al., 2006) and Notch signaling pathway is activated after infection with *Helicobacter pylori* in gastric cancer (Katoh, 2007b). Gastric cancer patients with Jagged1 expression in tumor tissues have more aggressive tumors and poor survival, suggesting an important role of this pathway in gastric cancer progression (Yeh et al., 2009). This aggressiveness seems to be correlated with the interaction between Notch signaling pathway and COX-2, an independent prognostic factor of gastric cancer (Shi et al., 2003). Notch signaling induces Cox-2 expression by directly binding to it through the intracellular domain of Notch1 receptor producing a stimulatory effect on cancer growth and invasion (Yeh et al., 2009). Nuclear factor-κB is also involved in Notch signaling and mediates COX-2 expression to regulate cell proliferation of human gastric cancer cells (Espinosa et al., 2003). Therefore, COX-2 inhibitors may be a new strategy to be used for treatment of gastric cancer in the future.

Twist, another transcription factor regulated by Notch signaling, was also shown to regulate cell motility and invasion in gastric cancer cell lines, probably through N-cadherin and fibronectin (Yang et al., 2007). Possibly, these EMT mediators induced by NICD could lead to an increased expression of COX-2. Whether N1ICD induces expression of COX-2 to modulate metastasis in gastric cancer through EMT mediators remains unknown.

Furthermore, activation of Notch signal pathway is involved in epithelial-mesenchymal transition (EMT), during development and tumorigenesis. Notch signaling increases Snail-1 expression and elevates EMT in cardiac development, kidney tubular cell differentiation, and hypoxia (Sahlgren et al., 2008; Timmerman et al., 2004; Zavadil et al., 2004). The Jagged1-activated Notch signaling also promotes EMT through E-cadherin repression by Slug (Leong et al., 2007). Jagged1 and Hey1, a target gene of Notch signal pathway, are also involved in mediating transforming growth factor-β–induced EMT (Zavadil et al., 2004). All these findings together indicate that Notch signaling plays a multitude of important roles in gastric carcinogenesis.

2.5 COX-2/PGE2 pathway

The regular use of nonsteroidal anti-inflammatory drugs (NSAIDs) is associated with a reduced risk of cancer development in the gastrointestinal tract (Thun et al., 1993; Farrow et al., 1998; Oshima et al., 2009). The major target of NSAIDs is cyclooxygenases (COXs), such as COX-2, which is a rate-limiting enzyme responsible for the conversion of arachidonic acid to prostaglandins (PGs) (Chan et al., 2007; Williams et al., 1999). The anticancer effect of these agents is thought to be caused by the inhibition of COX-2 and, consequently the reduction of PG synthesis (Wu et al., 2010). Regular use of NSAIDs is associated with a decreased incidence of gastric cancer (Oshima et al., 2009, as cited in Thun et al, 1993; Zaridze et al., 1999).

The over-expression of COX-2 was reported in several common human malignancies, such as in lung, colon, pancreas, bladder, head and neck cancers, being its main expression in gastrointestinal tract (Pereira et al., 2009, as cited by Fujimura et al., 2006 and van Rees & Ristimaki, 2001; Schuller et al., 2006). Several studies have shown that the treatment with NSAIDs or COX-2 selective inhibitors (COXIBs) suppressed chemically induced tumor formation and xenografted tumor growth, so these results show that the COX-2 pathway plays an essential role in cancer development (Oshima & Taketo, 2002; Oshima et al., 2009).

The inducible enzyme, COX-2 is responsible for catalyzing the biosynthesis of prostaglandin (PG) H2, which is further converted to PGE2 by microsomal PGE synthase-1 (mPGES-1), a PGE2 converting enzyme that is functionally coupled with COX-2 (Murakami et al., 2000; Seno et al, 2002). Cox-2-derived PGE2, a stable prostanoid synthesized by prostaglandin E synthase (PGES) can modulate inflammation (Huang & Chen, 2011, as cited in Harizi et al., 2000), relax vascular smooth muscles (Huang & Chen, 2011, as cited in Smyth et al., 2009) and act as a promoter of cancer progression (Huang & Chen, 2011, as cited in Iniguez, 2008). This molecule also has the ability to stimulate tumor-associated angiogenesis (formation of new blood vessels that supply oxygen and nutrients), promote cellular proliferation, inhibit apoptosis and enhance cellular invasiveness, facilitating the progression of cancers (Gross et al, 2005). Among the COX-2 downstream prostanoids, PGE2 is the one that is better studied, concerning its potential role in tumor progression (Huang & Chen, 2011) and mediates most, if not all, of the oncogenic effect of COX-2 in gastric cancer (Muller-Decker & Furstenberger, 2007). Such as for COX-2, an up-regulation of PGE2 in most of the gastrointestinal cancers also occurs (Huang & Chen, 2011). Therefore, it is crucial for gastric carcinogenesis an increased level of PGE2 through the induction of COX-2 and mPGES-1. Simultaneous induction of COX-2 and mPGES-1 is observed in gastric cancer tissues, which suggests the induction of PGE2 pathway in gastric tumors (Oshima et al., 2006). Several studies using mouse models have elucidated the roles of the PGE2 pathway in gastric tumorigenesis in the Wnt-activated and BMP-suppressed gastric mucosa (Oshima et al., 2009).

It is known that *Helicobacter pylori* infection causes chronic gastritis, as well as an over-expression of COX-2 and mPGES-1(Oshima et al., 2009). Concordantly, after eradication of *H. pylori*, COX-2 expression is suppressed (McCarthy et al., 1999), with correlation with decreased levels of mPGES-1, indicating that *H. pylori* infection induces the PGE2 pathway through induction of both COX-2 and mPGES-1. Several studies have found over-expression of COX-2 in gastric precancerous lesions and in gastric cancer (Tatsuguchi et al., 2000; Wambura et al., 2002). The molecular mechanism for COX-2 induction in tumors has not been totally elucidated, however there is a possibility that *H. pylori* can stimulate Toll-like receptors (TLRs) leading to the activation of the nuclear factor-κB (NF-κB) pathway that in turn induces the expression of COX-2. Another possibility is that the cytokine network can be activated by infection and, as a result, an induction of COX-2 expression occurs (Chang et al., 2004; Smith et al., 2003). Transgenic mice over-expressing COX-2 and mPGES-1 simultaneously develop intestinal metaplasia and hyperplastic tumors in the glandular stomach, which is associated with macrophage infiltration, so these results suggest that increased levels of PGE2 enhance infiltration of macrophages, whose activation by *H. pylori* may enhance gastric carcinogenesis (Oshima et al., 2004; Wu et al., 2010).

2.6 NF-κB pathway

NF-κB (Nuclear Factor kappa B) is a critical regulator of genes involved in cell survival and proliferation, cellular stress response, innate immunity and inflammation (Baeuerle & Baltimore, 1996; Barnes & Karin, 1997). The NF-κB family is composed by five closely related DNA binding proteins: RelA (p65), RelB, c-Rel, NF-κB1/p50 and NF-κB2/p52, which function as various homodimers and heterodimers. All share a highly conserved domain called the Rel homology domain (RHD), responsible for their dimerization, nuclear translocation, DNA binding and also interaction with the inhibitors of NF-κB (IκBs) (Gilmore, 2006). This family can be subdivided according to differences in synthesis and C-terminal sequences. While members of the "Rel subfamily" (RelA, RelB and c-Rel) have a transactivation domain (TAD) at their C-termini and are synthesized directly as mature forms, p50 and p52 from "NF-κB subfamily" are generated from large precursor proteins, p105 and p100, respectively, by limited proteolysis or arrested translation. Although lacking a TAD, the precursors of the second subfamily contain a C-terminal with multiple copies of ankyrin repeats - ankyrin repeat domain (ARD) - the typical domain of IκBs. Characteristic NF-κB dimmers usually involve one member from each subfamily, although all NF-κB members may form various homo- or heterodimers. p50 or p52 homodimers inhibit NF-κB target gene expression due to lack of a TAD, therefore, members of the NF-κB subfamily are generally not activators of transcription but function as IκB-like inhibitors of NF-κB, except when they form heterodimers with members of the Rel subfamily, participating in target gene transactivation (Li & Verma, 2002).

NF-κB is essencial in cellular response regulation being an example of transcription factors that are present in cells in an inactive state and do not require new protein synthesis to be activated. The activation of NF-κB requires phosphorylation of IκBs, resulting in their ubiquitin-dependent degradation. Therefore, NF-κB can enter the nucleus and activate the genes in response to certain stimuli, including reactive oxygen species (ROS), tumor necrosis factor alpha (TNFα), interleukin 1-beta (IL-1β) and bacterial lipopolysaccharides (LPS) - a component of the outer membrane of Gram-negative bacteria including *H. pylori* (Thanos & Maniatis, 1995). In unstimulated cells, the NF-κB dimers are sequestered in the cytoplasm by IκBs. There are two pathways leading to NF-κB activation: the canonical/classical and non-canonical/alternative. The canonical pathway can be activated by several stimuli including inflammation cytokines and antigens that induce the phosphorylation and activation of an IκB kinase (IKK) complex, consisting of catalytic kinase subunits (IKKα and/or IKKβ) and a scaffold, sensing protein termed NF-κB essential modulator (NEMO). The activated IKK promotes phosphorylation of IκBα and its ubiquitin-dependent degradation by the proteasome. The released NF-κB is able to enter the nucleus and regulate the expression of a wide range of genes including activation of its own repressor, IκBα (Nelson et al., 2004) (Figure 5).

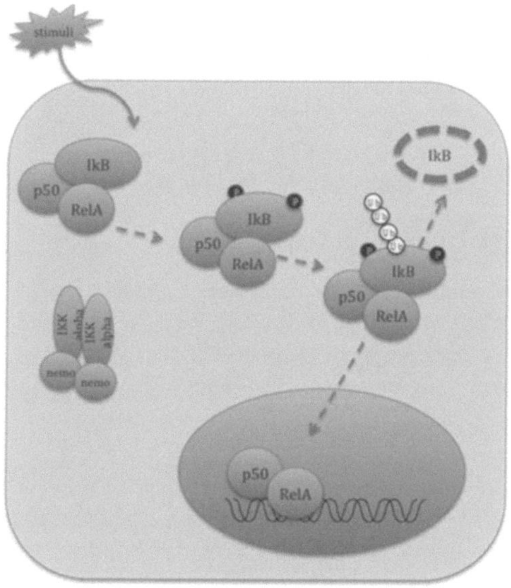

Fig. 5. NF-kB signaling pathway (canonical activation).

The non-canonical pathway is induced by certain receptor signals like B-cell activating factor (BAFF), Lymphotoxin β (LTβ), CD40 ligand, TNF-like weak inducer of apoptosis (TWEAK) and receptor activator of NF-κB ligand (RANKL) (Xiao et al., 2006). It is a slow process that depends on NF-κB-inducing kinase (NIK) protein synthesis. Despite the fact that its mRNA expression is abundant, protein levels are usually low due to its constitutive degradation by a TRAF3-dependent mechanism (Qing et al., 2005). When non-canonical NF-κB stimuli occur, the key components of this mechanism are degraded by the proteasome and NIK is activated and then able to activate an IKKα complex (an homodimer lacking NEMO), that consequentially phosphorylates p100, leading to its partial proteolysis (in the proteasome) and formation of p52. The p52/RelB complex then translocates into the nucleus to modulate gene expression (Zarnegar et al., 2008) (Figure 6).

There is evidence that NF-κB is constitutively activated in gastric cancer tissues, with higher levels in gastric carcinoma cells in comparison to normal adjacent epithelial cells (Sasaki et al., 2001) although it is RelA and not NF-κB that is used as a prognostic indicator of gastric carcinoma. It has also been reported that patients with highly activated NF-κB levels in cancer cells would have a lower survival potential when compared to those with low NF-κB activation (Yamanaka et al., 2004). In gastric cancer, abnormal NF-κB activation has been shown to lead to enhanced proliferation, evasion of apoptosis, genomic instability, increased rate of glycolysis and drug resistance (Cho et al., 2008; Kang et al., 2008; X. Liu et al., 2010).

Regarding drug resistance, a study has been performed in order to evaluate the effect of 5-Fluorouracil (5-FU) and irinotecan (CPT-11) in NF-κB activation. It led to the conclusion that these components are inducing two different pathways: apoptosis through direct effect on nucleic acids, and inhibition of apoptosis through activation of NF-κB. Moreover, the same authors used an inhibitor of NF-κB and predicted that its combination with 5-FU and CPT-11 may be a more effective treatment option instead of chemotherapy alone for gastric cancer (Camp et al., 2004).

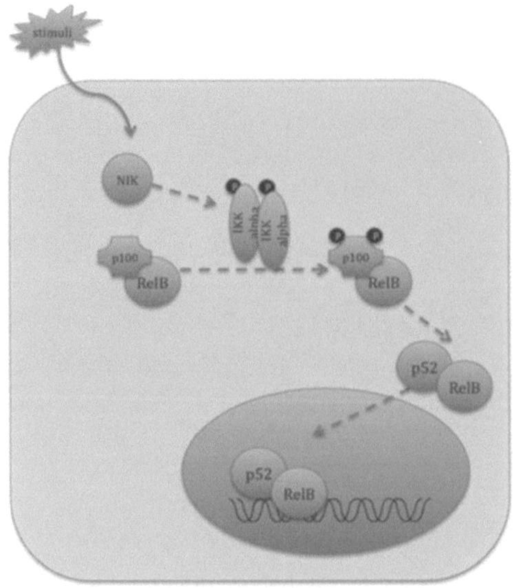

Fig. 6. NF-kB signaling pathway (non-canonical activation).

Since the discovery that blocking NF-κB can cause tumor cells to stop proliferating, to die, or enhance their sensitivity to the action of anti-tumor agents NF-κB has been widely used as a target for anti-cancer therapy (Escarcega et al., 2007). HIF-1α, one of the components of hypoxia-inducible factor 1 (HIF-1), has been directly implicated in tumorigenesis including angiogenesis, tumor cell proliferation, metastasis, as well as chemo- and radiotherapy response, particularly in gastric cancer (Liu et al., 2008; Weidemann & Johnson, 2008). Interestingly, a recent study showed that NF-κB inhibition in gastric cancer suppressed hypoxia-induced HIF-1α protein expression (but not at the mRNA level), suggesting that this protein is a downstream molecule of NF-κB in the angiogenesis pathway in gastric cancer. Also, NF-κB seems to be activated by hypoxia leading to HIF-1α protein accumulation at the translational level, but not at the transcriptional or post-translational levels. Thus, NF-κB/HIF-1α pathway may be a fitter candidate target for inhibition in gastric carcinoma therapy (Nam et al., 2011).

Using a different approach, other investigators described a new mechanism in gastric tumor cells associated with NF-κB inhibition responsible for impairment of cell proliferation and induction of apoptosis of cancer cells. By blocking NF-κB (with a RelA inhibitor, SN50) they achieved an increase in p53 expression, which led to the induction of pro-apoptotic and autophagic proteins. Thus, p53 contributes to NF-κB inhibitor-induced apoptosis of cancer cells by activation of autophagic mechanisms (Zhu et al., 2011).

2.7 Transforming growth factor- β, bone morphogenic protein pathway

Transforming growth factor (TGF)-β is a multifunctional cytokine that controls differentiation, apoptosis, cell growth and immune reactions (Roberts, 2002; Shi & Massagué, 2003). TGF-β1, -β2, and -β3 are three isoforms of TGF-β that are present in mammals. In most types of cells, TGF-β is a potent growth inhibitor, so alterations on TGF-β signaling lead to tumor progression by the induction of angiogenesis, extracellular matrix accumulation and immunosuppression (Blobe et al., 2000; Derynck et al., 2001; Wakefield & Roberts, 2002).

This pathway is considered to be a tumor suppressor pathway that negatively regulates cell growth and promotes apoptosis of epithelial cells (Siegel & Massagué, 2003). In early stages of cancer, TGF- β signaling acts as a tumor-suppressor and in later stages promotes invasion and metastasis (Wu et al., 2010). TGF-β signaling pathway is composed of two distinct receptors with intrinsic serine/threonine kinase activity, TGF-β type I and type II receptors (TbRI and TbRII) and Smad proteins. The binding of TGF-β to TbRII leads to recruitment and transphosphorylation of TbRI (heteromeric complex). Cytoplasmatic Smad2 and Smad3 are then phosphorylated by activated TbRI kinase, allowing them to form a heteromeric complex with Smad4, that is translocated into the nucleus acting as transcription factors. (Massagué, 1998; Miyazono et al., 2000; Miyazono et al., 2003) (Figure 7).

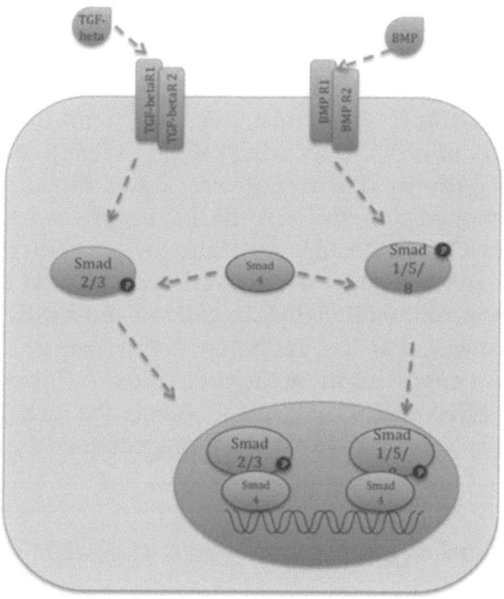

Fig. 7. Wnt signaling pathway (canonical).

Several studies demonstrated that the over-expression of TGF-β, in gastric cancer, is correlated with lymph node metastasis and poor prognosis (Maehara et al., 1999; Saito et al., 2000), as well as promotion of invasion and metastasis (via Smad3-, ERK- and JNK-dependent signal pathways) (Fu et al., 2009; Wang et al., 2006; Yoo et al., 2008). TGF-β induces RUNX3, a transcription factor that is involved in the formation of a variety of cancers (Ito, 2004). RUNX3 is expressed in glandular stomach epithelial cells, however, the loss of expression of this gene is associated with the progression, differentiation, metastasis and poor prognosis of gastric cancer (Li et al., 2002; Sugiura et al., 2008; Wei et al., 2005). Vogiatzi and colleagues (2006) demonstrated that RUNX3 interacts with FoxO3a /FKHRL1 to activate Bim and induce apoptosis in gastric cancer cells. *H. pylori* causes methylation of RUNX3 gene and its loss of expression in gastric epithelial cells (Katayama et al., 2009). Moreover, RUNX3, Smad4 inactivation has been documented in gastric cancer (Wu et al., 2010 as cited in Powell et al., 1997). Another study carried out by Shinto and colleagues (2011) demonstrated that the expression of p-Smad2 is associated with malignant phenotype and poor prognosis in patients with advanced gastric carcinoma.

Bone morphogenetic proteins (BMPs) are members of the TGF-β superfamily (von Bubnoff & Cho, 2001). They were originally identified as osteoinductive cytokines that regulate bone and cartilage formation (Balemans & Van Hul, 2002; Chen et al., 2004; Hogan, 1996). The BMPs mediate their effects by binding to type I and II serine–threonine kinase receptors (BMPR), leading to the phosphorylation of Smad1, Smad5 and Smad8. These phosphorylated Smads heterodimerize with Smad4 and this complex is translocated to the nucleus to activate the transcription of downstreams targets (Derynck et al., 1998; Kretzschmar et al., 1997; Heldin et al., 1997). Several studies have demonstrated that BMPs play important roles in the regulation of cell motility, proliferation, apoptosis, differentiation, self-renewal of embryonic stem cells and remodeling of the extracellular matrix (Hardwick et al., 2004; Hogan, 1996; Li et al., 1996; Massagué, 1996; Nissinen et al., 1997; Von Bubnoff, 2001). BMP proteins are expressed in adult stomach (Peek & Blaser, 2002; van den Brink et al., 2001).

BMP signaling in the stomach is down-regulated in cancer and upregulated during inflammation (Wu et al., 2010). *H. pylori* infection leads to an increase in BMP expression, mainly caused by an influx of BMP2-producing cells. The influx correlates with an increase in the activity of the BMP pathway (Bleumeing et al., 2006). A study carried out by Wen and colleagues (2004) demonstrated that BMP-2, a BMPR ligand, caused cell cycle arrest in the G1-phase in MKN74 and OUMS37 cells, and that this growth inhibitory action may be mediated by $p21^{Waf1/Cip1}$ (BMP-2 suppresses gastric cancer cells proliferation). Moreover, this BMP is suppressed by tumor methylation in gastric cancer cells (Wen et al., 2006). Taken together, these results suggest that the inhibition of BMP signaling contributes to gastric tumorigenesis through the suppression of differentiation. (Oshima et al., 2009). However, recent studies have discovered that BMP-2 can accelerate the migration and invasiveness of gastric cancer cells and may correlate with disease progression (Kang et al., 2010; Park et al., 2010).

3. MUC1 mucin-mediated signaling pathways in gastric cancer

The stomach is continuously subjected to a harsh acidic environment and several external aggressions. The mucus layer produced by the gastric epithelium has a crucial protective role against these adverse conditions. Three major heavily glycosylated proteins (mucins) line the stomach epithelium under normal conditions: one membrane associated mucin, MUC1, and two secreted mucins, MUC5AC and MUC6. They all contribute to the formation and maintenance of a cohesive "mucin net" that covers the entire epithelium, working as an efficient barrier. Abnormal expression and glycosylation have been described for these highly polymorphic mucins in gastric carcinoma and pre-neoplastic lesions (Reis et al., 1999; Teixeira et al., 2002). MUC1 polymorphism defines different susceptibility backgrounds associated with the development of conditions that precede gastric carcinoma: chronic atrophic gastritis and intestinal metaplasia (Silva et al., 2001).

MUC1 and MUC4 have been recently identified as participating in intracellular signaling pathways, by their cytoplasmic domains (Carraway et al., 2003; Hollingsworth and Swanson, 2004). The phosphorylation of MUC1 cytoplasmic domain (MUC1-CD) has been found to modulate its interaction with several molecules, such as EGFR, β-catenin, p53, ER-α, ICAM-1, among other molecules (for review see Singh & Hollingsworth , 2006). These interactions have been mainly found for breast, pancreatic and lung cancer cells and so far the data about MUC1-mediated signaling pathways or MUC1 signaling partners in gastric carcinoma cells is limited. MUC1-CD is known to interact with beta-catenin and upregulate the Wnt signaling pathway in CagA *Helicobacter pylori*-infected gastric carcinoma (Udhayakumar et al., 2007).

Our group has been studying the MUC1-dependent signaling pathways in gastric cancer cells. We have stably down-regulated MUC1 expression in MKN45 gastric carcinoma cell line by shRNA and we evaluated MUC1 down-regulation impact in potential MUC1-mediated signaling pathways. We observed that MUC1-downregulation leads to abnormal expression levels of ERK1/2 proteins and an increased phosphorylation of these kinases. We further characterized the association between MUC1 and ERK1/2 and we showed by proximity ligation assays that MUC1-CD directly interacts with ERK1/2 kinases in these cells. The impact of MUC1 in the transcription and stability of these kinases and the interaction with other signaling partners (e.g. EGFR) are being currently evaluated, nonethless this clearly suggests that MUC1-CD is involved at different levels in the regulation of the MAPK signaling pathway in gastric carcinoma cells (Figure 8).

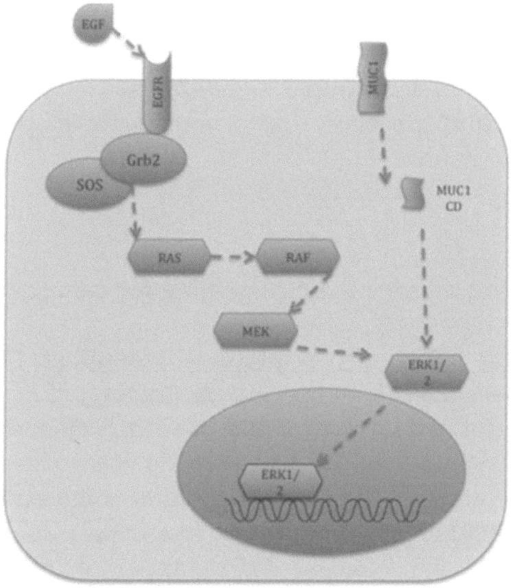

Fig. 8. MUC1 and EGFR/MAPK signaling pathway.

The kinases of EGFR/MAPK signaling pathway are crucial effectors responsible for cell proliferation and oncogenic transformation. Recent data from other tumor models further reinforce the relevance of MUC1 as a key player in cell-cell (microenvironment) signaling contexts (Behrens et al., 2010). Therefore, it assumes critical relevance an extensive characterization of MUC1-mediated signaling events in this pathway and their impact in gastric carcinoma phenotype. These results suggest MUC1 as a new and promising candidate to be targeted by therapies against gastric cancer.

4. Conclusions

Gastric cancer is a leading cause of cancer-related death worldwide. Given the limited options currently available for gastric cancer therapy and prevention, it becomes urgent to better understand the oncogenic signaling pathways beyond the emergence of the disease.

There is an increased knowledge about the alterations occurring in multiple signaling pathways and the acquisition of gastric cancer phenotype. The complex interplay between environmental factors and oncogenic signaling pathways involving cell proliferation, differentiation, apoptosis and invasion, remains however elusive. Emerging evidence in other models has brought new evidences on the complex interaction among different oncogenic signaling pathways. Whether such phenomena occur in gastric cancer, remains unclear.

The elucidation of individual interactions is thus required to develop a more consistent understanding of the gastric oncogenic signaling networks and will help to identify novel targets for anticancer drug development. The reviewed signaling pathways are relevant contributors for gastric carcinogenesis and encompass a multitude of potential therapeutic targets. In addition to these signaling-related targets we included new data on MUC1 mucin, previously described as being involved in gastric cancer susceptibility phenotype. The characterization of the complete spectrum of MUC1-dependent oncogenic signaling interactions in gastric cancer cells, will offer the molecular basis for the development of innovative therapies using MUC1 as an elective target. Furthermore an integrative perspective, of these MUC1-mediated signaling pathways, will be critical to design therapeutic strategies that inhibit multiple signaling pathways enhancing the efficacy of gastric cancer therapies and probably prevent the development of drug resistance phenotype.

5. References

Adjei, A. A. (2001). Blocking oncogenic Ras signaling for cancer therapy. *J Natl Cancer Inst,* 93, 1062–1074.

Androutsellis-Theotokis, A., Leker, R.R., Soldner, F., Hoeppner, D.J., Ravin, R., Poser, S.W., Rueger, M.A., Bae, S.K., Kittappa, R., & McKay, R.D. (2006). Notch signalling regulates stem cell numbers in vitro and in vivo. *Nature,* 442, 823-826.

Baeuerle, P. A., & Baltimore, D. (1996). NF-kappa B: ten years after. *Cell,* 87(1), 13-20.

Balemans, W., & Van Hul, W. (2002). Extracellular regulation of BMP signaling in vertebrates: a cocktail of modulators. *Dev Biol,* 250(2), 231-250.

Barnes, P. J., & Karin, M. (1997). Nuclear factor-kappaB: a pivotal transcription factor in chronic inflammatory diseases. *N Engl J Med,* 336(15), 1066-1071.

Berman, D.M., Karhadkar, S.S., Maitra, A., Montes De Oca, R., Gerstenblith, M.R., Briggs, K., Parker, A.R., Shimada, Y., Eshleman, J.R. & Watkins, D.N. (2003). Widespread requirement for Hedgehog ligand stimulation in growth of digestive tract tumours. *Nature,* 425, 846-851.

Behrens, M.E., Grandgenett, P.M., Bailey, J.M, Singh, P.K., Yi, C.H., Yu, F. & Hollingsworth M.A. (2010). The reactive tumor microenvironment: MUC1 signaling directly reprograms transciption of CTGF. *Oncogene,* 29(42), 5667-5677.

Blobe, G.C., Schiemann, W.P., & Lodish, H.F. (2000). Role of transforming growth factor-β in human disease. *N Engl J Med,* 342(3), 1350-1358.

Borggrefe, T., & Oswald, F. (2009). The Notch signaling pathway: transcriptional regulation at Notch target genes. *Cell Mol Life Sci,* 66, 1631-1646.

Bray, S.J. (2006). Notch signalling: a simple pathway becomes complex. *Nat Rev Mol Cell Biol,* 7, 678-689.

Bremm, A., Walch, A., Fuchs, M., Mages, J., Duyster, J., Keller, G., Hermannstädter, C., Becker, K.F., Rauser, S., Langer, R., von Weyhern, C.H., Höfler, H., & Luber, B. (2008). Enhanced activation of epidermal growth factor receptor caused by tumor-derived E-cadherin mutations. *Cancer Res,* 68(3),707-14.

Camp, E. R., Li, J., Minnich, D. J., Brank, A., Moldawer, L. L., MacKay, S. L., & Hochwald, S. N. (2004). Inducible nuclear factor-kappaB activation contributes to chemotherapy resistance in gastric cancer. *J Am Coll Surg,* 199(2), 249-258.

Carraway, K.L., Ramsauer, V.P., Haq, B., & Carothers Carraway, C.A. (2003). Cell signaling through membrane mucins. *Bioessays,* 25(1), 66-71.

Chan, A.T., Ogino, S. & Fuchs, C.S. (2007). Aspirin and the risk of colorectal cancer in relation to the expression of COX-2. *N Engl J Med,* 356(21), 2131-2142.

Chang, Y.J., Wu, M.S., Lin, J.T., Sheu, B.S., Muta, T., Inoue, H., & Chen, C. C. (2004). Induction of cyclooxygenase-2 overexpression in human gastric epithelial cells by Helicobacter pylori involves TLR2/TLR9 and c-Src-dependent nuclear factor-κB activation. *Mol Pharmacol,* 66(6), 1465-77.

Chen, D., Zhao, M., & Mundy, G.R. (2004). Bone morphogenetic proteins. *Growth factors,* 22(4), 233-241.

Chen, Y.C., Wang, Y., Li, J.Y., Xu, W.R., & Zhang, Y.L. (2006). H. pylori stimulates proliferation of gastric cancer cells through activating mitogen-activated protein kinase cascade. *World J Gastroenterol,* 12(37), 5972-7.

Cho, S. J., Park, J. W., Kang, J. S., Kim, W. H., Juhnn, Y. S., Lee, J. S., Kim, Y. H., Ko, Y. S., Nam, S. Y., & Lee, B. L. (2008). Nuclear factor-kappaB dependency of doxorubicin sensitivity in gastric cancer cells is determined by manganese superoxide dismutase expression. *Cancer Sci,* 99(6), 1117-1124.

Choi, J.S., Kim, M.A., Lee, H.E., Lee, H.S., & Kim W.H. (2009). Mucinous gastric carcinomas: clinicopathologic and molecular analyses. *Cancer,* 115(15),3581-90.

Clements, W.M., Wang, J., Sarnaik, A., Kim, O.J., MacDonald, .J, Fenoglio-Preiser, C., Groden, J., & Lowy, A.M.(2002). Beta-Catenin mutation is a frequent cause of Wnt pathway activation in gastric cancer. *Cancer Res,* 62(12),3503-6.

Correa, P., Haenszel, W., Cuello, C., Tannenbaum, S., & Archer, M. (1975). A model for gastric cancer epidemiology. *Lancet,* 2, 58-60.

Corso, G., Velho, S., Paredes, J., Pedrazzani, C., Martins, D., Milanezi, F., Pascale, V., Vindigni, C., Pinheiro, H., Leite, M., Marrelli, D., Sousa, S., Carneiro, F., Oliveira, C., Roviello, F., & Seruca, R. (2011). Oncogenic mutations in gastric cancer with microsatellite instability. *Eur J Cancer,* 47(3),443-51.

Derynck, R., Zhang, Y., & Feng, X.H. (1998). Smads: transcriptional activators of TGF-beta responses. *Cell,* 95(6), 737-40.

Derynck, R., Akhurst, R.J., & Balmain, A. (2001). TGF-β signaling in tumor suppression and cancer progression. *Nat Genet,* 29(2), 117-129.

Escarcega, R. O., Fuentes-Alexandro, S., Garcia-Carrasco, M., Gatica, A., & Zamora, A. (2007). The transcription factor nuclear factor-kappa B and cancer. *Clin Oncol (R Coll Radiol),* 19(2), 154-161.

Espinosa, L., Ingles-Esteve, J., Robert-Moreno, A., & Bigas, A. (2003). IkappaBalpha and p65 regulate the cytoplasmic shuttling of nuclear corepressors: cross-talk between Notch and NFkappaB pathways. *Mol Biol Cell,* 14, 491-502.

Farrow, D.C., Vaughan, T.L., Hansten, P.D., Stanford, J.L., Risch, H.A., Gammon, M.D., Chow, W.-H., Dubrow, R., Ahsan, H., Mayne, S.T., Schoenberg, J.B., West, A.B., Rotterdam, H., & Fraumeni, Jr. JF, Blot WJ (1998). Use of aspirin and other nonsteroidal anti-inflammatory drugs and risk of esophageal and gastric cancer. *Cancer Epidemiol Biomarkers Prev,* 7, 97-102.

Franco, A. T., Israel, D. A., Washington, M. K., Krishna, U., Fox, J. G., Rogers, A. B., Neish, A. S., Collier-Hyams, L., Perez-Perez, G. I., Hatakeyama, M., Whitehead, R., Gaus, K., O'Brien, D.P., Romero-Gallo, J., & Peek, R.M. Jr. (2005). Activation of beta-catenin by carcinogenic Helicobacter pylori. *Proc Natl Acad Sci USA,* 102, 10646-10651.

Fu, H., Hu, Z., Wen, J., Wang, K., & Liu, Y. (2009). TGF-beta promotes invasion and metastasis of gastric cancer cells by increasing fascin1 expression via ERK and JNK signal pathways. *Acta Biochim Biophys Sin* (Shanghai), 41(8), 648-656.

Fukaya, M., Isohata, N., Ohta, H., Aoyagi, K., Ochiya, T., Saeki, N., Yanagihara, K., Nakanishi, Y., Taniguchi, H., Sakamoto, H., Shimoda, T., Nimura, Y., Yoshida, T., & Sasaki, H. (2006). Hedgehog signal activation in gastric pit cell and in diffuse-type gastric cancer. *Gastroenterology,* 131, 14-29.

Gabbert, H.E., Mueller, W., Schneiders, A., Meier, S., Moll, R., Birchmeier, W., & Hommel, G. (1996). Prognostic value of E-cadherin expression in 413 gastric carcinomas. *Int J Cancer,* 69,184–9.

Gencer, S., Şen, G., Doğusoy, G., Bellı, A.K., Paksoy, M., & Yazicioğlu, M.B. (2010). β-Catenin-independent noncanonical Wnt pathway might be induced in gastric cancers. *Turk J Gastroenterol,* 21(3), 224-30.

Gilmore, T. D. (2006). Introduction to NF-kappaB: players, pathways, perspectives. *Oncogene,* 25(51), 6680-6684.

Goetz, J.A., Singh, S., Suber, L.M., Kull, F.J., & Robbins, D.J. (2006). A highly conserved amino-terminal region of sonic hedgehog is required for the formation of its freely diffusible multimeric form. *J Biol Chem,* 281, 4087-4093.

Gross, N.D., Boyle, J.O., Morrow, J.D., Williams, M.K., Moskowitz, C.S., Subbaramaiah, K., Dannenberg, A.J., & Duffield-Lillico, A.J. (2005). Levels of prostaglandin E metabolite, the major urinary metabolite of prostaglandin E2, are increased in smokers. *Clin Cancer Res,* 11(6), 6087-6093.

Hardwick, J.C., Van Den Brink, G.R., Bleuming, S.A., Ballester, I., Van Den Brande, J.M, Keller, J.J., Offerhaus, G.J., Van Deventer, S.J., & Peppelenbosch, M.P. (2004). Bone morphogenetic protein 2 is expressed by, and acts upon, mature epithelial cells in the colon. *Gastroenterology,* 126(1), 111-121.

Hatakeyama, M. (2006). The role of Helicobacter pylori CagA in gastric carcinogenesis. *Int J Hematol,* 84(4), 301-8.

Heldin, K., Miyazono, P. & ten Dijke, P. (1997). TGF-beta signaling from cell membrane to nucleus through SMAD proteins, *Nature,* 390 (6659) 465–471.

Hogan, B.L. (1996). Bone morphogenetic proteins: multifunctional regulators of vertebrate development. *Genes Dev,* 10(13), 1580-1594.

Hollingsworth, M.A., & Swanson, B. (2004). Mucins and cancer: protection and control of the cell surface. *Nat Rev Cancer,* 4(1), 45-60.

Houghton, J., & Wang, T.C. (2005). Helicobacter pylori and gastric cancer: a new paradigm for inflammation-associated epithelial cancers. *Gastroenterology,* 128, 1567–1578.

Huang, R.Y., & Chen, G.G. (2011). Cigarette smoking, cyclooxygenase-2 pathway and cancer. *Biochimica et Biophysica Acta,* 1815, 158-169.

Husain, S.S., Szabo, I.L., Pai, R., Soreghanb, B., Jones, M.K., & Tarnawskia, A.S. (2001). MAPK (ERK2) kinase—a key target for NSAIDs-induced inhibition of gastric cancer cell proliferation and growth. *Life Sciences,* 69, 3045–3054.

Ito, Y. (2004). Oncogenic potential of the RUNX gene family: 'overview'. *Oncogene,* 23(24), 4198-4208.

Kang, M. J., Ryu, B. K., Lee, M. G., Han, J., Lee, J. H., Ha, T. K., Byun, D. S., Chae, K. S., Lee, B. H., Chun, H. S., Lee, K. Y., Kim, H. J., & Chi, S. G. (2008). NF-kappaB activates transcription of the RNA-binding factor HuR, via PI3K-AKT signaling, to promote gastric tumorigenesis. *Gastroenterology,* 135(6), 2030-2042, 2042 e2031-2033.

Kang, M.H., Kim, J-S., Seo, J.E., Oh, S.C., & Yoo, Y.A. (2010). BMP2 accelerates the motility and invasiveness of gastric cancer cells via activation of the phosphatidylinositol 3-kinase (PI3K)/Akt pathway. *Exp Cell Res,* 316(1), 24-37.

Katayama, Y., Takahashi, M., & Kuwayama, H. (2009). Helicobacter pylori causes runx3 gene methylation its loss of expression in gastric epithelial cells which is mediated by nitric oxide produced by macrophages. *Biochem Biophys Res Commun,* 388(3), 496-500.

Katoh, M., Kirikoshi, H., Terasaki, H., & Shiokawa K. (2001). *WNT2B2* mRNA, Up-Regulated in Primary Gastric Cancer, Is a Positive Regulator of the WNT-b-Catenin–TCF Signaling Pathway. *Biochem Biophys Res Commun,* 289, 1093–1098

Katoh, Y., & Katoh, M. (2005). Comparative genomics on Sonic hedgehog orthologs. *Oncol Rep,* 14, 1087-1090.

Katoh, M. (2006). Notch ligand, JAG1, is evolutionarily conserved target of canonical WNT signaling pathway in progenitor cells. *Int J Mol Med,* 17, 681-685.

Katoh, M. (2007a). Notch signaling in gastrointestinal tract (review). *Int J Oncol,* 30, 247-251.

Katoh, M. (2007b). Dysregulation of stem cell signaling network due to germline mutation, SNP, Helicobacter pylori infection, epigenetic change and genetic alteration in gastric cancer. *Cancer Biol Ther,* 6, 832-839.

Kim, M.A., Lee, H.S., Lee, H.E., Jeon, Y.K., Yang, H.K., & Kim, W.H. (2008). EGFR in gastric carcinomas: prognostic significance of protein overexpression and high gene copy number. *Histopathology,* 52(6), 738-46.

Kim, E.K., & Choi, E. (2010). Pathological roles of MAPK signaling pathways in human diseases. *Biochem and Biophy Acta,* 1802, 396-405.

Koch, U., & Radtke, F. (2007). Notch and cancer: a double-edged sword. *Cell Mol Life Sci* 64, 2746-2762.

Kretzschmar, M., Liu, F., Hata, A., Doody, J., & Massagué, J. (1997). The TGF-beta family mediator Smad1 is phosphorylated directly and activated functionally by the BMP receptor kinase. *Genes Dev,* 11(8) 984-995.

Kubo, M., Nakamura, M., Tasaki, A., Yamanaka, N., Nakashima, H., Nomura, M., Kuroki, S., & Katano, M. (2004). Hedgehog signaling pathway is a new therapeutic target for patients with breast cancer. *Cancer Res,* 64, 6071-6074.

Kurayoshi, M., Oue, N., Yamamoto, H., Kishida, M., Inoue, A., Asahara, T., Yasui, W., & Kikuchi, A. (2006). Expression of Wnt-5a is correlated with aggressiveness of gastric cancer by stimulating cell migration and invasion. *Cancer Res,* 66,10439-10448.

Leckband, D., & Sivasankar, S. (2000). Mechanism of homophilic cadherin adhesion, Curr. Opin. *Cell Biol,* 12, 587–592.

Lee, S.Y., Han, H.S., Lee, K.Y., Hwang, T.S., Kim, J.H., Sung, I.K., Park, H.S., Jin, C.J., & Choi, K.W. (2007). Sonic hedgehog expression in gastric cancer and gastric adenoma. *Oncol Rep,* 17, 1051-1055.

Leong, K.G., & Karsan, A. (2006). Recent insights into the role of Notch signaling in tumorigenesis. *Blood,* 107, 2223-2233.

Leong, K.G., Niessen, K., Kulic, I., Raouf, A., Eaves, C., Pollet, I., & Karsan, A. (2007). Jagged1-mediated Notch activation induces epithelial-to-mesenchymal transition through Slug-induced repression of E-cadherin. *J Exp Med,* 204, 2935-2948.

Li, M., Eriksen, E.F., & Bunger, C. (1996). Bone morphogenetic protein-2 but not bone morphogenetic protein-4 and -6 stimulates chemotactic migration of human osteoblasts, human marrow osteoblasts, and U2-OS cells. *Bone,* 18(1), 53-57

Li, Q., & Verma, I. M. (2002). NF-kappaB regulation in the immune system. *Nat Rev Immunol,* 2(10), 725-734.

Li, Q.L., Ito, K., Sakakura, C., Fukamachi, H., Inoue, K., Chi, X.Z., Lee, K.Y., Nomura, S., Lee, C.W., Han, S.B., Kim, H.M., Kim, W.J., Yamamoto, H., Yamashita, N., Yano, T., Ikeda, T., Itohara, S., Inazawa, J., Abe, T., Hagiwara, A., Yamagishi, H., Ooe, A., Kaneda, A., Sugimura, T., Ushijima, T., Bae, S.C., & Ito, Y. (2002). Causal relationship between the loss of RUNX3 expression and gastric cancer. *Cell,* 109(1), 113-124.

Li, X., Deng, W., Nail, C.D., Bailey, S.K., Kraus, M.H., Ruppert, J.M., & Lobo-Ruppert, S.M. (2006). Snail induction is an early response to Gli1 that determines the efficiency of epithelial transformation. *Oncogene,* 25, 609-621.

Liang, B., Wang, S., Zhu, X.G., Yu, Y.X., Cui, Z.R., & Yu, Y.Z. (2005). Increased expression of mitogen-activated protein kinase and its upstream regulating signal in human gastric cancer. *World J Gastroenterol,* 11(5),623-8.

Liu, L., Ning, X., Sun, L., Zhang, H., Shi, Y., Guo, C., Han, S., Liu, J., Sun, S., Han, Z., Wu, K., & Fan, D. (2008). Hypoxia-inducible factor-1 alpha contributes to hypoxia-induced chemoresistance in gastric cancer. *Cancer Sci,* 99(1), 121-128.

Liu, X., Wang, X., Zhang, J., Lam, E. K., Shin, V. Y., Cheng, A. S., Yu, J., Chan, F. K., Sung, J. J., & Jin, H. C. (2010). Warburg effect revisited: an epigenetic link between glycolysis and gastric carcinogenesis. *Oncogene,* 29(3), 442-450.

Liu, X., Guo, W.J., Zhang, X.W., Cai, X., Tian, S., & Li, J. (2011). Cetuximab enhances the activities of irinotecan on gastric cancer cell lines through downregulating the EGFR pathway upregulated by irinotecan. *Cancer Chemother Pharmacol,* Feb 1.

Maehara, Y., Kakeji, Y., Kabashima, A., Emi, Y., Watanabe, A., Akazawa, K., Baba, H., Kohnoe, S., & Sugimachi K. (1999). Role of transforming growth factor-beta 1 in invasion and metastasis in gastric carcinoma. *J Clin Oncol,* 17(2), 607-614.

Martin, J., Donnelly, J.M., Houghton, J., & Zavros, Y. (2010). The role of sonic hedgehog reemergence during gastric cancer. *Dig Dis Sci,* 55, 1516-1524.

Massagué, J. (1996). TGF-beta signaling: receptors, transducers, and mad proteins. *Cell,* 85(7), 947-950.

Massagué, J. (1998). TGF-beta signal transduction. *Annu Rev Biochem,* 67, 753-791.

McCarthy, C.J., Crofford, L.J., Greenson, J. & Scheiman, J.M. (1999). Cyclooxygenase-2 expression in gastric antral mucosa before and after eradication of Helicobacter pylori infection. *Am J Gastroenterol,* 94, 1218–23.

Medici, D., Hay, E.D., & Olsen, B.R. (2008). Snail and Slug promote epithelial-mesenchymal transition through beta-catenin-T-cell factor-4-dependent expression of transforming growth factor-beta3. *Mol Biol Cell,* 19, 4875-4887.

Miele, L. (2006). Notch signaling. *Clin Cancer Res,* 12, 1074-1079.

Miyazono, K., ten Dijke, P., & Heldin, C.H. (2000). TGF-beta signaling by Smad proteins. *Adv Immunol,* 75(24), 115-157.

Miyazono, K., Suzuki, H., & Imamura, T. (2003). Regulation of TGF-β signaling and its roles in progression of tumors. *Cancer Sci,* 94(3), 230-4.

Muller-Decker, K., & Furstenberger, G. (2007). The cyclooxygenase-2- mediated prostaglandin signaling is causally related to epithelial carcinogenesis. *Mol Carcinogen,* 46(8), 705-710.

Murakami, M., Naraba, H., Tanioka, T. Semmyo, N., Nakatani, Y., Kojima, F., Ikeda, T., Fueki, M., Ueno, A., Oh, S., & Kudo, I. (2000). Regulation of prostaglandin E2 biosynthesis by inducible membrane-associated prostaglandin E2 synthase that acts in concert with cyclooxygenase-2. *J Biol Chem,* 275(42), 32783-32792.

Nabais, S., Machado, J.C., Lopes, C., Seruca, R., Carneiro, F., & Sobrinho-Simões, M. (2003). Patterns of beta-catenin expression in gastric carcinoma: clinicopathological relevance and mutation analysis. *Int J Surg Pathol,* 11(1),1-9.

Nam, S. Y., Ko, Y. S., Jung, J., Yoon, J., Kim, Y. H., Choi, Y. J., Park, J. W., Chang, M. S., Kim, W. H., & Lee, B. L. (2011). A hypoxia-dependent upregulation of hypoxia-inducible factor-1 by nuclear factor-kappaB promotes gastric tumour growth and angiogenesis. *Br J Cancer,* 104(1), 166-174.

Nelson, D. E., Ihekwaba, A. E., Elliott, M., Johnson, J. R., Gibney, C. A., Foreman, B. E., Nelson, G., See, V., Horton, C. A., Spiller, D. G., Edwards, S. W., McDowell, H. P., Unitt, J. F., Sullivan, E., Grimley, R., Benson, N., Broomhead, D., Kell, D. B., & White, M. R. (2004). Oscillations in NF-kappaB signaling control the dynamics of gene expression. *Science,* 306(5696), 704-708.

Nicholson, R.I., Gee, J.M., & Harper, M.E. EGFR and cancer prognosis. (2001). *Eur J Cancer,* 37 Suppl 4, S9-15.

Nicolas, M., Wolfer, A., Raj, K., Kummer, J.A., Mill, P., van Noort, M., Hui, C.C., Clevers, H., Dotto, G.P., & Radtke, F. (2003). Notch1 functions as a tumor suppressor in mouse skin. *Nat Genet,* 33, 416-421.

Nissinen, L., Pirila, L., & Heino, J. (1997). Bone morphogenetic protein-2 is a regulator of cell adhesion. *Exp Cell Res,* 230(2),377-385.

Oliveira, C., Seruca, R., & Carneiro, F. Genetics, pathology, and clinics of familial gastric cancer. (2006). *Int J Surg Pathol,* 14(1), 21-33.

Oshima, M., & Taketo, M.M. (2002). COX selectivity and animal models for colon cancer. *Curr Pharm Des,* 8(12), 1021–1034.

Oshima, H., Oshima, M., Inaba, K., & Taketo, M.M. (2004). Hyperplastic gastric tumors induced by activated macrophages in COX-2/mPGES-1 transgenic mice. *EMBO J,* 7, 23(7), 1669-1678.

Oshima, H., Matsunaga, A., Fujimura, T., Tsukamoto, T., Taketo, M.M., & Oshima, M. (2006). Carcinogenesis in Mouse Stomach by Simultaneous Activation of the Wnt Signaling and Prostaglandin E2 Pathway. *Gastroenterology*, 131(4), 1086-1095.

Oshima, H.; Oguma, K.; Du, Y.C. & Oshima, M. (2009). Prostaglandin E2, Wnt, and BMP in gastric tumor mouse models. *Cancer Sci*, 100(100), 1779-1785.

Park, Y., Kang, M.H., Seo, H.Y., Park, J.M., Choi, C.W., Kim, Y.H., Kim, I.S., Kim, J.S., & Oh, S.C. (2010). Bone morphogenetic protein-2 levels are elevated in the patients with gastric cancer and correlate with disease progression. *Med Oncol*, 27(4), 1192-1199.

Peek, R.M.Jr., & Blaser, M.J. (2002). Helicobacter pylori and gastrointestinal tract adenocarcinomas. *Nature Rev Cancer*, 2(1), 28-37.

Pereira, C., Medeiros, R.M., & Dinis-Ribeiro, M. (2009). Cyclooxygenase polymorphisms in gastric and colorectal carcinogenesis: are conclusive results available? *Eur J Gastroenterol Hepatol*, 21(1), 76-91.

Pinto, C., Di Fabio, F., Siena, S., Cascinu, S., Rojas Llimpe, F.L., Ceccarelli, C., Mutri, V., Giannetta, L., Giaquinta, S., Funaioli, C., Berardi, R., Longobardi, C., Piana, E., & Martoni, A.A. (2007). Phase II study of cetuximab in combination with FOLFIRI in patients with untreated advanced gastric or gastroesophageal junction adenocarcinoma (FOLCETUX study). *Ann Oncol*, 18, 510–517.

Polakis, P. (2007). The many ways of Wnt in cancer. *Curr Opin Gene Dev*, 17,45-51.

Power, D.G., Kelsen, D.P., & Shah, M.A. (2010). Advanced gastric cancer -Slow but steady progress. *Cancer Treat Rev*, 36, 384-392.

Qian, X., Karpova, T., Sheppard, A.M., McNally, J., & Lowy, D.R. (2004). E-cadherin-mediated adhesion inhibits ligand-dependent activation of diverse receptor tyrosine kinases. *EMBO J*, 23, 1739–1748.

Qing, G., Qu, Z., & Xiao, G. (2005). Stabilization of basally translated NF-kappaB-inducing kinase (NIK) protein functions as a molecular switch of processing of NF-kappaB2 p100. *J Biol Chem*, 280(49), 40578-40582.

Radtke, F., & Raj, K. (2003). The role of Notch in tumorigenesis: oncogene or tumour suppressor? *Nat Rev Cancer*, 3, 756-767.

Regalo, G., Resende, C., Wen, X., Gomes, B., Durães, C., Seruca, R., Carneiro, F., & Machado, J.C. (2010). C/EBP alpha expression is associated with homeostasis of the gastric epithelium and with gastric carcinogenesis. *Lab Invest*, 90(8),1132-9.

Reis, C.A., David, L., Correa, P., Carneiro, F., de Bolós, C., Garcia, E., Mandel, U., Clausen, H., & Sobrinho-Simões, M. (1999). Intestinal metaplasia of human stomach displays distinct patterns of mucin (MUC1,MUC2, MUC5AC, and MUC6) expression. *Cancer Res*, 59(5), 1003-1007.

Roberts, A.B. (2002). The ever-increasing complexity of TGF-beta signaling. *Cytokine Growth Factor Rev*, 13(1), 3-5.

Sahlgren, C., Gustafsson, M.V., Jin, S., Poellinger, L., & Lendahl, U. (2008). Notch signaling mediates hypoxia-induced tumor cell migration and invasion. *Proc Natl Acad Sci USA*, 105, 6392-6397.

Saito, H., Tsujitani, S., Oka, S., Kondo, A., Ikeguchi, M., Maeta, M., & Kaibara, N. (2000). An elevated serum level of transforming growth factor-beta 1 (TGF-beta 1) significantly correlated with lymph node metastasis and poor prognosis in patients with gastric carcinoma. *Anticancer Res*, 20(6B), 4489-4493.

Sander, G.R., & Powell, B.C. (2004). Expression of notch receptors and ligands in the adult gut. *J Histochem Cytochem*, 52, 509-516.
Saqui-Salces, M., & Merchant, J.L. (2010). Hedgehog signaling and gastrointestinal cancer. *Biochim Biophys Acta*, 1803, 786-795.
Sasaki, N., Morisaki, T., Hashizume, K., Yao, T., Tsuneyoshi, M., Noshiro, H., Nakamura, K., Yamanaka, T., Uchiyama, A., Tanaka, M., & Katano, M. (2001). Nuclear factor-kappaB p65 (RelA) transcription factor is constitutively activated in human gastric carcinoma tissue. *Clin Cancer Res*, 7(12), 4136-4142.
Schuller, H.M., Kabalka, G., Smith, G., Mereddy, A., Akula, M., & Cekanova, M. (2006) Detection of overexpressed COX-2 in precancerous lesions of hamster pancreas and lungs by molecular imaging: implications for early diagnosis and prevention. *Chem Med Chem*, 1(6), 603–610.
Sekine, A., Akiyama, Y., Yanagihara, K., & Yuasa, Y. (2006). Hath1 up-regulates gastric mucin gene expression in gastric cells. *Biochem Biophys Res Commun*, 344, 1166-1171.
Seno, H., Oshima, M., Ishikawa, T., Oshima, H., Takaku, K., Chiba, T., Narumiya, S., & Taketo, M. M. (2002). Cyclooxygenase-2 and prostaglandin E2 receptor EP2-dependent angiogenesis in Apc_716 mouse intestinal polyps. *Cancer Res*, 62(2), 506-511.
Shi, H., Xu, J.M., Hu, N.Z., & Xie, H.J. (2003). Prognostic significance of expression of cyclooxygenase-2 and vascular endothelial growth factor in human gastric carcinoma. *World J Gastroenterol*, 9, 1421-1426.
Shi, Y., & Massagué, J. (2003). Mechanisms of TGF-beta signaling from cell membrane to the nucleus. *Cell*, 113(6), 685-700.
Shino Y., Watanabe, A., Yamada, Y., Tanase, M., Yamada, T., Matsuda, M., Yamashita, J., Tatsumi, M., Miwa, T., & Nakano, H. (1995). Clinicopathologic evaluation of immunohistochemical E-cadherin expression in human gastric carcinomas. *Cancer*, 76, 2193–201.
Shinto, O., Yashiro, M., Toyokawa, T., Nishii, T., Kaizaki, R., Matsuzaki, T., Noda, S., Kubo, N., Tanaka, H., Doi, Y., Ohira, M., Muguruma, K., Sawada, T., & Hirakawa, K. (2011). Phosphorylated smad2 in advanced stage gastric carcinoma. *BMC Cancer*, 10, 652.
Shiotani, A., Iishi, H., Uedo, N., Ishiguro, S., Tatsuta, M., Nakae, Y., Kumamoto, M., & Merchant, J.L. (2005). Evidence that loss of sonic hedgehog is an indicator of Helicobater pylori-induced atrophic gastritis progressing to gastric cancer. *Am J Gastroenterol*, 100, 581-587.
Siegel, P. M. & Massagué, J. (2003). Cytostatic and apoptotic actions of TGF-β in homeostasis and cancer. *Nat Rev Cancer*, 3(11), 807-821.
Silva, F., Carvalho, F., Peixoto, A., Seixas, M., Almeida, R., Carneiro, F., Mesquita, P., Figueiredo, C., Nogueira, C., Swallow, D.M., Amorim, A., & David, L. (2001). MUC1 gene polymorphism in the gastric carcinogenesis pathway. *Eur J Hum Genet*, 9(7), 548-552.
Singh, P.K., & Hollingsworth, M.A. (2006). Cell surface-associated mucins in signal transduction. *Trends Cell Biol*, 16(9),467-76.
Smith, M.F.Jr., Mitchell, A., Li, G. Ding, G., Fitzmaurice, A.M., Ryan, K., Crowe, S., & Goldberg J.B. (2003). Toll-like receptor (TLR) 2 and TLR5, but not TLR4, are

required for Helicobacter pylori-induced NF-κB activation and chemokine expression by epithelial cells. *J Biol Chem,* 278(35), 552–60.

Sugiura, H., Ishiguro, H., Kuwabara, Y., Kimura, M., Mitsui, A., Mori, Y., Ogawa, R., Katada, T., Harata, K., & Fujii, Y. (2008). Decreased expression of RUNX3 is correlated with tumor progression and poor prognosis in patients with esophageal squamous cell carcinoma. *Oncol Rep,* 19(3), 713-719.

Suzuki, H., Minegishi, Y., Nomoto, Y., Ota, T., Masaoka, T., van den Brink, G.R., & Hibi, T. (2005). Down-regulation of a morphogen (sonic hedgehog) gradient in the gastric epithelium of Helicobacter pylori-infected Mongolian gerbils. *J Pathol,* 206, 186-197.

Tanaka, M., Kitajima, Y., Edakuni, G., Sato, S., & Miyazaki, K. (2002). Abnormal expression of E-cadherin and beta-catenin may be a molecular marker of submucosal invasion and lymph node metastasis in early gastric cancer. *Br J Surg,* 89, 236-244.

Tatsuguchi, A., Sakamoto, C., Wada, K., Akamatsu, T., Tsukui, T., Miyake, K., Futagami, S., Kishida, T., Fukuda, Y., Yamanaka, N., & Kobayashi M. (2000). Localization of cyclooxygenase-2 in Helicobacter pylori related gastritis and gastric ulcer tissue in human. *Gut,* 46(6), 782-789.

Teixeira, A., David, L., Reis, C.A., Costa, J., & Sobrinho-Simões, M. (2002). Expression of mucins (MUC1, MUC2, MUC5AC, and MUC6) and type 1 Lewis antigens in cases with and without Helicobacter pylori colonization in metaplastic glands of the human stomach. *J Pathol,* 197(1), 37-43.

Thanos, D., & Maniatis, T. (1995). NF-kappa B: a lesson in family values. *Cell,* 80(4), 529-532.

Thayer, S.P., di Magliano, M.P., Heiser, P.W., Nielsen, C.M., Roberts, D.J., Lauwers, G.Y., Qi, Y.P., Gysin, S., Fernandez-del Castillo, C., Yajnik, V., Antoniu, B., McMahon, M., Warshaw, A.L., & Hebrok, M. (2003). Hedgehog is an early and late mediator of pancreatic cancer tumorigenesis. *Nature,* 425, 851-856.

Thun, M.J., Namboodiri, M.M., Calle, E.E., Flanders, W.D., & Heath, C.W.Jr. (1993). Aspirin use and risk of fatal cancer. *Cancer Res,* 53(6),1322-7.

Timmerman, L.A., Grego-Bessa, J., Raya, A., Bertran, E., Perez-Pomares, J.M., Diez, J., Aranda, S., Palomo, S., McCormick, F., Izpisua-Belmonte, J.C., *&* de la Pompa, J.L. (2004). Notch promotes epithelial-mesenchymal transition during cardiac development and oncogenic transformation. *Genes Dev,* 18, 99-115.

Udhayakumar G., Jayanthi V., Devaraj N., & Devaraj H. (2007). Interaction of MUC1 with beta-catenin modulates the Wnt target gene cyclinD1 in H. pylori-induced gastric cancer. *Mol Carcinog,* 46(9), 807-17.

Uemura, N., Okamoto, S., Yamamoto, S., Matsumura, N., Yamaguchi, S., Yamakido, M., Taniyama, K., Sasaki, N., & Schlemper, R.J. (2001). Helicobacter pylori infection and the development of gastric cancer. *N Engl J Med,* 345, 784-789.

Van den Brink, G.R., Hardwick, J.C., Tytgat, G.N., Brink, M.A., Ten Kate, F.J., Van Deventer, S.J., & Peppelenbosch, M.P. (2001). Sonic hedgehog regulates gastric gland morphogenesis in man and mouse. *Gastroenterology,* 121(2), 317-328.

Van den Brink, G.R. (2007). Hedgehog signaling in development and homeostasis of the gastrointestinal tract. *Physiol Rev,* 87, 1343-1375.

Van Roy, F., & Berx, G. (2008). The cell-cell adhesion molecule E-cadherin. *Cell Mol Life Sci,* 65(23), 3756-88.

Velho, S., Corso, G., Oliveira, C., & Seruca, R. (2010). KRAS signaling pathway alterations in microsatellite unstable gastrointestinal cancers. *Adv Cancer Res,* 109,123-43.

Vogiatzi, P., De Falco, G., Claudio, P.P., & Giordano, A. (2006). How does the human RUNX3 gene induce apoptosis in gastric cancer? Latest data reflections and reactions. *Cancer Biol Ther,* 5(4), 371-374.

Von Bubnoff, A., & Cho, K.W. (2001). Intracellular BMP signaling regulation in vertebrates: pathway or network? *Dev Bio,* 239(1), 1-14.

Wakefield, L.M., & Roberts, A.B. (2002). TGF-β signaling: positive and negative effects on tumorigenesis. *Curr Opin Genet Dev,* 12(1), 22-29.

Wambura, C., Aoyama, N., Shirasaka, D., Sakai, T., Ikemura, T., Sakashita, M., Maekawa, S., Kuroda, K., Inoue, T., Ebara, S., Miyamoto, M., & Kasuga, M. (2002). Effect of Helicobacter pylori-induced cyclooxygenase-2 on gastric epithelial cell kinetics: implication for gastric carcinogenesis. *Helicobacter,* 7(2), 129-138.

Wang, K.S., Hu, Z.L., Li, J.H., Xiao, D.S., & Wen, J.F. (2006). Enhancement of metastatic and invasive capacity of gastric cancer cells by transforming growth factor-b1. *Acta Biochim Biophys Sin,* 38(3), 179-186.

Wang, Z., Li, Y., Banerjee, S., & Sarkar, F.H. (2009). Emerging role of Notch in stem cells and cancer. *Cancer Lett,* 279, 8-12.

Watkins, D.N., Berman, D.M., Burkholder, S.G., Wang, B., Beachy, P.A., & Baylin, S.B. (2003). Hedgehog signalling within airway epithelial progenitors and in small-cell lung cancer. *Nature,* 422, 313-317.

Wei, D., Gong, W., Oh, S.C., Li, Q., Kim, W.D., Wang, L., Le, X., Yao, J., Wu, T.T., Huang, S., & Xie, K. (2005). Loss of RUNX3 expression significantly affects the clinical outcome of gastric cancer patients and its restoration causes drastic suppression of tumor growth and metastasis. *Cancer Res,* 65(11), 4809-4816.

Weidemann, A., & Johnson, R. S. (2008). Biology of HIF-1alpha. *Cell Death Differ,* 15(4), 621-627.

Wen, X.Z., Miyake, S., Akiyama, Y., & Yuasa, Y. (2004). BMP-2 modulates the proliferation and differentiation of normal and cancerous gastric cells. *Biochem Biophys Res Commun,* 316(1), 100-106.

Wen, X.Z., Akiyama, Y., Baylin, S., & Yuasa, Y. (2006). Frequent epigenetic silencing of the bone morphogenetic protein 2 gene through methylation in gastric carcinomas. *Oncogene,* 25(18), 2666–73.

Williams, C. S., Mann, M., & DuBois, R. N. (1999). The role of cyclooxygenases in inflammation, cancer, and development. *Oncogene,* 18(55), 7908–7916.

Wu, W.K., Sung, J.J., Yu, L., Li, Z.J., Chu, K.M., & Cho, C.H. (2008). Constitutive hypophosphorylation of extracellular signal-regulated kinases-1/2 and down-regulation of c-Jun in human gastric adenocarcinoma. *Biochem Biophys Res Commun,* 373, 330–334.

Wu, W.K., Cho, C.H., Lee, C.W., Fan, D., Wu, K., Yu, J., & Sung, J.J. (2010). Dysregulation of cellular signaling in gastric cancer. *Cancer Lett,* 295(2), 144-153.

Xiao, G., Rabson, A. B., Young, W., Qing, G., & Qu, Z. (2006). Alternative pathways of NF-kappaB activation: a double-edged sword in health and disease. *Cytokine Growth Factor Rev,* 17(4), 281-293.

Xiao, C., Ogle, S.A., Schumacher, M.A., Orr-Asman, M.A., Miller, M.L., Lertkowit, N., Varro, A., Hollande, F., & Zavros, Y. (2010). Loss of parietal cell expression of Sonic hedgehog induces hypergastrinemia and hyperproliferation of surface mucous cells. *Gastroenterology,* 138, 550-561.e8.

Yamanaka, N., Sasaki, N., Tasaki, A., Nakashima, H., Kubo, M., Morisaki, T., Noshiro, H., Yao, T., Tsuneyoshi, M., Tanaka, M., & Katano, M. (2004). Nuclear factor-kappaB p65 is a prognostic indicator in gastric carcinoma. *Anticancer Res,* 24(2C), 1071-1075.

Yang, Z., Zhang, X., Gang, H., Li, X., Li, Z., Wang, T., Han, J., Luo, T., Wen, F., & Wu, X. (2007). Up-regulation of gastric cancer cell invasion by Twist is accompanied by N-cadherin and fibronectin expression. *Biochem Biophys Res Commun,* 358, 925-930.

Yang, L., Xie, G., Fan, Q., & Xie, J. (2010). Activation of the hedgehog-signaling pathway in human cancer and the clinical implications. *Oncogene,* 29, 469-481.

Yeh, T.S., Wu, C.W., Hsu, K.W., Liao, W.J., Yang, M.C., Li, A.F., Wang, A.M., Kuo, M.L., & Chi, C.W. (2009). The activated Notch1 signal pathway is associated with gastric cancer progression through cyclooxygenase-2. *Cancer Res,* 69, 5039-5048.

Yoo, Y.A., Kang, M.H., Kim, J.S., & Oh, S.C. (2008). Sonic hedgehog signaling promotes motility and invasiveness of gastric cancer cells through TGF-beta-mediated activation of the ALK5-Smad 3 pathway. *Carcinogenesis,* 29(3), 480–490.

Zaridze, D., Borisova, E., Maximovitch, D., & Chkhikvadze, V. (1999). Aspirin protects against gastric cancer: results of a case-control study from Moscow, Russia. Int J *Cancer,* 82(4), 473–6.

Zarnegar, B., Yamazaki, S., He, J. Q., & Cheng, G. (2008). Control of canonical NF-kappaB activation through the NIK-IKK complex pathway. *Proc Natl Acad Sci USA,* 105(9), 3503-3508.

Zavadil, J., Cermak, L., Soto-Nieves, N., & Bottinger, E.P. (2004). Integration of TGF-beta/Smad and Jagged1/Notch signalling in epithelial-to-mesenchymal transition. *EMBO J,* 23, 1155-1165.

Zavros, Y., Waghray, M., Tessier, A., Bai, L., Todisco, A., D, L.G., Samuelson, L.C., Dlugosz, A., & Merchant, J.L. (2007). Reduced pepsin A processing of sonic hedgehog in parietal cells precedes gastric atrophy and transformation. *J Biol Chem,* 282, 33265-33274.

Zavros, Y. (2008). The adventures of sonic hedgehog in development and repair. IV. Sonic hedgehog processing, secretion, and function in the stomach. *Am J Physiol Gastrointest Liver Physiol,* 294, G1105-1108.

Zhang H., & Xue Y. (2008). Wnt pathway is involved in advanced gastric carcinoma. *Hepatogastroenterology,* 55(84),1126-30.

Zhu, B. S., Xing, C. G., Lin, F., Fan, X. Q., Zhao, K., & Qin, Z. H. (2011). Blocking NF-kappaB nuclear translocation leads to p53-related autophagy activation and cell apoptosis. *World J Gastroenterol,* 17(4), 478-487.

2

Genetic Instability in Gastric Cancer

Petra Hudler, Matjaz Vogelsang and Radovan Komel
University of Ljubljana, Faculty of Medicine, Institute of Biochemistry, Medical Centre for Molecular Biology and Department for Biosynthesis and Biotransformation, National Institute of Chemistry
Slovenia

1. Introduction

Gastric cancer remains a worldwide burden as a second leading cause of cancer death in both sexes (Globocan, 2011; Nobili et al., 2011). Although its incidence is in decline in developed countries, it is still the fourth most common malignancy in the world, behind cancers of the lung, breast, colon, and rectum (Globocan, 2011). The fall in its incidence is attributed mainly to the decline of the intestinal type of stomach cancer, whereas the incidence of the diffuse type has remained constant over time (Yamashita et al., 2011). On the other hand, there has been a progressive increase in the cardia and gastroesophageal junction adenocarcinoma (Milne et al., 2009; Yamashita et al., 2011). The exact cause of this shift in location is not known. The general decrease of gastric cancer frequency in developed countries is attributed to the changes in dietary habits and food preservation methods (Crew & Neugut, 2006; Kufe et al., 2003). The prevalence of gastric cancer varies throughout the world, with the highest rates reported in Korea, Japan, Central and South America, and Eastern Europe, whereas Western Europe, North America, Africa, Australia, and New Zealand are low incidence areas (Crew & Neugut, 2006; Tahara, 2008; Yamashita et al., 2011). Despite the decrease in its incidence and improvements in diagnosis, curative surgery, and treatment, gastric cancer remains major health burden due to its poor prognosis (Smith et al., 2006; Yamashita et al., 2011).

Adenocarcinoma is the major histological type of gastric cancer; accounting for 90% to 95% of all gastric malignancies, and this chapter will focus only on this type of gastric tumours (Hamilton & Meltzer, 2006). Adenocarcinoma develops from the glandular cells of stomach mucosa, while other rare stomach cancers develop in lymph tissue (lymphoma), hormone - producing cells (carcinoid tumours), muscle cells (soft tissue sarcomas) or certain nerve cells (gastrointestinal stromal tumours or GIST) (Smith et al., 2006). Based on the widely used Lauren classification, adenocarcinomas are divided into two distinct pathological entities, intestinal and diffuse types, which have different clinicopathological and prognostic features (Yamashita et al., 2011). Intestinal type is associated with *Helicobacter pylori* infection, obesity and certain dietary factors, such as high intake of salt, smoked meats and food preserved with nitrites or nitrates, and is believed to arise through a long-term multistep progression from chronic gastritis to chronic atrophy to intestinal metaplasia to dysplasia (Crew & Neugut, 2006; Hamilton & Meltzer, 2006; Yamashita et al., 2011). Histologically it is well differentiated and occurs more commonly in older patients, males and blacks (Crew & Neugut, 2006). Diffuse type is poorly differentiated with infiltrating, non-cohesive cells and is more frequent in younger patients (Crew & Neugut, 2006; Panani, 2008). Studies showed that *Helicobacter pylori* infection also plays a role in the development of diffuse gastric cancer, through chronic inflammation, but without occurrence of intermediate steps, such as gastric atrophy and intestinal metaplasia (Milne et al., 2009).

It is believed that the pathogenesis of gastric cancer represents a classic example of gene-environment interactions (Panani, 2008). Epidemiologic studies have shown a reduction of its incidence in migrant populations, when they move from high-risk areas to low-incidence ones. Subsequent populations acquire risk levels similar to those in the host country, indicating the importance of environmental influences on its development (Crew & Neugut, 2006; Matysiak-Budnik & Megraud, 2006). Therefore, it is generally acknowledged that both, environmental and genetic factors are implicated in the pathogenesis of gastric cancer development (Milne et al., 2009). Furthermore, several researchers believe that environmental factors have a greater influence on the development of intestinal type, whereas diffuse type might have a stronger genetic background (Matysiak-Budnik & Megraud, 2006; Milne et al., 2009). Nevertheless, despite tremendous efforts in the past few decades, there is still no clear agreement on the genetic and epigenetic changes underlying the initiation and progression of both types of gastric adenocarcinoma (Milne et al., 2009; Panani, 2008).

This review is intended to focus on different molecular hypotheses of gastric carcinogenesis. New advances in the fields of high-throughput methodologies, functional genomics and molecular profiling will be discussed.

2. Molecular mechanisms of gastric carcinogenesis

Numerous cytogenetic and molecular genetic studies tested common cancer hypotheses, such as oncogene overexpression, suppressor, mutator, and methylator pathway hypotheses, but exact molecular mechanisms of gastric cancer development remain elusive. In nearly two decades of research a vast amount of articles referring to overexpression and silencing of genes was published (Resende et al., 2010). Several studies reported amplification and overexpression of growth factors, growth factor receptors, tyrosine kinases, nuclear factors, matrix metalloproteinases, cell cycle regulators cytokines and other genes (Panani, 2008; Tahara, 2008; Wu et al., 2010). Furthermore, other studies have shown that loss of heterozigosity (LOH) and inactivation of tumour suppressor genes seem to be involved in the development of gastric adenocarcinomas (Gazvoda et al., 2007; Juvan et al., 2007; Panani, 2008; Resende et al., 2010). The presence of spontaneous DNA replication errors in simple repetitive microsatellite sequences indicated a novel pathway of carcinogenesis, microsatellite instability (MSI) (Loeb, 2001; Panani, 2008; Simpson et al., 2001). It was found that it could be the consequence of defective DNA mismatch repair mechanism (MMR), caused by genetic alterations in *MLH1*, *MSH2*, *PMS1*, and *PMS2* genes (Hudler et al., 2004; Loeb, 2001; Panani, 2008; Simpson et al., 2001). In recent years, epigenetic changes, such as promoter methylation, hypomethylation and histone acetylation have been also recognized in gastric carcinogenesis (Hudler et al., 2004; Mitani et al., 2005; Schneider et al., 2010; Suzuki et al., 2006; Yamamoto et al., 2011).

In the 90's a model, describing genetic events of colorectal carcinogenesis, was suggested by Fearon and Vogelstein, which has shaped our understanding of the evolution of most types of malignancies today (Fearon & Vogelstein, 1990). The so-called 'Vogelgram' predicts that alterations in at least four to five cancer-related genes (oncogenes and tumour suppressor genes) are needed for malignancy to occur, and that the total accumulation of changes rather than the order of their appearance is responsible for progression of the cancer (Fearon & Vogelstein, 1990).

Although molecular mechanisms and alterations contributing to initiation and progression of gastric tumorigenesis are still not completely understood, it is now widely accepted that it is initiated by several genetic and epigenetic alterations that result in overexpression of oncogenes and growth factors, as well as impaired expression of tumour suppressor genes. It has also become evident that alterations in genome stability genes can initiate and accelerate these neoplastic processes (Nobili et al., 2011; Oda et al., 2005; Zheng et al., 2004). It is also important to note that the prevalence of these abnormalities varies between intestinal and diffuse types of gastric cancer (Hamilton & Meltzer, 2006).

Recently, another type of genetic instability has been recognized as the most common feature of gastric cancers, namely chromosomal instability (CIN), leading to aneuploidy (Buffart et al., 2011; Nobili et al., 2011). New advances in high-throughput methodologies have shown that majority of solid tumours are characterized by gross chromosomal abnormalities, such as gain and/or loss of whole chromosomes or chromosomal segments (Duesberg & Rasnick, 2000; Gollin, 2005).

2.1 Oncogenes

Cell proliferation is tightly regulated through signal transduction pathways, which are regulated by growth factors and their receptors. Alterations in growth factors and other oncogenes result in constantly active genes or active under conditions in which the wild-type genes are not. Oncogenes are mainly activated due to gene amplifications, intragenic mutations that regulate the activity of gene product or chromosomal translocations, all leading to overexpression of the oncoproteins. The occurrence and development of gastric cancer was found closely related to a variety of oncogenes, few of which are briefly discussed below.

Ras family oncogenes play an important role in the pathogenesis of colon and pancreatic cancers and were reported, though less frequently, in gastric carcinomas (Pellegata et al., 1992; Soh et al., 1993). The prevalence of alterations in *HRAS* (*K-ras*), which encodes a protein involved in cellular signal transduction pathways, appeared to be dependent of geographic and ethnic origins of gastric cancer cases. While *HRAS* mutations were rare in Western Europe and Japan, the prevalence in China was up to 30% (Deng et al., 1994; Hiyama et al., 2002; van Rees et al., 1999). Genetic changes in *HRAS* have been observed in gastric intestinal metaplasia and gastric adenomas, and could be an early event in the development of gastric cancer (Hirohashi & Sugimura, 1991; Osaki et al., 1996). Despite many studies focused on *HRAS* mutations, there is still some controversial data on the functional role of these mutations that needs to be elucidated.

Overexpression or activation, due to either amplification or mutation of genes of some tyrosine kinases (hepatocyte growth factor receptor (*MET* or *c-met*), fibroblast growth factor receptor 2 (*FGFR2* or K-sam), human epithelial growth factor receptor 2 (*HER2*), and epithelial growth factor receptor (*EGFR*)) could be associated with human gastric cancer. Both, *HER2* and *EGFR*, were found overexpressed in gastric cancer, with prevalence in the intestinal type cancers (Garcia et al., 2003). Receptors have an intracellular domain with tyrosine kinase activity and *EGFR* can bind ligands with its extracellular domain, which induces homodimerization of the receptor and generates autophosphorylation, initiating several signalling cascades that lead to DNA synthesis and cell proliferation. Overexpression of *EGFR* promotes cell migration, angiogenesis and inhibits apoptosis and has been observed in up to 47% of gastric cancers. Moreover, it was found to correlate with disease progression and poor clinical outcome (Malden et al., 1989; Yonemura et al., 1992; Yoshida et al., 1990). *HER2* does not bind to any known ligand, but it is known to heterodimerize with other members of the family, especially when it is overexpressed. The protein has been reported to be overexpressed or activated in 19% of gastric cancer cases. Studies suggest that overexpression of *HER2* might be prognostic factor for intestinal-type gastric cancer associated with shorter relapse-free survival and overall survival (Vizoso et al., 2004; Zhang et al., 2009).

Abnormalities in genes, such as *FGFR2* (*K-sam*), belonging to fibroblast growth factor receptor family, are associated with diffuse-type gastric cancer. Activation of *FGFR2* has been found in approximately 50% of diffuse type gastric cancers, and was associated with neoplastic progression and metastasis (Hara et al., 1998; Hattori et al., 1996; Werner et al., 2001).

The oncogene *MET* (*c-met*) encodes a receptor with tyrosine-kinase activity that binds hepatocyte growth factor. Aberrantly active receptor was preferentially found in intestinal-type gastric cancer tumours and was correlated with poor prognosis (Nakajima et al., 1999; Tsugawa et al., 1998). Employing a simple method of fluorescent multiplex RT-PCR assay and capillary electrophoresis separation we found overexpression of *MET* in 56% of Slovenian patients with gastric cancer (Rajcevic et al., 2007; Rajcevic et al., 2001). *MET* amplification could constitute an important biomarker for selecting patients for a targeted therapy, because it has been observed that a fraction of gastric cancer cell lines appeared to be exquisitely sensitive to a specific *MET* inhibitor (Smolen et al., 2006).

Vascular endothelial growth factor (*VEGF*), a pro-angiogenic molecule, was found frequently overexpressed in poorly differentiated gastric cancer (Brown et al., 1993; Scartozzi et al., 2004; Tian et al., 2001; Yamamoto et al., 1998). Recently, a *VEGF* +1612G/A gene polymorphism was found to be associated with gastric cancer in Chinese Han patients and was previously shown to affect *VEGF* plasma levels (Zhou et al., 2011). Several other oncogenes have been found overexpressed in gastric carcinomas (Nobili et al., 2011; Rajcevic et al., 2007; Tahara, 2004). Nevertheless, years of research have shown that overexpression of oncogenes is not the sole mechanism implicated in gastric cancer pathogenesis.

2.2 Suppressor phenotype

Tumour suppressor genes are targeted in the opposite way than oncogenes. Molecular abnormalities that result in a truncation of the proteins, deletions or insertions or epigenetic silencing, reduce the activity of the gene product. Generally, alterations in both alleles are required to confer impairment of the gene product, except in the case of haplo-insufficient genes (Dang et al., 2008; Vogelstein & Kinzler, 2004). Inactivation of the wild-type allele arises due to allelic loss, termed also loss of heterozygosity (LOH) or mutations (Knudson, 1993). The suppressor phenotype in gastric cancer is characterized by inactivation of suppressor genes, such as *TP53 (p53), APC, MCC, DCC, CDH1, Rb1, FHIT,* and other (Hamilton & Meltzer, 2006; Nobili et al., 2011).

In our study we evaluated LOH on loci associated with the following tumour suppressors: *TPp53, APC, nm23,* and *RB*) and found that 52% of all cases exhibited LOH in at least one locus (Gazvoda et al., 2007). The highest frequency of LOH was at APC locus (36%), followed by *TP53-1* (33%), *nm23* (33%), *TP53-2* (24%) and *RB* (24%). Interestingly, 5% of the samples exhibited MSI on all the evaluated loci (in LOH as well as in MSI evaluation). These samples were associated with clinicopathological features that differed from the rest. All tumours belonged to intestinal type, displayed expansive growth and were mostly tubular. Furthermore, we found that LOH on loci *TP53-1* and *TP53-2* was associated with more expansive growth and LOH on *TP53-1* locus tended to be associated with intestinal type tumours. In contrast, tumours without LOH on *TP53-1* locus were associated with ulcerating, infiltrating type of gastric adenocarcinoma (Gazvoda et al., 2007).

The *TP53* gene encodes a main regulator of cell growth and division, and its function in intestinal type of gastric cancer is mainly altered due to LOH and mutations. When protein p53 is impaired, the cells may not be able to induce apoptosis and control tumour growth (Vousden & Prives, 2005). Studies showed that mutations in *TP53* are present in a range of 40%-70% of early and advanced gastric cancers, and inactivation of *TP53* resulting from LOH is found in 60%-70% of intestinal-type gastric cancers, thus making this gene among the most frequently mutated genes in cancers (Hamilton & Meltzer, 2006; Werner et al., 2001). It was suggested that accumulation of mutations in *TP53* is involved in initiating carcinogenic processes, though not all studies are in agreement with this hypothesis (Liu et al., 2001; Zwick et al., 1997). The expression of p53 protein can be easily detected by immunohistochemical staining, because mutations in *TP53* gene increase the half-life of its product, and it was postulated that it could be used as a biomarker in a clinical setting (Zheng et al., 2004). However, there are conflicting results regarding the prevalence and of *TP53* mutations and its expression and their relationship to clinicopathological features of gastric cancer (Panani, 2008). We and some other researchers found that the *TP53* mutational status was not in association with p53 expression (Bataille et al., 2003; Juvan et al., 2007; Panani, 2008). Furthermore, we found that positive *TP53* expression was associated with poorer survival, which was accordance with some other studies (Bani-Hani et al., 2005; Lazar et al., 2010). On the other hand, other studies did not reveal this association, therefore, the prognostic value of *TP53* remains controversial (Panani, 2008).

Loss of *APC* gene function was first identified in 60%-80% of patients with familial adenomatous polyposis-associated colorectal cancers (Kinzler et al., 1991; Lynch & Lynch, 1998). Mutations and LOH of the gene were also reported in more than 50% of gastric cancers of intestinal type (Tahara, 1995; Wright & Williams, 1993). Functional product of *APC* gene targets β-catenin for ubiquitination, and thus prevents β-catenin associated induction of genes involved in growth control (Caca et al., 1999; Park et al., 1999).

E-cadherin, encoded by *CDH1* gene, is an adhesion molecule expressed from epithelial cells, which plays a crucial role in epithelial structural integrity and was found to be implicated in carcinogenesis. Germline mutations in *CDH1* were first described in patients with hereditary diffuse type gastric cancer, however the rate of *CDH1* mutations in sporadic gastric cancer was found to be as high as 50%, and reduced expression of E-cadherin protein was found in 51% of diffuse type gastric cancers (Becker et al., 1994; Guilford et al., 1998; Xiangming et al., 1999). Susceptible individuals with a germline mutation in tumour suppressor gene *CDH1* require the inactivation of the second allele due to somatic mutation or DNA methylation, rendering E-cadherin completely inactive (Becker et al., 2000). Abnormal expression of E-cadherin is thought to promote metastatic ability of gastric cancer cells (Kanai & Hirohashi, 1997).

2.3 Alterations in other genes

Genetic and epigenetic abnormalities have been found in numerous other genes that participate in proliferation, invasion and metastasis, such as cell cycle regulators, cell-adhesion molecules, growth factors, cytokines, nuclear factors, matrix metalloproteinases, DNA repair genes, and apoptosis regulators (Nobili et al., 2011; Tahara, 2004; Yokozaki et al., 2001). For example, cyclin E1 together with cyclin-dependent kinase, *CDK2*, promotes the entry into the S-phase of the cell cycle, and it was found overexpressed in one third of gastric cancer cases. Amplification of this gene was found to correlate with tumour aggressiveness (Jiaqing et al., 1998; Nobili et al., 2011; Xiangming et al., 2000). In our study we observed overexpression of cyclin E1 in 42% of patients with gastric cancer and in 57% of patients with precancerous lesions, indicating that abnormalities in this gene could be early event in gastric carcinogenesis (Rajcevic et al., 2007). Moreover, we also found overexpression of epidermal growth factor family members, such as *TDGF1* and *EGF*, and *NRG1*, signalling protein, that mediates cell-cell interactions and plays critical roles in the growth and development of multiple organ systems (Rajcevic et al., 2007). Several other genes have been reviewed extensively elsewhere (Nobili et al., 2011; Resende et al., 2010; Tahara, 2004; Wu et al., 2010; Yokozaki et al., 2001).

2.4 MSI and mutator phenotype

Molecular abnormalities in oncogenes and tumour suppressor genes drive the neoplastic process by increasing tumour growth. The increase is achieved by activating of genes that drive the cell cycle or by inhibiting normal apoptotic pathways (Vogelstein & Kinzler, 2004). The third class of genes that contribute to cancer development are the stability genes, which, when mutated, promote tumorigenesis in a completely different way. They keep genetic alterations to a minimum, and thus, when they are inactivated, mutations in oncogenes and tumour suppressor genes occur at a higher rate (Freiberg, 2003). As with tumour suppressor genes, both alleles must be inactivated for physiologic effect to result.

Mismatch repair (MMR) genes are an example of genome stability genes and molecular inactivation of these genes is a hallmark of so-called mutator pathway, which results in microsatellite instability (MSI) or mutator phenotype. Microsatellites are short tandem repeats abundant throughout the genome. They are polymorphic among individuals, but their length is stable in every noncancerous tissue within a given individual. Patients with MSI phenotype exhibit a high frequency of changes in length of microsatellites within a tumour tissue compared to normal tissue, due to slippage of DNA polymerase during DNA replication on repetitive sequences, which leads to insertion or deletion of nucleotides. In short, MSI phenotype is characterized by appearance of new alleles not present in the normal genotype. These postreplicational DNA errors are detected and repaired by a complex of MMR proteins, rather than proofreading activity of the polymerase. Inactivation or deficiency of one or more MMR genes, particularly *MLH1* or *MSH2*, leads to manifestation of MSI phenotype in gastric cancer. As shown in Figure 1, MSI often leads to additional genetic changes and allelic losses, due to frameshift mutations in coding repetitive sequences of genes involved in cell growth regulation, apoptosis and DNA repair (Buermeyer et al., 1999; Ottini et al., 2004). Remarkably, every human MMR gene except *MLH1* includes a mononucleotide repeats, suggesting that the MMR process becomes increasingly defective with subsequent losses of involved proteins (Perucho, 1996).

Impairment of MMR, eventually leading to cancer development, can occur: 1) by mutational inactivation of one or two MMR genes, or 2) by epigenetic inactivation of MMR genes. In gastric cancer, functional inactivation of MMR is mainly caused by latter. Epigenetic hypermethylation of *MLH1*promoter has been found to be responsible for the development of the majority, more than 50%, of MSI-H positive gastric cancers, whereas mutations in *MLH1* and *MSH2* are being reported in 12-15% of gastric cancer exhibiting MSI-H phenotype (Bacani et al., 2005; Wu et al., 2000; Yamamoto et al., 1999) (Figure 1). Silencing of multiple genes, including known tumour-related genes such as *CDKN2A (p16), hMLH1, THBS1,* and *CDH1,* due to promoter hypermethylation, is an important epigenetic event in stomach carcinogenesis and was shown to occur in early stages of gastric cancer development. This pathway of methylation of CpG islands characterizes alternative molecular phenotype of gastric cancer, referred to as the CpG island methylator phenotype (CIMP) (Nobili et al., 2011; Oue et al., 2001; Resende et al., 2010).

2.4.1 MSI analysis

MSI can be detected with polymerase chain reaction (PCR), where each microsatellite under investigation is amplified using specific primers. Lengths of PCR obtained products are usually assessed and compared between normal and tumour tissues from each individual using a simple and cost effective fluorescent multiplex PCR, followed by capillary electrophoresis separation (Gazvoda et al., 2007; Suraweera et al., 2002). Because of a huge number and diversity of microsatellite regions in the human genome, it is difficult to determine the prevalence of MSI in human cancers and its incidence varies depending on which loci are investigated (Lawes et al., 2003). To overcome this confusion, a standard panel of microsatellite markers, including mononucleotide repeats (BAT25 and BAT26) and dinucleotide repeats (D2S123, D5S346 and D17S250) has been recommended to identify MSI phenotype (Nobili et al., 2011). Cancers were subdivided in three groups based on the number of markers displaying instability: those demonstrating instability in > 30-40% of the loci investigated were classified as high-level MSI (MSI-H); those demonstrating instability in <30-40% of the loci investigated were classified as low level MSI (MSI-L); and stable cancers (MSS) showing no instability (Boland et al., 1998). Although these criteria were initially aimed at identifying MSI positive colorectal cancer, they were also successfully used for detecting MSI-H gastric cancers. Incidence of MSI-H has been observed in range 2-18% of gastric cancer cases, depending on the ethnic background. In Japan the incidence of MSI-H phenotype in patients with gastric cancer was reported in 5% of cases, whereas in Western populations it was ranging from 2 to 15% (Gu et al., 2009; Hudler et al., 2004; Leung et al., 1999; Pedrazzani et al., 2009; Schneider et al., 2000; Zhou et al., 1998). Moreover, studies reported 3-fold higher prevalence of MSI-H status in intestinal rather than diffuse-type gastric cancers (Leite et al., 2011). As reviewed by Lawes et al., patients with gastric cancer that exhibit MSI-H phenotype were associated with a better survival (64-88%) when compared to MSS counterparts (39-53%) (Lawes et al., 2003). Furthermore, we and other researchers have found that MSI-H phenotype was not associated with LOH-H phenotype, which is in agreement with other studies proposing that the mutator and suppressor pathways are independent of each other at least in the early stages of gastric carcinogenesis (Gazvoda et al., 2007; Kim et al., 2001). Likewise, patients with LOH-H were associated with MSI-L or did not show MSI (microsatellite stable, MSS) on evaluated loci. In our study we evaluated MSI on loci BAT25, BAT26, BAT40, D2S123, D3S1277, and D10S107, and as mentioned before, LOH on loci, associated with tumour suppressors. Interestingly, the highest frequency of MSI was found at RB locus (21%), which was initially tested for LOH, followed by BAT25 (15%), D3S1277 (14%), D2S123 (13%), D10S107 (13%), BAT40 (12%) and BAT26 (10%) (Gazvoda et al., 2007). We observed that in our study BAT26 was the most informative locus. We also correlated MSI with clinicopathological features and found that MSI-L phenotype was associated with diffuse or mixed types of gastric cancers.

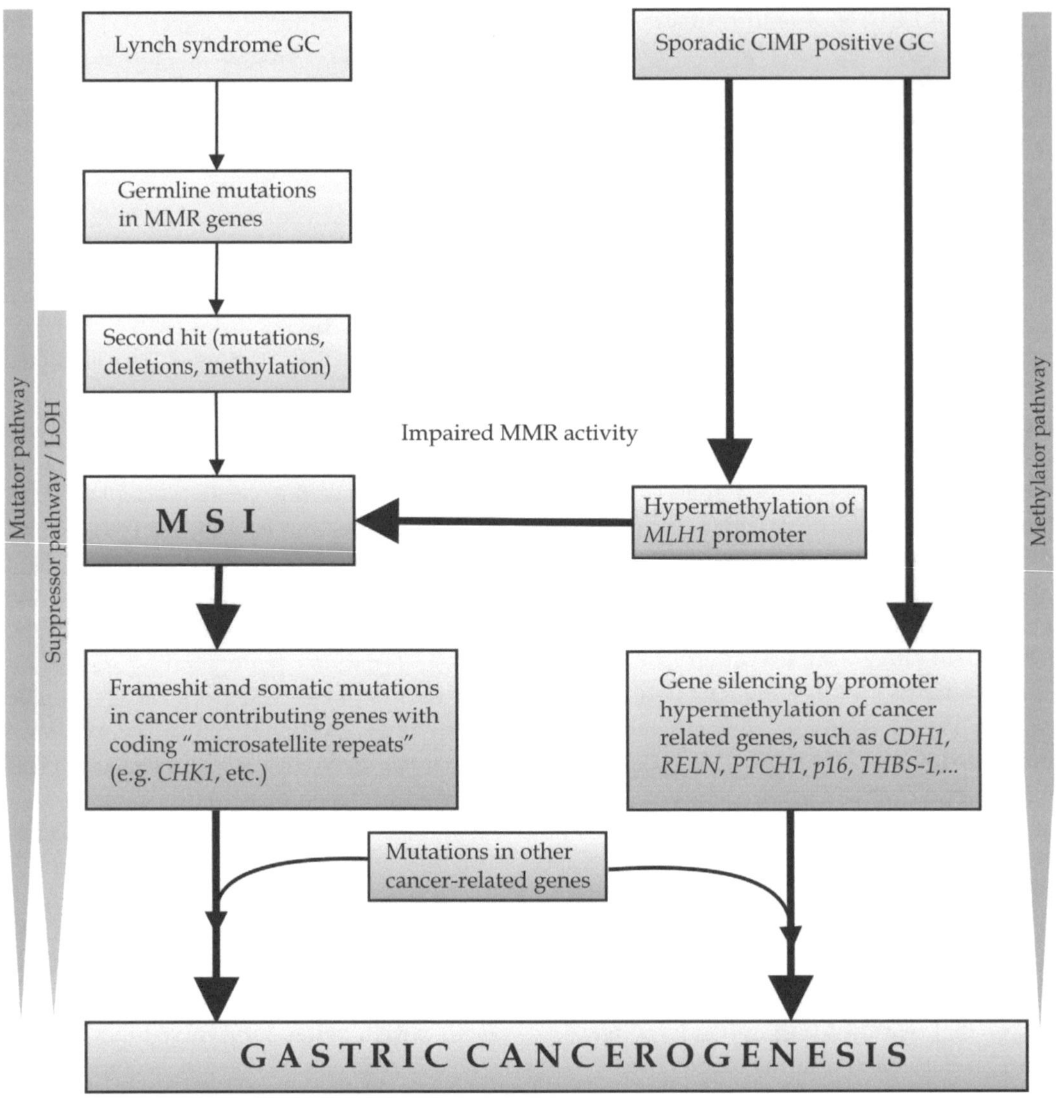

Fig. 1. Mutator pathway overlapping with suppressor and methylator pathways in gastric tumorigenesis. These changes should not be considered a specific sequence of alterations, but rather an overall collection of abnormalities that contribute to the pathogenesis of gastric cancer (Adopted from Boland & Goel, 2010).

It has recently become evident that dinucleotide repeats are less sensitive than mononucleotide repeats for detection of MSI-H, therefore revised criteria proposes the use of a mononucleotide markers in order to define MSI-H instability (Umar et al., 2004). A panel of five mononucleotide repeats (BAT25, BAT26, NR-21, NR-22 and NR-24) that may be more instrumental for detecting MSI-H status in humans has been suggested (Buhard et al., 2004). It has been further demonstrated that these markers are quasimonomorphic in 1206 studied individuals from 55 different populations worldwide, and can therefore be used for MSI-H determination without the requirement for matching normal DNA (Buhard et al., 2006). By adopting the panel, MSI-H phenotype was reported in a range from 5% to 50% of all gastric carcinomas with significant differences in various population groups (Leite et al., 2011; Ottini et al., 2004; Simpson et al., 2001).

2.4.2 Mutational impairment of MMR activity and pathogenic significance of observed alterations

The most common inherited condition that gives rise to MSI positive cancers is Lynch syndrome, an autosomal dominant disease, also referred to as Hereditary Non-polyposis Colorectal Cancer (HNPCC), where gastric cancer is a common neoplasia, occurring in 6% of Lynch syndrome cases (Percesepe et al., 2001; Samowitz et al., 2001). Predisposed individuals carry a recessive, first-hit germline mutation in the MMR genes, including large genomic rearrangement, which account for 5-20% of all mutations. In reference of Knudson's hypothesis, the MSI-H phenotype requires the "second hit" inactivation of the responsible MMR gene for development of malignant phenotype.

In Lynch syndromes, somatic inactivation of the remaining wild-type allele can occur due to different mechanisms: loss of heterozygosity (LOH), somatic mutation and promoter methylation (Imai & Yamamoto, 2008). The relative risk of gastric cancer development in Lynch syndrome individuals has been reported to be 4-19-fold higher, compared to general population, suggesting that screening for MMR mutations in predisposed carriers could be of importance for the detection of predisposed individuals (Gylling et al., 2007). Particularly, patients with MSI-positive gastric carcinomas, but lacking *MLH1* promoter hypermethylation are regarded as potential germline MMR-related mutation carriers.

Majority of MMR alterations, found in patients with Lynch syndrome are known to be pathogenic as they result in premature termination of protein synthesis and thus loss of MMR activity. However, hundreds of MMR variants that do not lead to truncation of the respective MMR protein have been identified in Lynch cancer cases and their pathogenic significance is often difficult to establish on clinical samples alone.

Information on functional nature of MMR alterations is essential for accurate early diagnosis and prognosis as well as for proper genetic counselling for members from affected families. Therefore in the past decade, many functional assays have been developed to ease the interpretation of pathogenicity of unclassified variants (UVs). Recent and some of the most recognized *in vivo* and *in vitro* assays together with available *in silico* algorithms are summarised in Table 1.

While many *in vitro* assays characterize specific biological functions of MMR proteins, *in vivo* tests strive to assess the MMR repair capacity as a complex cellular process (Ou et al., 2007). Since efficiency of MMR repair relies on several successfully completed biochemical events of involved proteins (e.g. protein expression levels and stability, localization of MMR protein to the nucleus, heterodimerization ability and effective recognition and repair of the DNA lesions, etc.), *in vivo* approaches are preferable and are either cell line- or yeast-based. However, all assays have their limitations and problems, mostly concerning toxic episomal overexpression of MMR proteins and lack of evolutionary conserved regions between yeast and human MMR proteins at the regions of interest. Moreover, since variety of strategies have been used, it is difficult to establish and compare clinical significance of analysed variants. Finally, it is also not easy to determine sensitivity and specificity of these tests, therefore results should still be utilized with caution and interpreted alongside clinical data of the affected carriers.

Assay type	Biochemical feature analysed	Assay	References
In vitro	Protein-protein interaction	GST pull-down	Raevaara, 2005; Guerette, 1999; Belvederesi, 2006; Perera, 2008
		Expression of MMR genes in human cell lines	Trojan, 2002
	Protein expression	Western blotting	Takahashi, 2007
	mRNA splicing	pCAS minigene	Tournier, 2008
	MMR activity	Cell-free assay w/ protein extracts	Takahashi, 2007; Raevaara, 2005;
In vivo	Protein-protein interaction	Human-yeast hybrid MLH1 in yeast	Kondo, 2003;
	Protein expression	Immunohistochemical staining	Leite, 2011
	Intracellular localization	Fluorescence microscopy	Raevaara, 2005
	mRNA splicing	*In vivo* splicing assay in human cells	Auclair, 2006; Sharp, 2004; Arnold, 2009
	MMR activity	Yeast-based chromosome-integrated hMMR gene	Vogelsang, 2009; Vogelsang, 2010
		Dominant mutator effect	Raevara, 2005;Takahashi, 2007; Shimodaira, 1998
		Functional assay using yeast	Ellison, 2001;Wanat, 2007
		Utility of *MLH1*-deficient cells	Blasi, 2006
In silico	Effect of amino acid substitution on protein functions	SIFT	Kumar, 2009; Ng, 2003
		PolyPhen	Ramensky, 2002
		MAPP-MMR	Chao, 2008
		Align GVDV	Tavgtigian, 2006; Mathe, 2006
	mRNA splicing	NNSPLICE	Sharp, 2004

Table 1. Compilation of functional assays used in characterizing pathogenic significance of MMR variants found in Lynch syndrome patients.

We have recently described an *in vivo* yeast-based functional approach, expressing human MMR genes in yeast, enabling all variants found within the coding region of the MMR gene to be analysed. With chromosomal integration of relevant human MMR genes we obtained their stable expression throughout the experiment (Vogelsang et al., 2009). With our approach we have functionally characterized four missense *MLH1* variants, which we previously identified in MSI-H positive gastric cancers with limited *MLH1* hypermethylation. We also assessed two of the variants, which were described for the first time in our study (Hudler et al., 2004). We have shown that identified missense mutations were not causally associated with MSI-H phenotype in analysed gastric cancer tissues (Vogelsang & Komel, 2010).

2.5 Chromosomal instability (CIN) and aneuploidy

In contrast to MSI, CIN is characterized by gross chromosomal abnormalities, such as gain or loss of whole chromosomes and/or fractions of chromosomes (LOH, amplifications, translocations) (Martin et al., 2010). Aneuploidy is the state of altered chromosome number in malignant cells (Pino & Chung, 2010). Studies showed that MSI phenotype is characteristic for hereditary type of gastric cancer, developed in the context of Lynch syndrome, and a smaller subset of sporadic cancers ranging from 15% to 35% (Panani, 2008). CIN, however, has been recently recognized as the most common feature of sporadic gastric cancers, and has been reported in up to 84% of gastrointestinal tumours (Grabsch et al., 2004; Ottini et al., 2006).

Several techniques, such as karyotyping, cytometry, detection of LOH, and fluorescent *in situ* hybridization (FISH) have been developed to measure CIN and some of them have already been successfully transferred to clinical practice. New methods, such as CGH arrays and copy number variation analysis (CNV), have advanced the field, due to their ability to detect chromosomal abnormalities with higher resolution and accuracy (Pino & Chung, 2010).

CIN has been recognized as valuable prognostic factor and tumour stage indicator in gastric cancers, although in the study of Birkbak et al. it has been found that intermediate CIN had more impact on poor prognosis than extreme CIN phenotype (Birkbak et al., 2011; Suzuki et al., 2003). Furthermore, it has been found that DNA copy number changes are not uniform in gastric cancers and subgroups with different patterns of DNA copy number alterations have been recognized, which have been associated with prognosis, lymph node status and metastasis (Buffart et al., 2007b; Kang et al., 2006; Morohara et al., 2005; Panani, 2008; Weiss et al., 2004; Wu et al., 2002).

Buffart et al. explored the differences in DNA copy number by CGH arrays and reported that the mean number of chromosomal events was lower in adenomas compared to gastric carcinomas, suggesting that distinct losses and gains on chromosomes likely represent early events in carcinogenesis (Buffart et al., 2007b). In another study they compared CGH profiles of gastric cancers in young and old patients (Buffart et al., 2007a). They found out that chromosome regions 11q23.3 and 19p13.3 contributed most to age-related differences in tumour profiles and that tumours of younger patients showed gains in chromosomal regions 6p21, 9p34, 11p15, 11q23, 17p13, 19p13, and 22q13, whereas in the majority of older patients normal copy status was observed. They concluded that these differences in genomic profiles likely reflect different pathogenic mechanisms of the disease.

Varis et al., similarly observed that the most frequent cytogenetic aberrations were gains seen at 17q, 19q, and 20q in younger patients (Varis et al., 2003). They also found that DNA copy number changes were mostly detected in intestinal or mixed types of tumours.

Tsukamoto et al. observed higher frequencies of DNA copy number aberrations, especially in the case of 20q13 chromosome gain, which was detected in 97% of cases, compared to other studies (Tsukamoto et al., 2008). They used laser microdissection method to isolate tumour cells, therefore their samples contained fewer cells from tumour microenvironment. They also identified 114 upregulated candidate genes located in regions of amplification and 11 down-regulated genes located in regions of deletion.

Several other studies reported different DNA copy number changes in patients with gastric cancer (Buffart et al., 2007b; Hou et al., 2008; Junnila et al., 2010; Kimura et al., 2004). Hou et al., for example, used an integrated approach using CGH and 100K SNP arrays, FISH, reverse transcription PCR, Western immunoblotting, and siRNA-mediated gene knockdown to determine and identify potential overexpressed genes in region 6p11p12, which they found to be amplified in their study (Hou et al., 2008). They identified *RAB23*, which could be implicated in invasion.

Despite the remarkable effort made by researchers to identify significant chromosomal aberrations in gastric cancers and to correlate them with clinicopathological features, the results are still inconclusive and not consistent with each other (reviewed in Nobili et al., 2011; Panani, 2008).

2.5.1 LOH

As stated before, LOH studies have already revealed several chromosomal loci with significant allelic losses, facilitating the identification of tumour suppressor genes, which could be important in gastric tumorigenesis (Gazvoda et al., 2007; Juvan et al., 2007; Kim et al., 1991; Kondo et al., 2005; Panani, 2008; Tamura, 2006). LOH is also a marker of chromosomal instability and might indicate a second inactivational hit of a cancer suppressor gene. Allelic losses are typically detected by using highly polymorphic microsatellite sequences that are dispersed throughout the human genome. Several LOH studies demonstrated that the extent of chromosomal loss appeared to be of prognostic significance (French et al., 2004; Gazvoda et al., 2007; Koo et al., 2004). It was established that there was a trend of two distinct subtypes, high-level LOH (named LOH-H) and low-level LOH (named LOH-L), being correlated with intestinal or mixed and diffuse growth patterns, respectively (Hong et al., 2010). In our study we also found out that LOH-H was associated with intestinal type of gastric cancer (Gazvoda et al., 2007). LOH has been shown to relate to cancer progression, where a transition from LOH-L to LOH-H is thought to reflect an increase in chromosomal instability during tumour advancement. These findings on LOH events suggest that the degrees of allelic loss may have an influence on the clinical course of gastric cancer.

2.5.2 Aneuploidy

Although some opinions still diverge regarding the clinical impact of aneuploidy alone (mostly measured by FISH, flow cytometry or image cytometry), recently there are reports pointing out that it could be of importance as a predictive marker in gastric cancer, and its potential clinical practicability in pre-malignant disease to stratify patients by their cancer risk. It is important to note recent evidence supporting the hypothesis of stepwise ploidy progression: from diploid or minor aneuploid in most early cancers to aneuploid in most advanced cancers (Duesberg et al., 2005). As a progressive increase in the severity of aneuploidy with neoplastic progression has been observed, it has thus been shown to be a

useful prognostic indicator for patient classification as low or high-risk cases for cancer development (Russo et al., 2000; Yasa et al., 2005).
Interestingly, aneuploidy was found in human tumours more than 100 years ago by von Hansenmann and Boveri (Duesberg & Rasnick, 2000; Ricke et al., 2008). However, in the last decades, the research was oriented towards oncogenes and tumour suppressors' hunt, and in identifying mutator and methylator pathways of gastric carcinogenesis. Yet to date, not one subtype of gastric adenocarcinomas has been completely described and no cancer-causing genes or combination of genes have been found to be specific for gastric cancers, although a number of mutations and other genetic changes have been described (Duesberg & Rasnick, 2000; Nobili et al., 2011; Panani, 2008; Weber, 2002).
Recently, it has been found that aneuploidy, either in the form of LOH or gross chromosomal copy number changes, stands out as the most consistent marker of neoplastic cells in solid tumours (Duesberg & Li, 2003; Ottini et al., 2006). Indeed, several studies confirmed a high frequency of aneuploidy in sporadic gastric cancers, even up to 84% (Belien et al., 2009; Buffart et al., 2007b; Buffart et al., 2011; Grabsch et al., 2004; Russo et al., 2000).

2.5.3 Mechanisms leading to chromosomal instability

The mechanisms leading to abnormal chromosome content and other chromosomal abnormalities are poorly understood, although it is now believed that CIN might, through stepwise clonal progression, lead to oncogene activation, tumour suppressor inactivation and alterations in other crucial genes, implicated in establishing the malignant phenotype of cells. Several different mechanisms have been proposed by researchers, such as telomere dysfunction, defective DNA damage response, impaired chromosomal segregation, and aberrations in cell cycle regulators (Castro et al., 2007; Gollin, 2005; Grabsch et al., 2004; Yasui et al., 1999).
Lately, the attention of researchers in the field of epithelial tumours, including gastric adenocarcinomas, has focused on genetic changes in mitotic genes, with emphasis on chromosome segregation. Segregation is one of the fundamental processes in cells, which are rapidly dividing, such as gastric epithelial cells. Therefore, if regulation mechanisms, governing this process are damaged, the cells might proceed through cytokinesis with DNA or spindle errors and thus could inherit unrepaired mutations or gain an abnormal number of chromosomes (aneuploidy) (Schmit & Ahmad, 2007). However, the molecular defects underlying CIN and aneuploidy and weather it is a cause or consequence of tumour phenotype are not completely clear. At least two possible mechanisms for CIN development have been suggested: mutations and/or polymorphisms in mitotic genes, implicated in chromosome segregation, or the activity of carcinogens on susceptible genetic background of individuals. (Duesberg et al., 2005; Iovino et al., 2006).
Studies on several animal species and humans showed that certain genetic mutations and polymorphisms in genes involved in segregation of chromosomes might cause an increased incidence of a particular tumour type (Shepard et al., 2007; Tomonaga & Nomura, 2007). Kim et al. analysed expression of *MAD2L1*, a component of the mitotic spindle assembly checkpoint, and kinase gene *BUB1*, involved in activating the spindle checkpoint. They found mutations in *MAD2L*, whereas they did not detect any mutations in *BUB1*.
Grabsch et al., on other hand, observed overexpression of BUB1 protein in gastric cancers, which was significantly higher in tissues of patients with diffuse type adenocarcinomas

(Grabsch et al., 2004). However, their study did not reveal any association between BUB1 protein expression level and DNA ploidy status of examined tumour types.

Aurora kinase A (*AURKA* or *STK15*) located at 20q13, a region that is frequently amplified in gastric cancer, has been found overexpressed in stomach adenocarcinomas (Dar et al., 2008). Functional analysis of upregulated *AURKA* gene, done by the same researchers, revealed a possible novel oncogenic pathway, involved in gastric carcinogenesis. *AURKA* overexpression led to a significant increase in mRNA levels of several direct targets of the β-catenin/TCF transcription complex (cyclin D1, *MYC*, *MYC*-binding protein, *CLDN1*, *FGF18*, and *VEGF*).

However, these and several other studies, explored overexpression and/or mutations of these genes, which could already be the consequence of CIN. Therefore, it has been proposed that minor alterations in mitotic genes could contribute to the onset of cancer (Frank, 2004). The mounting evidence is suggesting that subtle variations, such as single-nucleotide polymorphisms (SNPs) or non-lethal mutations, might induce CIN and aneuploidy. This hypothesis of low-penetrance allelic variants or risk alleles is further supported by the fact that non-heritable cancers usually develop in elderly, whereas dominant mutations in oncogenes and tumour suppressors usually induce the disease early in life (Duesberg & Rasnick, 2000; Frank, 2004). Minor genetic variants in mitotic genes could in combination with environmental factors modulate mitotic pathways, and could thus exert minor changes in the DNA of replicating epithelial cells. The search for these changes has begun only recently, and further investigations are needed to clarify these aberrations and their involvement in carcinogenesis.

In our study, we genotyped two polymorphic sites, T91A (F31I) and G169A (V57I) in serine-threonine-kinase *STK15* (*AURKA*), which is involved in the regulation of several cell cycle events (Hudler et al., 2009). It is responsible for the functioning of centrosome, for microtubule formation and stabilization at the spindle pole throughout all phases of segregation, and for chromosome segregation during anaphase. We found a putative protective role of the genotype A/T (F31I) in examined population of gastric cancer patients. We also found a weak protective association between homozygotes A/A, heterozygotes A/G (V57I) and A/T (F31I) genotype and reduced risk for perineural invasion. In another study we performed the case-control study of selected polymorphisms rs151658 and rs239559, rs1031963 and rs1801376 in mitotic segregation genes, TTK and BUB1B, respectively (Hudler et al., 2010). We found a significant interaction between patients and control cases for genotype A/G in rs151658 polymorphism. We also observed a statistically important difference in genotype frequencies between female patients and control cases for polymorphism rs1801376. Our results showed that this difference was significant only for female population of patients. Polymorphisms rs151658, rs1031963 and rs1801376 showed significant associations with certain clinicopathological factors, such as differentiation of tumours, infiltration, and intestinal type of gastric cancers. This study provides new support for the role of mitotic genes in gastric cancer development, suggesting that smaller changes could be associated with genetically unstable gastric tumours. However, the biological basis for the role of risk alleles of mitotic genes in cancers of the upper gastrointestinal tract needs to be established to understand its consequences and role during carcinogenesis.

Carcinogens are a second probable cause of CIN and particular agents, such as *Helicobacter pylori* infection, tobacco, nitrates, and nitrites have an important impact on gastric tumorigenesis in genetically susceptible individuals (Matysiak-Budnik & Megraud, 2006). In addition, a combination of SNPs within pro-inflammatory genes IL-1β, IL-1RA, TNFα, and IL-10 conferred even greater risk for gastric cancer development in combination with CIN causing *Helicobacter pylori* infection (El-Omar et al., 2003).

3. Future directions

Recent advances in high-throughput methods revealed the lack of consistency regarding the number and species of genes mutated in all subtypes of gastric adenocarcinomas, or even from one cell to another within the same tumour, which points to amazing genetic diversity of cancer cells. The idea that mutations in a few specific genes are necessary and sufficient to cause the disease in any of the most common human cancer forms was opposed by observation that random mutations accumulate much faster inside genetically unstable malignant cells and that genome instability might be a critical early event that leads to the mutation of oncogenes and suppressor genes. Furthermore, in contrast to gene mutation hypotheses neoplastic transformation of normal epithelial cells is a slow process, which explains the fact that majority of cancers appear at an advanced age. All these facts make relevant molecular cancer diagnosis and treatment extremely complex and difficult to fulfil. Therefore, in the future we suggest performing combined analyses of gene expression profiles, genetic polymorphisms in mitotic genes, and functional analyses of these polymorphisms. Studies should be expanded on candidate genes by employing genome-wide association studies in order to identify novel genetic variants associated with gastric cancer.

4. Conclusion

It is apparent that majority of gastric cancers are characterized by genetic instability, either MSI or CIN. Whereas MSI is characterized by changes in short repeat sequences, the hallmark of CIN are gross chromosomal rearrangements, such as the gain or loss of whole chromosomes (Martin et al., 2010). Accumulating evidence shows that CIN and aneuploidy are the most common characteristics of sporadic gastric adenocarcinomas, accounting for more than 60% of cases, whereas MSI is characteristic for hereditary type of gastric cancer, developed in the context of Lynch syndrome, and a smaller subset of sporadic cancers, ranging from 15% to 35% (Panani, 2008). The newly formed chromosomal/aneuploidy hypothesis (aneuploidy could be the consequence of carcinogens or genetic changes in certain mitotic genes) could answer several questions remaining from the currently established classic oncogene overexpression model, mutator and suppressor theories, which postulate that cancer is caused by clonal expansion of one single cell, which has accumulated 4-7 mutations during the lifetime of a patient. (Castro et al., 2007; Duesberg et al., 2005; Duesberg et al., 2000). However, these theories do not explain the long latent periods in cancer development and more importantly, despite more than two decades of effort, they have failed to identify a particular sets of gene mutations that occur in every instance of gastric tumour development.

It is evident that gastric cancer is the consequence of a multistep process involving different genetic and epigenetic changes in numerous genes. Host genetic background and environmental factors also play an important role in the pathogenesis of the disease. The majority of genetic alterations contributing to the malignant transformation were observed in growth regulatory genes, and in genes involved in cell cycle progression and arrest.

However, exact genetic steps involved in the stomach carcinogenesis still remain uncertain. Different histological forms, as well as different aetiologies point to different genetic pathways for intestinal and diffuse tumours. To date, no single genomic abnormality is known to be specific to sporadic gastric cancer, or to any of its histological subtypes. Some of the genetic changes occur commonly in both major types, intestinal and diffuse, but some differ depending on the histological type. Even more, recent studies supported the idea that there are subgroups where MSI, CIN, suppressor, and methylator pathways overlap during the development of malignant phenotype. In conclusion, further research is required, with emphasis on collecting as many genetic changes as possible, which could aid in deciphering the molecular mechanisms of gastric cancer and in the development of suitable methods for screening, risk assessment and prognostic evaluation.

5. References

Arnold, S., Buchanan, D. D., Barker, M., Jaskowski, L., Walsh, M. D., Birney, G., Woods, M. O., Hopper, J. L., Jenkins, M. A., Brown, M. A., Tavtigian, S. V., Goldgar, D. E., Young, J. P. & Spurdle, A. B. (2009). Classifying MLH1 and MSH2 variants using bioinformatic prediction, splicing assays, segregation, and tumor characteristics. *Hum Mutat*, 30, (5), pp. 757-770, ISSN 1098-1004

Auclair, J., Busine, M. P., Navarro, C., Ruano, E., Montmain, G., Desseigne, F., Saurin, J. C., Lasset, C., Bonadona, V., Giraud, S., Puisieux, A. & Wang, Q. (2006). Systematic mRNA analysis for the effect of MLH1 and MSH2 missense and silent mutations on aberrant splicing. *Hum Mutat*, 27, (2), pp. 145-154, ISSN 1098-1004

Bacani, J., Zwingerman, R., Di Nicola, N., Spencer, S., Wegrynowski, T., Mitchell, K., Hay, K., Redston, M., Holowaty, E., Huntsman, D., Pollett, A., Riddell, R. & Gallinger, S. (2005). Tumor microsatellite instability in early onset gastric cancer. *J Mol Diagn*, 7, (4), pp. 465-477

Bani-Hani, K. E., Almasri, N. M., Khader, Y. S., Sheyab, F. M. & Karam, H. N. (2005). Combined evaluation of expressions of cyclin E and p53 proteins as prognostic factors for patients with gastric cancer. *Clin Cancer Res*, 11, (4), pp. 1447-1453, ISSN 1078-0432

Bataille, F., Rummele, P., Dietmaier, W., Gaag, D., Klebl, F., Reichle, A., Wild, P., Hofstadter, F. & Hartmann, A. (2003). Alterations in p53 predict response to preoperative high dose chemotherapy in patients with gastric cancer. *Mol Pathol*, 56, (5), pp. 286-292

Becker, K. F., Atkinson, M. J., Reich, U., Becker, I., Nekarda, H., Siewert, J. R. & Hofler, H. (1994). E-cadherin gene mutations provide clues to diffuse type gastric carcinomas. *Cancer Res*, 54, (14), pp. 3845-3852, ISSN 0008-5472

Belvederesi, L., Bianchi, F., Loretelli, C., Gagliardini, D., Galizia, E., Bracci, R., Rosati, S., Bearzi, I., Viel, A., Cellerino, R. & Porfiri, E. (2006). Assessing the pathogenicity of MLH1 missense mutations in patients with suspected hereditary nonpolyposis colorectal cancer: correlation with clinical, genetic and functional features. *Eur J Hum Genet*, 14, (7), pp. 853-859, ISSN 1018-4813

Becker, K. F., Keller, G. & Hoefler, H. (2000). The use of molecular biology in diagnosis and prognosis of gastric cancer. *Surg Oncol*, 9, (1), pp. 5-11, ISSN 0960-7404

Belien, J. A., Buffart, T. E., Gill, A. J., Broeckaert, M. A., Quirke, P., Meijer, G. A. & Grabsch, H. I. (2009). Gross genomic damage measured by DNA image cytometry independently predicts gastric cancer patient survival. *Br J Cancer*, 101, (6), pp. 1011-1018, ISSN 1532-1827

Birkbak, N. J., Eklund, A. C., Li, Q., McClelland, S. E., Endesfelder, D., Tan, P., Tan, I. B., Richardson, A. L., Szallasi, Z. & Swanton, C. (2011). Paradoxical relationship between chromosomal instability and survival outcome in cancer. *Cancer Res*, pp., ISSN 1538-7445

Blasi, M. F., Ventura, I., Aquilina, G., Degan, P., Bertario, L., Bassi, C., Radice, P. & Bignami, M. (2006). A human cell-based assay to evaluate the effects of alterations in the MLH1 mismatch repair gene. *Cancer Res*, 66, (18), pp. 9036-9044, ISSN 0008-5472

Boland, C. R., Thibodeau, S. N., Hamilton, S. R., Sidransky, D., Eshleman, J. R., Burt, R. W., Meltzer, S. J., Rodriguez-Bigas, M. A., Fodde, R., Ranzani, G. N. & Srivastava, S. (1998). A National Cancer Institute Workshop on Microsatellite Instability for cancer detection and familial predisposition: development of international criteria for the determination of microsatellite instability in colorectal cancer. *Cancer Res*, 58, (22), pp. 5248-5257, ISSN 0008-5472

Boland, C. R. & Goel, A. (2010). Microsatellite instability in colorectal cancer. *Gastroenterology*, 138, (6), pp. 2073-2087 e2073, ISSN 1528-0012

Brown, L. F., Berse, B., Jackman, R. W., Tognazzi, K., Manseau, E. J., Senger, D. R. & Dvorak, H. F. (1993). Expression of vascular permeability factor (vascular endothelial growth factor) and its receptors in adenocarcinomas of the gastrointestinal tract. *Cancer Res*, 53, (19), pp. 4727-4735, ISSN 0008-5472

Buermeyer, A. B., Deschenes, S. M., Baker, S. M. & Liskay, R. M. (1999). Mammalian DNA mismatch repair. *Annu Rev Genet*, 33, pp. 533-564, ISSN 0066-4197

Buffart, T. E., Carvalho, B., Hopmans, E., Brehm, V., Kranenbarg, E. K., Schaaij-Visser, T. B., Eijk, P. P., van Grieken, N. C., Ylstra, B., van de Velde, C. J. & Meijer, G. A. (2007a). Gastric cancers in young and elderly patients show different genomic profiles. *J Pathol*, 211, (1), pp. 45-51, ISSN 0022-3417

Buffart, T. E., Carvalho, B., Mons, T., Reis, R. M., Moutinho, C., Silva, P., van Grieken, N. C., Vieth, M., Stolte, M., van de Velde, C. J., Schrock, E., Matthaei, A., Ylstra, B., Carneiro, F. & Meijer, G. A. (2007b). DNA copy number profiles of gastric cancer precursor lesions. *BMC Genomics*, 8, pp. 345, ISSN 1471-2164

Buffart, T. E., Louw, M., van Grieken, N. C., Tijssen, M., Carvalho, B., Ylstra, B., Grabsch, H., Mulder, C. J., van de Velde, C. J., van der Merwe, S. W. & Meijer, G. A. (2011). Gastric cancers of Western European and African patients show different patterns of genomic instability. *BMC Med Genomics*, 4, pp. 7, ISSN 1755-8794

Buhard, O., Suraweera, N., Lectard, A., Duval, A. & Hamelin, R. (2004). Quasimonomorphic mononucleotide repeats for high-level microsatellite instability analysis. *Dis Markers*, 20, (4-5), pp. 251-257, ISSN 0278-0240

Buhard, O., Cattaneo, F., Wong, Y. F., Yim, S. F., Friedman, E., Flejou, J. F., Duval, A. & Hamelin, R. (2006). Multipopulation analysis of polymorphisms in five mononucleotide repeats used to determine the microsatellite instability status of human tumors. *J Clin Oncol*, 24, (2), pp. 241-251, ISSN 1527-7755

Caca, K., Kolligs, F. T., Ji, X., Hayes, M., Qian, J., Yahanda, A., Rimm, D. L., Costa, J. & Fearon, E. R. (1999). Beta- and gamma-catenin mutations, but not E-cadherin inactivation, underlie T-cell factor/lymphoid enhancer factor transcriptional deregulation in gastric and pancreatic cancer. *Cell Growth Differ*, 10, (6), pp. 369-376, ISSN 1044-9523

Castro, d. I. P., Carcer, d. G. & Malumbres, M. (2007). A Census of Mitotic Cancer Genes: New Insights into Tumor Cell Biology and Cancer Therapy. *Carcinogenesis*, 28, (5), pp. 899-912

Chao, E. C., Velasquez, J. L., Witherspoon, M. S., Rozek, L. S., Peel, D., Ng, P., Gruber, S. B., Watson, P., Rennert, G., Anton-Culver, H., Lynch, H. & Lipkin, S. M. (2008). Accurate classification of MLH1/MSH2 missense variants with multivariate analysis of protein polymorphisms-mismatch repair (MAPP-MMR). *Hum Mutat*, 29, (6), pp. 852-860, ISSN 1098-1004

Crew, K. D. & Neugut, A. I. (2006). Epidemiology of gastric cancer. *World J Gastroenterol*, 12, (3), pp. 354-362

Dang, V. T., Kassahn, K. S., Marcos, A. E. & Ragan, M. A. (2008). Identification of human haploinsufficient genes and their genomic proximity to segmental duplications. *Eur J Hum Genet*, 16, (11), pp. 1350-1357, ISSN 1018-4813

Dar, A. A., Zaika, A., Piazuelo, M. B., Correa, P., Koyama, T., Belkhiri, A., Washington, K., Castells, A., Pera, M. & El-Rifai, W. (2008). Frequent overexpression of Aurora Kinase A in upper gastrointestinal adenocarcinomas correlates with potent antiapoptotic functions. *Cancer*, 112, (8), pp. 1688-1698

Deng, G., Eh, Z., Xu, Y. & Lu, Y. (1994). Activation of oncogene c-Ha-ras in gastric cancer of Chinese patients. *Semin Surg Oncol*, 10, (2), pp. 83-87, ISSN 8756-0437

Duesberg, P., Li, R., Rasnick, D., Rausch, C., Willer, A., Kraemer, A., Yerganian, G. & Hehlmann, R. (2000). Aneuploidy precedes and segregates with chemical carcinogenesis. *Cancer Genet Cytogenet*, 119, (2), pp. 83-93, ISSN 0165-4608

Duesberg, P. & Rasnick, D. (2000). Aneuploidy, the somatic mutation that makes cancer a species of its own. *Cell Motil Cytoskeleton*, 47, (2), pp. 81-107, ISSN 0886-1544

Duesberg, P. & Li, R. (2003). Multistep carcinogenesis: a chain reaction of aneuploidizations. *Cell Cycle*, 2, (3), pp. 202-210, ISSN 1538-4101

Duesberg, P., Li, R., Fabarius, A. & Hehlmann, R. (2005). The chromosomal basis of cancer. *Cell Oncol*, 27, (5-6), pp. 293-318

El-Omar, E. M., Rabkin, C. S., Gammon, M. D., Vaughan, T. L., Risch, H. A., Schoenberg, J. B., Stanford, J. L., Mayne, S. T., Goedert, J., Blot, W. J., Fraumeni, J. F., Jr. & Chow, W. H. (2003). Increased risk of noncardia gastric cancer associated with proinflammatory cytokine gene polymorphisms. *Gastroenterology*, 124, (5), pp. 1193-1201, ISSN 0016-5085

Ellison, A. R., Lofing, J. & Bitter, G. A. (2001). Functional analysis of human MLH1 and MSH2 missense variants and hybrid human-yeast MLH1 proteins in Saccharomyces cerevisiae. *Hum Mol Genet*, 10, (18), pp. 1889-1900

Fearon, E. R. & Vogelstein, B. (1990). A genetic model for colorectal tumorigenesis. *Cell*, 61, (5), pp. 759-767, ISSN 0092-8674

Frank, S. A. (2004). Genetic predisposition to cancer - insights from population genetics. *Nat Rev Genet*, 5, (10), pp. 764-772, ISSN 1471-0056

Freiberg, E. C. (2003). DNA damage and repair. *Nature*, 421, pp. 436-440

French, A. J., Petroni, G., Thibideau, S. N., Smolkin, M., Bissonette, E., Roviello, F., Harper, J. C., Koch, B. R., Anderson, S. A., Hebbring, S. J. & Powell, S. M. (2004). Allelic imbalance of 8p indicates poor survival in gastric cancer. *J Mol Diagn*, 6, (3), pp. 243-252, ISSN 1525-1578

Garcia, I., del Casar, J. M., Corte, M. D., Allende, M. T., Garcia-Muniz, J. L. & Vizoso, F. (2003). Epidermal growth factor receptor and c-erbB-2 contents in unresectable (UICC R1 or R2) gastric cancer. *Int J Biol Markers*, 18, (3), pp. 200-206, ISSN 0393-6155

Gazvoda, B., Juvan, R., Zupanic-Pajnic, I., Repse, S., Ferlan-Marolt, K., Balazic, J. & Komel, R. (2007). Genetic changes in Slovenian patients with gastric adenocarcinoma evaluated in terms of microsatellite DNA. *Eur J Gastroenterol Hepatol*, 19, (12), pp. 1082-1089

Globocan, I. A. f. R. o. C. (2011). Available from: http://globocan.iarc.fr/.

Gollin, S. M. (2005). Mechanisms leading to chromosomal instability. *Semin Cancer Biol*, 15, (1), pp. 33-42

Grabsch, H. I., Askham, J. M., Morrison, E. E., Pomjanski, N., Lickvers, K., Parsons, W. J., Boecking, A., Gabbert, H. E. & Mueller, W. (2004). Expression of BUB1 protein in gastric cancer correlates with the histological subtype, but not with DNA ploidy or microsatellite instability. *J Pathol*, 202, (2), pp. 208-214, ISSN 0022-3417

Gu, M., Kim, D., Bae, Y., Choi, J., Kim, S. & Song, S. (2009). Analysis of microsatellite instability, protein expression and methylation status of hMLH1 and hMSH2 genes in gastric carcinomas. *Hepatogastroenterology*, 56, (91-92), pp. 899-904, ISSN 0172-6390

Guilford, P., Hopkins, J., Harraway, J., McLeod, M., McLeod, N., Harawira, P., Taite, H., Scoular, R., Miller, A. & Reeve, A. E. (1998). E-cadherin germline mutations in familial gastric cancer. *Nature*, 392, (6674), pp. 402-405, ISSN 0028-0836

Guerrette, S., Acharya, S. & Fishel, R. (1999). The interaction of the human MutL homologues in hereditary nonpolyposis colon cancer. *J Biol Chem*, 274, (10), pp. 6336-6341, ISSN 0021-9258

Gylling, A., Abdel-Rahman, W. M., Juhola, M., Nuorva, K., Hautala, E., Jarvinen, H. J., Mecklin, J. P., Aarnio, M. & Peltomaki, P. (2007). Is gastric cancer part of the tumour spectrum of hereditary non-polyposis colorectal cancer? A molecular genetic study. *Gut*, 56, (7), pp. 926-933, ISSN 0017-5749

Hamilton, J. P. & Meltzer, S. J. (2006). A review of the genomics of gastric cancer. *Clin Gastroenterol Hepatol*, 4, (4), pp. 416-425, ISSN 1542-3565

Hara, T., Ooi, A., Kobayashi, M., Mai, M., Yanagihara, K. & Nakanishi, I. (1998). Amplification of c-myc, K-sam, and c-met in gastric cancers: detection by fluorescence in situ hybridization. *Lab Invest*, 78, (9), pp. 1143-1153, ISSN 0023-6837

Hattori, Y., Itoh, H., Uchino, S., Hosokawa, K., Ochiai, A., Ino, Y., Ishii, H., Sakamoto, H., Yamaguchi, N., Yanagihara, K., Hirohashi, S., Sugimura, T. & Terada, M. (1996). Immunohistochemical detection of K-sam protein in stomach cancer. *Clin Cancer Res*, 2, (8), pp. 1373-1381, ISSN 1078-0432

Hirohashi, S. & Sugimura, T. (1991). Genetic alterations in human gastric cancer. *Cancer Cells*, 3, (2), pp. 49-52, ISSN 1042-2196

Hiyama, T., Haruma, K., Kitadai, Y., Masuda, H., Miyamoto, M., Tanaka, S., Yoshihara, M., Shimamoto, F. & Chayama, K. (2002). K-ras mutation in helicobacter pylori-associated chronic gastritis in patients with and without gastric cancer. *Int J Cancer*, 97, (5), pp. 562-566, ISSN 0020-7136

Hong, S. J., Jeon, E. J., Oh, J. H., Seo, E. J., Choi, S. W. & Rhyu, M. G. (2010). The gene-reduction effect of chromosomal losses detected in gastric cancers. *BMC Gastroenterol*, 10, pp. 138

Hou, Q., Wu, Y. H., Grabsch, H., Zhu, Y., Leong, S. H., Ganesan, K., Cross, D., Tan, L. K., Tao, J., Gopalakrishnan, V., Tang, B. L., Kon, O. L. & Tan, P. (2008). Integrative genomics identifies RAB23 as an invasion mediator gene in diffuse-type gastric cancer. *Cancer Res*, 68, (12), pp. 4623-4630, ISSN 1538-7445

Hudler, P., Vouk, K., Liovic, M., Repse, S., Juvan, R. & Komel, R. (2004). Mutations in the hMLH1 gene in Slovenian patients with gastric carcinoma. *Clin Genet*, 65, (5), pp. 405-411

Hudler, P., Kastelic, S., Frkovic-Grazio, S. & Komel, R. (2009). Polymorphisms in AURKA gene in Slovenian patients with gastric cancer. (Preliminary report). *Proceedings of* Joint Congress of the Slovenian Biochemical Society and the Genetic Society of Slovenia with International Participation, Otocec, September, 2009

Hudler, P., Simic, M., Frkovic-Grazio, S. & Komel, R. (2010). Polymorphisms in TTK and BUB1B genes in Slovenian patients with gastric cancer. (Preliminary report). *Proceedings of* 5th CFGBC Symposium, Ljubljana, June 2010

Imai, K. & Yamamoto, H. (2008). Carcinogenesis and microsatellite instability: the interrelationship between genetics and epigenetics. *Carcinogenesis*, 29, (4), pp. 673-680, ISSN 1460-2180

Iovino, F., Lentini, L., Amato, A. & Di Leonardo, A. (2006). RB acute loss induces centrosome amplification and aneuploidy in murine primary fibroblasts. *Mol Cancer*, 5, pp. 38, ISSN 1476-4598

Jiaqing, L., Hokita, S., Xiangming, C., Natsugoe, S., Tanabe, G., Baba, M., Takao, S. & Aikou, T. (1998). Role of cyclin E and p53 expression in progression of early gastric cancer. *Gastric Cancer*, 1, (2), pp. 160-165, ISSN 1436-3291

Junnila, S., Kokkola, A., Karjalainen-Lindsberg, M. L., Puolakkainen, P. & Monni, O. (2010). Genome-wide gene copy number and expression analysis of primary gastric tumors and gastric cancer cell lines. *BMC Cancer*, 10, pp. 73, ISSN 1471-2407

Juvan, R., Hudler, P., Gazvoda, B., Repse, S., Bracko, M. & Komel, R. (2007). Significance of genetic abnormalities of p53 protein in Slovenian patients with gastric carcinoma. *Croat Med J*, 48, (2), pp. 207-217, ISSN 1332-8166

Kanai, Y. & Hirohashi, S. (1997). Invasion and metastasis, In: *Gastric cancer*, T. Sugimura, pp. 109, Oxford University Press, Oxford.

Kang, J. U., Kang, J. J., Kwon, K. C., Park, J. W., Jeong, T. E., Noh, S. M. & Koo, S. H. (2006). Genetic alterations in primary gastric carcinomas correlated with clinicopathological variables by array comparative genomic hybridization. *J Korean Med Sci*, 21, (4), pp. 656-665, ISSN 1011-8934

Kim, H. S., Lee, B. L., Woo, D. K., Bae, S. I. & Kim, W. H. (2001). Assessment of markers for the identification of microsatellite instability phenotype in gastric neoplasms. *Cancer Lett*, 164, (1), pp. 61-68, ISSN 0304-3835

Kim, J. H., Takahashi, T., Chiba, I., Park, J. G., Birrer, M. J., Roh, J. K., De Lee, H., Kim, J. P., Minna, J. D. & Gazdar, A. F. (1991). Occurrence of p53 gene abnormalities in gastric carcinoma tumors and cell lines. *J Natl Cancer Inst*, 83, (13), pp. 938-943

Kimura, Y., Noguchi, T., Kawahara, K., Kashima, K., Daa, T. & Yokoyama, S. (2004). Genetic alterations in 102 primary gastric cancers by comparative genomic hybridization:

gain of 20q and loss of 18q are associated with tumor progression. *Mod Pathol*, 17, (11), pp. 1328-1337, ISSN 0893-3952

Kinzler, K. W., Nilbert, M. C., Su, L. K., Vogelstein, B., Bryan, T. M., Levy, D. B., Smith, K. J., Preisinger, A. C., Hedge, P., McKechnie, D. & et al. (1991). Identification of FAP locus genes from chromosome 5q21. *Science*, 253, (5020), pp. 661-665, ISSN 0036-8075

Knudson, A. G. (1993). Antioncogenes and human cancer. *Proc Natl Acad Sci U S A*, 90, (23), pp. 10914-10921, ISSN 0027-8424

Kondo, T., Oue, N., Mitani, Y., Kuniyasu, H., Noguchi, T., Kuraoka, K., Nakayama, H. & Yasui, W. (2005). Loss of heterozygosity and histone hypoacetylation of the PINX1 gene are associated with reduced expression in gastric carcinoma. *Oncogene*, 24, (1), pp. 157-164, ISSN 0950-9232

Kondo, E., Suzuki, H., Horii, A. & Fukushige, S. (2003). A yeast two-hybrid assay provides a simple way to evaluate the vast majority of hMLH1 germ-line mutations. *Cancer Res*, 63, (12), pp. 3302-3308, ISSN 0008-5472

Koo, S. H., Jeong, T. E., Kang, J., Kwon, K. C., Park, J. W. & Noh, S. M. (2004). Prognostic implications for gastric carcinoma based on loss of heterozygosity genotypes correlation with clinicopathologic variables. *Cancer Genet Cytogenet*, 153, (1), pp. 26-31, ISSN 0165-4608

Kumar, P., Henikoff, S. & Ng, P. C. (2009). Predicting the effects of coding non-synonymous variants on protein function using the SIFT algorithm. *Nat Protoc*, 4, (7), pp. 1073-1081

Kufe, D. W., Holland, J. F., Frei, E., Abramson, D. H., Dang, C. T., DeAngelis, L. M., Dolphin, K. W., Gilewski, T. A., Holland, J. C., Silver, R. T. & American Cancer Society. (2003). *Cancer medicine 6*, BC Decker, ISBN 1550092138, Hamilton, Ont.

Lawes, D. A., SenGupta, S. & Boulos, P. B. (2003). The clinical importance and prognostic implications of microsatellite instability in sporadic cancer. *Eur J Surg Oncol*, 29, (3), pp. 201-212, ISSN 0748-7983

Lazar, D., Taban, S., Sporea, I., Dema, A., Cornianu, M., Lazar, E., Goldis, A., Ratiu, I. & Vernic, C. (2010). The immunohistochemical expression of the p53-protein in gastric carcinomas. Correlation with clinicopathological factors and survival of patients. *Rom J Morphol Embryol*, 51, (2), pp. 249-257, ISSN 1220-0522

Leite, M., Corso, G., Sousa, S., Milanezi, F., Afonso, L. P., Henrique, R., Soares, J. M., Castedo, S., Carneiro, F., Roviello, F., Oliveira, C. & Seruca, R. (2011). MSI phenotype and MMR alterations in familial and sporadic gastric cancer. *Int J Cancer*, 128, (7), pp. 1606-1613, ISSN 1097-0215

Leung, S. Y., Yuen, S. T., Chung, L. P., Chu, K. M., Chan, A. S. & Ho, J. C. (1999). hMLH1 promoter methylation and lack of hMLH1 expression in sporadic gastric carcinomas with high-frequency microsatellite instability. *Cancer Res*, 59, (1), pp. 159-164, ISSN 0008-5472

Liu, X. P., Tsushimi, K., Tsushimi, M., Oga, A., Kawauchi, S., Furuya, T. & Sasaki, K. (2001). Expression of p53 protein as a prognostic indicator of reduced survival time in diffuse-type gastric carcinoma. *Pathol Int*, 51, (6), pp. 440-444

Loeb, L. A. (2001). A mutator phenotype in cancer. *Cancer Res*, 61, (8), pp. 3230-3239, ISSN 0008-5472

Lynch, H. T. & Lynch, J. F. (1998). Genetics of colonic cancer. *Digestion*, 59, (5), pp. 481-492, ISSN 0012-2823

Malden, L. T., Novak, U. & Burgess, A. W. (1989). Expression of transforming growth factor alpha messenger RNA in the normal and neoplastic gastro-intestinal tract. *Int J Cancer*, 43, (3), pp. 380-384, ISSN 0020-7136

Mathe, E., Olivier, M., Kato, S., Ishioka, C., Hainaut, P. & Tavtigian, S. V. (2006). Computational approaches for predicting the biological effect of p53 missense mutations: a comparison of three sequence analysis based methods. *Nucleic Acids Res*, 34, (5), pp. 1317-1325, ISSN 1362-4962

Martin, S. A., Hewish, M., Lord, C. J. & Ashworth, A. (2010). Genomic instability and the selection of treatments for cancer. *J Pathol*, 220, (2), pp. 281-289, ISSN 1096-9896

Matysiak-Budnik, T. & Megraud, F. (2006). Helicobacter pylori infection and gastric cancer. *Eur J Cancer*, 42, (6), pp. 708-716, ISSN 0959-8049

Milne, A. N., Carneiro, F., O'Morain, C. & Offerhaus, G. J. (2009). Nature meets nurture: molecular genetics of gastric cancer. *Hum Genet*, 126, (5), pp. 615-628, ISSN 1432-1203

Mitani, Y., Oue, N., Hamai, Y., Aung, P. P., Matsumura, S., Nakayama, H., Kamata, N. & Yasui, W. (2005). Histone H3 acetylation is associated with reduced p21(WAF1/CIP1) expression by gastric carcinoma. *J Pathol*, 205, (1), pp. 65-73, ISSN 0022-3417

Morohara, K., Nakao, K., Tajima, Y., Nishino, N., Yamazaki, K., Kaetsu, T., Suzuki, S., Tsunoda, A., Kawamura, M., Aida, T., Tachikawa, T. & Kusano, M. (2005). Analysis by comparative genomic hybridization of gastric cancer with peritoneal dissemination and/or positive peritoneal cytology. *Cancer Genet Cytogenet*, 161, (1), pp. 57-62, ISSN 0165-4608

Nakajima, M., Sawada, H., Yamada, Y., Watanabe, A., Tatsumi, M., Yamashita, J., Matsuda, M., Sakaguchi, T., Hirao, T. & Nakano, H. (1999). The prognostic significance of amplification and overexpression of c-met and c-erb B-2 in human gastric carcinomas. *Cancer*, 85, (9), pp. 1894-1902

Ng, P. C. & Henikoff, S. (2003). SIFT: Predicting amino acid changes that affect protein function. *Nucleic Acids Res*, 31, (13), pp. 3812-3814, ISSN 1362-4962

Nobili, S., Bruno, L., Landini, I., Napoli, C., Bechi, P., Tonelli, F., Rubio, C. A., Mini, E. & Nesi, G. (2011). Genomic and genetic alterations influence the progression of gastric cancer. *World J Gastroenterol*, 17, (3), pp. 290-299, ISSN 1007-9327

Oda, S., Zhao, Y. & Maehara, Y. (2005). Microsatellite instability in gastrointestinal tract cancers: a brief update. *Surg Today*, 35, (12), pp. 1005-1015, ISSN 0941-1291

Osaki, M., Miyata, H., Hayashi, A., Gomyo, Y., Tatebe, S. & Ito, H. (1996). Lack of rearranged Tpr-met mRNA expression in human gastric cancer cell lines and gastric mucosa and carcinoma. *Anticancer Res*, 16, (5A), pp. 2881-2884, ISSN 0250-7005

Ottini, L., Falchetti, M., Saieva, C., De Marco, M., Masala, G., Zanna, I., Paglierani, M., Giannini, G., Gulino, A., Nesi, G., Mariani Costantini, R. & Palli, D. (2004). MRE11 expression is impaired in gastric cancer with microsatellite instability. *Carcinogenesis*, 25, (12), pp. 2337-2343, ISSN 0143-3334

Ottini, L., Falchetti, M., Lupi, R., Rizzolo, P., Agnese, V., Colucci, G., Bazan, V. & Russo, A. (2006). Patterns of genomic instability in gastric cancer: clinical implications and perspectives. *Ann Oncol*, 17, (suppl_7), pp. vii97-vii102

Ou, J., Niessen, R. C., Lutzen, A., Sijmons, R. H., Kleibeuker, J. H., de Wind, N., Rasmussen, L. J. & Hofstra, R. M. (2007). Functional analysis helps to clarify the clinical importance of unclassified variants in DNA mismatch repair genes. *Hum Mutat*, 28, (11), pp. 1047-1054, ISSN 1098-1004

Oue, N., Sentani, K., Yokozaki, H., Kitadai, Y., Ito, R. & Yasui, W. (2001). Promoter methylation status of the DNA repair genes hMLH1 and MGMT in gastric carcinoma and metaplastic mucosa. *Pathobiology*, 69, (3), pp. 143-149, ISSN 1015-2008

Panani, A. D. (2008). Cytogenetic and molecular aspects of gastric cancer: clinical implications. *Cancer Lett*, 266, (2), pp. 99-115, ISSN 0304-3835

Park, W. S., Oh, R. R., Park, J. Y., Lee, S. H., Shin, M. S., Kim, Y. S., Kim, S. Y., Lee, H. K., Kim, P. J., Oh, S. T., Yoo, N. J. & Lee, J. Y. (1999). Frequent somatic mutations of the beta-catenin gene in intestinal-type gastric cancer. *Cancer Res*, 59, (17), pp. 4257-4260, ISSN 0008-5472

Pedrazzani, C., Corso, G., Velho, S., Leite, M., Pascale, V., Bettarini, F., Marrelli, D., Seruca, R. & Roviello, F. (2009). Evidence of tumor microsatellite instability in gastric cancer with familial aggregation. *Fam Cancer*, 8, (3), pp. 215-220, ISSN 1573-7292

Pellegata, N. S., Losekoot, M., Fodde, R., Pugliese, V., Saccomanno, S., Renault, B., Bernini, L. F. & Ranzani, G. N. (1992). Detection of K-ras mutations by denaturing gradient gel electrophoresis (DGGE): a study on pancreatic cancer. *Anticancer Res*, 12, (5), pp. 1731-1735, ISSN 0250-7005

Perera, S. & Bapat, B. (2008). The MLH1 variants p.Arg265Cys and p.Lys618Ala affect protein stability while p.Leu749Gln affects heterodimer formation. *Hum Mutat*, 29, (2), pp. 332, ISSN 1098-1004

Percesepe, A., Borghi, F., Menigatti, M., Losi, L., Foroni, M., Di Gregorio, C., Rossi, G., Pedroni, M., Sala, E., Vaccina, F., Roncucci, L., Benatti, P., Viel, A., Genuardi, M., Marra, G., Kristo, P., Peltomaki, P. & Ponz de Leon, M. (2001). Molecular screening for hereditary nonpolyposis colorectal cancer: a prospective, population-based study. *J Clin Oncol*, 19, (19), pp. 3944-3950

Perucho, M. (1996). Microsatellite instability: the mutator that mutates the other mutator. *Nat Med*, 2, (6), pp. 630-631, ISSN 1078-8956

Pino, M. S. & Chung, D. C. (2010). The chromosomal instability pathway in colon cancer. *Gastroenterology*, 138, (6), pp. 2059-2072, ISSN 1528-0012

Rajcevic, U., Juvan, R., Gazvoda, B., Repse, S. & Komel, R. (2001). Assessment of differential expression of oncogenes in gastric adenocarcinoma by fluorescent multiplex RT-PCR assay. *Pflugers Arch*, 442, (6 Suppl 1), pp. R190-192, ISSN 0031-6768

Rajcevic, U., Hudler, P., Mijovski, G., Gorjanc, G., Hoelzl, G., Repse, S., Juvan, R., Kovac, M., Huber, C. G. & Komel, R. (2007). Assessment of differential expression of oncogenes in adenocarcinoma of stomach with fluorescent labeling and simultaneous amplification of gene transcripts. *Radiol Oncol*, 41, (4), pp. 174-182

Raevaara, T. E., Korhonen, M. K., Lohi, H., Hampel, H., Lynch, E., Lonnqvist, K. E., Holinski-Feder, E., Sutter, C., McKinnon, W., Duraisamy, S., Gerdes, A. M., Peltomaki, P., Kohonen-Ccorish, M., Mangold, E., Macrae, F., Greenblatt, M., de la

Chapelle, A. & Nystrom, M. (2005). Functional significance and clinical phenotype of nontruncating mismatch repair variants of MLH1. *Gastroenterology*, 129, (2), pp. 537-549, ISSN 0016-5085

Ramensky, V., Bork, P. & Sunyaev, S. (2002). Human non-synonymous SNPs: server and survey. *Nucleic Acids Res*, 30, (17), pp. 3894-3900, ISSN 1362-4962

Resende, C., Ristimaki, A. & Machado, J. C. (2010). Genetic and epigenetic alteration in gastric carcinogenesis. *Helicobacter*, 15 Suppl 1, pp. 34-39, ISSN 1523-5378

Ricke, R. M., van Ree, J. H. & van Deursen, J. M. (2008). Whole chromosome instability and cancer: a complex relationship. *Trends Genet*, 24, (9), pp. 457-466, ISSN 0168-9525

Russo, A., Bazan, V., Migliavacca, M., Zanna, I., Tubiolo, C., Tumminello, F. M., Dardanoni, G., Cajozzo, M., Bazan, P., Modica, G., Latteri, M., Tomasino, R. M., Colucci, G., Gebbia, N. & Leto, G. (2000). Prognostic significance of DNA ploidy, S-phase fraction, and tissue levels of aspartic, cysteine, and serine proteases in operable gastric carcinoma. *Clin Cancer Res*, 6, (1), pp. 178-184, ISSN 1078-0432

Samowitz, W. S., Curtin, K., Lin, H. H., Robertson, M. A., Schaffer, D., Nichols, M., Gruenthal, K., Leppert, M. F. & Slattery, M. L. (2001). The colon cancer burden of genetically defined hereditary nonpolyposis colon cancer. *Gastroenterology*, 121, (4), pp. 830-838, ISSN 0016-5085

Scartozzi, M., Galizia, E., Freddari, F., Berardi, R., Cellerino, R. & Cascinu, S. (2004). Molecular biology of sporadic gastric cancer: prognostic indicators and novel therapeutic approaches. *Cancer Treat Rev*, 30, (5), pp. 451-459, ISSN 0305-7372

Schmit, T. L. & Ahmad, N. (2007). Regulation of mitosis via mitotic kinases: new opportunities for cancer management. *Mol Cancer Ther*, 6, (7), pp. 1920-1931, ISSN 1535-7163

Schneider, B. G., Bravo, J. C., Roa, J. C., Roa, I., Kim, M. C., Lee, K. M., Plaisance, K. T., Jr., McBride, C. M. & Mera, R. (2000). Microsatellite instability, prognosis and metastasis in gastric cancers from a low-risk population. *Int J Cancer*, 89, (5), pp. 444-452, ISSN 0020-7136

Schneider, B. G., Peng, D. F., Camargo, M. C., Piazuelo, M. B., Sicinschi, L. A., Mera, R., Romero-Gallo, J., Delgado, A. G., Bravo, L. E., Wilson, K. T., Peek, R. M., Jr., Correa, P. & El-Rifai, W. (2010). Promoter DNA hypermethylation in gastric biopsies from subjects at high and low risk for gastric cancer. *Int J Cancer*, 127, (11), pp. 2588-2597, ISSN 1097-0215

Sharp, A., Pichert, G., Lucassen, A. & Eccles, D. (2004). RNA analysis reveals splicing mutations and loss of expression defects in MLH1 and BRCA1. *Hum Mutat*, 24, (3), pp. 272, ISSN 1098-1004

Shepard, J. L., Amatruda, J. F., Finkelstein, D., Ziai, J., Finley, K. R., Stern, H. M., Chiang, K., Hersey, C., Barut, B., Freeman, J. L., Lee, C., Glickman, J. N., Kutok, J. L., Aster, J. C. & Zon, L. I. (2007). A mutation in separase causes genome instability and increased susceptibility to epithelial cancer. *Genes Dev*, 21, (1), pp. 55-59

Shimodaira, H., Filosi, N., Shibata, H., Suzuki, T., Radice, P., Kanamaru, R., Friend, S. H., Kolodner, R. D. & Ishioka, C. (1998). Functional analysis of human MLH1 mutations in Saccharomyces cerevisiae. *Nat Genet*, 19, (4), pp. 384-389

Simpson, A. J., Caballero, O. L. & Pena, S. D. (2001). Microsatellite instability as a tool for the classification of gastric cancer. *Trends Mol Med*, 7, (2), pp. 76-80, ISSN 1471-4914

Smith, M. G., Hold, G. L., Tahara, E. & El-Omar, E. M. (2006). Cellular and molecular aspects of gastric cancer. *World J Gastroenterol*, 12, (19), pp. 2979-2990

Smolen, G. A., Sordella, R., Muir, B., Mohapatra, G., Barmettler, A., Archibald, H., Kim, W. J., Okimoto, R. A., Bell, D. W., Sgroi, D. C., Christensen, J. G., Settleman, J. & Haber, D. A. (2006). Amplification of MET may identify a subset of cancers with extreme sensitivity to the selective tyrosine kinase inhibitor PHA-665752. *Proc Natl Acad Sci U S A*, 103, (7), pp. 2316-2321, ISSN 0027-8424

Soh, K., Yanagisawa, A., Hiratsuka, H., Sugano, H. & Kato, Y. (1993). Variation in K-ras codon 12 point mutation rate with histological atypia within individual colorectal tumors. *Jpn J Cancer Res*, 84, (4), pp. 388-393, ISSN 0910-5050

Suraweera, N., Duval, A., Reperant, M., Vaury, C., Furlan, D., Leroy, K., Seruca, R., Iacopetta, B. & Hamelin, R. (2002). Evaluation of tumor microsatellite instability using five quasimonomorphic mononucleotide repeats and pentaplex PCR. *Gastroenterology*, 123, (6), pp. 1804-1811, ISSN 0016-5085

Suzuki, K., Ohnami, S., Tanabe, C., Sasaki, H., Yasuda, J., Katai, H., Yoshimura, K., Terada, M., Perucho, M. & Yoshida, T. (2003). The genomic damage estimated by arbitrarily primed PCR DNA fingerprinting is useful for the prognosis of gastric cancer. *Gastroenterology*, 125, (5), pp. 1330-1340, ISSN 0016-5085

Suzuki, K., Suzuki, I., Leodolter, A., Alonso, S., Horiuchi, S., Yamashita, K. & Perucho, M. (2006). Global DNA demethylation in gastrointestinal cancer is age dependent and precedes genomic damage. *Cancer Cell*, 9, (3), pp. 199-207

Tahara, E. (1995). Genetic alterations in human gastrointestinal cancers. The application to molecular diagnosis. *Cancer*, 75, (6 Suppl), pp. 1410-1417

Tahara, E. (2004). Genetic pathways of two types of gastric cancer. *IARC Sci Publ*, (157), pp. 327-349

Tahara, E. (2008). Abnormal growth factor/cytokine network in gastric cancer. *Cancer Microenviron*, 1, (1), pp. 85-91, ISSN 1875-2292

Takahashi, M., Shimodaira, H., Andreutti-Zaugg, C., Iggo, R., Kolodner, R. D. & Ishioka, C. (2007). Functional analysis of human MLH1 variants using yeast and in vitro mismatch repair assays. *Cancer Res*, 67, (10), pp. 4595-4604, ISSN 0008-5472

Tamura, G. (2006). Alterations of tumor suppressor and tumor-related genes in the development and progression of gastric cancer. *World J Gastroenterol*, 12, (2), pp. 192-198

Tavtigian, S. V., Greenblatt, M. S., Lesueur, F. & Byrnes, G. B. (2008). In silico analysis of missense substitutions using sequence-alignment based methods. *Hum Mutat*, 29, (11), pp. 1327-1336, ISSN 1098-1004

Tian, X., Song, S., Wu, J., Meng, L., Dong, Z. & Shou, C. (2001). Vascular endothelial growth factor: acting as an autocrine growth factor for human gastric adenocarcinoma cell MGC803. *Biochem Biophys Res Commun*, 286, (3), pp. 505-512

Tomonaga, T. & Nomura, F. (2007). Chromosome instability and kinetochore dysfunction. *Histol Histopathol*, 22, (2), pp. 191-197

Tournier, I., Vezain, M., Martins, A., Charbonnier, F., Baert-Desurmont, S., Olschwang, S., Wang, Q., Buisine, M. P., Soret, J., Tazi, J., Frebourg, T. & Tosi, M. (2008). A large fraction of unclassified variants of the mismatch repair genes MLH1 and MSH2 is associated with splicing defects. *Hum Mutat*, 29, (12), pp. 1412-1424

Trojan, J., Zeuzem, S., Randolph, A., Hemmerle, C., Brieger, A., Raedle, J., Plotz, G., Jiricny, J. & Marra, G. (2002). Functional analysis of hMLH1 variants and HNPCC-related mutations using a human expression system. *Gastroenterology*, 122, (1), pp. 211-219

Tsugawa, K., Yonemura, Y., Hirono, Y., Fushida, S., Kaji, M., Miwa, K., Miyazaki, I. & Yamamoto, H. (1998). Amplification of the c-met, c-erbB-2 and epidermal growth factor receptor gene in human gastric cancers: correlation to clinical features. *Oncology*, 55, (5), pp. 475-481, ISSN 0030-2414

Tsukamoto, Y., Uchida, T., Karnan, S., Noguchi, T., Nguyen, L. T., Tanigawa, M., Takeuchi, I., Matsuura, K., Hijiya, N., Nakada, C., Kishida, T., Kawahara, K., Ito, H., Murakami, K., Fujioka, T., Seto, M. & Moriyama, M. (2008). Genome-wide analysis of DNA copy number alterations and gene expression in gastric cancer. *J Pathol*, 216, (4), pp. 471-482, ISSN 1096-9896

Umar, A., Boland, C. R., Terdiman, J. P., Syngal, S., de la Chapelle, A., Ruschoff, J., Fishel, R., Lindor, N. M., Burgart, L. J., Hamelin, R., Hamilton, S. R., Hiatt, R. A., Jass, J., Lindblom, A., Lynch, H. T., Peltomaki, P., Ramsey, S. D., Rodriguez-Bigas, M. A., Vasen, H. F., Hawk, E. T., Barrett, J. C., Freedman, A. N. & Srivastava, S. (2004). Revised Bethesda Guidelines for hereditary nonpolyposis colorectal cancer (Lynch syndrome) and microsatellite instability. *J Natl Cancer Inst*, 96, (4), pp. 261-268, ISSN 1460-2105

van Rees, B. P., Musler, A., Caspers, E., Drillenburg, P., Craanen, M. E., Polkowski, W., Chibowski, D. & Offerhaus, G. J. (1999). K-ras mutations in gastric stump carcinomas and in carcinomas from the non-operated stomach. *Hepatogastroenterology*, 46, (27), pp. 2063-2068, ISSN 0172-6390

Varis, A., van Rees, B., Weterman, M., Ristimaki, A., Offerhaus, J. & Knuutila, S. (2003). DNA copy number changes in young gastric cancer patients with special reference to chromosome 19. *Br J Cancer*, 88, (12), pp. 1914-1919, ISSN 0007-0920

Vizoso, F. J., Corte, M. D., Alvarez, A., Garcia, I., del Casar, J. M., Bongera, M., Gonzalez, L. O., Garcia-Muniz, J. L. & Allende, M. T. (2004). Membranous levels of c-erbB-2 oncoprotein in gastric cancer: their relationship with clinicopathological parameters and their prognostic significance. *Int J Biol Markers*, 19, (4), pp. 268-274, ISSN 0393-6155

Vogelsang, M., Comino, A., Zupanec, N., Hudler, P. & Komel, R. (2009). Assessing pathogenicity of MLH1 variants by co-expression of human MLH1 and PMS2 genes in yeast. *BMC Cancer*, 9, pp. 382, ISSN 1471-2407

Vogelsang, M. & Komel, R. (2010). Non-truncating hMLH1 variants identified in Slovenian gastric cancer patients are not associated with Lynch Syndrome: a functional analysis report. *Fam Cancer*, pp., ISSN 1573-7292

Vogelstein, B. & Kinzler, K. W. (2004). Cancer genes and the pathways they control. *Nat Med*, 10, (8), pp. 789-799

Vousden, K. H. & Prives, C. (2005). P53 and prognosis: new insights and further complexity. *Cell*, 120, (1), pp. 7-10, ISSN 0092-8674

Wanat, J. J., Singh, N. & Alani, E. (2007). The effect of genetic background on the function of Saccharomyces cerevisiae mlh1 alleles that correspond to HNPCC missense mutations. *Hum Mol Genet*, 16, (4), pp. 445-452, ISSN 0964-6906

Weber, B. L. (2002). Cancer genomics. *Cancer Cell*, 1, (1), pp. 37-47, ISSN 1535-6108

Weiss, M. M., Kuipers, E. J., Postma, C., Snijders, A. M., Pinkel, D., Meuwissen, S. G., Albertson, D. & Meijer, G. A. (2004). Genomic alterations in primary gastric adenocarcinomas correlate with clinicopathological characteristics and survival. *Cell Oncol*, 26, (5-6), pp. 307-317, ISSN 1570-5870

Werner, M., Becker, K. F., Keller, G. & Hofler, H. (2001). Gastric adenocarcinoma: pathomorphology and molecular pathology. *J Cancer Res Clin Oncol*, 127, (4), pp. 207-216, ISSN 0171-5216

Wright, P. A. & Williams, G. T. (1993). Molecular biology and gastric carcinoma. *Gut*, 34, (2), pp. 145-147, ISSN 0017-5749

Wu, C. W., Chen, G. D., Fann, C. S., Lee, A. F., Chi, C. W., Liu, J. M., Weier, U. & Chen, J. Y. (2002). Clinical implications of chromosomal abnormalities in gastric adenocarcinomas. *Genes Chromosomes Cancer*, 35, (3), pp. 219-231, ISSN 1045-2257

Wu, M. S., Lee, C. W., Shun, C. T., Wang, H. P., Lee, W. J., Chang, M. C., Sheu, J. C. & Lin, J. T. (2000). Distinct clinicopathologic and genetic profiles in sporadic gastric cancer with different mutator phenotypes. *Genes Chromosomes Cancer*, 27, (4), pp. 403-411, ISSN 1045-2257

Wu, W. K., Cho, C. H., Lee, C. W., Fan, D., Wu, K., Yu, J. & Sung, J. J. (2010). Dysregulation of cellular signaling in gastric cancer. *Cancer Lett*, 295, (2), pp. 144-153, ISSN 1872-7980

Xiangming, C., Hokita, S., Natsugoe, S., Tanabe, G., Baba, M., Takao, S., Kuroshima, K. & Aikou, T. (1999). Cooccurrence of reduced expression of alpha-catenin and overexpression of p53 is a predictor of lymph node metastasis in early gastric cancer. *Oncology*, 57, (2), pp. 131-137, ISSN 0030-2414

Xiangming, C., Natsugoe, S., Takao, S., Hokita, S., Tanabe, G., Baba, M., Kuroshima, K. & Aikou, T. (2000). The cooperative role of p27 with cyclin E in the prognosis of advanced gastric carcinoma. *Cancer*, 89, (6), pp. 1214-1219

Yamamoto, E., Suzuki, H., Takamaru, H., Yamamoto, H., Toyota, M. & Shinomura, Y. (2011). Role of DNA Methylation in the Development of Diffuse-Type Gastric Cancer. *Digestion*, 83, (4), pp. 241-249, ISSN 1421-9867

Yamamoto, H., Perez-Piteira, J., Yoshida, T., Terada, M., Itoh, F., Imai, K. & Perucho, M. (1999). Gastric cancers of the microsatellite mutator phenotype display characteristic genetic and clinical features. *Gastroenterology*, 116, (6), pp. 1348-1357, ISSN 0016-5085

Yamamoto, S., Yasui, W., Kitadai, Y., Yokozaki, H., Haruma, K., Kajiyama, G. & Tahara, E. (1998). Expression of vascular endothelial growth factor in human gastric carcinomas. *Pathol Int*, 48, (7), pp. 499-506, ISSN 1320-5463

Yamashita, K., Sakuramoto, S. & Watanabe, M. (2011). Genomic and epigenetic profiles of gastric cancer: potential diagnostic and therapeutic applications. *Surg Today*, 41, (1), pp. 24-38, ISSN 1436-2813

Yasa, M. H., Bektas, A., Yukselen, V., Akbulut, H., Camci, C. & Ormeci, N. (2005). DNA analysis and DNA ploidy in gastric cancer and gastric precancerous lesions. *Int J Clin Pract*, 59, (9), pp. 1029-1033, ISSN 1368-5031

Yasui, W., Tahara, E., Tahara, H., Fujimoto, J., Naka, K., Nakayama, J., Ishikawa, F. & Ide, T. (1999). Immunohistochemical detection of human telomerase reverse transcriptase in normal mucosa and precancerous lesions of the stomach. *Jpn J Cancer Res*, 90, (6), pp. 589-595, ISSN 0910-5050

Yokozaki, H., Yasui, W. & Tahara, E. (2001). Genetic and epigenetic changes in stomach cancer. *Int Rev Cytol*, 204, pp. 49-95, ISSN 0074-7696

Yonemura, Y., Takamura, H., Ninomiya, I., Fushida, S., Tsugawa, K., Kaji, M., Nakai, Y., Ohoyama, S., Yamaguchi, A. & Miyazaki, I. (1992). Interrelationship between transforming growth factor-alpha and epidermal growth factor receptor in advanced gastric cancer. *Oncology*, 49, (2), pp. 157-161, ISSN 0030-2414

Yoshida, K., Yasui, W., Ito, H. & Tahara, E. (1990). Growth factors in progression of human esophageal and gastric carcinomas. *Exp Pathol*, 40, (4), pp. 291-300, ISSN 0232-1513

Zhang, X. L., Yang, Y. S., Xu, D. P., Qu, J. H., Guo, M. Z., Gong, Y. & Huang, J. (2009). Comparative study on overexpression of HER2/neu and HER3 in gastric cancer. *World J Surg*, 33, (10), pp. 2112-2118, ISSN 1432-2323

Zheng, L., Wang, L., Ajani, J. & Xie, K. (2004). Molecular basis of gastric cancer development and progression. *Gastric Cancer*, 7, (2), pp. 61-77

Zhou, X. P., Hoang, J. M., Li, Y. J., Seruca, R., Carneiro, F., Sobrinho-Simoes, M., Lothe, R. A., Gleeson, C. M., Russell, S. E., Muzeau, F., Flejou, J. F., Hoang-Xuan, K., Lidereau, R., Thomas, G. & Hamelin, R. (1998). Determination of the replication error phenotype in human tumors without the requirement for matching normal DNA by analysis of mononucleotide repeat microsatellites. *Genes Chromosomes Cancer*, 21, (2), pp. 101-107, ISSN 1045-2257

Zhou, Y., Li, N., Zhuang, W. & Wu, X. (2011). Vascular endothelial growth factor (VEGF) gene polymorphisms and gastric cancer risk in a chinese han population. *Mol Carcinog*, 50, (3), pp. 184-188, ISSN 1098-2744

Zwick, A., Munir, M., Ryan, C. K., Gian, J., Burt, R. W., Leppert, M., Spirio, L. & Chey, W. Y. (1997). Gastric adenocarcinoma and dysplasia in fundic gland polyps of a patient with attenuated adenomatous polyposis coli. *Gastroenterology*, 113, (2), pp. 659-663, ISSN 0016-5085

3

The Epigenetic Aspect of Gastric Cancer

Xian Wang and Hongchuan Jin
Laboratory of Cancer Epigenetics, Biomedical Research Center, Sir Runrun Shaw Hospital, School of Medicine, Zhejiang University, Hangzhou, China

1. Introduction

Genetic susceptibility seems to play an important role in some gastric cancers. In some rare cases, gastric cancer can be one part of familial cancer syndromes. A well-known example is the family of Napoleon since the Emperor himself as well as his father and his grandfather had gastric cancer. Generally, hereditary factors include germline mutations of E-cadherin, APC, p53 or mismatch repair genes like hMLH1 or hMSH2. Gatekeeper genes like E-cadherin and APC encode signaling proteins important to cellular proliferation and differentiation while protein products from caretaker genes like p53 or mismatch repair genes are important to maintain the integrality and fidelity of the genome. In addition to gene mutations, gene polymorphisms have been shown to be associated with the susceptibility of gastric cancer (El-Omar et al., 2000; Persson et al., 2011). Interestingly, most of these genes are encoding proinflammatory cytokines, strongly indicating the importance of inflammation to the initiation and progression of gastric cancer.

Environment factors play important roles in the pathogenesis of gastric cancer by affecting the inflammation in the stomach. The infection of Helicobacter pylori is apparently one of the primary risk factors of gastric cancer. In 1994, the World Health Organization and the International Agency for Research on Cancer Consensus group classified H. pylori as a type I carcinogen in human beings. Although numerous studies reported the growth promoting effect of H. pylori or its derived proteins in vitro, no direct evidence about the interaction of H. pylori with cancer initiating or stem cells have been presented. In contrast, accumulating reports indicated that the inflammation induced by H. pylori infection is the key to gastric carcinogenesis. Thus, it was believed that H. pylori infection is the initial step in the stepwise process of gastric carcinogenesis starting from chronic gastritis, gastric atrophy, intestinal metaplasia, dysplasia to gastric carcinoma. Consistently, diets rich in fruit and vegetables is protective factors of gastric cancer since vitamin C are helpful to attenuate inflammation while inflammation-promoting factors such as smoking, foods with high salts and nitrite could facilitate the development of gastric cancer by promoting chronic inflammation.

Microenvironments in chronic inflammatory tissues are rich in growth factors and cytokines important to promote the perpetuation of tumor growth by epigenetically reprogramming cancer stem cells. In addition, there are some DNA damage inducing agents such as reactive oxygen and nitrogen species (RONS) that can cause genomic alterations, promoting the accumulation of mutations in proliferating cancer stem cells (Meira et al., 2008). On the other

hand, cancer cells during their progression can not only circumvent inhibitory signals from immune cells in inflammatory microenvironments but also suppress the anti-tumor immune response, eventually transforming the inflammation microenvironment into tumor permissive microenvironment, the niche for the survival and expansion of cancer stem cells (Wang and Jin, 2010).
Tumor promoting factors in tumor-permissive microenvironments can reprogram epigenetic regulatory network in cancer cells through various signaling pathways that deregulated in both inflammation and carcinogenesis, such as NF-kB pathway and IL6-STAT3 pathway (Pikarsky et al., 2004; Yu et al., 2009a). However, epigenetic changes directly controlled by intracellular signaling pathways can immediately reform cellular response to extracellular signals and therefore most likely precede genetic changes that take several cell divisions to be fixed. Similar to genetic changes, epigenetic changes can also affect the activity of many signaling pathways critical to cancer development. By doing so, epigenetic trans-generation of extracellular signals plays important roles in the initiation of many sporadic cancers (Figure 1).

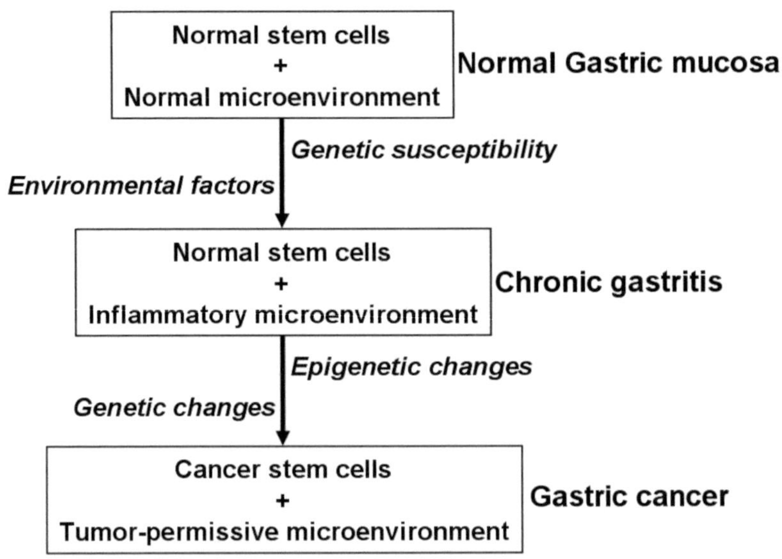

Fig. 1. Gastric cancer is resulting from the accumulation of genetic and epigenetic changes. Genetic factors such as polymorphism of genes encoding cytokines affect the pathogenesis of inflammation induced by environmental factors such as H. Pylori infection. Bioactive factors enriched in inflammatory microenvironments such as IL-6, INF-α and other prosurvival and anti-apoptotic signals could reprogram epigenetic regulatory network to promote genetic changes and the subsequent malignant transformation of stem or progenitor cells. The interaction of transformed stem cells with microenvironment gradually transformed microenvironment into tumor permissive microenvironment and stem cells into cancer stem cells.

2. Epigenetic view of gastric carcinogenesis

Epigenetic information is defined as cellular information heritable during cell division in addition to DNA sequence. Epigenetic network regulates the expression or function but not the sequence of genes. Up to date, the major components of epigenetic regulatory network include DNA methylation, non-coding RNAs mainly microRNAs and histone modifications. Similar to genetic changes, some of epigenetic changes are important to maintain the malignant phenotypes of cancer cells and thereby could be named as driver epigenetic changes while the others are passenger epigenetic changes since they are passively altered during cancer development.

Mechanism	Name	Scale
Bisulfite dependent	MS-PCR	Single Gene
	BGS	Single Gene
	MDFS	Single Gene
	Cobra	Single Gene
Bisulfite independent	Enzyme digestion-Southern Blot	Single Gene
	Enzyme digestion-PCR	Single Gene
	RLGS	Genome wide
	aPRIMES	Genome wide
	MB-PCR	Single Gene
	MB-Array/-sequencing	Genome wide

Table 1. Methods to detect DNA methylation

3. Aberrant DNA methylation in gastric carcinogenesis

DNA methylation is a type of chemical modification with the covalent addition of a methyl group to the fifth position of cytosine predominantly within the CpG dinucleotides. As one of the major mechanisms of epigenetic regulation, DNA methylation is involved in a number of important biological processes including linage-specific gene expression, parental or maternal imprinting and tumor suppressor gene silencing in carcinogenesis (Bird, 1986; Jones, 2002). Aberrant DNA methylation is deeply involved in gastric carcinogenesis by affecting various cellular processes including signal transduction, cell cycle regulation and gene expression. In addition to driver methylations, there are passenger methylations that could be used as the biomarkers for the detection or monitoring of cancer development and progression instead of the screening or defining of novel tumor suppressor genes. The genes silenced by DNA methylation in gastric cancer have been intensively discussed and thus will not be included here (Choi and Wu, 2005; Tamura, 2006). Instead, the potential application of DNA methylation in the detection of gastric cancer will be overviewed after the brief introduction of general approaches to detect DNA methylation.

3.1 General approaches to detect DNA methylation

In general, the approaches to detect DNA methylation could be grouped into two classes: bisulfite-dependent methods and bisulfite-independent methods (Table 1). Methylated DNA could be differentiated from unmethylated DNA by bisulfite DNA modification or restriction enzyme digestion. Bisulfite treatment could change unmethylated cytosine into uracil while left methylated cytosine unchanged. DNAs with different methylation status respond to the digestion of methylation-sensitive restriction enzymes differently, making it possible to detect DNA methylation indirectly by analyzing the products of enzyme digestion.

After the conversion of unmethylated cytosine into uracil by bisulfite treatment, methylated DNA could be amplified by methylation specific-PCR (MS-PCR) with specifically designed primers (Herman et al., 1996). The advantage of this method includes the fast detection of DNA methylation with high sensitivity and specificity. The main disadvantage is the low level of resolution to determine the methylation of particular CpG sites only in the 3'-terminus of primers. The pattern of multiple methylated CpG sites could be determined by bisulfite genome sequencing in which PCR products with methylation non-selective primers will be directly sequenced or sequenced indirectly after TA cloning. Alternatively, methylation could be quantified by MethyLight in which methylation or unmethylation specific probes were used in PCR amplification (Eads et al., 2000). Other quantitative methods include MS-HRM (Methylation-sensitive high resolution melting) which takes the advantage of the differences in melting of PCR products from methylated and unmethylated DNA while methylation-dependent fragment separation (MDFS) could detect DNA methylation by comparing differential migration times of PCR products in electrophoresis (Boyd et al., 2006; Wojdacz and Dobrovic, 2007). In the method termed Cobra (combined Bisulfite Restriction Analysis), PCR products from bisulfite-treated DNAs will be digested by restriction enzymes like BstUI and the resulting fraction could directly reflect the percentage of methylated and unchanged CpGs at sites that will be cut by the enzymes. It is relatively sensitive and small amount of DNAs from tiny tissues could be used for Cobra analysis (Xiong and Laird, 1997). However, it is semi-quantitative and restricted to analyze CpGs only in special sites of particular restriction enzymes. Overall, the efficiency of bisulfite conversion which is a complicated and time consuming procedure with relatively low sensitivity and high false positive rate is the critical factor for bisulfite dependent approaches to quantify DNA methylation.

In bisulfite independent groups, methylated DNAs are differentiated from unmethylated DNA by either enzyme digestion or affinity enrichment. In contrast to other quantification methods like MSP, enzyme digestion based methods could analyze the methylation pattern of multiple CpGs sites. The resulting products from methylation-sensitive restriction enzymes could be further analyzed by Souther blot or PCR at the single gene level and RLGS (restriction landmark genomic scanning) or aPRIMES (array based profiling of reference independent methylation status) in genome-wide level to screening novel methylated sites. The influence of digestion efficiency could be adjusted by the internal control which could not be cut by the particular enzyme irrespective of DNA methylation. Methylated DNA could also be analyzed by PCR, sequencing or array based hybridization after being enriched by anti-5-methylcytosine antibody or methylation binding domain (MBD) containing proteins. It could yield the information including both the level and pattern of DNA methylation with physiological relevance.

3.2 DNA methylation as biomarkers for gastric cancer

Although there are many studies reporting that methylation of particular genes could be useful to predict the prognosis of gastric cancer, few of them were validated to be superior to classical prognosis prediction factors such as TNM staging (Liu et al., 2010; Yu et al., 2009b). Therefore, the clinical application of DNA methylation in prognosis predication of gastric cancer remains uncertain. In contrast, the detection of methylated DNA markers is believed to be useful to detect newly and relapsed gastric cancer, thus representing a promising approach of developing non-invasive detection for gastric cancer progression (Corvalan and Maturana, 2010; Laird, 2003).

Biomarker detection in peritoneal fluid is clinically important and feasible to determine the micrometastesis to the peritoneum of gastric cancer which is the most frequent event in recurrent gastric cancer and often associated with resistance to chemotherapy and poor prognosis. The detection of peritoneal micrometastasis is critical for patients to take timely and correct treatment based on an accurate diagnosis. Based on the quantitatively detection of methylated DNAs with the MethyLight method, DNA methylation in peritoneal fluids was found to be able to detect occult neoplastic cells in the peritoneum (Hiraki et al., 2011; Hiraki et al., 2010). Among 11 genes reported to be methylated in gastric cancer, BNIP3, CHFR, CYP1B1, MINT25, SFRP2, and RASSF2 were specifically methylated in tumor tissues but not adjacent non-tumor tissues. Interestingly, the methylation status of all six genes were significantly different among three different groups: patients with tumor invasion under muscularis propria (MP) (n=42, methylation percentage: 0-5%), patients with tumor invasion beyond the MP (n=45, methylation percentage: 0-15%) and patients with histologically or cytologically confirmed peritoneal metastasis (n = 20, methylation percentage: 15-45%). Among 45 patients with tumor invasion beyond the MP, 3 of 9 patients with methylation in any of 6 genes were diagnosed as peritoneal recurrence later while only 1 out of 35 patients without methylation in any of 6 genes developed peritoneal metastasis at least 8 months after surgery (Hiraki et al., 2011). Other potential methylation markers of peritoneal metastasis of gastric cancer include RUNX3 which was silenced by DNA methylation in 100% of peritoneal metastases of gastric cancers and 75% of primary gastric cancers but not normal gastric mucosa (Sakakura et al., 2005).

In addition to detect methylated DNA in peritoneal fluids, researchers have endeavored to develop sensitive methods to quantify methylated DNA in peripheral bloods. It is promising to identify sensitive circulating biomarkers to detect early gastric cancer at a curable stage.

In a qualitative analysis of methylated p16, E-cadherin, and retinoic acid receptor-1 (RARbeta) in serum, 52 patients (48%) of the 109 preoperative gastric cancer patients showed hypermethylation of at least one gene while no methylation of any of three genes was detected in control sera (Ikoma et al., 2007). Furthermore, methylation of three genes was detected in 2 of the 3 patients with recurrence, indicating that the detection of the methylated DNA in circulation could facilitate the early detection of newly and recurrent gastric cancer. The methylations of p16, Reprimo as well as RASSF1A were also proposed as potential biomarkers for early detection of gastric cancer (Abbaszadegan et al., 2008; Bernal et al., 2008; Wang et al., 2008).

The quantitative analysis of RUNX3 methylation in serum revealed that methylated RUNX3 was detected in 29% (19/65) of gastric cancer patients and the serum level of methylated RUNX3 was concordant with tumor burden as well as disease stage, histology, lymphatic and vascular invasion (Sakakura et al., 2009). In addition, it seems to be more sensitive than serum level of carcinoembryonic antigen (CEA) as a biomarker for the detection of gastric cancer. However, the methylation of RUNX3 is not specific to gastric cancer and methylated RUNX3 could be detected in patients with various cancers such as breast cancer and lung cancer, indicating that methylation of RUNX3 could be more useful in monitoring the progression or recurrence of gastric cancer than in screening asymptomatic patients with early gastric cancer (Tan et al., 2007). Similarly, preferential methylation in the serum DNA of gastric cancer patients was noted in APC (17%), E-cadherin (13%), hMLH1 (41%) and TIMP3 (17%) genes and patients with advanced gastric cancer tended to have higher concentrations of methylated APC, TIMP3 and hMLH1 in the serum (Leung et al., 2005). Overall, methylations in at least one of these markers were detected in the serum of 33 patients (55%) while no methylation was detected in normal subjects. The combined use of APC and E-cadherin methylation markers identified a subgroup of gastric cancer patients with worse prognosis (Leung et al., 2005).

Similar to diver mutations, methylations in critical or driver genes are most likely not specific to gastric cancer. The value of driver methylation in the screening of gastric cancer is certainly controversial. Most of potential biomarkers, however, are usually transformed from functional studies. Many passenger methylations were, thus, discarded for further validation of their potential as indicators of gastric cancer development. Many biomarkers currently used in clinic, such as AFP, CEA and CA-125, are not functional oncogenes or tumor suppressors per se. To identify biomarkers for clinical application, more attention should be paid to those passenger methylations instead of driver methylations although they are probably not important to the development or progression of gastric cancer in function. In addition, quantitative MSP is currently the most often used approach to detect DNA methylated in blood. It would be more interesting to see the progress on the biomarkers identified by methods based on affinity enrichment since methylation contents with physiological relevance instead of single or few methylated sites could be determined.

4. MicroRNAs deregulated in gastric carcinogenesis

Although there are some discrepancies in the microRNA profiling of cell lines and primary tissues, microRNAome as a whole is downregulated in human carcinogenesis. It was believed that the general downregulation of microRNAs in cancer cells is mainly caused by the impaired post-transcriptional maturation of microRNAs starting from primary microRNA transcripts rather than the transcriptional of microRNA genes (Croce, 2009; Lee et al., 2008; Slezak-Prochazka et al., 2010; Thomson et al., 2006; White et al., 2005; Winter et al., 2009). The functions of microprocessors necessary and sufficient for processing microRNA precursors are generally suppressed in cancer cells partially due to the reduced expression of Drosha and Dicer, two major enzymes responsible for the maturation of microRNAs (Dedes et al., 2011; Hwang et al., 2009; Karube et al., 2005; Lee et al., 2008; Lin et al., 2010; Merritt et al., 2008). In addition, proteins with tumor suppressing functions like p53 were found to participate in the maturation of microRNAs (Bikkavilli and Malbon, 2010; Davis et al., 2008; Suzuki et al., 2009).

In contrast to genome-wide downregulation of microRNAs, some microRNAs are specifically upregulated in cancer cells. MicroRNAs have been implicated in the control of many fundamental cellular and physiological processes such as cellular differentiation and proliferation, stem cell maintenance and tissue development. By acting as oncogenes or tumor suppressors, microRNAs also play a significant role in cellular transformation and carcinogenesis (Inui et al., 2010; Wiemer, 2007; Wu et al., 2010). In the next, we will briefly overview the very recent studies on the relevance of microRNAs deregulated in gastric carcinogenesis to signal transduction, cell cycle and apoptosis control, and transcriptional regulation.

4.1 MicroRNAs in signal transduction

MiR-204 and probably miR-211 are downregulated in gastric cancer, contributing to the aberrant Ras activation by inhibiting the expression of ezrin (Lam et al., 2011). As a membrane-cytoskeleton linker protein, ezrin can promote Ras activation by stimulating the assembly of SOS-Ras complex (Morrison et al., 2007). Therefore, downregulation of miR-204 in gastric cancer represents a new mechanism of aberrant Ras activation which was often attributed to Ras mutations in many other cancers. CDC42, one Ras-related small G protein that plays important roles in the regulation of cell motility and tumor metastasis, was found to be targeted by miR-137 in gastric cancer cells (Chen et al., 2011). MiR-137 was downregulated in many cancers including gastric cancer probably due to the hypermethylation of its promoter. As the upstream regulator of MAPK signaling, EGF receptor ERBB2 was found as the direct target of miR-125a-5p (Nishida et al., 2011). While miR-125a-5p could potently suppress the proliferation of gastric cancer cells, low expression levels of miR-125a-5p were associated with enhanced malignant potential such as tumor size, tumor invasion and liver metastasis. By blocking apoptosis and promoting cell survival, NF-kappaB pathway plays important roles in both inflammation and cancer and is often activated in gastric carcinogenesis. NF-kappaB1 is directly targeted by miR-9 which was downregulated in gastric carcinomas (Wan et al., 2010). MiR-516a-3p can block metastatic dissemination of gastric cancer cells and was downregulated in highly metastatic gastric carcinoma cells. It can suppress the expression of sulfatase 1 which is known to promote the activation of wnt/beta-catenin signaling pathway by removing 6-O-sulfates from heparan sulfate proteoglycans on the cell surface and causing the release of membrane-bound wnt ligands from plasma membrane (Takei et al., 2011). The G-protein coupled receptor of gastrin, cholecystokinin B receptor (CCKBR), is regulated by miR-148b which was downregulated in gastric cancer (Song et al., 2011). Restored expression of miR-148b in gastric cancer cells inhibited cell growth both in vitro and in vivo.

4.2 MicroRNAs in cell cycle and apoptosis control

Cell cycle checkpoints consist of many proteins including cyclins, cyclin dependent kinases (CDKs) and CDK inhibitors (CKIs) to secure the integrity and fidelity of genome during cell mitosis. It was found that members of same family of CKIs could be regulated by microRNAs in one cluster. For example, miR-25 targeted p57 (Kip2) and the other two microRNAs in this cluster suppressed the expression of p21 (Cip1); while miR-222 and miR-221 cluster regulated both p27 (Kip1) and p57 (Kim et al., 2009). MicroRNAs in one cluster usually display similar pattern of expression, therefore ensuring the effect to attenuate the function of targeted proteins by interacting with different regions in 3'-UTR of the same gene. Cyclin G1 was targeted by miR-122 which was downregulated in gastric cancer and colorectal cancer probably due to aberrant activation of wnt signaling (Fornari et al., 2009; Wang et al., 2009).

As a direct target of p53, miR-34 was downregulated in gastric cancer. MiR-34 could inhibit the growth of gastric cancer cells by targeting anti-apoptotic oncoprotein Bcl-2 (Ji et al., 2008). Bcl-2 was also targeted by miR-181b, which was downregulated in multidrug-resistant human gastric cancer cell line SGC7901/vincristine (VCR). Enforced miR-181b expression reduced Bcl-2 protein level and sensitized SGC7901/VCR to VCR-induced apoptosis (Zhu et al., 2010). The novel tumor suppressor protein programmed cell death 4 (PDCD4) was downregulated in several human solid cancer types. PDCD4 was the target of miR-21 which was upregulated in gastric cancer in response to the activation of NF-kB signaling by smoking and many other factors such as inflammation (Motoyama et al., 2010).

4.3 MicroRNAs in transcription regulation

SRY (sex-determining region Y)-box 2 (SOX2) is a crucial transcription factor for the maintenance of stem cell pluripotency and the determination of cell fate. Its expression was reduced in gastric cancer cells due to the upregulation of miR-126 (Otsubo et al., 2011). Enhanced expression of miR-126 significantly promoted both anchorage-dependent and -independent growth of gastric cancer cells by reducing SOX2 expression. Similarly, SOX4 was upregulated in gastric cancers compared with benign gastric tissues probably resulting from the epigenetic silencing of miR-129-2 (Shen et al., 2010). Restoration of miR-129-2 induced apoptosis of gastric cancer cells.

In addition to transcription factors that regulate gene expression through direct interaction with DNA, many other proteins especially in the epigenetic regulatory network are also targeted by microRNAs. As one component in the polycomb complex, EZH2 plays important roles in stem cell homeostasis as well as cancer development. It has been proven to be upregulated in many cancers including gastric cancer. Such an upregulation is at least partially caused by the downregulation of miR-101 (Varambally et al., 2008; Wang et al., 2010). Restoration of miR-101 expression in gastric cancer cells led to the significant inhibition of cellular proliferation, migration and invasion as well as tumorigenicity. Another chromatin remodeling protein ING4 (Inhibitor of growth family, member 4) was targeted by miR-650 which was downregulated in gastric cancer and could promote tumorigenesis and proliferation of gastric cancer cells (Zhang et al., 2010). Methyl-CpG-binding protein MeCP2 could promote cancer development by initiating the assembly of transcription inhibitory complex to silence the expression of tumor suppressors. It was found to be the direct target of miR-212 which was downregulated in gastric cancer (Wada et al., 2010). Transfection of the miR-212 precursor into gastric cancer cells induced significant decrease of cell growth in vitro. In addition to methylated DNA binding proteins and histone modification related proteins, DNA methyltransferases (DNMTs) were directly targeted by microRNAs as well (Ng et al., 2009b). MiR-143 was frequently downregulated in gastric cancer and many other cancers and one target directly regulated by miR-143 was turned out to be DNA methyltranserase-3A (DNMT-3A) (Takagi et al., 2009). The transcription of DNMT-3A was resulted from aberrant Ras activation. Therefore, downregulation of miR-143 could be in concert with Ras activation to promote carcinogenesis by increasing the expression of DNMTs to promote hypermethylation-mediated silencing of tumor suppressors.

4.4 Deregulated microRNAs as biomarkers for gastric cancer

The number of microRNAs deregulated in gastric cancer is still increasing (Hou et al., 2011; Lee and Dutta, 2009; Wu et al., 2010). Many other microRNAs important to gastric carcinogenesis were not included due to the limitation of the space. For example, macrophage migration inhibitory factor (MIF) which plays important roles in the transformation of tumor-permissive microenvironment was targeted by miR-451 and miR-451 was downregulated in gastric cancer. The downregulation of miR-451 was associated with worse prognosis and restoration of miR-451 expression in gastric cancer cells reduced cell proliferation and increased sensitivity to radiation (Bandres et al., 2009). Microsatellite instability (MSI) was believed to be one important feature of some gastric cancers. MSI was usually caused by the mutations in mismatch repair (MMR) genes or reduced expression of

MMRs. A microRNA contribution to MSI was recently identified. MiR-155 which was overexpressed in gastric cancers could target the expression of several MMR genes, such as hMSH2, hMSH6, and hMLH1 (Valeri et al., 2010).

The clarification of their biological relevance will certainly deepen our understanding of carcinogenesis so that new and effective therapeutics could be developed. Different microRNAs could regulate gene expression by targeting different sites in the 3′-UTR of the same gene and a single microRNA could target more than one gene. Computational predictions indicate over 50% of human protein-coding genes might be regulated by microRNAs although there are only several hundred of microRNAs in human genome. In addition, microRNA could regulate gene expression by interacting with 5′-UTR even other elements in the gene, making it challenging to understand the biological relevance of microRNAs.

Interestingly, microRNAs were also recognized as the next generation of biomarkers for the diagnosis and prognosis prediction of cancers due to the development of methods to quantify microRNA expression in both tissues and bloods. Realtime RT-PCR and in situ hybridization could detect the expression of microRNA in tissues quantitatively or semi-quantitatively. Many studies have confirmed that microRNAs could be used for prognosis prediction (Iorio et al., 2008). For example, miR-125a-5p expression was found to be an independent prognostic factor and its lower expression in tumor tissues was often associated with shorter survival (Nishida et al., 2011). In a screening with a large cohort of 353 gastric samples, miR-125b, miR-199a and miR-100 were found to be related with the progression of gastric cancer while the downregulation of let-7g and miR-433 and the upregulation of miR-214 were associated with unfavorable outcome in overall survival independent of clinical covariates, including depth of invasion, lymph-node metastasis, and stage (Ueda et al., 2010). Based on the study of a relative small scale cohort of 160 gastric cancer patients, a signature consisting of miR-10b, miR-21, miR-223, miR-338, let-7a, miR-30a-5p and miR-126 was found as an independent predictor of overall survival and relapse-free survival (Li et al., 2010). Six microRNAs including miR-103, miR-21, miR-145, miR-106b, miR-146a and miR-148a were screened out from a total of 857 microRNA probes to separate node-positive from node-negative gastric cancers, indicating that these six miRNAs may be useful for the decision-making of doctors by the prediction of potential lymph node metastasis (Tchernitsa et al., 2010). Other microRNAs such as miR-27a was also related with the lymph node metastasis of gastric cancer (Katada et al., 2009). However, no microRNA signature was commonly accepted to predict the prognosis of gastric cancer since results from different labs were usually different. This could be due to the different methods used in different labs. Alternatively, the ethnic variation could be one of the reasons. Large scale multi-centered clinical trials will be warranted to validate the relevance of microRNA based signature to the prognosis predication of gastric cancer.

Given the stability in nature, microRNAs in peripheral blood or other body fluids were recognized as the ideal biomarkers for various cancers (Ng et al., 2009a). The plasma miRNA levels usually reflected the expression level of microRNAs in tumor tissues (Tsujiura et al., 2010). Microarray and new generations of sequencing platforms have been widely used to screen circulating microRNAs for the diagnosis of gastric cancer. Solexa sequencing of microRNAs in serum from 20 patients with gastric cancer and 20 age- and gender-matched tumour-free controls revealed 19 miRNAs specifically upregulated in gastric cancer. Five of them including miR-1, miR-20a, miR-27a, miR-34 and miR-423-5p were confirmed by qRT-PCR analysis. In a validation set consisting of 142 serum samples from gastric cancer patients and 105 control serum samples, the quantification of serum level of these five microRNAs could successfully separate gastric cancer cases from normal donors. The areas under the receiver operating characteristic (ROC) curve of this five-microRNA signature was even markedly higher than these of widely used biomarkers such as serum carcinoembryonic antigen (CEA) and carbohydrate antigen 19-9 (CA19-9), indicating that expression levels of this serum miRNA-based biomarker could be potential biomarkers for the detection of gastric cancer (Liu et al., 2011). Other reports indicated that plasma level of miR-17, miR-106b, and miR-106a could also be useful for the detection of gastric cancer (Tsujiura et al., 2010; Zhou et al., 2010). Currently, the detection of circulating microRNAs has received a great deal of attention for its potential application for the early detection and postoperative recurrence prediction of gastric cancer. Although approaches based on the detection of circulating nucleic acid have been approved for the clinical application, microRNAs based methods are still in their infancy. The stability of microRNAs and the sensitivity of microRNA detection certainly make microRNAs promising biomarkers for cancer detection or monitoring. More clinical trials will be needed to confirm the values of microRNA biomarkers in screening high-risk individuals for early detection of gastric cancer by further invasive examinations such as gastroendoscopy.

5. Conclusions and perspectives

In recent years, it has become apparent that gastric cancer is resulting from the accumulation of both genetic and epigenetic changes. Chronic inflammation gradually renders inflammatory microenvironment into tumor permissive, allowing the survival and growth of cancer initiating cells with reprogrammed epigenetic regulatory network. As the major components of epigenetic regulatory network, DNA methylation and microRNA are deregulated in cancer initiating cells. Although the mechanisms underlying aberrant DNA methylation as well as dysregulated microRNA expression are largely unknown, changes in patterns of DNA methylation and microRNA expression are believed to contribute to the initiation and progression of gastric cancer by altering the expression of genes important to control apoptosis, cellular proliferation and differentiation. Approaches to renormalize methylation patterns in both global levels such as DNA methyltransferases inhibitors or histone deacetyltransferases inhibitors (HDACi) or targeted therapeutics have been developed as novel strategies to treat cancer. Despite its promising future in cancer prevention and intervention, the great promise of cancer epigenetics currently lies in the potential in diagnostics in which epigenetic biomarkers would be helpful for risk assessment, early detection, prognosis prediction and monitoring of treatment response as well as disease relapse. The quantification of DNA methylation and microRNAs in peripheral blood has received a great deal of attention recently. With the progress in the technology of genome-wide analysis such as new generation of sequencing, more and more epigenetic biomarkers specific to gastric cancer will be identified in the peripheral blood, allowing the development of epigenetic biomarker panel alone or in combination with other biochemical biomarkers for the detection and monitoring of gastric cancer.

6. References

Abbaszadegan, M.R., Moaven, O., Sima, H.R., Ghafarzadegan, K., A'Rabi, A., Forghani, M.N., Raziee, H.R., Mashhadinejad, A., Jafarzadeh, M., Esmaili-Shandiz, E., *et al.* (2008). p16 promoter hypermethylation: a useful serum marker for early detection of gastric cancer. World J Gastroenterol *14*, 2055-2060.

Bandres, E., Bitarte, N., Arias, F., Agorreta, J., Fortes, P., Agirre, X., Zarate, R., Diaz-Gonzalez, J.A., Ramirez, N., Sola, J.J., *et al.* (2009). microRNA-451 regulates macrophage migration inhibitory factor production and proliferation of gastrointestinal cancer cells. Clin Cancer Res *15*, 2281-2290.

Bernal, C., Aguayo, F., Villarroel, C., Vargas, M., Diaz, I., Ossandon, F.J., Santibanez, E., Palma, M., Aravena, E., Barrientos, C., *et al.* (2008). Reprimo as a potential biomarker for early detection in gastric cancer. Clin Cancer Res *14*, 6264-6269.

Bikkavilli, R.K., and Malbon, C.C. (2010). Dishevelled-KSRP complex regulates Wnt signaling through post-transcriptional stabilization of beta-catenin mRNA. J Cell Sci *123*, 1352-1362.

Bird, A.P. (1986). CpG-rich islands and the function of DNA methylation. Nature *321*, 209-213.

Boyd, V.L., Moody, K.I., Karger, A.E., Livak, K.J., Zon, G., and Burns, J.W. (2006). Methylation-dependent fragment separation: direct detection of DNA methylation by capillary electrophoresis of PCR products from bisulfite-converted genomic DNA. Anal Biochem *354*, 266-273.

Chen, Q., Chen, X., Zhang, M., Fan, Q., Luo, S., and Cao, X. (2011). miR-137 Is Frequently Down-Regulated in Gastric Cancer and Is a Negative Regulator of Cdc42. Dig Dis Sci.

Choi, I.S., and Wu, T.T. (2005). Epigenetic alterations in gastric carcinogenesis. Cell Res *15*, 247-254.

Corvalan, A.H., and Maturana, M.J. (2010). Recent patents of DNA methylation biomarkers in gastrointestinal oncology. Recent Pat DNA Gene Seq *4*, 202-209.

Croce, C.M. (2009). Causes and consequences of microRNA dysregulation in cancer. Nat Rev Genet *10*, 704-714.

Davis, B.N., Hilyard, A.C., Lagna, G., and Hata, A. (2008). SMAD proteins control DROSHA-mediated microRNA maturation. Nature *454*, 56-61.

Dedes, K.J., Natrajan, R., Lambros, M.B., Geyer, F.C., Lopez-Garcia, M.A., Savage, K., Jones, R.L., and Reis-Filho, J.S. (2011). Down-regulation of the miRNA master regulators Drosha and Dicer is associated with specific subgroups of breast cancer. Eur J Cancer *47*, 138-150.

Eads, C.A., Danenberg, K.D., Kawakami, K., Saltz, L.B., Blake, C., Shibata, D., Danenberg, P.V., and Laird, P.W. (2000). MethyLight: a high-throughput assay to measure DNA methylation. Nucleic Acids Res *28*, E32.

El-Omar, E.M., Carrington, M., Chow, W.H., McColl, K.E., Bream, J.H., Young, H.A., Herrera, J., Lissowska, J., Yuan, C.C., Rothman, N., *et al.* (2000). Interleukin-1 polymorphisms associated with increased risk of gastric cancer. Nature *404*, 398-402.

Fornari, F., Gramantieri, L., Giovannini, C., Veronese, A., Ferracin, M., Sabbioni, S., Calin, G.A., Grazi, G.L., Croce, C.M., Tavolari, S., *et al.* (2009). MiR-122/cyclin G1 interaction modulates p53 activity and affects doxorubicin sensitivity of human hepatocarcinoma cells. Cancer Res *69*, 5761-5767.

Herman, J.G., Graff, J.R., Myohanen, S., Nelkin, B.D., and Baylin, S.B. (1996). Methylation-specific PCR: a novel PCR assay for methylation status of CpG islands. Proc Natl Acad Sci U S A *93*, 9821-9826.

Hiraki, M., Kitajima, Y., Koga, Y., Tanaka, T., Nakamura, J., Hashiguchi, K., Noshiro, H., and Miyazaki, K. (2011). Aberrant Gene Methylation Is a Biomarker for the Detection of Cancer Cells in Peritoneal Wash Samples from Advanced Gastric Cancer Patients. Ann Surg Oncol.

Hiraki, M., Kitajima, Y., Sato, S., Nakamura, J., Hashiguchi, K., Noshiro, H., and Miyazaki, K. (2010). Aberrant gene methylation in the peritoneal fluid is a risk factor predicting peritoneal recurrence in gastric cancer. World J Gastroenterol *16*, 330-338.

Hou, Z., Xie, L., Yu, L., Qian, X., and Liu, B. (2011). MicroRNA-146a is down-regulated in gastric cancer and regulates cell proliferation and apoptosis. Med Oncol.

Hwang, H.W., Wentzel, E.A., and Mendell, J.T. (2009). Cell-cell contact globally activates microRNA biogenesis. Proc Natl Acad Sci U S A *106*, 7016-7021.

Ikoma, H., Ichikawa, D., Daito, I., Nobuyuki, T., Koike, H., Okamoto, K., Ochiai, T., Ueda, Y., Yamagishi, H., and Otsuji, E. (2007). Clinical application of methylation specific-polymerase chain reaction in serum of patients with gastric cancer. Hepatogastroenterology *54*, 946-950.

Inui, M., Martello, G., and Piccolo, S. (2010). MicroRNA control of signal transduction. Nat Rev Mol Cell Biol *11*, 252-263.

Iorio, M.V., Casalini, P., Tagliabue, E., Menard, S., and Croce, C.M. (2008). MicroRNA profiling as a tool to understand prognosis, therapy response and resistance in breast cancer. Eur J Cancer *44*, 2753-2759.

Ji, Q., Hao, X., Meng, Y., Zhang, M., Desano, J., Fan, D., and Xu, L. (2008). Restoration of tumor suppressor miR-34 inhibits human p53-mutant gastric cancer tumorspheres. BMC Cancer *8*, 266.

Jones, P.A. (2002). DNA methylation and cancer. Oncogene *21*, 5358-5360.

Karube, Y., Tanaka, H., Osada, H., Tomida, S., Tatematsu, Y., Yanagisawa, K., Yatabe, Y., Takamizawa, J., Miyoshi, S., Mitsudomi, T., *et al.* (2005). Reduced expression of Dicer associated with poor prognosis in lung cancer patients. Cancer Sci *96*, 111-115.

Katada, T., Ishiguro, H., Kuwabara, Y., Kimura, M., Mitui, A., Mori, Y., Ogawa, R., Harata, K., and Fujii, Y. (2009). microRNA expression profile in undifferentiated gastric cancer. Int J Oncol *34*, 537-542.

Kim, Y.K., Yu, J., Han, T.S., Park, S.Y., Namkoong, B., Kim, D.H., Hur, K., Yoo, M.W., Lee, H.J., Yang, H.K., *et al.* (2009). Functional links between clustered microRNAs: suppression of cell-cycle inhibitors by microRNA clusters in gastric cancer. Nucleic Acids Res *37*, 1672-1681.

Laird, P.W. (2003). The power and the promise of DNA methylation markers. Nat Rev Cancer *3*, 253-266.

Lam, E.K., Wang, X., Shin, V.Y., Zhang, S., Morrison, H., Sun, J., Ng, E.K., Yu, J., and Jin, H. (2011). A microRNA contribution to aberrant Ras activation in gastric cancer. Am J Transl Res *3*, 209-218.

Lee, E.J., Baek, M., Gusev, Y., Brackett, D.J., Nuovo, G.J., and Schmittgen, T.D. (2008). Systematic evaluation of microRNA processing patterns in tissues, cell lines, and tumors. RNA *14*, 35-42.

Lee, Y.S., and Dutta, A. (2009). MicroRNAs in cancer. Annu Rev Pathol *4*, 199-227.

Leung, W.K., To, K.F., Chu, E.S., Chan, M.W., Bai, A.H., Ng, E.K., Chan, F.K., and Sung, J.J. (2005). Potential diagnostic and prognostic values of detecting promoter hypermethylation in the serum of patients with gastric cancer. Br J Cancer *92*, 2190-2194.

Li, X., Zhang, Y., Ding, J., Wu, K., and Fan, D. (2010). Survival prediction of gastric cancer by a seven-microRNA signature. Gut *59*, 579-585.

Lin, R.J., Lin, Y.C., Chen, J., Kuo, H.H., Chen, Y.Y., Diccianni, M.B., London, W.B., Chang, C.H., and Yu, A.L. (2010). microRNA signature and expression of Dicer and Drosha can predict prognosis and delineate risk groups in neuroblastoma. Cancer Res *70*, 7841-7850.

Liu, R., Zhang, C., Hu, Z., Li, G., Wang, C., Yang, C., Huang, D., Chen, X., Zhang, H., Zhuang, R., *et al.* (2011). A five-microRNA signature identified from genome-wide serum microRNA expression profiling serves as a fingerprint for gastric cancer diagnosis. Eur J Cancer *47*, 784-791.

Liu, X., Wang, X., Zhang, J., Lam, E.K., Shin, V.Y., Cheng, A.S., Yu, J., Chan, F.K., Sung, J.J., and Jin, H.C. (2010). Warburg effect revisited: an epigenetic link between glycolysis and gastric carcinogenesis. Oncogene *29*, 442-450.

Meira, L.B., Bugni, J.M., Green, S.L., Lee, C.W., Pang, B., Borenshtein, D., Rickman, B.H., Rogers, A.B., Moroski-Erkul, C.A., McFaline, J.L., *et al.* (2008). DNA damage induced by chronic inflammation contributes to colon carcinogenesis in mice. J Clin Invest *118*, 2516-2525.

Merritt, W.M., Lin, Y.G., Han, L.Y., Kamat, A.A., Spannuth, W.A., Schmandt, R., Urbauer, D., Pennacchio, L.A., Cheng, J.F., Nick, A.M., *et al.* (2008). Dicer, Drosha, and outcomes in patients with ovarian cancer. N Engl J Med *359*, 2641-2650.

Morrison, H., Sperka, T., Manent, J., Giovannini, M., Ponta, H., and Herrlich, P. (2007). Merlin/neurofibromatosis type 2 suppresses growth by inhibiting the activation of Ras and Rac. Cancer Res *67*, 520-527.

Motoyama, K., Inoue, H., Mimori, K., Tanaka, F., Kojima, K., Uetake, H., Sugihara, K., and Mori, M. (2010). Clinicopathological and prognostic significance of PDCD4 and microRNA-21 in human gastric cancer. Int J Oncol *36*, 1089-1095.

Ng, E.K., Chong, W.W., Jin, H., Lam, E.K., Shin, V.Y., Yu, J., Poon, T.C., Ng, S.S., and Sung, J.J. (2009a). Differential expression of microRNAs in plasma of patients with colorectal cancer: a potential marker for colorectal cancer screening. Gut *58*, 1375-1381.

Ng, E.K., Tsang, W.P., Ng, S.S., Jin, H.C., Yu, J., Li, J.J., Rocken, C., Ebert, M.P., Kwok, T.T., and Sung, J.J. (2009b). MicroRNA-143 targets DNA methyltransferases 3A in colorectal cancer. Br J Cancer *101*, 699-706.

Nishida, N., Mimori, K., Fabbri, M., Yokobori, T., Sudo, T., Tanaka, F., Shibata, K., Ishii, H., Doki, Y., and Mori, M. (2011). MicroRNA-125a-5p is an independent prognostic factor in gastric cancer,and inhibits the proliferation of human gastric cancer cells in combination with trastuzumab. Clin Cancer Res.

Otsubo, T., Akiyama, Y., Hashimoto, Y., Shimada, S., Goto, K., and Yuasa, Y. (2011). MicroRNA-126 inhibits SOX2 expression and contributes to gastric carcinogenesis. PLoS One *6*, e16617.

Persson, C., Canedo, P., Machado, J.C., El-Omar, E.M., and Forman, D. (2011). Polymorphisms in inflammatory response genes and their association with gastric cancer: A HuGE systematic review and meta-analyses. Am J Epidemiol *173*, 259-270.

Pikarsky, E., Porat, R.M., Stein, I., Abramovitch, R., Amit, S., Kasem, S., Gutkovich-Pyest, E., Urieli-Shoval, S., Galun, E., and Ben-Neriah, Y. (2004). NF-kappaB functions as a tumour promoter in inflammation-associated cancer. Nature *431*, 461-466.

Sakakura, C., Hamada, T., Miyagawa, K., Nishio, M., Miyashita, A., Nagata, H., Ida, H., Yazumi, S., Otsuji, E., Chiba, T., *et al.* (2009). Quantitative analysis of tumor-derived methylated RUNX3 sequences in the serum of gastric cancer patients. Anticancer Res *29*, 2619-2625.

Sakakura, C., Hasegawa, K., Miyagawa, K., Nakashima, S., Yoshikawa, T., Kin, S., Nakase, Y., Yazumi, S., Yamagishi, H., Okanoue, T., *et al.* (2005). Possible involvement of RUNX3 silencing in the peritoneal metastases of gastric cancers. Clin Cancer Res *11*, 6479-6488.

Shen, R., Pan, S., Qi, S., Lin, X., and Cheng, S. (2010). Epigenetic repression of microRNA-129-2 leads to overexpression of SOX4 in gastric cancer. Biochem Biophys Res Commun *394*, 1047-1052.

Slezak-Prochazka, I., Durmus, S., Kroesen, B.J., and van den Berg, A. (2010). MicroRNAs, macrocontrol: regulation of miRNA processing. RNA *16*, 1087-1095.

Song, Y.X., Yue, Z.Y., Wang, Z.N., Xu, Y.Y., Luo, Y., Xu, H.M., Zhang, X., Jiang, L., Xing, C.Z., and Zhang, Y. (2011). MicroRNA-148b is frequently down-regulated in gastric cancer and acts as a tumor suppressor by inhibiting cell proliferation. Mol Cancer *10*, 1.

Suzuki, H.I., Yamagata, K., Sugimoto, K., Iwamoto, T., Kato, S., and Miyazono, K. (2009). Modulation of microRNA processing by p53. Nature *460*, 529-533.

Takagi, T., Iio, A., Nakagawa, Y., Naoe, T., Tanigawa, N., and Akao, Y. (2009). Decreased expression of microRNA-143 and -145 in human gastric cancers. Oncology *77*, 12-21.

Takei, Y., Takigahira, M., Mihara, K., Tarumi, Y., and Yanagihara, K. (2011). The Metastasis-Associated microRNA miR-516a-3p Is a Novel Therapeutic Target for Inhibiting Peritoneal Dissemination of Human Scirrhous Gastric Cancer. Cancer Res *71*, 1442-1453.

Tamura, G. (2006). Alterations of tumor suppressor and tumor-related genes in the development and progression of gastric cancer. World J Gastroenterol *12*, 192-198.

Tan, S.H., Ida, H., Lau, Q.C., Goh, B.C., Chieng, W.S., Loh, M., and Ito, Y. (2007). Detection of promoter hypermethylation in serum samples of cancer patients by methylation-specific polymerase chain reaction for tumour suppressor genes including RUNX3. Oncol Rep *18*, 1225-1230.

Tchernitsa, O., Kasajima, A., Schafer, R., Kuban, R.J., Ungethum, U., Gyorffy, B., Neumann, U., Simon, E., Weichert, W., Ebert, M.P., *et al.* (2010). Systematic evaluation of the miRNA-ome and its downstream effects on mRNA expression identifies gastric cancer progression. J Pathol *222*, 310-319.

Thomson, J.M., Newman, M., Parker, J.S., Morin-Kensicki, E.M., Wright, T., and Hammond, S.M. (2006). Extensive post-transcriptional regulation of microRNAs and its implications for cancer. Genes Dev *20*, 2202-2207.

Tsujiura, M., Ichikawa, D., Komatsu, S., Shiozaki, A., Takeshita, H., Kosuga, T., Konishi, H., Morimura, R., Deguchi, K., Fujiwara, H., *et al.* (2010). Circulating microRNAs in plasma of patients with gastric cancers. Br J Cancer *102*, 1174-1179.

Ueda, T., Volinia, S., Okumura, H., Shimizu, M., Taccioli, C., Rossi, S., Alder, H., Liu, C.G., Oue, N., Yasui, W., *et al.* (2010). Relation between microRNA expression and progression and prognosis of gastric cancer: a microRNA expression analysis. Lancet Oncol *11*, 136-146.

Ushijima, T., and Sasako, M. (2004). Focus on gastric cancer. Cancer Cell *5*, 121-125.

Valeri, N., Gasparini, P., Fabbri, M., Braconi, C., Veronese, A., Lovat, F., Adair, B., Vannini, I., Fanini, F., Bottoni, A., *et al.* (2010). Modulation of mismatch repair and genomic stability by miR-155. Proc Natl Acad Sci U S A *107*, 6982-6987.

Varambally, S., Cao, Q., Mani, R.S., Shankar, S., Wang, X., Ateeq, B., Laxman, B., Cao, X., Jing, X., Ramnarayanan, K., *et al.* (2008). Genomic loss of microRNA-101 leads to overexpression of histone methyltransferase EZH2 in cancer. Science *322*, 1695-1699.

Wada, R., Akiyama, Y., Hashimoto, Y., Fukamachi, H., and Yuasa, Y. (2010). miR-212 is downregulated and suppresses methyl-CpG-binding protein MeCP2 in human gastric cancer. Int J Cancer *127*, 1106-1114.

Wan, H.Y., Guo, L.M., Liu, T., Liu, M., Li, X., and Tang, H. (2010). Regulation of the transcription factor NF-kappaB1 by microRNA-9 in human gastric adenocarcinoma. Mol Cancer *9*, 16.

Wang, H.J., Ruan, H.J., He, X.J., Ma, Y.Y., Jiang, X.T., Xia, Y.J., Ye, Z.Y., and Tao, H.Q. (2010). MicroRNA-101 is down-regulated in gastric cancer and involved in cell migration and invasion. Eur J Cancer.

Wang, X., and Jin, H. (2010). The epigenetic basis of Warburg effect. Epigenetics *5*.

Wang, X., Lam, E.K., Zhang, J., Jin, H., and Sung, J.J. (2009). MicroRNA-122a functions as a novel tumor suppressor downstream of adenomatous polyposis coli in gastrointestinal cancers. Biochem Biophys Res Commun *387*, 376-380.

Wang, Y.C., Yu, Z.H., Liu, C., Xu, L.Z., Yu, W., Lu, J., Zhu, R.M., Li, G.L., Xia, X.Y., Wei, X.W., *et al.* (2008). Detection of RASSF1A promoter hypermethylation in serum from gastric and colorectal adenocarcinoma patients. World J Gastroenterol *14*, 3074-3080.

White, P.S., Thompson, P.M., Gotoh, T., Okawa, E.R., Igarashi, J., Kok, M., Winter, C., Gregory, S.G., Hogarty, M.D., Maris, J.M., *et al.* (2005). Definition and characterization of a region of 1p36.3 consistently deleted in neuroblastoma. Oncogene *24*, 2684-2694.

Wiemer, E.A. (2007). The role of microRNAs in cancer: no small matter. Eur J Cancer *43*, 1529-1544.

Winter, J., Jung, S., Keller, S., Gregory, R.I., and Diederichs, S. (2009). Many roads to maturity: microRNA biogenesis pathways and their regulation. Nat Cell Biol *11*, 228-234.

Wojdacz, T.K., and Dobrovic, A. (2007). Methylation-sensitive high resolution melting (MS-HRM): a new approach for sensitive and high-throughput assessment of methylation. Nucleic Acids Res *35*, e41.

Wu, W.K., Lee, C.W., Cho, C.H., Fan, D., Wu, K., Yu, J., and Sung, J.J. (2010). MicroRNA dysregulation in gastric cancer: a new player enters the game. Oncogene *29*, 5761-5771.

Xiong, Z., and Laird, P.W. (1997). COBRA: a sensitive and quantitative DNA methylation assay. Nucleic Acids Res *25*, 2532-2534.

Yu, H., Pardoll, D., and Jove, R. (2009a). STATs in cancer inflammation and immunity: a leading role for STAT3. Nat Rev Cancer *9*, 798-809.

Yu, J., Cheng, Y.Y., Tao, Q., Cheung, K.F., Lam, C.N., Geng, H., Tian, L.W., Wong, Y.P., Tong, J.H., Ying, J.M., *et al.* (2009b). Methylation of protocadherin 10, a novel tumor suppressor, is associated with poor prognosis in patients with gastric cancer. Gastroenterology *136*, 640-651 e641.

Zhang, X., Zhu, W., Zhang, J., Huo, S., Zhou, L., Gu, Z., and Zhang, M. (2010). MicroRNA-650 targets ING4 to promote gastric cancer tumorigenicity. Biochem Biophys Res Commun *395*, 275-280.

Zhou, H., Guo, J.M., Lou, Y.R., Zhang, X.J., Zhong, F.D., Jiang, Z., Cheng, J., and Xiao, B.X. (2010). Detection of circulating tumor cells in peripheral blood from patients with gastric cancer using microRNA as a marker. J Mol Med *88*, 709-717.

Zhu, W., Shan, X., Wang, T., Shu, Y., and Liu, P. (2010). miR-181b modulates multidrug resistance by targeting BCL2 in human cancer cell lines. Int J Cancer *127*, 2520-2529.

4

Molecular Features and Their Clinical Implications on Gastric Adenocarcinoma

Yves Dittmar and Utz Settmacher
University Hospital Jena
Germany

1. Introduction

Gastric cancer is one of the most frequent malignant tumors worldwide. It is known to have a poor prognosis leading to more than 600.000 fatalities every year. This dilemma is caused mainly by the late onset of clinical symptoms. Thus, when gastric cancer is diagnosed, more than 50% of patients cannot be cured.

Even in those cases where cure by surgery can be achieved, the prognosis is poor due to the high incidence of early recurrence of the primary tumor as well as the development of metachronous metastases. The attempt to improve survival by extended surgical procedures, such as extensive lymph node removal did not have a significant impact on survival leading medical professionals to regard advanced gastric cancer as a systemic rather than a locally confined disease. Therefore, over the last two decades the importance of chemotherapy as a part of the curative treatment strategy was became more evident. The findings of molecular research show that gastric cancer has a very heterogenous biology with a broad variety of signalling pathways and chromosomal imbalances involved. With the growing insight into the molecular biology of gastric cancer it became clear that every single gastric cancer has to be regarded as an individual entity which can change its molecular behavior over time. This chapter presents the current knowledge of the molecular profile of gastric cancer. The most important basic signalling pathways that are known to play critical roles in the development as well as the progression of gastric cancer are discussed. Furthermore, the currently available molecular targets and their clinical relevance are reviewed in this chapter.

2. Chromosomal imbalances in gastric cancer

To date, the TNM system and the classification according to Lauren are the "gold standard" tools to predict survival and to define the treatment strategy in patients with gastric cancer. However, there is a wide range of clinical outcomes in patients with similar TNM stages. Therefore, it seems to be important to improve the characterization of gastric cancer by using molecular criteria [1].

The development as well as the progression of gastric cancer is the result based on the interplay between the host genetic profile and the environment. The precise transfer of genetic information requires accurate replication, DNA mismatch repair and the segregation of replicated DNA strands. Whereas an impaired replication is not compatible with cellular survival, the uneven distribution of chromosomes in tumor cells is termed aneuploidia and can be frequently observed in gastric cancer tissue. Defects in the mismatch repair system can gradually lead to chromosomal imbalances. Functional losses of MLH1 and MSH2 are known to cause multiple somatic mutations which may present microsatellite instability and may lead to tumor formation at multiple locations at a younger age in the colon /rectum (Lynch syndrome). Most frequently, the hypermethylation of CpG islands in the promoter region of these mismatch repair genes is the underlying mechanism of loss of function. This type of tumor development is called microsatellite mutator phenotype and has also been described in gastric cancer by several authors [2,3]. The other type of tumor development based on chromosomal imbalances is the chromosomal/ intrachromosomal instability type leading to amplifications and deletions of whole chromosomes as well as chromosome cytobands potentially harbouring tumor suppressor genes or oncogenes. The following locations have been observed to be frequently amplified in gastric cancer: 3p22, 4q25, 8q24, 11p13, and 20q13. Losses have been documented most commonly at 1p36 and 9p21 [4]. Furthermore, it has been reported that intestinal type gastric cancer according to Lauren´s classification has a higher degree of chromosomal aberrations than the diffuse type. Furthermore, a relationship between clinical outcome and the degree of chromosomal aberrations in intestinal type gastric cancer was observed [5].

Another level of chromosomal assessment is the detection of gross chromosomal imbalances by using flow cytometry. The loss or amplification of complete chromosomes is known to be a frequently occurring event in cancer development [6]. Non-diploid status of chromosomes has been shown to be present in about 20% of gastric cancer cases. Patients with a non-diploid chromosome status have a significantly poorer survival than those who present with a diploid status [1].

Additionally, there is a growing body of evidence that the epigenetic level of regulation of gene expression plays an important role in cancer development. The chromatine remodelling machinery contains in particular enzymes that modify histons [7]. Recently, it has been shown that the histone demethylase RBP2 is upregulated in gastric cancer and that depletion of that enzyme causes senescence of resident tumor cells [8].

3. Hereditary gastric cancer

In 10% of all gastric cancer cases, a familial clustering of the disease can be observed but only 1 -3% are of hereditary origin. In those cases where no histological finding is available the term "familial gastric cancer" is used [9]. The following syndromes include patients with available histology and are known to be associated with both familial clustering and certain germline mutations: hereditary diffuse gastric cancer, familial diffuse gastric cancer and familial intestinal gastric cancer. Furthermore, there are several syndromes which may include early onset gastric cancer in addition to other tumor manifestations: Lynch syndrome, Li-Fraumeni syndrome, Li-Fraumeni-like syndrome. Peutz-Jeghers syndrome and the familial adenomatous polyposis (FAP).

Hereditary diffuse gastric cancer develops from germline mutations in the *CDH-1* gene (about one third of cases) coding for E-cadherin, an important cell adhesion molecule on the lateral surface of the cellular membrane, whereas in two thirds of the cases the underlying mutation cannot be identified [9,10]. The inactivation of the *CDH-1* gene may be triggered by epigenetic mechanisms (hypermethylation of the promoter region) as well as by a genetic mechanism (loss of heterocygosity plus *CDH-1* mutation). The syndrome is associated with early onset and gastric cancer lesions growing in multiple locations as well as with lobular breast carcinoma. The International Gastric Cancer Linkage Consortium defined two main criteria to identify patients susceptible for hereditary diffuse gastric cancer from the population: 2 cases of diffuse gastric cancer in first or second degree relatives (at least one of them to be younger than 50 years at the time of diagnosis) or 3 cases of diffuse gastric cancer in first or second degree relatives independently of the age at the time of diagnosis. Families with numerous cases of diffuse gastric cancer who do not fulfil these abovementioned criteria are considered to be familial diffuse gastric cancer [11].

The majority of cases of familial intestinal gastric cancer is associated with Lynch syndrome which is also termed hereditary non-polyposis colorectal cancer (HNPCC) [12,13]. Therefore, Caldas and co-workers suggested to identify patients with risk for familial intestinal gastric cancer by using the HNPCC-related Amsterdam criteria in countries with a high incidence of gastric cancer. In contrast, countries with a lower incidence should use the criteria analogous to hereditary diffuse gastric cancer [13].

Lynch syndrome is caused by germline mutations in genes associated to the mismatch repair (MMR) machinery. Most frequently, alterations of the *MLH* gene family (MutL-homolog) or the *MSH* gene family (MutS-homolog) are responsible for the defective MMR. These two proteins form heterodimers that recognize mismatched bases selectively within the newly synthesized daughter DNA strand which can be removed subsequently by exonucleases. Appoximately 5 - 8% (depending on gender and the mutated gene) of patients with Lynch syndrome develop gastric cancer during their life time [12,14].

The Li-Fraumeni syndrome as well as the Li-Fraumeni-like syndrome originate from germline mutations of the *TP53* gene. About 250 different mutations of that gene have been identified to cause a broad variety of tumor diseases, the majority of them being missense mutations leading to a molecule that cannot bind to the DNA [15]. There is a broad variety of tumor diseases which can develop based on that syndrome including breast cancer, adrenal tumors, sarcomas and gastric cancer. The Li-Fraumeni syndrome and the Li-Fraumeni-like syndrome are distinguished by several clinical based criteria. Recently it has been demonstrated that the DNA repair gene *BRCA2* might be another molecular mechanism of causing these syndromes [16].

Peutz-Jeghers syndrome (*STK11* gene, coding for serin-threonin kinase 11) and the FAP (associated to the *APC* gene) can are associated with gastric cancer in rare cases.

4. Dysregulation of signalling pathways

Non-hereditary gastric cancer has a complex and multistep carcinogenesis in which - among numerous other factors - signalling pathways are involved. The dysregulation of these signalling pathways may lead to activation of genes that code for proteins regulating growth processes, such as cell division, differentiation, epithelial-mesenchymal transition and proliferation. Several studies on the molecular development as well as the progression of gastric cancer show clearly that there are differences in the biological behavior between young and elderly people. According to the classification of Lauren, intestinal gastric cancer with differentiated glandular growth pattern presents with a profile of dysregulated signalling pathways that can be distinguished from the diffuse type gastric cancer. Furthermore, there appears to be a difference between cancer of the upper stomach as compared to that of the lower stomach.

4.1 Tyrosine kinase signalling

4.1.1 The epidermal growth factor receptor (EGFR) family and downstream signalling

Epidermal growth factor receptor is a member of the ErbB receptor family and normally regulates gastric mucosa proliferation. Under normal conditions, two receptor molecules form dimers as a result of ligand binding and phosphorylate each other via their tyrosin kinase activity. Every heterodimer has its own effector molecule (see Fig. 1). One important pathway is the activation of the guanine exchange factor SOS which subsequently activates the MEK-ERK MAP kinase pathway leading to the expression of proliferation-promoting transcription factors, such as AP-1, ELK-1 and c-fos. Alternative signal transduction pathways downstream of the EGF receptor family are STAT and PKB (protein kinase B). An important downstream effector of PKB is the mTOR complex 1. Active mTOR complex 1 leads via expression of specific mRNA stabilizing proteins and of ribosomal subunit S6 to increased proliferation.

In summary, EGFR related signals promote many cellular activities towards tumor growth, in particular proliferation, migration, adhesion, apoptosis and differentiation [17].

EGFR	7p11.2	EGFR	EGF TGFα
ERBB2	17q12	HER2/NEU	none
ERBB3	12q13.2	HER3	neuregulin1 neuregulin2
ERBB4	2q34	HER4	neuregulin1 neuregulin2

Fig. 1. The members of the EGF receptor family and their typical ligands

Dysregulation of signalling pathways downstream of the EGFR is frequently observed in gastric cancer. Therefore, currently two main subgroups of targeted drugs exist: first the inhibition of the receptor by blocking the ligand binding site and second the inhibition of the intracellular tyrosin kinase activity of the receptor molecule. For the first-mentioned mechanism the monoclonal antibodies cetuximab, matuzumab and panitumumab have been developed. Gefitinib and erlotinib are tyrosin kinase inhibitors.

The ErbB2 receptor (Her2/Neu) can dimerize without a binding ligand and, thus, cannot be inhibited by antibodies against the ligand binding site. About one third of all tumors express ErbB2. In up to 27% of gastric cancer cases an overexpressed ErBB2 can be detected [18]. ErbB2 is overexpressed more frequently in intestinal type gastric cancers as compared to diffuse type gastric cancer. Furthermore, younger patients show less frequent ErbB2 overexpression than elderly patients [19]. The humanized antibody trastuzumab inhibits the ErbB2 receptor and has been shown to provide a significant survival benefit in ErbB2-positive cases [20].

Recently, it has been shown in vivo and in vitro on gastric cancer cell lines that the mTOR specific inhibitor rapamycin is effective in those cases which are resistant to EGFR inhibitors. Moreover, when administered in combination with cetuximab it can restore the anticancer effects of EGFR inhibition. Thus, rapamycin alone or in combination with other agents may provide a new target for the clinical use in the future [21].

K-ras, BRAF and SOS mutations are detected only in few gastric cancer cases [22]. Nevertheless the novel k-ras inhibitor tipifernib should be mentioned. K-ras mutations result in a continuosly active k-ras protein. Tipifernib inhibits the enzyme farnesyltransferase which forms an essential step in the posttranscriptional modification and thereby downregulates the k-ras signal. The clinical outcome of tipifernib administration in advanced gastric cancer is currently investigated in a phase 2 trial and might be a potential target-specific therapy for selected gastric cancer cases in the future, too [23].

4.1.2 Vascular endothelial growth factor (VEGF) and tumor angiogenesis

When tumors grow larger than 1-2mm in diameter, further tumor growth requires the development of new blood vessels in the tumor environment. This tumor-related angiogenesis is different from physiological angiogenesis in terms of distinct vessel architecture, vascular permeability as well as a different interplay between endothelial cells and perivascular cells. One of the most potent angiogenesis-promoting factors is VEGF. VEGF is expressed as a result of tissue hypoxia. It promotes its biological effects (inhibition of apoptosis and proliferation of endothelial cells, increased endothelial cell migration) via binding to the VEGF receptor. Synchronously with the once initiated tumor angiogenesis the development of metastases is promoted.

Overexpression of VEGF has been reported in gastric cancer cases.

Currently, 4 different mechanisms of VEGF signalling inhibition can be distinguished: VEGF-inhibiting antibodies (bevacizumab), soluble VEGF receptors (aflibercept), VEGFR-inhibiting antibodies (IMC-1121B) and VEGFR tyrosin kinase inhibitors (vatalinib, cediranib, sunitinib, sorafenib).

To date, for gastric cancer no angiogenesis-inhibiting agent has been approved worldwide. But a growing experience with angiogenesis-inhibiting agents in colorectal cancer demonstrates a survival benefit with acceptable adverse effects [24].

4.1.3 Hepatocellular growth factor (HGF) and gastric cancer

HGF signals induce a broad variety of biological features, such as morphogenesis, adhesion, migration, remodelling of extracellular matrix and are also involved in tumor angiogenesis [25]. It is known to be one of the key players in tissue regeneration following injury. Under physiological conditions, HGF is secreted in a paracrine manner most commonly by mesenchymal cells. Its target, the HGF receptor (HGFR or MET) is usually present on the surface of epithelial cells. Several cytokines, such as interleukin-1 and -6, tumour necrosis factor-α and transforming growth factor-β (TGFβ) that are released into the reactive interstitium (wound healing, cancer) induce the upregulation of HGF and HGFR expression. Furthermore, HGF is a strong antagonist of liver fibrosis by inhibiting the TGFβ signal as well as by pro-apoptotic effects on myofibroblasts. [26]. Intracellular signal transduction is similar to the EGFR signalling pathways.

In gastric cancer, the upregulation of the HGF signalling is an event which predominantly occurs at advanced stages, in particular in those who have liver metastases [27]. About 23% of patients with gastric cancer have an overexpression of c-met [28].

There are currently no substances available for clinical use that inhibit the HGF signalling pathway but the effect of the novel agent XL880 (a tyrosin kinase inhibitor) on poorly differentiated gastric cancer is currently investigated. Furthermore, antibodies against HGF and MET are planned [29].

4.1.4 Fibroblast growth factor and its receptor FGFR in gastric cancer

Like EGFR and HGFR, the fibroblast growth factor receptor belongs to the large family of receptor tyrosin kinases. To date, 23 different isoforms (FGF 1-23) and 4 receptor subtypes (FGFR 1-4) have been identified. FGFR2 or k-sam has been reported to be overexpressed in poorly differentiated gastric cancer The MAP-kinase pathway, the AKT pathway as well as NFAT signalling and activation of protein kinase C are the most prominent subsequent intracellular transduction pathways. Recently it has been shown that the receptor of keratinocyte growth factor on epithelial cells is identical with FGFR2. The amplification of the k-sam gene has been detected in poorly differentiated diffuse gastric cancer in about 50% of cases resulting in a poor prognosis [30,31]. In contrast, it is rarely present in intestinal type gastric cancer.

The novel FGFR2 inhibitor Ki23057 showed considerable antiproliferative effects in the mouse model and might become an effective target-specific agent in the future.

4.1.5 Vascular endothelial growth factor (VEGF), platelet derived growth factor (PDGF) and its receptor PDGFR in gastric cancer

VEGF and PDGF are key players of angiogenesis. Whereas VEGF promotes neoangiogenesis, PDGF has its impacts on the maintainance of microvessels. Both factors are secreted by tumor cells and act on the surrounding tumor microenvironment. There are protein families for both factors, the most important subtypes in gastric cancer are VEGF-A and PDGF-B. The signals are mediated via binding to VEGF- and PDGF receptors which have an autophosphorylating tyrosin kinase activity and subsequently initiate intracellular signal cascades that result in migration, proliferation and angiogenesis.

The overexpression of both signal molecules has been shown to be correlating to each other in gastric cancer. PDGF-B seems to play a more important role in intestinal type gastric cancer whereas VEGF-A is more important for angiogenesis in diffuse type gastric cancer [32].

The PDGF receptor can be inhibited by imatinib. Imatinib is a specific tyrosin kinase inhibitor that is frequently used in gastrointestinal stroma tumors. A potential treatment option in the future might be the novel multiple receptor tyrosine kinase inhibitor LY2457546 which has been shown to have anti-tumor effects in animal models recently.[33]

4.2 Proteinase-activated receptors (PAR) in gastric cancer

Proteinase-activated receptors belong to the family of G-protein coupled receptors. The receptor is activated by serin-proteases, such as thrypsin and thrombin by removing an N-terminal segment on the extracellular space. The thus created neo-N-terminal end subsequently serves as an intramolecular ligand that binds to the binding domaine. The signal is then transferred to the intracellular space leading to activation of several signal transduction pathways. In gastric cancer cell lines, PAR2 has been shown to trans-activate the EGF receptor. This effect could not be blocked by EGFR inhibitors [34]. To date, there are no inhibitors of PAR evaluated for clinical use.

4.3 WNT signalling and the involvement of E-caherin

The WNT signalling pathway belongs to the most important signalling systems and is evolutionary highly conserved. It plays a central role in embryonic differentiation processes. In adults, WNT activity can be detected within the stem cell niche of the gastrointestinal tract. Furthermore, there is a growing body of evidence that the WNT signalling pathway is a key player in the progression of tumors. The signal originates in the extracellular space with the binding of WNT (several subtypes exist) to its receptor frizzled. In co-operation with the co-receptor LRP the signal is then transduced to the intracellular space. From here, 4 different signalling cascades can be activated, which is shown in more detail in Tab. 1. In the classical or canonical WNT pathway the WNT signal leads to the destabilization of the multiprotein complex consisting of Axin, GSK3B and APC. GSK3b normally phosphorylizes beta catenin which in turn leads to the degradation of beta catenin. Intact beta catenin moves to the nucleus and binds to TCF/ LEF complex which constitutes a transcription factor with the subsequent expression of specific genes.

WNT sub-pathway	Targets	Biological effects
Canonical WNT/ beta catenin pathway	Cyclin D1, c-myc, MMP-7, FGF 20, DKK 1	Embryonic development, differentiation, tumor progression
WNT/JNK Pathway = planar cell polarity pathway (PCP)	Cytosceleton	Cytosceletal remodelling, cell polarity
WNT/ calcium pathway	PKC, PLC	Cell adhesion
Asymmetric cell division pathway	Mitotic spindle	Asymmetric cell division

Table 2. Several pathways downstream to the WNT signal

It is of importance to know that the WNT signalling pathway is part of a complex network of signal transduction which is controlled and regulated by a multitude of factors belonging to different pathways. In particular, a complex crosstalk between WNT, E-cadherin and beta-catenin has been described. E-cadherin inhibits dimerisation and activation of the EGFR via binding to EGFR monomers. On the other hand, activation of EGFR leads to the internalization of E-cadherin-beta-catenin complexes which in turn induces expression of WNT dependent target genes [35].

About 30% of gastric cancer cases show an overexpression of beta-catenin which is associated with poorer prognosis than beta-catenin-negative gastric cancer. The loss of APC function which is essential for the beta-catenin degradation is observed in about 20% of gastric cancer cases. The downregulation of SFRP - an inhibitor of the WNT receptor - by methylation of the promoter region has been described to occur in gastric cancer, too [17,36]. To date, there are no WNT specific anticancer drugs available. Recently, it has been demonstrated that differentiation-inducing factors downregulate the WNT pathway by activating the GSK3B in several cancer cell lines [37].

4.4 Sonic hedgehog signalling pathway (SHH)

The basic structure of SHH shows some similarity with the WNT pathway: An extracellular ligand (SHH) binds to a receptor at the cell surface (patched) which transduces the signal into the cell. Thereby, an intracellular signal transducer (smoothened) is activated which in turn deactivates a multiprotein complex (fused, suppressor of fused, coastal and others).

This deactivation leads to accumulation of a nuclear factor (Gli) which is normally degraded by the functional multiprotein complex. Eventually, specific genes encoding proteins, such as cyclin D2, patched and Gli (positive feedback) are activated. There is a ample crosstalk with other signalling pathways, in particular the expression of TGF-beta (TGF-beta pathway), the expression of SFRP1 (WNT pathway) and FOXL1 (bone morphogenic pathway).

The sonic hedgehog signalling plays a central role in embryonic development and has been shown to be upregulated in a broad variety of malignant tumors [38]. The overexpression of both Gli and the receptor patched have been reported in two thirds of gastric cancer cases. It has been shown that SHH expression is stronger in intestinal type gastric cancer and tubular growth pattern than in diffuse type gastric cancer and mucinous or undifferentiated growth pattern [39]. SHH is also overexpressed in non-malignant lesions, such as gastric adenomas or intestinal metasplasia. Due to the upregulation of SHH signalling at an early stage of cancer development it might serve as an early diagnostic tool in patients who have an increased risk for the development of gastric cancer.

The SHH signalling pathway theoretically could be blocked by cyclopamine. This substance was first discovered on sheep that fed on a certain lilieaceous plant (veratrum californicum) and delivered lambs with only one eye, reflecting the crucial role of SHH in the differentiation of embryonic body axes. Currently the design of a fully synthetic cyclopamine analogon is underway. Another potential inhibitor of SHH signal might be HMG reductase inhibitors, such as statins. HMG reductase inhibitors are necessary to process the functional SHH molecule. To date, there are no studies available on the effect of statin-dependent downregulation of SHH signals by statins and its effects on clinical outcome in the field of gastric cancer.

4.5 Notch signalling pathway and gastric cancer

Notch signalling belongs to the morphogenic embryonic signalling pathways. Notch is involved in the regulation of cellular proliferation, apoptosis and differentiation. It participates in organ development and mediates lateral inhibition of neighboring cells. The receptor (notch) and its activating ligand (delta) are located on the cell surface of two different cells. The binding of delta to its receptor notch leads to a two-step cleavage of the receptor. The intracellular receptor residue then moves to the nucleus where it forms a complex with other proteins and in turn promotes specific gene expression. Notch-specific target genes encode for several members of the Hes-family (regulation of embryonic neurodermal development), CD 25 (interleukin receptor 2, parts of the T-cell receptor), GATA3 (transcription factor for T-cell maturation), c-myc, cyclin D1, p21 bcl-2 [40-46].

Upregulated notch signalling by the ligand Jagged1 has been reported to occur frequently in gastric cancer. This upregulation was associated with poorer survival. To date, there is no target-specific treatment introduced in the current literature.

4.6 The transforming growth factor beta (TGFbeta)/ bone morphogenic protein (BMP) family and signalling pathways in gastric cancer

TGFbeta-signalling is another member of the family of embryonic developmental pathways. In cancers, TGFbeta signalling has a bivalent function: at an early tumor stage it serves as a tumor suppressor by inhibiting proliferation and promoting cellular differentiation as well as apoptosis. These processes are regulated via theRunx3 and the SMAD4 protein [17].

During cancer progression, the corresponding genes are silenced by methylation or otherwise undergo loss of function. The tumor suppressive function changes dramatically in advanced tumor stages where BMP promotes tumor angiogenesis, cell motility and the interaction of tumor cells with the interstitium. Furthermore, the immune response is suppressed by BMP [47,48]. The tumor promoting function is realized via several MAP kinase signalling pathways.

Similarly, BMP signals have bivalent functions: whereas BMP is upregulated in gastric inflammation it is downregulated in gastric cancer. On the other hand, BMP2 has been shown to promote tumor cell motility and, thus, invasiveness of gastric cancer. Furthermore, activins that constitute another subgroup of the TGFbeta/ BMP superfamily have tumor suppressive effects via activation of several caspases (pro-apoptotic), activation of p21 (cell cycle arrest) and downregulation of bcl-2 (anti-apoptotic) [49]. In summary, TGFbeta, BMP and activin signals can be regarded as a tumor suppressive mechanism restricted to certain stages of tumor progression [17].

In scirrhous gastric cancer cell lines it has been observed that treatment with two novel TGFbeta receptor 1 inhibitors (Ki26894 and A-77) decreases biological tumor progression features, such as invasiveness and epithelial-mesenchymal transition. These compounds are potential targeted drugs for metastatic scirrhous gastric cancer in the future [17,50,51].

4.7 Cell cycle dysregulation in gastric cancer

The cell cycle is strictly regulated by a broad variety of controlling factors. To move the cell cycle machinery forward, several checkpoints that control the entry to the next cell cycle phase have to be passed [52]. The most important checkpoint is the G1/S-checkpoint which regulates the initiation of cell division [53]. Under physiological conditions growth factors and other signals are needed to open the gate but in cancer cells the cell cycle can be active without the presence of activating signals and furthermore might be accelerated by overexpressed growth factors as mentioned above. Figure 2 illustrates the different checkpoints as an overview.

Both cyclin D and E in combination with the corresponding cyclin dependent kinase CDK 4/6 and CDK2 are essential for the S phase entry and the subsequent activation of the retinoblastoma protein [54]. Both cyclin D1 and 2 are known to be frequently upregulated in gastric cancer [17,54]. Cyclin D subtypes are downstream targets of several signalling pathways (Notch, SHH, WNT) whereas cyclin E has been reported to be upregulated by gene amplification in about 15% of gastric cancer cases [55].

The *TP-53* tumor suppressor gene is due to its various functions also called the "guardian of the genome". The protein p53 recognizes signals that point to DNA damage, initiates cell cycle arrest for damage repair (by activating target genes that encode for p21), functions as a transcription factor that activates expression of DNA repair genes and also can promote cell death via apoptosis in cases of irreparable DNA damage [56]. About 50% of all tumors and 40% of gastric cancer cases present with *TP-53* mutations resulting in a loss of p53 function. Loss of p53 is frequently associated with advanced tumor stages and undifferentiated tumors reflecting the increased accumulation of mutations within the tumor cell genome [57].

The loss of function of the tumor suppressor p21 occurs in 60% of gastric cancer cases and is associated with increased invasiveness, metastasis and poor prognosis. Moreover, the incidence of that loss increases with advancing tumor stages. The p27 which is an inhibitor of the CDK4-cyclinD complex and the CDK2-cyclinE complex as well arrest the cell cycle at the restriction checkpoint [58]. The loss of p27 similarly to p21, occurs in gastric cancer in dependence of tumor stage and predicts poor prognosis [59].

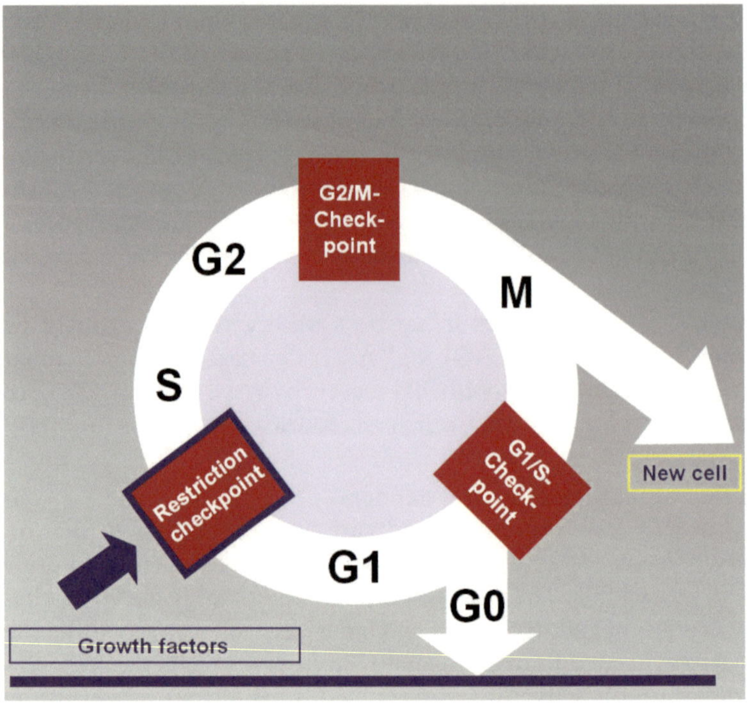

Fig. 2. Checkpoints of cell cycle

4.8 Nuclear factor kappa B in gastric cancer

Nuclear factor kappa B (NFkappaB) is a quick-time transcription factor that modulates the immune reaction and regulates proliferation and apoptosis. Extracellular signals (interleukin 1beta, tumor necrosis factor alpha via their receptors) as well as free radicals, bacterial and viral antigens are transmitted to the nucleus within minutes. This is accomplished by storing NFkappaB bound to a complex (IkappaB) in the cytoplasma from which NFkappa B is mobilized via inactivation of IkappaB by a IkappaB specific kinase (IKK). The free NFkappaB molecule can then move within the nucleus and activate specific genes like cytokines (IL-6, IL-1beta, TNF), chemokines (IL-8, CCL2, CCL3), enzymes (iNOS, COX-2) and adhesion molecules (VCAM-1, ICAM-1, CEACAM-1) which in turn promote inflammatory processes [60].

NFkappaB plays a central role in inflammatory cancers. Dysregulation of the NFkappaB has been observed in gastric cancer to be associated with increased proliferation, genomic instability and drug resistance [61,62].

There is a variety of phytochemicals, such as silibinin, resveratrol and catechins which are known to suppress the activation of NFkappaB. Also, several poly-phenol bonds (green tea) can act as anti-cancer drugs. Furthermore, inhibitors of IKK are studied at a preclinical stage [60].

4.9 S-100 proteins in gastric cancer

The S-100 protein family currently counts 21 members which are responsible for various cellular functions, in particular they are assumed to be second messenger molecules which interact with numerous different molecules. S-100A2, 3, 4, 7 and 10 have been observed to be overexpressed in gastric cancer.

S-100A4 is regulated by epigenetic mechanisms and by beta-catenin. Overexpressed S-100A4 was associated with advanced tumor stages, diffuse type gastric cancer and increased incidence of tumor lymph node involvement [63]. S-100A4 has been demonstrated to be upregulated predominantly in early stages of gastric cancer [64], other studies associated this protein to metastasis in several tumors and, therefore, it is also named metastasin. S-100A4 has a multitude of binding partners, such as E-cadherin, p53, actin and p37 among many others. Interestingly, S-100A4 is one of the strongest molecular based predictors of survival in patients with ovarian carcinoma, pancreatic cancer and gastric cancer [65].

Moreover, calcyclin-binding protein has been shown to inhibit proliferation and invasiveness in gastric cancer by promoting S-100-protein ubiquitinylation which might be a potential target-specific treatment option in the future [66].

4.10 Dysregulated DNA repair mechanisms

The accurate transfer of genetic information through the DNA replication and cell division machinery is dependent on both, exact DNA synthesis procedure and sufficient DNA damage repair systems. Moreover, the DNA is permanently exposed to toxic metabolites, such as oxygen radicals and to physical stress, such as ultraviolet radiation. In addition, spontaneous mutations and DNA methylation occur. In particular, 4 basic mechanisms of DNA repair exist: 1.) the single base excision system, 2.) mismatch repair system, 3.) the nucleotide excision repair system and 4.) the double strand break repair system.

The single base excision system removes defective and modified bases. Therefore, two mechanisms exist: either the aberrant base is recognized and selectively removed by specific DNA glycosylases resulting in an apurinic or apyrimidic ribosyl residue which is in turn cleaved by a AP endonuclease; or the base is repaired directly without removing.

The mismatch repair system recognizes mismatched single bases, small single strand loops and the recombination of non-homologous sequences. Heterodimers from MLH2, 3 and 6 recognize and bind to those DNA loci which in turn leads to the recruitment of further proteins (helicase, single strand binding protein, MSH, and others) forming a protein complex. Hereditary defects in this system are known as as the Lynch syndrome.

The nucleotide excision repair system in particular is responsible for recognizing and repairing DNA damage that is caused by solar radiation. As a logical consequence those patients who have genetic defects concerning this system primarily present with dermal diseases due to the direct exposition of the skin to solar radiation (e.g. xeroderma pigmentosum). It is the only one repair system that is able to remove bulky adducts (dimers of pyrimidin and cyclobutan) and remove up to 32 nucleotides. More than 30 genes are involved in that repair mechanism system.

The double strand break repair system can either act with homologous recombination (HR) immediately behind the replication fork or can act with non-homologous endjoining (NHEJ). The first mechanism requires a sister chromatide which is not available during G0 and G1 phase, therefore in these phases of cell cycle only NHEJ can be performed. The frequently discussed tumor suppessor proteins BRCA1 and 2 are involved in the HR repair system [67,68].

Defective DNA repair systems cause the accumulation of mutations which can lead to transformation provided that the mutation provides a selection benefit. Therefore, it is not surprising that genetic defects in DNA repair are associated with the development of malignant tumors, as it is the case in about 15% of all colorectal cancer cases as well as in other tumor entities like ovarian carcinoma and endometrial carcinoma. For gastric cancer it has been reported that about 8% of sporadic cases show microsatellite instability pointing to defective DNA mismatch repair [69].

PARP inhibitors which block the enzyme poly(ADP-ribose) polymerase might a become potential target specific therapy in cases of mutated BRCA1 and 2. The substance psoralen that induces interstrand crosslinks is investigated in preclinical studies [67].

5. Conclusion

A growing body of knowledge about the biological behavior as well as the molecular nature of gastric cancer is available in the current literature. Although there are only few targeted treatment strategies implemented in the clinical routine a large number of studies dedicated to molecular based strategies is currently underway.

This chapter also implicates that there is a complex pattern of molecular mechanisms that extend the interpretation of gastric cancer in addition to classifications that are exclusively based on macroscopic and histological findings. The pattern of genetic imbalances and of dysregulated pathways is of essential importance to treat patients in a more individualized fashion.

6. References

[1] Belien JA, Buffart TE, Gill AJ, et al.: Gross genomic damage measured by DNA image cytometry independently predicts gastric cancer patient survival. Br J Cancer 2009;101:1011-1018.

[2] Nardone G: Review article: molecular basis of gastric carcinogenesis. Aliment Pharmacol Ther 2003;17 Suppl 2:75-81.

[3] Yamamoto H, Imai K, Perucho M: Gastrointestinal cancer of the microsatellite mutator phenotype pathway. J Gastroenterol 2002;37:153-163.

[4] Zhang D, Wang Z, Luo Y, et al.: Analysis of DNA copy number aberrations by multiple ligation-dependent probe amplification on 50 intestinal type gastric cancers. J Surg Oncol;103:124-132.

[5] Dittmar Y, Posorski N, Rauchfuss F, et al.: Relationship between degree of chromosomal aberration and survival in intestinal-type gastric cancer - a preliminary report based on three cases of hepatic metastasized gastric cancer with long-time survival. Onkologie;33:591-596.

[6] Lengauer C, Kinzler KW, Vogelstein B: Genetic instabilities in human cancers. Nature 1998;396:643-649.

[7] Resende C, Ristimaki A, Machado JC: Genetic and epigenetic alteration in gastric carcinogenesis. Helicobacter;15 Suppl 1:34-39.

[8] Zeng J, Ge Z, Wang L, et al.: The histone demethylase RBP2 Is overexpressed in gastric cancer and its inhibition triggers senescence of cancer cells. Gastroenterology;138:981-992.

[9] Carneiro F, Oliveira C, Seruca R: Pathology and genetics of familial gastric cancer. Int J Surg Pathol;18:33S-36S.
[10] Corso G, Marrelli D, Roviello F: Familial gastric cancer: update for practice management. Fam Cancer.
[11] Wolf EM, Geigl JB, Svrcek M, et al.: [Hereditary gastric cancer]. Pathologe;31:423-429.
[12] Leite M, Corso G, Sousa S, et al.: MSI phenotype and MMR alterations in familial and sporadic gastric cancer. Int J Cancer;128:1606-1613.
[13] Caldas C, Carneiro F, Lynch HT, et al.: Familial gastric cancer: overview and guidelines for management. J Med Genet 1999;36:873-880.
[14] Capelle LG, Van Grieken NC, Lingsma HF, et al.: Risk and epidemiological time trends of gastric cancer in Lynch syndrome carriers in the Netherlands. Gastroenterology;138:487-492.
[15] Varley JM: Germline TP53 mutations and Li-Fraumeni syndrome. Hum Mutat 2003;21:313-320.
[16] Evans DG, Wu CL, Birch JM: BRCA2: a cause of Li-Fraumeni-like syndrome. J Med Genet 2008;45:62-63.
[17] Wu WK, Cho CH, Lee CW, et al.: Dysregulation of cellular signaling in gastric cancer. Cancer Lett;295:144-153.
[18] Gravalos C, Jimeno A: HER2 in gastric cancer: a new prognostic factor and a novel therapeutic target. Ann Oncol 2008;19:1523-1529.
[19] Moelans CB, Milne AN, Morsink FH, et al.: Low frequency of HER2 amplification and overexpression in early onset gastric cancer. Cell Oncol (Dordr).
[20] Meza-Junco J, Au HJ, Sawyer MB: Trastuzumab for gastric cancer. Expert Opin Biol Ther 2009;9:1543-1551.
[21] Bianco R, Garofalo S, Rosa R, et al.: Inhibition of mTOR pathway by everolimus cooperates with EGFR inhibitors in human tumours sensitive and resistant to anti-EGFR drugs. Br J Cancer 2008;98:923-930.
[22] Wu M, Semba S, Oue N, et al.: BRAF/K-ras mutation, microsatellite instability, and promoter hypermethylation of hMLH1/MGMT in human gastric carcinomas. Gastric Cancer 2004;7:246-253.
[23] Waldner MJ, Neurath MF: The molecular therapy of colorectal cancer. Mol Aspects Med;31:171-178.
[24] Iwasaki J, Nihira S: Anti-angiogenic therapy against gastrointestinal tract cancers. Jpn J Clin Oncol 2009;39:543-551.
[25] Lesko E, Majka M: The biological role of HGF-MET axis in tumor growth and development of metastasis. Front Biosci 2008;13:1271-1280.
[26] Trusolino L, Bertotti A, Comoglio PM: MET signalling: principles and functions in development, organ regeneration and cancer. Nat Rev Mol Cell Biol;11:834-848.
[27] Amemiya H, Kono K, Takahashi A, et al.: c-Met expression in a gastric cancer cell line producing alpha-fetoprotein. Surg Today 2004;34:115-122.
[28] Kuniyasu H, Yasui W, Kitadai Y, et al.: Frequent amplification of the c-met gene in scirrhous type stomach cancer. Biochem Biophys Res Commun 1992;189:227-232.
[29] Arkenau HT: Gastric cancer in the era of molecularly targeted agents: current drug development strategies. J Cancer Res Clin Oncol 2009;135:855-866.
[30] Ming SC: Cellular and molecular pathology of gastric carcinoma and precursor lesions: A critical review. Gastric Cancer 1998;1:31-50.

[31] Hattori Y, Itoh H, Uchino S, et al.: Immunohistochemical detection of K-sam protein in stomach cancer. Clin Cancer Res 1996;2:1373-1381.
[32] Suzuki S, Dobashi Y, Hatakeyama Y, et al.: Clinicopathological significance of platelet-derived growth factor (PDGF)-B and vascular endothelial growth factor-A expression, PDGF receptor-beta phosphorylation, and microvessel density in gastric cancer. BMC Cancer;10:659.
[33] Burkholder TP, Clayton JR, Rempala ME, et al.: Discovery of LY2457546: a multi-targeted anti-angiogenic kinase inhibitor with a novel spectrum of activity and exquisite potency in the acute myelogenous leukemia-Flt-3-internal tandem duplication mutant human tumor xenograft model. Invest New Drugs.
[34] Caruso R, Pallone F, Fina D, et al.: Protease-activated receptor-2 activation in gastric cancer cells promotes epidermal growth factor receptor trans-activation and proliferation. Am J Pathol 2006;169:268-278.
[35] Hu T, Li C: Convergence between Wnt-beta-catenin and EGFR signaling in cancer. Mol Cancer;9:236.
[36] Tahara E: Molecular biology of gastric cancer. World J Surg 1995;19:484-488; discussion 489-490.
[37] Takahashi-Yanaga F, Sasaguri T: Drug development targeting the glycogen synthase kinase-3beta (GSK-3beta)-mediated signal transduction pathway: inhibitors of the Wnt/beta-catenin signaling pathway as novel anticancer drugs. J Pharmacol Sci 2009;109:179-183.
[38] Yang L, Xie G, Fan Q, Xie J: Activation of the hedgehog-signaling pathway in human cancer and the clinical implications. Oncogene;29:469-481.
[39] Lee SY, Han HS, Lee KY, et al.: Sonic hedgehog expression in gastric cancer and gastric adenoma. Oncol Rep 2007;17:1051-1055.
[40] Borggrefe T, Oswald F: The Notch signaling pathway: transcriptional regulation at Notch target genes. Cell Mol Life Sci 2009;66:1631-1646.
[41] Iso T, Kedes L, Hamamori Y: HES and HERP families: multiple effectors of the Notch signaling pathway. J Cell Physiol 2003;194:237-255.
[42] Fischer A, Gessler M: Delta-Notch--and then? Protein interactions and proposed modes of repression by Hes and Hey bHLH factors. Nucleic Acids Res 2007;35:4583-4596.
[43] Satoh Y, Matsumura I, Tanaka H, et al.: Roles for c-Myc in self-renewal of hematopoietic stem cells. J Biol Chem 2004;279:24986-24993.
[44] Palomero T, Lim WK, Odom DT, et al.: NOTCH1 directly regulates c-MYC and activates a feed-forward-loop transcriptional network promoting leukemic cell growth. Proc Natl Acad Sci U S A 2006;103:18261-18266.
[45] Ronchini C, Capobianco AJ: Induction of cyclin D1 transcription and CDK2 activity by Notch(ic): implication for cell cycle disruption in transformation by Notch(ic). Mol Cell Biol 2001;21:5925-5934.
[46] Deftos ML, He YW, Ojala EW, Bevan MJ: Correlating notch signaling with thymocyte maturation. Immunity 1998;9:777-786.
[47] Mishra L, Derynck R, Mishra B: Transforming growth factor-beta signaling in stem cells and cancer. Science 2005;310:68-71.
[48] Miyazono K, Suzuki H, Imamura T: Regulation of TGF-beta signaling and its roles in progression of tumors. Cancer Sci 2003;94:230-234.

[49] Kim YI, Lee HJ, Khang I, et al.: Selective inhibition of cell growth by activin in SNU-16 cells. World J Gastroenterol 2006;12:3000-3005.
[50] Shinto O, Yashiro M, Kawajiri H, et al.: Inhibitory effect of a TGFbeta receptor type-I inhibitor, Ki26894, on invasiveness of scirrhous gastric cancer cells. Br J Cancer;102:844-851.
[51] Kawajiri H, Yashiro M, Shinto O, et al.: A novel transforming growth factor beta receptor kinase inhibitor, A-77, prevents the peritoneal dissemination of scirrhous gastric carcinoma. Clin Cancer Res 2008;14:2850-2860.
[52] O'Connor PM: Mammalian G1 and G2 phase checkpoints. Cancer Surv 1997;29:151-182.
[53] Schwartz GK, Shah MA: Targeting the cell cycle: a new approach to cancer therapy. J Clin Oncol 2005;23:9408-9421.
[54] Boonstra J: Progression through the G1-phase of the on-going cell cycle. J Cell Biochem 2003;90:244-252.
[55] Akama Y, Yasui W, Yokozaki H, et al.: Frequent amplification of the cyclin E gene in human gastric carcinomas. Jpn J Cancer Res 1995;86:617-621.
[56] Menendez D, Inga A, Resnick MA: The expanding universe of p53 targets. Nat Rev Cancer 2009;9:724-737.
[57] Fenoglio-Preiser CM, Wang J, Stemmermann GN, Noffsinger A: TP53 and gastric carcinoma: a review. Hum Mutat 2003;21:258-270.
[58] Yasui W, Akama Y, Kuniyasu H, et al.: Expression of cyclin-dependent kinase inhibitor p21WAF1/CIP1 in non-neoplastic mucosa and neoplasia of the stomach: relationship with p53 status and proliferative activity. J Pathol 1996;180:122-128.
[59] Le TV, Seo Y, Ryu CJ, et al.: Increased expression of p27 is associated with the cisplatin resistance in gastric cancer cell line YCC-3. Arch Pharm Res;33:1127-1132.
[60] Schneider G, Kramer OH: NFkappaB/p53 crosstalk-a promising new therapeutic target. Biochim Biophys Acta;1815:90-103.
[61] Liu CA, Wang MJ, Chi CW, et al.: Rho/Rhotekin-mediated NF-kappaB activation confers resistance to apoptosis. Oncogene 2004;23:8731-8742.
[62] Cho SJ, Park JW, Kang JS, et al.: Nuclear factor-kappaB dependency of doxorubicin sensitivity in gastric cancer cells is determined by manganese superoxide dismutase expression. Cancer Sci 2008;99:1117-1124.
[63] Yoon CS, Hyung WJ, Lee JH, et al.: Expression of S100A4, E-cadherin, alpha- and beta-catenin in gastric adenocarcinoma. Hepatogastroenterology 2008;55:1916-1920.
[64] Huang HL, Wu BY, Zhu XD, et al.: [Expression of S100A6 in primary and metastatic human gastric cancer]. Zhonghua Zhong Liu Za Zhi 2008;30:506-510.
[65] Boye K, Maelandsmo GM: S100A4 and metastasis: a small actor playing many roles. Am J Pathol;176:528-535.
[66] Ning X, Sun S, Hong L, et al.: Calcyclin-binding protein inhibits proliferation, tumorigenicity, and invasion of gastric cancer. Mol Cancer Res 2007;5:1254-1262.
[67] Fackenthal JD, Olopade OI: Breast cancer risk associated with BRCA1 and BRCA2 in diverse populations. Nat Rev Cancer 2007;7:937-948.
[68] Liang Y, Lin SY, Brunicardi FC, et al.: DNA damage response pathways in tumor suppression and cancer treatment. World J Surg 2009;33:661-666.

[69] Huang YQ, Yuan Y, Ge WT, et al.: Comparative features of colorectal and gastric cancers with microsatellite instability in Chinese patients. J Zhejiang Univ Sci B;11:647-653.

5

miRNAs in Gastric Cancer

Yu-Lun Liao[1*], Kuo-Wang Tsai[2*] and Wen-chang Lin[1]
[1]*Institute of Biomedical Sciences, Academia Sinica, Taipei;*
[2]*Department of Medical Education and Research, Kaohsiung Veterans General Hospital, Kaohsiung, Taiwan, Republic of China*

1. Introduction

Gastric cancer (GC) is the most of common cancers, and is especially common in the Andean region of South America and in the Far East (Parkin, Pisani and Ferlay 1999). It can spread throughout the stomach and to other organs, including the esophagus, lungs, lymph nodes or liver. Therefore, gastric cancer is the second leading cause of cancer-related death in the world (Kim et al. 2011). Currently, it remains as one of common cancer types and still be a leading cause of cancer-related death. The development and progression of gastric cancer have been characterized by multiple genetic mutations of proto-oncogenes and tumor-suppressor genes (Wu et al. 2010, Wang et al. 2010).

MicroRNAs (miRNAs) are endogenous non-protein-coding short RNAs of 21-23 nucleotides (Kim, 2005; Bartel, 2004). It was initially discovered in *Caenorhabditis elegans* and thousands have been identified in many organisms, including human, mammals, invertebrates, insects, plants and viruses. In humans, miRNAs play important roles in cellular physiology, development, and disease by negatively regulating gene expression (Kim, 2005; Bartel, 2004). miRNAs regulate their target genes through targeting 3-UTR region of the gene. While miRNA is imperfect pairing with target gene mRNAs, it may lead to translational repression. Therefore, when perfectly paired with targeting genes, the result was cleavage of the target mRNAs. Depending on their respective target genes, miRNAs could act as tumor-suppressive or in an oncogenesis role. Tumor suppressive miRNAs have usually repressed growth-promoting genes, and oncogenic miRNAs targeted cell growth inhibiting genes.

Previous studies have used an miRNA profiling approach to investigate the function of the miRNA in gastric cancer, showing many miRNAs aberrantly overexpressed or downregulated in gastric cancer progression. Various mechanisms contribute to miRNA aberrant expression during gastric carcinogenesis, including genetic mutation, epigenetic silencing and deregulated transcriptional activity. In this review, we will discuss the detailed mechanisms of miRNA deregulation, such as epigenetic alteration and transcriptional activity in gastric cancer progression. Based on their target genes, we further discuss miRNAs involved in important biological process related to cell growth, cell cycles, apoptosis and cell

---

[*] Equal contribution

migration. These miRNA candidates can be used as candidate biomarkers for the detection of gastric cancer and monitoring recurrence.

2. Alteration of miRNA in gastric cancer

Since miRNA had been shown as a significant factor during gastric cancer progress, global miRNA expression profiles have been performed using microarray, real-time PCR, or next-generation sequencing approaches. The identified dysregulated miRNAs in gastric cancer are listed in Table 1 (Katada et al., 2009a; Guo et al., 2009; Ueda et al., 2010; Ribeiro-dos-Santos et al., 2010; Luo et al., 2009; Tsukamoto et al., 2010).

Upregulation in gastric cancer			Downregulation in gastric cancer		
miR-7	miR-9	miR-10a	miR-9	miR-19b	miR-29b/c
miR-15a/b	miR-16	miR-17	miR-30a/b/c/d/e	miR-31	miR-128b
miR-18a/b	miR-19a/b	miR-20a/b	miR-129	miR-133b	miR-139
miR-21	miR-23a	miR-24	miR-148a/b	miR-152	miR-155
miR-25	miR-26b	miR-27a	miR-188	miR-195	miR-197
miR-30a	miR-34a/b/c	miR-92	miR-218	miR-338	miR-370
miR-93	miR-103	miR-106a/b	miR-375	miR-378	miR-383
miR-107	miR-128	miR-128	miR-422b	miR-433	miR-451
miR-135a/b	miR-146a	miR-181a/b/c/d	miR-490	miR-497	miR-503
miR-191	miR-192	miR-194	miR-545	miR-551a	miR567
miR-200b	miR-212	miR-215	miR-575	miR-611	miR-630
miR-222	miR-223	miR-224	miR-638	miR-649	miR-652
miR-320	miR-345	miR-379	miR768		
miR-409	miR-425	miR-429			
miR-518b					

Table 1. Summary of the dysregulation of miRNAs in gastric cancer

However, the factors causing miRNA dysregulation are very complex. The process is composed of multiple steps, including (1) pri-miRNA transcriptional regulation; (2) miRNA maturation process; (3) genetic alteration. The miRNAs serve as tumor suppressors or oncogenes depending on their target genes. Therefore, we have reviewed previous studies which have elucidated the mechanism of dysregulated miRNAs and their confirmed targets during gastric cancer progress, and we have listed these important studies in Table 2.

3. Mechanism of miRNA deregulation in gastric cancer

There is a lot of information on aberrantly expressed miRNAs and their tumorigenic effect in gastric cancers, but the clear mechanisms of such miRNA deregulation remain poorly understood. Recent studies have identified some possible mechanisms including epigenetic alteration and deregulated transcription.

3.1 Epigenetic regulation of miRNAs expression in gastric cancer

Epigenetic regulation includes histone modification and DNA methylation, processes which are involved in regulation of cell growth and development in mammals. DNA methylation

Tumor suppressive microRNAs

microRNA	Regulator	Function	Target genes	References
Let-7 family		cell migration	RAS , HMGA2,RAB40C	(Motoyama, Inoue et al. 2008; Ohshima, Inoue et al. 2010; Yang, Jie et al. 2011)
miR-9	hypermethylation	cell growth, cell cycle	NF-kB1; CDX2; RAB34	(Luo, Zhang et al. 2009; Wan, Guo et al. 2010; Rotkrua, Akiyama et al. 2011)
miR-29		cell growth, cell migration	Cdc42	(Lang, Liu et al. 2010)
miR-34	hypermethylation	cell growth, cell cycle, apoptosis	Bcl-2, Notch, HMGA2	(Ji, Hao et al. 2008; Suzuki, Yamamoto et al. 2010; Tsai, Wu et al. 2011)
miR-101		cell growth, cell migration	EZH2, Cox-2, Mcl-1 and Fos	(Varambally, Cao et al. 2008; Wang, Ruan et al. 2010)
miR-107		cell growth, cell cycle	CDK6;DRCE1	(Li, Zhang et al. 2010; Feng, Xie et al. 2011)
miR-126		cell growth, cell migration	SOX2;Crk	(Feng, Chen et al. 2010; Otsubo, Akiyama et al. 2011)
miR-125a		cell growth	ERBB2	(Nishida, Mimori et al. 2011)
miR-129	hypermethylation	cell growth	SOX4; Cdk6	(Shen, Pan et al. 2010; Wu, Qian et al. 2010; Tsai, Wu et al. 2011)
miR-137	hypermethylation	cell cycle, apoptosis	Cdc42	(Chen, Chen et al. 2011)
miR-141		cell growth	FGFR2	(Du, Xu et al. 2009)
miR-148		cell growth	CCKBR	(Song, Yue et al. 2011)
miR-181c	hypermethylation	cell growth	NOTCH4, KRAS	(Hashimoto, Akiyama et al. 2010)
miR-200 family	BARF0,EBNA1,LMP2A	cell growth		(Shinozaki, Sakatani et al. 2010)
miR-212	hypermethylation	cell growth	myc, MeCP2	(Wada, Akiyama et al. 2010; Xu, Wang et al. 2010)
miR-218		cell migration	Robo1, NFkB	(Gao, Zhang et al. 2010; Tie, Pan et al. 2010)
miR-331		cell growth	E2F1	(Guo, Guo et al. 2010)
miR-375		cell growth	JAK2; PDK1, 14-3-3zeta	(Ding, Xu et al. 2010; Tsukamoto, Nakada et al. 2010)
miR-433			GRB2	(Luo, Zhang et al. 2009)
miR-512	hypermethylation	cell growth, apoptosis	PTEN,Mcl-1	(Saito, Suzuki et al. 2009)
miR-516a	hypermethylation	cell migration	sulfatase 1	(Takei, Takigahira et al. 2011)
Oncogenesis microRNA				
miR-16	NF-kB	cell growth	Bcl2	(Xia, Zhang et al. 2008; Shin, Jin et al. 2011)
miR-21	NF-kB	cell growth	PDCG4,	(Motoyama, Inoue et al. 2010; Shin, Jin et al. 2011)
miR-27a		cell growth	prohibitin	(Liu, Tang et al. 2009)
miR-43c		cell cycle	VEZT	(Guo, Jing et al. 2011)
miR-106b/93/25	E2F1	cell growth, cell cycle	p57,p21	(Petrocca, Visone et al. 2008; Kim, Yu et al. 2009)
miR-130b		cell growth	RUNX3	(Lai, Koh et al. 2010)
miR-150		cell growth, apoptosis	EGR2	(Wu, Jin et al. 2010)
miR-181b		apoptosis	Bcl2	(Zhu, Shan et al. 2010)
miR-192		cell growth; cell migration	ALCAM	(Jin, Selaru et al. 2010)
miR-199a		cell growth, cell migration	MAP3K11	(Song, Zeng et al. 2010)
miR-221/222		cell growth, cell cycle	p27, p57	(Kim, Yu et al. 2009; Chun-Zhi, Lei et al. 2010)
miR-372		cell growth, cell cycle, apoptosis	LAS2	(Cho, Shin et al. 2009)
miR-421		cell growth	CBX7,RBMXL1	(Jiang, Guo et al. 2010)
miR-497		apoptosis	BCL2	(Zhu, Zhu et al. 2011)
miR-650		cell growth, cell migration	ING4	(Zhang, Zhu et al. 2010)

Table 2. Studies confirming aberrant miRNAs expressed in gastric carcinoma

plays an important role in regulation of gene expression through establishing and maintaining the DNA methylation status of gene promoters. Previous studies have demonstrated that abnormal methylation patterns lead to gastric carcinogenesis through the hypermethylated promoter of tumor suppressor genes (Watanabe & Maekawa, 2010). The basic transcription mechanism of miRNA is fundamentally similar to that of classic protein-coding genes, hence, the hypermethylated promoter region of tumor-suppressive miRNAs may result in gastric cancer formation and progression. Recently, we identified the 48 methylation-regulated miRNAs in AGS cells using a real-time PCR microRNA expression profile (Tsai et al., 2009). In this profile, our laboratory first identified a primate-specific miRNA cluster (C19MC) comprising 46 pre-miRNAs, C19MC, which could be co-regulated in placenta tissue by methylating its distal CpG-rich domain (Tsai et al., 2009; Noguer-Dance et al., 2010). A recent study showed that C19MC displays a maternal-specific methylation imprint acquired in oocytes (Noguer-Dance et al., 2010). Saito et al. reported that epigenetic activation of miR-512-5p induces suppression of Mcl-1, resulting in apoptosis of gastric cancer cells (Saito et al., 2009). Accumulating evidence indicates that several tumor-suppressive miRNAs have been shown to contain the aberrant hypermethylation of their promoter regions in human cancers, including miR-9, miR-34b/c, miR-129, miR-137, miR-181C, miR-199a, miR-212, miR-512 and miR-516 (Cheung et al., 2011; Luo et al., 2009; Saito et al., 2009; Shen et al., 2010; Suzuki et al., 2010; Tsai et al., 2009; Tsai et al., 2011; Xu et al., 2010) (Figure 1).

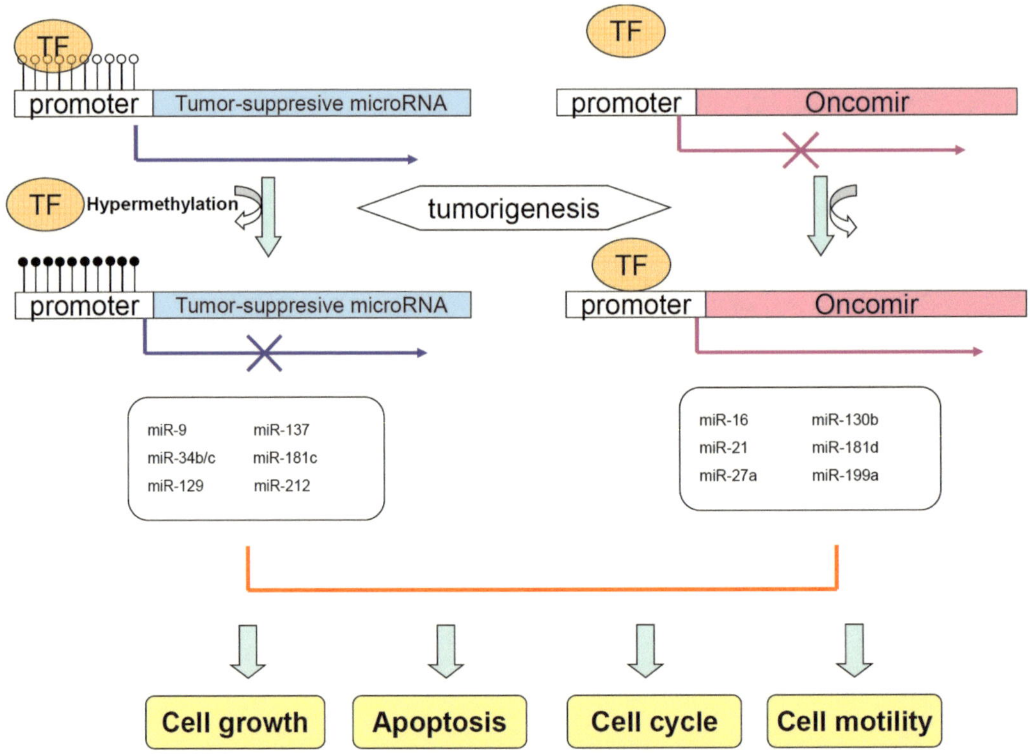

Fig. 1. Schematic diagram depicting miRNA dysregulation and its function in gastric carcinogenesis.

Hypermethylation silencing miR-129 expression is associated with a poor clinical outcome in gastric cancer, and restoration of miR-129 downregulated SOX4 and Cdk6 expression. Overexpression of miR-129-2 could inhibit cell growth and induce apoptosis through suppression of its target genes in gastric cancer cells (Shen et al., 2010; Tsai et al., 2011; Wu et al., 2010a). Hypermethylation leads miR-9 underexpression and affects cell growth and the cell cycle through regulating NF-κB1, CDX2, RAB34 (Luo et al., 2009; Rotkrua et al., 2011; Wan et al., 2010). Transfection of an anti-miR-9 molecule significantly inhibited cell growth by promoting G1 cell cycle arrest in MKN45 cells similarly to the effect of CDX2 (Rotkrua et al., 2011).

Tumor-specific transcriptional repression via promoter hypermethylation is often associated with the silencing of tumor suppressive miRNA. Interestingly, a DNA-methylation-dependent transcriptional regulation of oncomir, miR-196b, was dramatically overexpressed in gastric cancer tissue samples with a hypomethylated promoter (Tsai et al., 2010). Therefore, DNA methylation plays a critical role in gastric cancer, and involved in the control of the imprinting genes during developmental stages, or tumor-suppressive miRNAs / oncomirs in gastric tumor development (Figure 2).

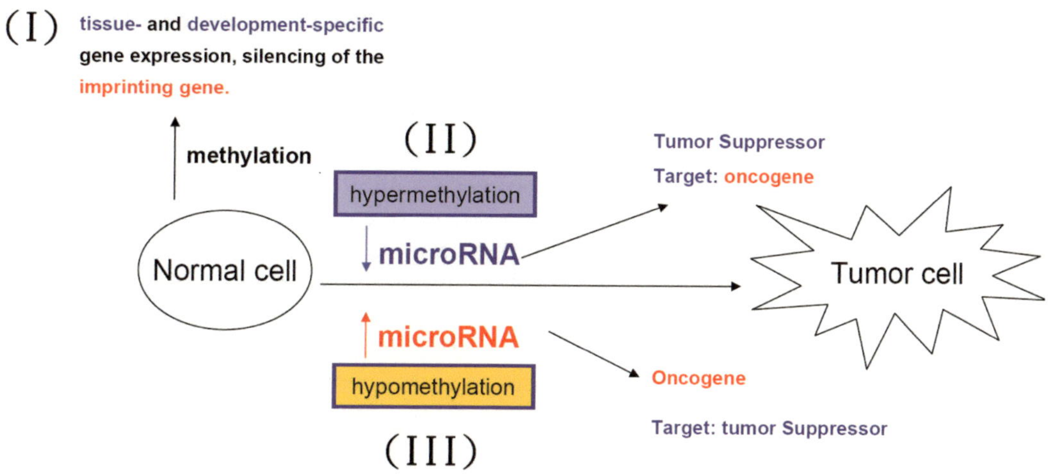

Fig. 2. Schematic diagram depicting miRNA regulation by DNA methylation in gastric carcinogenesis.

3.2 Deregulated transcription of miRNAs in gastric cancer

Like the classic protein-coding genes, the possibility of up- or downregulation of miRNAs could also be controlled by transcription factors. E2F1 transcription factor could directly upregulate the transcription of miR-106b-25 cluster in gastric cancer cells. Conversely, miR-106b and miR-93 regulate E2F1 expression, establishing a miRNA-directed negative feedback loop (Petrocca et al., 2008). Shin et al. found that miR-16 and miR-21 are directly regulated by the transcription factor NF-κB in nicotine-treated gastric cancer cells (Shin et al., 2011). miR-34 was thereby demonstrated to be involved in the network and tumor suppressing pathways of p53 as a downstream target of p53 (Ji et al., 2008). Alteration of genes involved in miRNA processing could also contribute to miRNA deregulation. Recent studies reported that both Ago2 and TNRC6A are related to the execution of the gene-silencing function of miRNA, and are observed in gastric cancer with high microsatellite instability (Kim et al., 2010). It has been reported the expression of Dicer1 and Drosha are different in non-neoplastic and neoplastic gastric tissues (Tchernitsa et al., 2010).

4. Putative role of miRNAs in gastric cancer

Previous studies revealed a broad variety of oncogenes and tumor suppressor genes regulated by different miRNAs in gastric cancer cells. Recent research has revealed evidence showing that miRNAs play roles in the initiation and progression of cancer (Volinia et al., 2006). Some of these miRNAs modulate expression of known oncogenes or tumor suppressor genes, whereas others function as so-called onco-miRs or tumor-suppressor-miRs. Furthermore, evidence for regulation of carcinogenesis by miRNAs has been obtained, including promotion of proliferation, migration, invasion and anti-apoptosis.

4.1 miRNAs and the cell cycle

Increased cell proliferation is a common feature of gastric carcinogenesis. The miR-222-221 and miR-106b-25 clusters have been found abnormally upregulated in gastric cancer tissues and reported to suppress the p21 family of CDK inhibitors (p57Kip2, p21Cip1, and p27Kip1) (Kim et al., 2009). Ectopic expression of miR-222-221 and miR-106b-25 clusters result in activation of CDK2 activity and facilitates the G1/S phase transition. Inhibition of miR-372-suppressed proliferation, arrested the cell cycle at G2/M phase, and increased apoptosis through downregulation of a tumor suppressor gene, LATS2 in gastric cancer cells (Cho et al., 2009). Deregulation of E2F1 activity is characteristic of gastric tumorigenesis and Guo et al. found that overexpression of miR-331-3p blocked G1/S transition in gastric cancer cell lines. miR-331-3p functions in cell cycle control by targeting cell cycle-related molecule E2F1 (Guo et al., 2010). A previous study provided evidence that downregulation of miR-663 in tumor cells may contribute to aberrant cell hyperplasia by indirectly affected upregulation of cyclin B, leading to the development of gastric cancer. Therefore, miR-663 might function as a potent suppressor of tumor growth (Pan et al., 2010). miR-126 was significantly downregulated in gastric cancer tissues. Ectopic expression of miR-126 potently inhibited cell growth by inducing cell cycle arrest in G0/G1 phase in gastric cancer cells. miR-126 may function as a tumor suppressor, and was capable of regulating Crk in gastric cancer (Feng et al., 2010). Restoration of the miR-137 expression downregulated the Cdc42 expression and induced cell cycle G1 arrest in gastric cancer cells. The miR-137 expression was found to be inversely correlated with CDC42 expression in gastric cancer. miR-137 is downregulated in gastric cancer and is a indirectly negative regulator of Cdc42 (Chen et al., 2011). Cyclin-dependent kinase 6 (CDK6) is found to be upregulated in gastric cancer and has been implicated in tumor initiation and progression. Feng et al. have identified miR-107 as a potential regulator of CDK6 expression. Ectopic expression of miR-107 reduced both mRNA and protein expression levels of CDK6, inhibited proliferation, induced G1 cell cycle arrest. miR-107 may have a tumor suppressor function by directly targeting CDK6 to inhibit the proliferation in gastric cancer cells (Feng et al., 2011). Otsubo et al. demonstrated that SRY (sex determining region Y)-box 2 (SOX2) plays important roles in growth inhibition through cell cycle arrest and apoptosis, and that SOX2 expression is frequently downregulated in gastric cancers. They found miR-126 targets SOX2 in gastric cancer cells. Aberrant overexpression of miR-126 and consequent SOX2 downregulation may contribute to gastric carcinogenesis (Otsubo et al., 2011). These findings suggest that aberrant miRNA expression may enhance cell-cycle progression through direct or indirect regulation of cell-cycle regulators.

4.2 miRNAs and apoptosis

Escape from the process of apoptosis is a hallmark of cellular transformation. miRNA dysregulation has been shown to regulate apoptosis by altering the expression of Bcl-2 family members in gastric cancer. Disturbances in apoptotic pathways lead to uncontrolled cell proliferation which indicates a critical step in tumor development.

Forced expression of miR-21 significantly promoted cell proliferation and inhibited apoptosis in gastric cancer cells. Zhang et al. have identified RECK as the direct target of miR-21. RECK is a tumor-suppressor gene in gastric cancer and the oncogenic effect of miR-21 may be mediated by regulation of RECK (Zhang et al., 2008). miR-218 expression was reduced significantly in gastric cancer tissues and overexpression of miR-218 inhibited cell proliferation and induced apoptosis in gastric cancer cells through direct targeting of Epidermal growth factor receptor-coamplified and overexpressed protein (ECOP), a positive regulator of NF-κB transcriptional activity. Overexpression of miR-218 also inhibited NF-κB transcriptional activation and transcription of cyclooxygenase-2, a proliferative and anti-apoptotic gene regulated by NF-κB (Gao et al., 2010). Overexpression of miR-150 in gastric cancer could promote proliferation and growth of cancer cells through directly targeting the tumor-suppressor EGR2, whose activation induces apoptosis (Wu et al., 2010b).

RUNX3 is an important tumor suppressor that is inactivated in many cancer types. miR-130b expression was significantly higher in gastric tumors, and overexpression of miR-130b has also been reported to suppress TGFβ-mediated Bim expression and apoptosis by targeting RUNX3 in gastric cancer cells (Lai et al., 2010). miR-375 was greatly downregulated in gastric cancer tissues, and its ectopic expression in gastric carcinoma cells reduced cell viability via the caspase dependent apoptosis pathway. miR-375 suppresses the Akt phosphorylation pathway through direct targeting of PDK1, a kinase that phosphorylates Akt. In addition to PDK1, miR-375 also targets 14-3-3zeta, a potent anti-apoptotic gene, indicating that miR-375 is a candidate tumor suppressor miRNA in gastric carcinoma (Tsukamoto et al., 2010).

Chen et al. previously found that miRNA-200c could not only induce the expression of E-cadherin, but also increase the sensitivity of gastric cancer cells to cisplatin. miRNA-200c can indirectly regulate apoptosis through E-cadherin in gastric cancer cells, which may be a possible mechanism of miRNA-200c in inhibiting proliferation (Chen et al., 2010). SOX2 plays important roles in growth inhibition through cell cycle arrest and apoptosis, and that SOX2 expression is downregulated in gastric cancers. Otsubo et al. revealed that miR-126 inhibited SOX2 expression by targeting two binding sites in the 3'-untranslated region (3'-UTR) of SOX2 mRNA. In addition, the authors found that expression of the placenta-specific 1 (PLAC1) gene was significantly downregulated by SOX2. These results indicate that miR-126 is a novel miRNA that targets SOX2, and PLAC1 may be a novel downstream target gene of SOX2 in gastric cancer cells (Otsubo et al., 2011). Hou et al. showed decreased expression of miR-146a in gastric cancer and low expression of miR-146a was correlated with increased tumor size and poor differentiation. Overall survival time of patients with high miR-146a expression was significantly longer than that of patients with low expression of miR-146a. Overexpression of miR-146a inhibited cell proliferation and induced apoptosis in gastric cancer cells. miR-146a has potential as a novel suppressor gene in gastric cancer (Hou et al., 2011).

4.3 miRNAs and proliferation

miR-27a is upregulated in human gastric adenocarcinoma and was identified as an oncogenic miRNA in a gastric cancer cell line, in which it targets the tumor suppressor prohibitin, an evolutionary conserved and ubiquitous protein interacting with pRb and its family members. Downregulation of prohibitin by miR-27a may explain why suppression of miR-27a can inhibit gastric cancer cell growth (Liu et al., 2009). In p53-mutant human gastric cancer cells, overexpression of miR-34 increases caspase-3 activation and impairs the tumorsphere formation and growth, accumulating the cells in G1 phase. Restoration of miR-34 expression resulted in a downregulation of Bcl-2, Notch1 and HMGA2, indicating that miR-34 may be involved in gastric cancer stem cell self-renewal/differentiation pathways (Ji et al., 2008). The expression of oncogene macrophage migration inhibitory factor (MIF) has been shown to be targeted by miR-451, whose expression is downregulated in gastric cancer. Bandres and colleagues show that the restoration of miR-451 in gastric cancer cells led to downregulation of the MIF gene, which is accompanied by reduction in cell proliferation and increased sensitivity to radiotherapy. In addition, a significant inverse correlation was found between miR-451 and MIF expression in gastric cancer biopsies (Bandres et al., 2009). Human miR-141, a member of the miR-200 family, has been reported to be associated with various tumorigenesis processes. Du et al. found that miR-141 was expressed at significantly low levels in primary gastric cancer, and overexpression of miR-141 could inhibit the proliferation of gastric cancer cell lines. These results suggest that miR-141 may be involved in the development of gastric cancer through its inhibitory effect on cell proliferation (Du et al., 2009).

miR-9 was downregulated in gastric cancer and targeted NF-κB1 and thereby suppressing NF-κB transcriptional activity. Restoration of miR-9 expression suppressed the proliferation of gastric cancer cells. NF-κB has been shown to be directly targeted by miRNA in gastric cancer. Aberrant activation of NF-κB signaling as a result of miRNA dysregulation may be an important molecular event in gastric tumorigenesis (Wan et al., 2010). Besides PDK1 and 14-3-3zeta, forced expression of miR-375 in gastric cancer cells significantly reduced the protein level of Janus kinase 2 (JAK2), indicating that JAK2 may be a miR-375 target gene. Moreover, ectopic expression of JAK2 can partially reverse the inhibition of cell proliferation caused by miR-375 and a significant inverse correlation between miR-375 expression and JAK2 protein level in gastric cancer (Ding et al., 2010).

Zhang et al. show that miR-650 is involved in lymphatic and distant metastasis in human gastric cancer. Ectopic expression of miR-650 promotes tumorigenesis and proliferation of gastric cancer cells through directly targeting the Inhibitor of Growth 4 (ING4) protein (Zhang et al., 2010). Ectopic expression of miR-29s significantly reduced the expression of Cdc42 and its downstream molecular PAK1 phosphorylation levels, and inhibited proliferation and migration in gastric cancer cells (Lang et al., 2010). miR-221 and miR-222 were discovered to induce cell growth and cell cycle progression via direct targeting of p27Kip1 in various human cancers. Upregulation of miR-221 and miR-222 induced the malignant phenotype of gastric cancer cells, in addition, knockdown of miR-221 and miR-222 inhibited cell growth and invasion and increased the radiosensitivity of gastric cancer cells. These results demonstrate that miR-221 and miR-222 regulate radiosensitivity, and cell growth and invasion, possibly via direct modulation of PTEN expression (Chun-Zhi et al., 2010). Previous study showed that miR-23a was significantly upregulated in gastric adenocarcinoma tissues and miR-23a has been found to function as a growth-promoting factor in gastric cancer cells. Zhu et al. identified IL6R as a direct target gene for miR-23a and demonstrated that miR-23a can target IL6R and promote the growth activity of gastric adenocarcinoma cells *in vitro* (Zhu et al., 2010a). Song et al. found that miR-199a is highly expressed in gastric cancer tissues. miR-199a positively regulated gastric cancer cell proliferation through directly targeting the mitogen-activated protein kinase kinase kinase 11. The level of miR-199a expression in gastric cancer significantly correlated with clinical progression (Song et al., 2010). Expression of miR-203 was not significant in gastric cancer tissues compared to non-tumor counterparts, but miR-203 was correlated with tumor size, macroscopic type, and pT stage and miR-203 can inhibit the cell proliferation in gastric cancer cells. miR-203 may be associated with the proliferation of gastric cancers (Chiang et al., 2011).

Ectopic miR-16 or miR-21 expression has exhibited an effect on cell proliferation, and is mediated via EP2/4 receptors (Shin et al., 2011). MicroRNA microarray analyses revealed that miR-192 and -215 were significantly more upregulated in gastric carcinomas than in non-neoplastic stomach. In addition, expression levels of ALCAM were significantly lower in gastric cancers. Western blotting and luciferase assays were performed to confirm direct activated leukocyte cell adhesion molecule (ALCAM) targeting by miR-192 and -215. Both miR-192 and -215 are overexpressed *in vivo* and exert cell growth -promoting effects *in vitro* (Jin et al., 2010). Previous studies have revealed that miR-148a and miR-152 are significantly downregulated in gastrointestinal cancers. The purpose of this study was to elucidate the molecular mechanisms by which miR-148b acts as a tumor suppressor in gastric cancer. Song et al. showed significant downregulation of miR-148b in gastric cancer tissues and four gastric cancer cell lines. The authors also found that miR-148b could inhibit cell proliferation *in vitro* and suppress tumorigenicity *in vivo*. CCKBR was identified as a target of miR-148b in cells, and inverse correlation was observed between the expression of CCKBR protein and miR-148b in gastric cancer tissues. These findings indicated that miR-148b targets CCKBR and is significant in suppressing gastric cancer cell growth (Song et al., 2011). Ectopic expression of CDX2, a caudal-related homeobox protein, is known to be associated with the development of gastric tumorigenesis. The inverse correlation between the miR-9 and CDX2 protein levels was demonstrated in gastric cancer cell lines. Inhibition of miR-9 significantly inhibited cell growth by promoting G1 cell cycle arrest in gastric cancer cells. Therefore, miR-9 might directly repress CDX2 expression resulting in the promotion of cell proliferation in gastric cancers (Rotkrua et al., 2011).

4.4 miRNA and metastasis

Migration and invasion are essential aspects of cancer cells metastasis. The high mobility group A2 (HMGA2) overexpression is a hallmark of gastric cancer. Motoyama and colleagues demonstrated that HMGA2 is negatively regulated by the let-7 miRNA family in gastric cancer cell lines. There is an inverse relationship between the expression of let-7 and HMGA2 in gastric cancer cell lines and primary gastric cancer tissues. High expression of HMGA2 in gastric cancer correlates with tumor invasion and is an independent prognostic factor (Motoyama et al., 2008). Zhang et al. also demonstrated that knockdown of miR-21 significantly decreased cell invasion and migration of gastric cancer cells (Zhang et al., 2008). miR-27a was found correlated between the tumor size and lymph node metastasis and may be associated with the prognosis in undifferentiated gastric cancer patients (Katada et al., 2009b). Downregulation of miR-218 is also implicated in metastatic gastric cancer. Robo1, one of several Slit receptors, is negatively regulated by miR-218. It has been shown that reduced expression of miR-218 in gastric cancer results in upregulation of its target Robo1, one of several Slit receptors, enhancing Slit/Robo1 signaling. Tie et al. demonstrated that restoration of miR-218 expression inhibits invasion and metastasis of gastric cancer cells *in vitro* and *in vivo* (Tie et al., 2010). Lang et al. found that ectopic expression of miRNA-29s inhibited migration in gastric cancer cells. Members of the miR-29 family can obviously inhibit migration and invasion of gastric cancer cells by targeting Cdc42 (Lang et al., 2010). The expression of let-7a was significantly lower in gastric carcinomas with lymph node metastasis than in those without metastasis (Zhu et al., 2010c). let-7 miRNAs generally play a tumor-suppressive role as shown in targeting oncogenes such as RAS and HMGA2 (Ohshima et al., 2010). The expression of miR-101 is downregulated in gastric cancer tissues and cells, and ectopic expression of miR-101 significantly inhibits cellular migration and invasion of gastric cancer cells. miR-101 may inversely regulate EZH2, Cox-2, Mcl-1 and Fos. These might indicate that miR-101 may function as a tumor suppressor in gastric cancer, as it has an inhibitory role in cellular proliferation and metastasis (Wang et al., 2010). Li et al. demonstrate that miR-107 is frequently upregulated in gastric cancers and its overexpression is significantly associated with gastric cancer metastasis. Furthermore, subsequent investigation characterized DRCE1 as a direct target of miR-107. These results suggested that miR-107 is an oncogene miRNA promoting gastric cancer metastasis through downregulation of DRCE1 (Li et al., 2010). miR-199a is highly expressed in metastatic gastric cancer tissues. MiR-199a positively regulated gastric cancer migration and invasion. Further studies showed that mitogen-activated protein kinase kinase kinase 11 was significantly downregulated by miR-199a and the level of miR-199a expression in gastric cancer significantly correlated with clinical progression (Song et al., 2010). Expression levels of both miR-192 and -215 were significantly higher in gastric cancer. miR-215 inhibits activated leukocyte cell adhesion molecule (ALCAM) expression at the posttranscriptional level. In addition, expression levels of ALCAM were significantly lower in gastric cancer. Overexpression of miR-192or -215 and ALCAM knockdown significantly increased the migration of gastric cancer cells (Jin et al., 2010). Takei et al. defined miR-516a-3p involved in cancer metastasis as a candidate anti-metastatic miRNA. Sulfatase1 is known to remove 6-O-sulfates from heparan sulfate proteoglycans on the cell surface, causing release of membrane-bound Wnt ligands from cells. The authors documented that Sulfatase1 as a direct target of miR-516a-3p (Takei et al., 2011). Feng et al. identified miR-107 as a regulator of CDK6 expression. Expression of miR-107 in gastric cancer cell lines was found inversely correlated with CDK6 expression. Ectopic expression of miR-107 reduced expression of CDK6 and blocked invasion in the gastric cancer cells (Feng et al., 2011)..

4.5 Multidrug resistance (MDR)

Xia and colleagues demonstrated significant correlations between miRNA expression patterns and multidrug resistance, suggesting that miRNAs may play a role in chemoresistance. Up- or downregulation of several miRNAs can lead to modified sensitivity to anticancer treatments. miR-15b and miR-16 were downregulated in a multidrug resistant gastric cancer cell line. Enforced overexpression of miR-15b or miR-16 caused a significant increase of apoptosis after vincristine (VCR) therapy. The chemotherapy-sensitizing effect of miR-15b and miR-16 were mediated by modulation of apoptosis via targeting BCL2 (Xia et al., 2008). Zhu et al. investigated the role of miR-181b in the development of multidrug resistance in human the gastric cancer cell line. miR-181b was downregulated in the multidrug resistant human gastric cancer cell line. Enforced miR-181b expression reduced

BCL2 protein level and sensitized gastric cancer cells to VCR-induced and cisplatin (CDDP)-induced apoptosis. These findings suggest that miR-181b could play a role in the development of MDR in gastric cancer cells by targeting BCL2 (Zhu et al., 2010b).

5. miRNAs as biomarkers in gastric cancer

Most patients have advanced gastric cancer at diagnosis, resulting in a high frequency cause of death. The survival and prognosis of gastric cancer patients depends on stage of gastric cancer (Fujita, 2009). Unfortunately, highly sensitive and specific biomarkers for diagnosis and detection of gastric cancer in early stages are lacking. Therefore, it is essential to identify molecular biomarkers for early diagnosis and effective monitoring of the progression of gastric cancer, as well as for prospective development of therapeutic pharmacological reagents. miRNA is a putative candidate to improve diagnostic sensitivity of tumor markers for early stage tumors is beneficial for improving the survival rate of gastric cancer patients. Accumulating studies have shown the diagnostic and prognostic values of miRNAs in gastric cancer. In our study, clinicopathological analysis indicated that low expression of miR-34b and miR-129 is associated with a poor clinical prognosis feature (Tsai et al., 2011). Ueda et al. reported that low expression of let-7g and miR-433 and high expression of miR-214 were associated with poor outcome (Ueda et al., 2010). Katada et al. indicated that miR-20b or 150 overexpression in undifferentiated gastric cancer, and high level expression is associated with poor survival in patients (Katada et al., 2009a). A recent study analyzed the miRNA expression profile in 65 gastric cancer patients, 29 patients with recurrence and 36 patients without recurrence. Their results indicated that the combination of miR-375 and miR-142 could predict recurrence risk for GC patients (Zhang et al., 2011).

Recent studies have shown that quantities of circulating miRNAs exist in body fluids, including blood, and these miRNAs are derived generally from cell debris or transporting exosomes (Chen et al., 2008; Gilad et al., 2008). Chim et al. and Gilad et al. both demonstrate that the high abundance of placental miRNA in serum could reflect pregnancy conditions in maternal blood (Chim et al., 2008; Gilad et al., 2008). Mitchell et al. demonstrated that circulating miRNAs in serum are released from solid tumor, which could serve as a means for cancer detection (Mitchell et al., 2008). This cumulative evidence indicated that circulating miRNAs in blood might show promise as useful non-invasive biomarkers for diagnosis of gastric cancers. Liu et al. (Liu et al., 2011) identified a profile of five serum miRNAs (miR-1, miR-20a, miR-27a, miR-34 and miR-423-5p) as a biomarker for GC detection and their expression level was well correlated to tumor stage. In large-scale analysis, the plasma concentrations of miRNAs (miR-17-5p, miR-21, miR-106a, miR-106b) were significantly higher in GC patients, and significantly decreased in pre-operative serum compared with post-operative serum (Tsukamoto et al., 2010). Concluding above result, circulating miRNAs have a good potential to be novel biomarkers for the detection of gastric cancer and monitoring recurrence.

6. Conclusion

miRNAs represent a recently identified class of small, noncoding RNA molecules which control gene expression at post-transcriptional levels. In the past decade, there is a lot of evidence on the critical role of deregulated miRNAs in the pathogenesis and progression of human tumors, dysregulation of miRNA occurs in gastric cancer as well as other malignant

diseases. The mechanisms by which miRNA takes part in tumor promotion and progression are various and complex. Most of researchers focus on common signaling mechanisms that control cell proliferation, apoptosis and metastasis. The association of miRNA deregulation explains great potential of utilizing miRNAs as targets for therapeutic intervention.
Gene profiling studies have demonstrated a number of significantly deregulated miRNAs and identified signatures of both diagnostic and prognostic value in gastric cancer. It has been shown that alterations in miRNA expression profiles can be used to estimate and monitor the success of potential therapeutic modalities. miRNAs play a role in the complicated gene regulation networks, and regulate the expression of multiple genes. Using miRNAs in combination with existing therapeutic strategies may synergistically affect the results of cancer treatment and improve survival of patients. Therefore, additional studies have to be carried out in future to verify the safety and efficiency of such treatment combinations in clinical therapies.

7. References

Bandres, E., N. Bitarte, F. Arias, J. Agorreta, P. Fortes, X. Agirre, R. Zarate, J. A. Diaz-Gonzalez, N. Ramirez, J. J. Sola, P. Jimenez, J. Rodriguez & J. Garcia-Foncillas (2009) microRNA-451 regulates macrophage migration inhibitory factor production and proliferation of gastrointestinal cancer cells. *Clinical cancer research : an official journal of the American Association for Cancer Research,* Vol.15, pp. 2281-90, ISSN 1078-0432

Bartel, D. P. (2004) MicroRNAs: genomics, biogenesis, mechanism, and function. *Cell,* Vol.116, 281-97.

Chen, Q., X. Chen, M. Zhang, Q. Fan, S. Luo & X. Cao (2011) miR-137 Is Frequently Down-Regulated in Gastric Cancer and Is a Negative Regulator of Cdc42. *Dig Dis Sci.* Vol.116, pp. 281-97, ISSN 0092-8674

Chen, X., Y. Ba, L. Ma, X. Cai, Y. Yin, K. Wang, J. Guo, Y. Zhang, J. Chen, X. Guo, Q. Li, X. Li, W. Wang, Y. Zhang, J. Wang, X. Jiang, Y. Xiang, C. Xu, P. Zheng, J. Zhang, R. Li, H. Zhang, X. Shang, T. Gong, G. Ning, J. Wang, K. Zen, J. Zhang & C. Y. Zhang (2008) Characterization of microRNAs in serum: a novel class of biomarkers for diagnosis of cancer and other diseases. *Cell Res,* Vol.18, pp. 997-1006, ISSN 1748-7838

Chen, Y., J. Zuo, Y. Liu, H. Gao & W. Liu (2010) Inhibitory effects of miRNA-200c on chemotherapy-resistance and cell proliferation of gastric cancer SGC7901/DDP cells. *Chinese journal of cancer,* Vol.29, pp. 1006-11, ISSN 1944-446X

Cheung, H. H., A. J. Davis, T. L. Lee, A. L. Pang, S. Nagrani, O. M. Rennert & W. Y. Chan (2011) Methylation of an intronic region regulates miR-199a in testicular tumor malignancy. *Oncogene.*, Vol.15, pp. 63-70, ISSN 1476-5594

Chiang, Y., Y. Song, Z. Wang, Y. Chen, Z. Yue, H. Xu, C. Xing & Z. Liu (2011) Aberrant expression of miR-203 and its clinical significance in gastric and colorectal cancers. *Journal of gastrointestinal surgery : official journal of the Society for Surgery of the Alimentary Tract,* Vol.15, pp. 63-70, ISSN

Chim, S. S., T. K. Shing, E. C. Hung, T. Y. Leung, T. K. Lau, R. W. Chiu & Y. M. Lo (2008) Detection and characterization of placental microRNAs in maternal plasma. *Clin Chem,* Vol.54, pp. 482-90, ISSN 0009-9147

Cho, W. J., J. M. Shin, J. S. Kim, M. R. Lee, K. S. Hong, J. H. Lee, K. H. Koo, J. W. Park & K. S. Kim (2009) miR-372 regulates cell cycle and apoptosis of ags human gastric cancer cell line through direct regulation of LATS2. *Mol Cells,* Vol.28, pp. 521-7, ISSN 0219-1032

Chun-Zhi, Z., H. Lei, Z. An-Ling, F. Yan-Chao, Y. Xiao, W. Guang-Xiu, J. Zhi-Fan, P. Pei-Yu, Z. Qing-Yu & K. Chun-Sheng (2010) MicroRNA-221 and microRNA-222 regulate gastric carcinoma cell proliferation and radioresistance by targeting PTEN. *BMC Cancer,* Vol.10, pp. 367, ISSN

Ding, L., Y. Xu, W. Zhang, Y. Deng, M. Si, Y. Du, H. Yao, X. Liu, Y. Ke, J. Si & T. Zhou (2010) MiR-375 frequently downregulated in gastric cancer inhibits cell proliferation by targeting JAK2. *Cell Res,* Vol.20, pp. 784-93, ISSN 1748-7838

Du, Y., Y. Xu, L. Ding, H. Yao, H. Yu, T. Zhou & J. Si (2009) Down-regulation of miR-141 in gastric cancer and its involvement in cell growth. *J Gastroenterol,* Vol.44, pp. 556-61, ISSN 0944-1174

Feng, L., Y. Xie, H. Zhang & Y. Wu (2011) miR-107 targets cyclin-dependent kinase 6 expression, induces cell cycle G1 arrest and inhibits invasion in gastric cancer cells. *Med Oncol.* ISSN 1559-131X

Feng, R., X. Chen, Y. Yu, L. Su, B. Yu, J. Li, Q. Cai, M. Yan, B. Liu & Z. Zhu (2010) miR-126 functions as a tumour suppressor in human gastric cancer. *Cancer Lett,* Vol.298, pp. 50-63, ISSN 1872-7980

Fujita, T. (2009) Gastric cancer. *Lancet,* Vol.374, pp. 1593-4; author reply pp. 1594-5, ISSN 1474-547X

Gao, C., Z. Zhang, W. Liu, S. Xiao, W. Gu & H. Lu (2010) Reduced microRNA-218 expression is associated with high nuclear factor kappa B activation in gastric cancer. *Cancer,* Vol.116, pp. 41-9, ISSN 0008-543X

Gilad, S., E. Meiri, Y. Yogev, S. Benjamin, D. Lebanony, N. Yerushalmi, H. Benjamin, M. Kushnir, H. Cholakh, N. Melamed, Z. Bentwich, M. Hod, Y. Goren & A. Chajut (2008) Serum microRNAs are promising novel biomarkers. *PLoS One,* Vol.3, pp. e3148, ISSN 1932-6203

Guo, J., Y. Miao, B. Xiao, R. Huan, Z. Jiang, D. Meng & Y. Wang (2009) Differential expression of microRNA species in human gastric cancer versus non-tumorous tissues. *J Gastroenterol Hepatol,* Vol.24, pp. 652-7, ISSN 1440-1746

Guo, X., L. Guo, J. Ji, J. Zhang, J. Zhang, X. Chen, Q. Cai, J. Li, Q. Gu, B. Liu, Z. Zhu & Y. Yu (2010) miRNA-331-3p directly targets E2F1 and induces growth arrest in human gastric cancer. *Biochem Biophys Res Commun,* Vol.398, pp. 1-6, ISSN 1090-2104

Guo, X., C. Jing, L. Li, L. Zhang, Y. Shi, J. Wang, J. Liu & C. Li (2011) Down-regulation of VEZT gene expression in human gastric cancer involves promoter methylation and miR-43c. *Biochem Biophys Res Commun,* Vol.404, pp. 622-7, ISSN 1090-2104

Hashimoto, Y., Y. Akiyama, T. Otsubo, S. Shimada & Y. Yuasa (2010) Involvement of epigenetically silenced microRNA-181c in gastric carcinogenesis. *Carcinogenesis,* Vol.31, pp. 777-84, ISSN 1460-2180

Hou, Z., L. Xie, L. Yu, X. Qian & B. Liu (2011) MicroRNA-146a is down-regulated in gastric cancer and regulates cell proliferation and apoptosis. *Med Oncol.* ISSN 1559-131X

Ji, Q., X. Hao, Y. Meng, M. Zhang, J. Desano, D. Fan & L. Xu (2008) Restoration of tumor suppressor miR-34 inhibits human p53-mutant gastric cancer tumorspheres. *BMC Cancer,* Vol.8, pp.266, ISSN 1471-2407

Jiang, Z., J. Guo, B. Xiao, Y. Miao, R. Huang, D. Li & Y. Zhang (2010) Increased expression of miR-421 in human gastric carcinoma and its clinical association. *J Gastroenterol,* Vol.45, pp. 17-23, ISSN 1435-5922

Jin, Z., F. M. Selaru, Y. Cheng, T. Kan, R. Agarwal, Y. Mori, A. V. Olaru, J. Yang, S. David, J. P. Hamilton, J. M. Abraham, J. Harmon, M. Duncan, E. A. Montgomery & S. J. Meltzer (2010) MicroRNA-192 and -215 are upregulated in human gastric cancer in vivo and suppress ALCAM expression in vitro. *Oncogene.* Vol. pp. , ISSN 1476-5594

Katada, T., H. Ishiguro, Y. Kuwabara, M. Kimura, A. Mitui, Y. Mori, R. Ogawa, K. Harata & Y. Fujii (2009) microRNA expression profile in undifferentiated gastric cancer. *International journal of oncology,* Vol.34, pp. 537-42, ISSN 1019-6439

Kim, J., S. Y. Min, H. E. Lee & W. H. Kim (2011) Aberrant DNA methylation and tumor suppressive activity of the EBF3 gene in gastric carcinoma. *International journal of cancer. Journal international du cancer,* ISSN 1097-0215

Kim, M. S., J. E. Oh, Y. R. Kim, S. W. Park, M. R. Kang, S. S. Kim, C. H. Ahn, N. J. Yoo & S. H. Lee (2010) Somatic mutations and losses of expression of microRNA regulation-related genes AGO2 and TNRC6A in gastric and colorectal cancers. *The Journal of pathology,* Vol.221, pp. 139-46, ISSN 1096-9896

Kim, V. N. (2005) Small RNAs: classification, biogenesis, and function. *Mol Cells,* Vol.19, pp. 1-15, ISSN 1016-8478

Kim, Y. K., J. Yu, T. S. Han, S. Y. Park, B. Namkoong, D. H. Kim, K. Hur, M. W. Yoo, H. J. Lee, H. K. Yang & V. N. Kim (2009) Functional links between clustered microRNAs: suppression of cell-cycle inhibitors by microRNA clusters in gastric cancer. *Nucleic Acids Res,* Vol.37, pp. 1672-81, ISSN 1362-4962

Lai, K. W., K. X. Koh, M. Loh, K. Tada, M. M. Subramaniam, X. Y. Lim, A. Vaithilingam, M. Salto-Tellez, B. Iacopetta, Y. Ito & R. Soong (2010) MicroRNA-130b regulates the tumour suppressor RUNX3 in gastric cancer. *Eur J Cancer,* Vol.46, pp. 1456-63, ISSN 1879-0852

Lang, N., M. Liu, Q. L. Tang, X. Chen, Z. Liu & F. Bi (2010) Effects of microRNA-29 family members on proliferation and invasion of gastric cancer cell lines. *Chin J Cancer,* Vol.29, pp. 603-10, ISSN 1944-446X

Li, X., Y. Zhang, Y. Shi, G. Dong, J. Liang, Y. Han, X. Wang, Q. Zhao, J. Ding, K. Wu & D. Fan (2010) MicroRNA-107, an Oncogene MicroRNA that Regulates Tumor Invasion and Metastasis By Targeting DICER1 in Gastric Cancer: MiR-107 promotes gastric cancer invasion and metastasis. *J Cell Mol Med.* Vol. pp. , ISSN 1582-4934

Liu, R., C. Zhang, Z. Hu, G. Li, C. Wang, C. Yang, D. Huang, X. Chen, H. Zhang, R. Zhuang, T. Deng, H. Liu, J. Yin, S. Wang, K. Zen, Y. Ba & C. Y. Zhang (2011) A five-microRNA signature identified from genome-wide serum microRNA expression profiling serves as a fingerprint for gastric cancer diagnosis. *Eur J Cancer,* Vol.47, pp. 784-91, ISSN 1879-0852

Liu, T., H. Tang, Y. Lang, M. Liu & X. Li (2009) MicroRNA-27a functions as an oncogene in gastric adenocarcinoma by targeting prohibitin. *Cancer Lett,* Vol.273, pp. 233-42, ISSN 1872-7980

Luo, H., H. Zhang, Z. Zhang, X. Zhang, B. Ning, J. Guo, N. Nie, B. Liu & X. Wu (2009) Down-regulated miR-9 and miR-433 in human gastric carcinoma. *J Exp Clin Cancer Res,* Vol.28, pp. 82, ISSN 1756-9966

Mitchell, P. S., R. K. Parkin, E. M. Kroh, B. R. Fritz, S. K. Wyman, E. L. Pogosova-Agadjanyan, A. Peterson, J. Noteboom, K. C. O'Briant, A. Allen, D. W. Lin, N. Urban, C. W. Drescher, B. S. Knudsen, D. L. Stirewalt, R. Gentleman, R. L. Vessella, P. S. Nelson, D. B. Martin & M. Tewari (2008) Circulating microRNAs as stable blood-based markers for cancer detection. *Proc Natl Acad Sci U S A,* Vol.105, pp. 10513-8, ISSN 1091-6490

Motoyama, K., H. Inoue, K. Mimori, F. Tanaka, K. Kojima, H. Uetake, K. Sugihara & M. Mori (2010) Clinicopathological and prognostic significance of PDCD4 and microRNA-21 in human gastric cancer. *Int J Oncol,* Vol.36, pp. 1089-95, ISSN 1791-2423

Motoyama, K., H. Inoue, Y. Nakamura, H. Uetake, K. Sugihara & M. Mori (2008) Clinical significance of high mobility group A2 in human gastric cancer and its relationship to let-7 microRNA family. *Clin Cancer Res,* Vol.14, pp. 2334-40, ISSN 1078-0432

Nishida, N., K. Mimori, M. Fabbri, T. Yokobori, T. Sudo, F. Tanaka, K. Shibata, H. Ishii, Y. Doki & M. Mori (2011) MicroRNA-125a-5p is an independent prognostic factor in gastric cancer,and inhibits the proliferation of human gastric cancer cells in combination with trastuzumab. *Clin Cancer Res.* ISSN 1078-0432

Noguer-Dance, M., S. Abu-Amero, M. Al-Khtib, A. Lefevre, P. Coullin, G. E. Moore & J. Cavaille (2010) The primate-specific microRNA gene cluster (C19MC) is imprinted in the placenta. *Hum Mol Genet,* Vol.19, pp. 3566-82, ISSN 1460-2083

Ohshima, K., K. Inoue, A. Fujiwara, K. Hatakeyama, K. Kanto, Y. Watanabe, K. Muramatsu, Y. Fukuda, S. Ogura, K. Yamaguchi & T. Mochizuki (2010) Let-7 microRNA family is selectively secreted into the extracellular environment via exosomes in a metastatic gastric cancer cell line. *PLoS One,* Vol.5, pp. e13247, ISSN 1932-6203

Otsubo, T., Y. Akiyama, Y. Hashimoto, S. Shimada, K. Goto & Y. Yuasa (2011) MicroRNA-126 Inhibits SOX2 Expression and Contributes to Gastric Carcinogenesis. *PLoS One,* Vol.6, pp. e16617, ISSN 1932-6203

Pan, J., H. Hu, Z. Zhou, L. Sun, L. Peng, L. Yu, J. Liu, Z. Yang & Y. Ran (2010) Tumor-suppressive mir-663 gene induces mitotic catastrophe growth arrest in human gastric cancer cells. *Oncology reports,* Vol.24, pp. 105-12, ISSN 1791-2431

Parkin, D. M., P. Pisani & J. Ferlay (1999) Global cancer statistics. *CA: a cancer journal for clinicians,* Vol.49, pp. 33-64, ISSN 0007-9235

Petrocca, F., R. Visone, M. R. Onelli, M. H. Shah, M. S. Nicoloso, I. de Martino, D. Iliopoulos, E. Pilozzi, C. G. Liu, M. Negrini, L. Cavazzini, S. Volinia, H. Alder, L. P. Ruco, G. Baldassarre, C. M. Croce & A. Vecchione (2008) E2F1-regulated microRNAs impair TGFbeta-dependent cell-cycle arrest and apoptosis in gastric cancer. *Cancer Cell,* Vol.13, pp. 272-86, ISSN 1878-3686

Ribeiro-dos-Santos, A., A. S. Khayat, A. Silva, D. O. Alencar, J. Lobato, L. Luz, D. G. Pinheiro, L. Varuzza, M. Assumpcao, P. Assumpcao, S. Santos, D. L. Zanette, W. A. Silva, Jr., R. Burbano & S. Darnet (2010) Ultra-deep sequencing reveals the microRNA expression pattern of the human stomach. *PLoS One,* Vol.5, pp. e13205, ISSN 1932-6203

Rotkrua, P., Y. Akiyama, Y. Hashimoto, T. Otsubo & Y. Yuasa (2011) MiR-9 down-regulates CDX2 expression in gastric cancer cells. *Int J Cancer.* Vol. pp. , ISSN 1097-0215

Saito, Y., H. Suzuki, H. Tsugawa, I. Nakagawa, J. Matsuzaki, Y. Kanai & T. Hibi (2009) Chromatin remodeling at Alu repeats by epigenetic treatment activates silenced microRNA-512-5p with downregulation of Mcl-1 in human gastric cancer cells. *Oncogene,* Vol.28, pp. 2738-44, ISSN 1476-5594

Shen, R., S. Pan, S. Qi, X. Lin & S. Cheng (2010) Epigenetic repression of microRNA-129-2 leads to overexpression of SOX4 in gastric cancer. *Biochem Biophys Res Commun,* 394, pp. 1047-52, ISSN 1090-2104

Shin, V. Y., H. Jin, E. K. Ng, A. S. Cheng, W. W. Chong, C. Y. Wong, W. K. Leung, J. J. Sung & K. M. Chu (2011) NF-kappaB targets miR-16 and miR-21 in gastric cancer: involvement of prostaglandin E receptors. *Carcinogenesis,* Vol.32, pp. 240-5, ISSN 1460-2180

Shinozaki, A., T. Sakatani, T. Ushiku, R. Hino, M. Isogai, S. Ishikawa, H. Uozaki, K. Takada & M. Fukayama (2010) Downregulation of microRNA-200 in EBV-associated gastric carcinoma. *Cancer Res,* Vol.70, pp. 4719-27, ISSN 1538-7445

Song, G., H. Zeng, J. Li, L. Xiao, Y. He, Y. Tang & Y. Li (2010) miR-199a regulates the tumor suppressor mitogen-activated protein kinase kinase kinase 11 in gastric cancer. *Biol Pharm Bull,* Vol.33, pp. 1822-7, ISSN 1347-5215

Song, Y. X., Z. Y. Yue, Z. N. Wang, Y. Y. Xu, Y. Luo, H. M. Xu, X. Zhang, L. Jiang, C. Z. Xing & Y. Zhang (2011) MicroRNA-148b is frequently down-regulated in gastric cancer and acts as a tumor suppressor by inhibiting cell proliferation. *Mol Cancer,* Vol.10, pp. 1, ISSN 1476-4598

Suzuki, H., E. Yamamoto, M. Nojima, M. Kai, H. O. Yamano, K. Yoshikawa, T. Kimura, T. Kudo, E. Harada, T. Sugai, H. Takamaru, T. Niinuma, R. Maruyama, H. Yamamoto, T. Tokino, K. Imai, M. Toyota & Y. Shinomura (2010) Methylation-associated silencing of microRNA-34b/c in gastric cancer and its involvement in an epigenetic field defect. *Carcinogenesis,* Vol.31, pp. 2066-73, ISSN 1460-2180

Takei, Y., M. Takigahira, K. Mihara, Y. Tarumi & K. Yanagihara (2011) The Metastasis-Associated microRNA miR-516a-3p Is a Novel Therapeutic Target for Inhibiting Peritoneal Dissemination of Human Scirrhous Gastric Cancer. *Cancer Res,* Vol.71, pp. 1442-1453, ISSN 1538-7445

Tchernitsa, O., A. Kasajima, R. Schafer, R. J. Kuban, U. Ungethum, B. Gyorffy, U. Neumann, E. Simon, W. Weichert, M. P. Ebert & C. Rocken (2010) Systematic evaluation of the miRNA-ome and its downstream effects on mRNA expression identifies gastric cancer progression. *The Journal of pathology,* Vol.222, pp. 310-9, ISSN 1096-9896

Tie, J., Y. Pan, L. Zhao, K. Wu, J. Liu, S. Sun, X. Guo, B. Wang, Y. Gang, Y. Zhang, Q. Li, T. Qiao, Q. Zhao, Y. Nie & D. Fan (2010) MiR-218 inhibits invasion and metastasis of gastric cancer by targeting the Robo1 receptor. *PLoS Genet,* Vol. 6, pp. e1000879, ISSN 1553-7404

Tsai, K. W., L. Y. Hu, C. W. Wu, S. C. Li, C. H. Lai, H. W. Kao, W. L. Fang & W. C. Lin (2010) Epigenetic regulation of miR-196b expression in gastric cancer. *Genes Chromosomes Cancer,* Vol.49, pp. 969-80, ISSN 1098-2264

Tsai, K. W., H. W. Kao, H. C. Chen, S. J. Chen & W. C. Lin (2009) Epigenetic control of the expression of a primate-specific microRNA cluster in human cancer cells. *Epigenetics,* 4, pp. 587-92, ISSN 1559-2308

Tsai, K. W., C. W. Wu, L. Y. Hu, S. C. Li, Y. L. Liao, C. H. Lai, H. W. Kao, W. L. Fang, K. H. Huang, W. C. Chan & W. C. Lin (2011) Epigenetic regulation of miR-34b and miR-129 expression in gastric cancer. *Int J Cancer.* ISSN 1097-0215

Tsukamoto, Y., C. Nakada, T. Noguchi, M. Tanigawa, L. T. Nguyen, T. Uchida, N. Hijiya, K. Matsuura, T. Fujioka, M. Seto & M. Moriyama (2010) MicroRNA-375 is downregulated in gastric carcinomas and regulates cell survival by targeting PDK1 and 14-3-3zeta. *Cancer Res,* Vol.70, pp. 2339-49, ISSN 1538-7445

Ueda, T., S. Volinia, H. Okumura, M. Shimizu, C. Taccioli, S. Rossi, H. Alder, C. G. Liu, N. Oue, W. Yasui, K. Yoshida, H. Sasaki, S. Nomura, Y. Seto, M. Kaminishi, G. A. Calin & C. M. Croce (2010) Relation between microRNA expression and progression and prognosis of gastric cancer: a microRNA expression analysis. *Lancet Oncol,* Vol.11, pp. 136-46, ISSN 1474-5488

Varambally, S., Q. Cao, R. S. Mani, S. Shankar, X. Wang, B. Ateeq, B. Laxman, X. Cao, X. Jing, K. Ramnarayanan, J. C. Brenner, J. Yu, J. H. Kim, B. Han, P. Tan, C. Kumar-Sinha, R. J. Lonigro, N. Palanisamy, C. A. Maher & A. M. Chinnaiyan (2008) Genomic loss of microRNA-101 leads to overexpression of histone methyltransferase EZH2 in cancer. *Science,* Vol.322, pp. 1695-9, ISSN 1095-9203

Volinia, S., G. A. Calin, C. G. Liu, S. Ambs, A. Cimmino, F. Petrocca, R. Visone, M. Iorio, C. Roldo, M. Ferracin, R. L. Prueitt, N. Yanaihara, G. Lanza, A. Scarpa, A. Vecchione, M. Negrini, C. C. Harris & C. M. Croce (2006) A microRNA expression signature of human solid tumors defines cancer gene targets. *Proceedings of the National Academy of Sciences of the United States of America,* Vol.103, pp. 2257-61, ISSN 0027-8424

Wada, R., Y. Akiyama, Y. Hashimoto, H. Fukamachi & Y. Yuasa (2010) miR-212 is downregulated and suppresses methyl-CpG-binding protein MeCP2 in human gastric cancer. *Int J Cancer,* Vol.127, pp. 1106-14, ISSN 1097-0215

Wan, H. Y., L. M. Guo, T. Liu, M. Liu, X. Li & H. Tang (2010) Regulation of the transcription factor NF-kappaB1 by microRNA-9 in human gastric adenocarcinoma. *Mol Cancer,* Vol.9, pp. 16, ISSN 1476-4598

Wang, H. J., H. J. Ruan, X. J. He, Y. Y. Ma, X. T. Jiang, Y. J. Xia, Z. Y. Ye & H. Q. Tao (2010) MicroRNA-101 is down-regulated in gastric cancer and involved in cell migration and invasion. *Eur J Cancer*. ISSN 1879-0852

Wang, J., Q. Wang, H. Liu, B. Hu, W. Zhou & Y. Cheng (2010) MicroRNA expression and its implication for the diagnosis and therapeutic strategies of gastric cancer. *Cancer letters,* Vol.297, pp.137-43, ISSN 1872-7980

Watanabe, Y. & M. Maekawa (2010) Methylation of DNA in cancer. *Adv Clin Chem,* Vol.52, pp. 145-67, ISSN 0065-2423

Wu, J., J. Qian, C. Li, L. Kwok, F. Cheng, P. Liu, C. Perdomo, D. Kotton, C. Vaziri, C. Anderlind, A. Spira, W. V. Cardoso & J. Lu (2010a) miR-129 regulates cell proliferation by downregulating Cdk6 expression. *Cell Cycle,* Vol.9, pp. 1809-18, ISSN 1551-4005

Wu, Q., H. Jin, Z. Yang, G. Luo, Y. Lu, K. Li, G. Ren, T. Su, Y. Pan, B. Feng, Z. Xue, X. Wang & D. Fan (2010b) MiR-150 promotes gastric cancer proliferation by negatively regulating the pro-apoptotic gene EGR2. *Biochem Biophys Res Commun,* Vol.392, pp. 340-5, ISSN 1090-2104

Wu, W. K., C. W. Lee, C. H. Cho, D. Fan, K. Wu, J. Yu & J. J. Sung (2010) MicroRNA dysregulation in gastric cancer: a new player enters the game. *Oncogene,* Vol.29, pp. 5761-71, ISSN 1476-5594

Xia, L., D. Zhang, R. Du, Y. Pan, L. Zhao, S. Sun, L. Hong, J. Liu & D. Fan (2008) miR-15b and miR-16 modulate multidrug resistance by targeting BCL2 in human gastric cancer cells. *Int J Cancer,* Vol.123, pp. 372-9, ISSN 1097-0215

Xu, L., F. Wang, X. F. Xu, W. H. Mo, Y. J. Xia, R. Wan, X. P. Wang & C. Y. Guo (2010) Down-regulation of miR-212 expression by DNA hypermethylation in human gastric cancer cells. *Med Oncol.* ISSN 1559-131X

Yang, Q., Z. Jie, H. Cao, A. R. Greenlee, C. Yang, F. Zou & Y. Jiang (2011) Low-level expression of let-7a in gastric cancer and its involvement in tumorigenesis by targeting RAB40C. *Carcinogenesis.* ISSN 1460-2180

Zhang, X., Z. Yan, J. Zhang, L. Gong, W. Li, J. Cui, Y. Liu, Z. Gao, J. Li, L. Shen & Y. Lu (2011) Combination of hsa-miR-375 and hsa-miR-142-5p as a predictor for recurrence risk in gastric cancer patients following surgical resection. *Ann Oncol.* ISSN 1569-8041

Zhang, X., W. Zhu, J. Zhang, S. Huo, L. Zhou, Z. Gu & M. Zhang (2010) MicroRNA-650 targets ING4 to promote gastric cancer tumorigenicity. *Biochem Biophys Res Commun,* Vol.395, pp. 275-80, ISSN 1090-2104

Zhang, Z., Z. Li, C. Gao, P. Chen, J. Chen, W. Liu, S. Xiao & H. Lu (2008) miR-21 plays a pivotal role in gastric cancer pathogenesis and progression. *Laboratory investigation; a journal of technical methods and pathology,* Vol.88, pp. 1358-66, ISSN 1530-0307

Zhu, L. H., T. Liu, H. Tang, R. Q. Tian, C. Su, M. Liu & X. Li (2010a) MicroRNA-23a promotes the growth of gastric adenocarcinoma cell line MGC803 and downregulates interleukin-6 receptor. *The FEBS journal,* Vol.277, pp. 3726-34, ISSN 1742-4658

Zhu, W., X. Shan, T. Wang, Y. Shu & P. Liu (2010b) miR-181b modulates multidrug resistance by targeting BCL2 in human cancer cell lines. *Int J Cancer,* Vol.127, pp. 2520-9, ISSN 1097-0215

Zhu, W., D. Zhu, S. Lu, T. Wang, J. Wang, B. Jiang, Y. Shu & P. Liu (2011) miR-497 modulates multidrug resistance of human cancer cell lines by targeting BCL2. *Med Oncol.* Vol. pp, ISSN 1559-131X

Zhu, Y. M., Z. X. Zhong & Z. M. Liu (2010c) Relationship between let-7a and gastric mucosa cancerization and its significance. *World journal of gastroenterology : WJG,* Vol.16, pp. 3325-9, ISSN 1007-9327

6

Integrin and E-Cadherin Expression Alterations as a Possible Reason of Undifferentiated-Type Gastric Carcinoma Diversity

Natalia Yanchenko and Hiroyuki Sugihara
Shiga University of Medical Science, Department of Pathology (Division of Molecular and Diagnostic Pathology) Japan

1. Introduction

Undifferentiated-type gastric carcinoma (UGC), according to the Japanese classification of gastric carcinoma (GC) (Japanese Gastric Cancer Association, 1998), is a type that poorly develops a tubular component. Relationship between Japanese and other classifications was discussed previously (Natsagdorj et al., 2008). The etiology and histogenetic pathways of UGC are still less elucidated than in GC with predominant tubular component (differentiated type GC, DGC), despite the notable advances of molecular technology and remarkable increase of percentage of UGC in the whole GC pool due to decrease of DGC and growth of UGC incidence worldwide in the last two decades (Crew & Neugut 2006; Kaneko & Yoshimura, 2001; Sidoni, 2005).

Histological structure of UGCs is also more complicated than that of DGC and trends to display remarkable diversity due to combination of signet-ring cells, poorly differentiated, tubular and mucinous components; cohesive and dissociative cell arrangement; areas with scirrhous and non-scirrhous stroma. Additionally, cancer cells are intermingled with inflammatory cells (especially in mucosal area of early UGC) and stromal cells (especially in extramucosal areas).

Possible reason of UGCs histological diversity is contribution of at least two processes to UGC local growth and invasion, i.e. individual migration of dissociative cells and cohort-type migration of cell-clusters (Friedl & Wolf, 2003; Nabeshima et al., 1999). It could be supposed, that both individual and cohort migrations depend on cell-extracellular matrix (ECM) interaction and could be studied from the position of cell-ECM receptors integrins. Cohort-type migration demands, additionally, "localized modulation of cell-cell adhesion" (Friedl & Wolf, 2003; Nabeshima et al., 1999), which could be changed allowing cell groups or scanty tubular structures to penetrate environmental tissues. Such cell-cell adhesion could be studied from the position of cadherin-phenotype alteration.

Integrin and E-cadherin phenotype was proved to undergo remarkable changes during tumor progression of GC and other carcinomas, being related to various clinicopathological tumor features linked with tumors invasive properties (Choi et al., 2009; Hazan et al., 2004; Stefansson et al., 2004; Yanchenko et al., 2009; Yang et al., 2008). However, most studies were performed at the tumors array without specification of their individual features and the precise interrelationship between integrin and cadherin phenotype alteration and UGCs histopathological diversity has not been elucidated yet.

Why is the precise analysis of UGCs histology so important? Tumor invasion and growth is a process, however in pathology we commonly deal with its result, i.e. tumor with its individual features. Some of those features, e.g. scirrhous stroma, were already proved to be linked with high invasiveness and poor prognosis (Guszczyn & Sobolewski, 2004).
However, the role and prognostic significance of other tumor components, for example signet-ring cell (SRC) component in tumor progression is still unclear. Whereas early SRC carcinomas are rather dormant tumors with predominantly spreading growth, advanced SRC are linked with LN prominent LN metastazing and poor outcome (Humar et al., 2007; Hyung et al., 2002; Kim et al., 1997; Li et al. 2007).
One more example is the area of layer arrangement of SRC and poorly differentiated cells, called layered structures (LS), in mucosal areas of some UGCs. LSs have been proved to be the only one reliable histological sign of primary genesis of UGC from early SRC carcinomas. UGCs aroused from dedifferentiated tubular GC lack LS (Humar et al., 2007; Natsagdorj et al., 2008; Sugihara et al., 1987). Biological behavior of advanced GC arisen from early SRC (primary UGC) and via tubular GC dedifferentiation was proved to be different (Natsagdorj et al., 2008), and it could be supposed that presence and extension of LS could predict tumor aggressiveness.
To clarify the invasive potential of UGC and interrelationship between tumor histology and cell-cell and cell-ECM interaction alterations we introduce precise quantitated analysis of histological structure of each individual UGC case, supplemented by integrated immunohistochemical analysis of integrin and E-cadherin phenotype alterations.

2. Materials and methods

2.1 Materials

We used 30 randomly selected cases with fresh resection specimens of UGC (13 early and 17 advanced). In early UGC group 10 cases were diagnosed as signet-ring cell carcinomas (SIG) and demonstrated LS in the mucosa; 3 cases were poorly differentiated adenocarcinoma (POR), one of them with remarkable tubular component. In advanced UGC group 1 case was diagnosed as SIG and 16 as POR, most of which were accompanied with some SRCs and/or tubular component. Nine of advanced UGC had remnants of LS in the mucosa.
To study integrin expression, tissue samples were snap-frozen in liquid nitrogen and then stored at –80°C until sectioning. Serial 4-µm-thick sections were cut at –22°C and placed in plastic boxes for storage at –80°C until further processing. To study expression of other antigens, we used 10% formalin-fixed paraffin-embedded tissues and cut them into 2-µm-thick sections.

2.2 Method

2.2.1 Quantitative tumor structure analysis

To analyze tumor histotype, each tumor was cut through into 0.5×2-3 cm blocks (Fig. 1A), the entire HE (hematoxylin and eosin) stained 2 µm-thick slices (one from each block) was scanned using Nikon Super COOLSCAN 5000 ED film scanner at a resolution of 2000 dpi. Scanned slice area was mapped at the microscope control (Fig. 1A, B, C) according to: (1) invasion depth (mucosal, submucosal [sm], muscularis propria [mp] and subserosal /adventitial [ss] areas); (2) tumor histotype (signet-ring cell, poorly differentiated, tubular and mucinous components); (3) cell cohesiveness (cohesive and dissociative component); (4) stromal development (scirrhous and non-scirrhous areas). Lymphatic and venous invasion areas were marked separately. Different tumor areas were assessed using analysis/measuring feature of Adobe Photoshop CS4 Extended Edition (Adobe Systems,

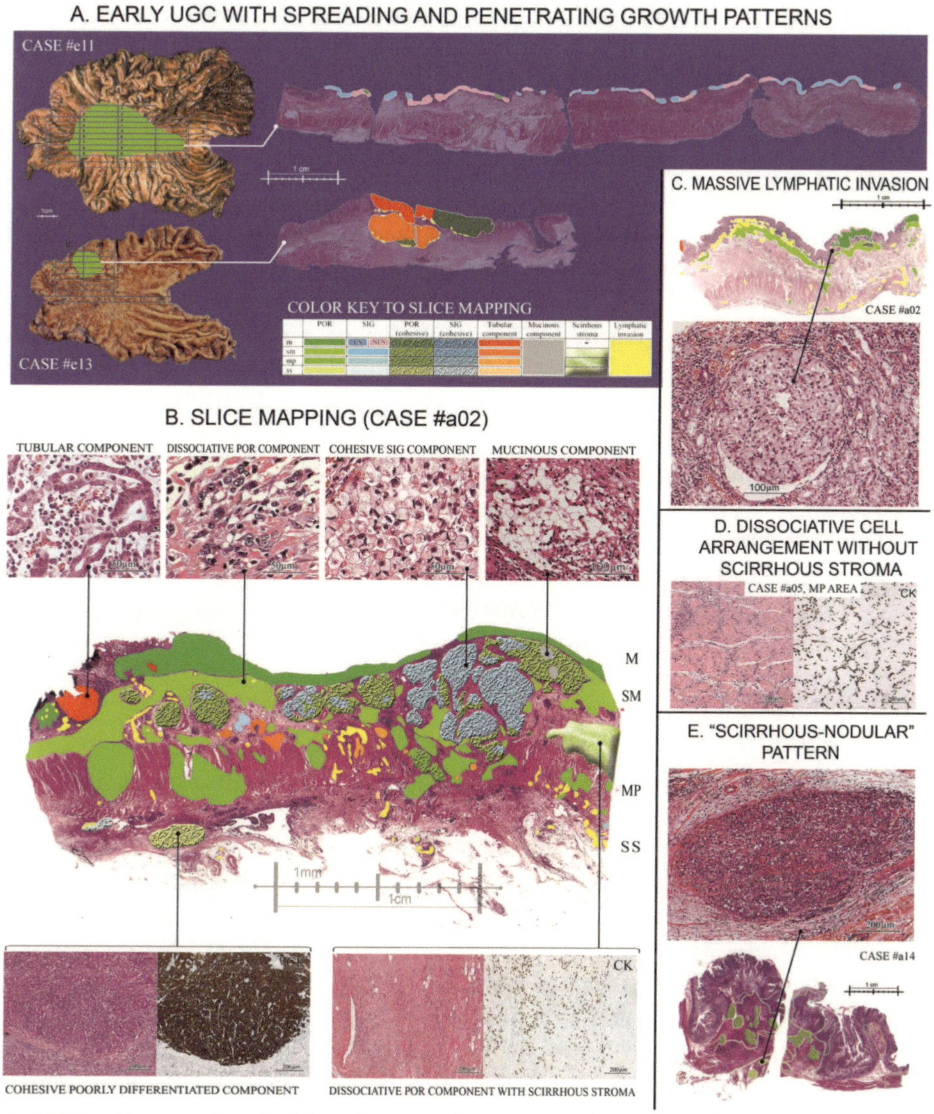

A - Early UGC with spreading (#e11) and penetrating pattern of invasion. Green areas at the photos of stomachs at the left designate tumor invasion areas. Mapped slices at the right demonstrate superficial (mucosal) spreading of relatively dormant case #e11, vs. rapid sm penetration of case #e13. Color key to slices mapping refer to all pictures (A, B, C, E). **B** - example of slices mapping demonstrate the histological structures designated as tubular, poorly differentiated (POR), cohesive signet-ring cell (SIG) and other components. Cytokeratin (CK) staining (as well as in picture D) supplemented HE slices when identity of tumor cells is not obvious. M, SM, MP, SS - invasion depth. **C** - unusually extensive lymphatic penetration (mapped in yellow). Cells in the lymphatic vessels are SRC (lower microphoto), although tumor consists mostly of POR component (mapped in green). **D** - case demonstrating that dissociative cell arrangement is not always means scirrhous stroma development. **E** - case demonstrating rather rare mixture of nodules with cohesive cell arrangement and areas with scirrhous stroma.

Fig. 1. Blocks and slices mapping; examples of UGCs structure.

Mountain View, CA). "Vertical" invasion area (Area V) was calculated as a sum of all slices areas. The percentage of each area was calculated as a percentage of the corresponded area in the whole tumor area at this slice, e.g.

$$Percentage\ of\ mucosal\ area = \frac{mucosal\ area}{\sum mucosal,\ sm,\ mp\ and\ ss\ areas}$$

We also assessed some other clinicopathological UGC features related to tumor invasiveness, such as: (1) "horizontal" spreading area (Area H); the spreading area at each slice was mapped at stomach wall photograph and then assessed using analysis/measuring feature of Adobe Photoshop (Fig. 1A); (2) the number of lymph node (LN) metastasis, (3) invasion front shape (α, β, γ-invasion according to Japanese classification of GC) (Japanese Gastric Cancer Association, 1998).

2.2.2 Immunohistochemical study of integrin expression (frozen section processing)

To study integrin expression we used double APAAP staining with subsequent image analysis, which was introduced earlier (Yanchenko et al., 2009). Briefly, acetone fixed frozen sections were stained for integrin and, after heating, for cytokeratin (CK) to discriminate cancer cell from inflammatory and stromal cells. Microphotos were taken after first and second steps and processed with Adobe Photoshop. For the estimation of the fraction of positive cells, cancer cells positive for integrin were counted within 100 cytokeratin-positive cancer cells, in mucosal, submucosal and deeper areas.

2.2.3 Immunohistochemical study of integrin expression (paraffin-embedded section processing)

Automated staining using Ventana Discovery XT autostainer (Ventana Japan, Yokohama, Japan) was performed for staining of E-cadherins. As HECD-1 antibody, often used for E-cadherin extracellular domain staining, could not be used for automated staining, it was replaced by G-10 (Table 1), the results were comparative with HECD-1 manual staining with autoclave-based antigen retrieval in citric acid.

To discriminate cancerous cells from non-cancerous cells in UGC, where cancerous calls are often intermingled with stromal and inflammatory cells, we used an epithelial marker cytokeratin, as was described previously for integrin study (Yanchenko et al., 2009). After automated cadherin staining slices underwent 15 minute trypsin-based antigen retrieval (trypsin was obtained from Histofine, Tokyo, Japan) with subsequent overnight anti-cytokeratin antibody incubation.

Since E-cadherin was expressed only by epithelial cells, we could omit image processing, necessary for study of mesenchymal and ubiquitous proteins (Yanchenko et al., 2009), and it was possible to estimate the fraction of cadherin-positive cells within 100 cytokeratin-positive cancer cells in mucosal, submucosal and deeper areas without taking intermediate microphotograph.

Antibodies, used for integrins and E-cadherin staining are listed in Table 1.

Controls. For a positive control we used: (1) normal tissue of the same stomach sample (for proteins which normally occur in stomach tissue), (2) specimen from our collection, proved to be positive for this protein (for abnormal proteins). For a negative control, every processed glass contained one serial section of the same sample (frozen tissues) or we used separate slice of the same sample (paraffin-embedded tissues), which was stained with an omission of the primary antibody.

Antigen	Clone	Dilution	Manufacturer
α1 IS	TS2/7	1:50	Santa Cruz Biotechnology, Inc, Santa Cruz, CA
α2 IS	P1E6	1:200	Chemicon International, Inc., Temecula, CA
α3 IS	J143	1:40	GeneTex, Inc., San Antonio, TX
α5 IS	SAM-1	1:10	Chemicon International, Inc., Temecula, CA
α6 IS	4F10	1:20	Chemicon International, Inc., Temecula, CA
αV IS	LM142 13C2	1:1000 1:20	Chemicon International, Inc., Temecula, CA
β1 IS	K-20 DF5	1:50 1:100	Santa Cruz Biotechnology, Inc, Santa Cruz, CA BIOMOL International, L.P., Plymouth Meeting, PA
β4 IS	3E1	1:2500	Chemicon International, Inc., Temecula, CA
αVβ3 integrin	P1F6	1:1000	Chemicon International, Inc., Temecula, CA
αVβ5 integrin	LM609	1:200	Chemicon International, Inc., Temecula, CA
αVβ6 integrin	E7P6	1:200	Chemicon International, Inc., Temecula, CA
E-cadherin ^{ID}	AEC-36	1:1500	BD Biosciences, San Jose, CA
E-cadherin^{ED}	HECD-1	1:500 1:50	Takara Shuzo CO., LND, Otsu, Japan Abcam, Cambridge, MA
E-cadherin^{ED}	G-10	1:100	Santa Cruz Biotechnology, Inc, Santa Cruz, CA
Cytokeratins (1-8,10, 14-16, 19)	AE1/AE3	prediluted	Histofine, Tokyo, Japan

Table 1. Primary mouse antibodies. IS – integrin subunit, ID - intracellular domain; ED - extracellular domain.

2.3 Calculation and statistical analysis

"Normal" or "preserved" expression means that more than 95% of tumor cells expressed this receptor at the same manner as NN epithelium (positive for normal proteins and negative for abnormal). "Weak alteration" means that no more than 1/3 (0-33%) of tumor cells demonstrated altered expression pattern. "Moderate alteration" designates alteration in 34-66% of tumor cells, and in cases with "strong alteration" the percentage of abnormally expressing cells is more than 2/3 (>67%).

Descriptive statistical parameters, including means and standard errors, were calculated with the standard method (using descriptive statistics package, Microsoft Excel). To compare early and advanced UGCs, the statistical significance of differences between means was calculated using Student's unpaired t-test. To prove the mutual correlation between protein expression and UGC features, correlation coefficient R was calculated (using the same statistics package, Microsoft Excel). Mean values throughout this report are expressed as means ± standard error. A probability (P-value) less than 0.05 was considered significant in all methods, including correlation analysis.

3. Results

3.1 Histological structure of UGC: UGC diversity analysis

3.1.1 Invasion depth

According to the invasion depth pattern, UGC could be divided into several groups (Fig. 2): Early UGC: 1) E(m) – intramucosal tumors, submucosal (sm) involvement less than 1% of the total tumor Area V (12 cases); 2) E(sm) – predominantly intramucosal with some submucosal invasion (1 case).

Advanced UGC: 3) A(sm) - mostly submucosal (3 cases), 4) A(sm/mp) - with equal submucosal and muscularis propria (mp) portions (9 cases), 5) A(mp) - with prominent muscularis propria portion (5 cases).

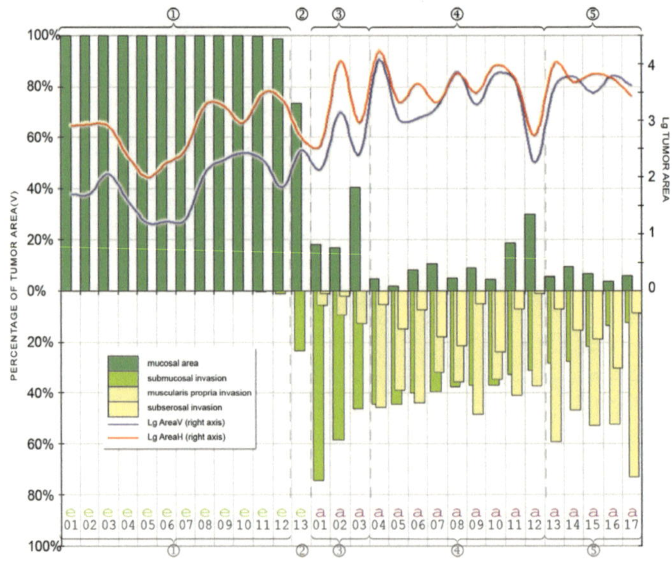

Fig. 2. Invasion depth patterns All UGC cases are arranged along x-axis. Cases are divided into 5 groups according to the proportion of m, sm, and mp component in their structure. Bars depict the percentage of correspondent components in whole tumor. Bars are arranged above and below x-axis only for better representation, i.e. location below the axis does not mean negative values. Line graphs depict tumor size and are plotted at secondary (right) y-axis.

3.1.2 UGCs histotype

3.1.2.1 Signet-ring cell and poorly differentiated components, layer structures

Histotype of tumor was as follows (Fig. 3): (1) SIG – predominantly signet-ring cell (SRC) tumors, were SRC comprised more than 55% of carcinoma area: 11 cases, among them 10 early and 1 advanced cases (77% of early and 6% of advanced UGC, respectively); (2) POR - predominantly poorly differentiated tumors (poorly differentiated cells comprised more than 55% of carcinoma area): 19 cases, 3 early and 16 advanced (23% of early and 94% of advanced UGC, respectively).

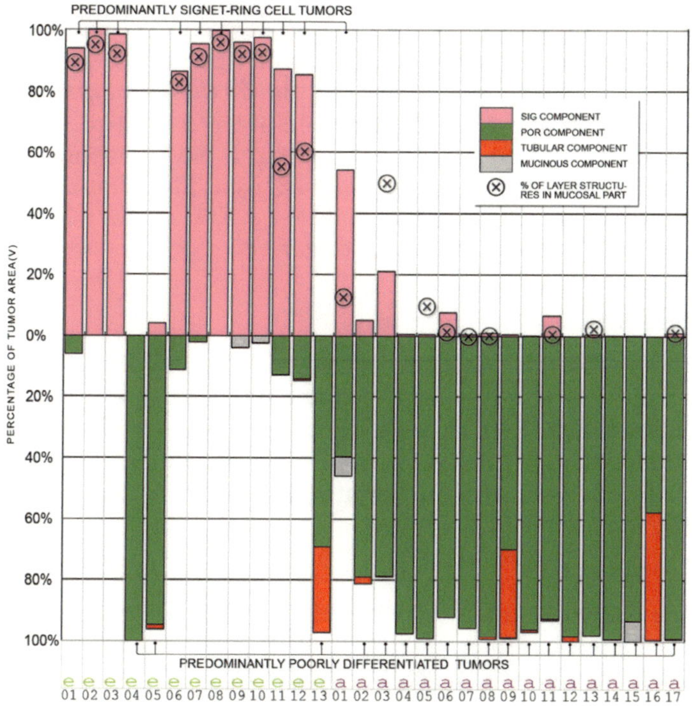

Fig. 3. UGCs histotypes (for explanation see Fig. 2). Enclosed crosses depict percentage of LS in mucosal part.

Ten (77%) early UGCs and 9 (53%) advanced UGCs demonstrated layer structures (LS) in the mucosa (Fig. 3). However, in early carcinomas LS formed the most part (88%±5%) of tumor area, whereas in advanced carcinomas they were replaced by poorly differentiated component and remained only in 5% ± 3% of mucosal part.

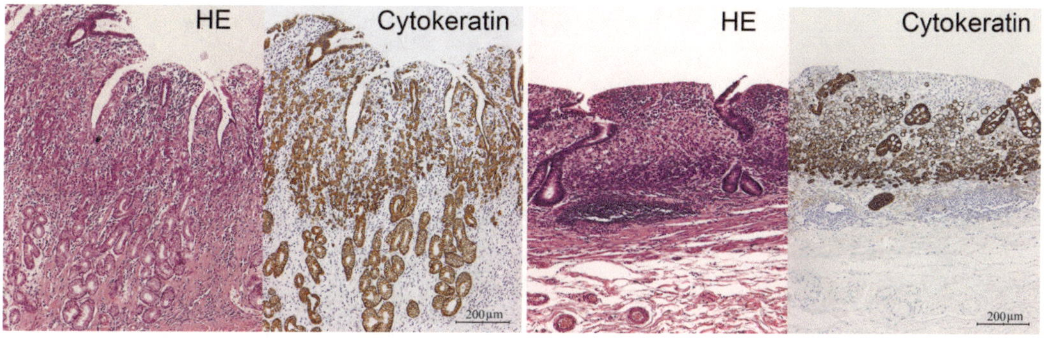

Fig. 4. Variants of layered structures in early carcinomas.

A SRC component percentage correlated in early UGC with bigger tumor horizontal invasion area (R=0.58) and spreading growth (R=0.71) (see Fig. 1A, case #e11) submucosal invasion risk in such tumors was lower (R=0.55). On the other hand, in advanced UGC SRC was linked to smaller tumor size (R=0.60), and spreading in the submucosa (R=0.71), but not to the muscularis propria (R=0.64) (compare Fig. 2 and Fig. 3, cases #a01, #a03).

In advanced UGC LS remnants percentage in mucosa correlated with smaller tumor size (Area V, R=0.54) and mucosal vs extramucosal portion prevalence (R=0.76), those tumors had smaller tendency to invade muscularis propria (R=0.49) (compare cases #a03, #a05, a#06 with LS remnants and cases #a14-16 without LS at Fig. 2 and Fig. 3)

Only in advanced UGC without LS in the mucosa, a SRC component correlated with lymphatic invasion (R=0.99), venous invasion (R=0.82) and LN metastasis number (R=0.71). In one of such tumors lymphatic invasion comprised 13% of the whole tumor area and consisted mostly of SRC, whereas the whole tumor was mostly poorly differentiated (Fig. 1C, Fig. 3 case #02).

3.1.2.2 Tubular component

A tubular component (TC) was found in 5 (38%) early and 10 (59%) advanced UGC and ranged from 0.01% to 41.46% of the whole tumor area (Area V) (Fig. 3). In early UGC TC was higher in bigger tumors (R=0.55), with tendency to submucosal and lymphatic vessel invasion (R=1.00), and less layer structures portion (R=0.55). In advanced UGC presence of TC did not correlate with local invasion features, but was linked to bigger number of LN metastasis (R=0.54).

3.1.2.3 Mucinous component

A mucinous component was found in 2 (15%) early and 7 (41%) advanced UGC ranged from 0.03% to 6.62% of the whole tumor area (Area V) (Fig. 3). In advanced UGC it appeared mostly in tumors with developed SRC component (R=0.57).

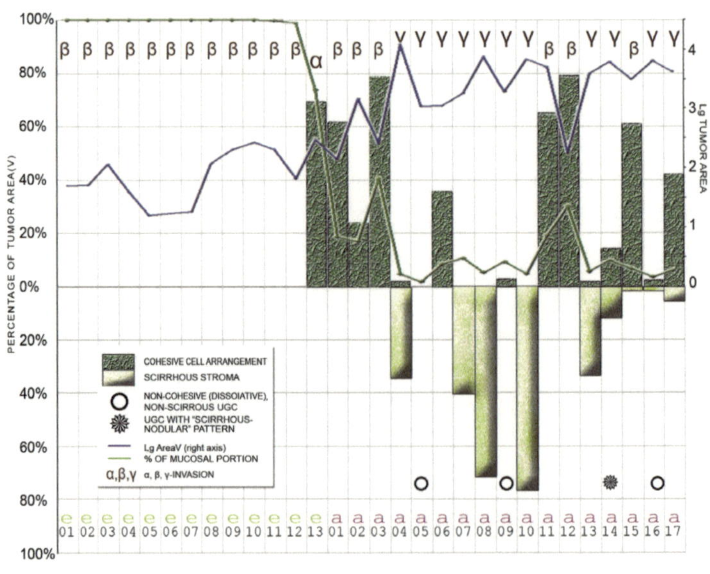

Fig. 5. Cohesive cell arrangement, scirrhous stroma, and invasion front (for explanation see Fig. 2)

3.1.3 Cell cohesiveness

Areas with cohesive cell arrangement were observed in 2 (15%) of early and 15 (88%) of advanced UGC, ranging from 1% to 79% of the whole tumor area. 1 (8%) early and 5 (29%) advanced UGC were predominantly (>60% of Area V) cohesive (Fig. 5). As could be expected, advanced UGC with bigger cohesive component were smaller in size (Area V; R=0.64), had higher mucosal (vs extramucosal) portion (R=0.77) (at Fig. 5 compare sizes and mucosal portion of cases a#03 and a#12 with "pure dissociative" cases #a08 and #a10). The only early case #e13 with cohesive poorly differentiated growth had the highest percentage of tubular component (Fig. 3), and demonstrated the biggest submucosal invasion portion (Fig. 2), despite rather small horizontally spreading area (Fig. 1A).

3.1.4 Stromal component

Scirrhous component was present in 10 (59%) advanced UGC and was prominent (>30% of the whole tumor area) in 5 of them, correlating with bigger tumor size (Area V; R=0.50) (Fig. 5, compare cases #a04, #a07, #a08 and #a10 with other advanced UGC).

Despite scirrhous component inversely correlated with cohesive growth pattern (R=0.55), and it could be seen from the Fig. 5 that in most tumor of cohesive cell arrangement and scirrhous stroma were mutually exclusive components, non-cohesive cell arrangement did not always mean scirrhous stroma development, and 3 of advanced UGC were mostly (>98%) non-cohesive, but did not demonstrate scirrhous stroma (Fig. 1D, Fig. 5, cases a#05, a#09, a#16). Additionally, case #a14 partially demonstrated a pattern that could be named "scirrhous-nodular", where nodules of cohesive tumor cells were surrounded by scirrhous stroma. (Fig. 1E, Fig. 5).

3.1.5 Invasion front

Invasion front was clearly seen in all slices (α-INF) only case #e13, mostly cohesive tumor, other early UGC demonstrated fuzzy infiltration front (β-INF) (Fig. 5). 6 (35%) of advanced UGC, mostly with prevailed cohesive component, had clearly seen invasive front in cohesive areas and fuzzy or indistinguishable front in non-cohesive areas (β-INF). Other advanced UGC exhibited γ-INF and most of their borders were unclear (Fig. 5).

Less distinct borders / invasion fronts correlated not only with dissociative growth pattern (in advanced UGC), but with such signs of local invasion tendency as bigger tumor size (R=0.60); and extramucosal (vs mucosal) growth prevalence (R=0.66) (Fig. 5).

3.2 E-cadherin expression and UGC histopathological features

Average percentage of E-cadherin positive cells (Table 2) had no significant difference in early and advanced UGC.

	E-cadherin (internal domain)	E-cadherin (external domain)
NN expression pattern	strongly positive	moderately positive, except some surface cells
Early UGC	0.84±0.08	0.44±0.08
Advanced UGC	0.56±0.11	0.28±0.07
T-test	NS	NS

Table 2. Percentage of cancer cells positive for internal and external domains of E-cadherin

However, the pool of UGC was rather heterogenous in E-cadherin preservation or loss (Fig. 6). Around a half of UGC (early and advanced) preserved normal expression of internal domain, and around a quarter of them preserved normal pattern of external domain expression (Fig. 6, see first bars at graphs). On the other hand, almost quarter of cases (23%: 1 (8%) early, 6 (35%) advanced) showed strong loss of internal E-cadherin domain expression and almost half of cases (47%: 4 (31%) early, 10 (59%) advanced) demonstrated strong loss of external domain (Fig. 6, see last bars at graphs).

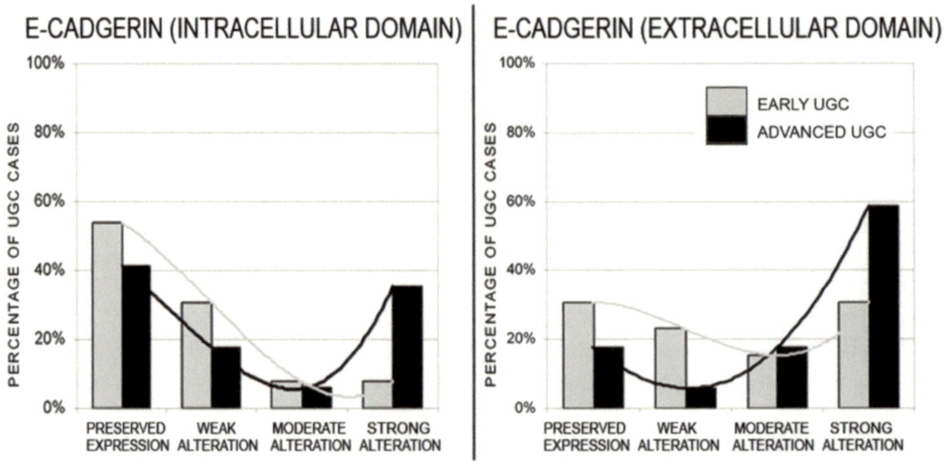

Fig. 6. UGC distribution according E-cadherin expression pattern. All UGC cases are arranged along x-axis. Bars represent percentage of UGC cases in the whole UGC group (e.g. 7 of 13 early UGC demonstrate normal expression of external E-cadherin domain, so the correspondent bar equals 54%). Lines are trends of cadherin and integrin distribution.

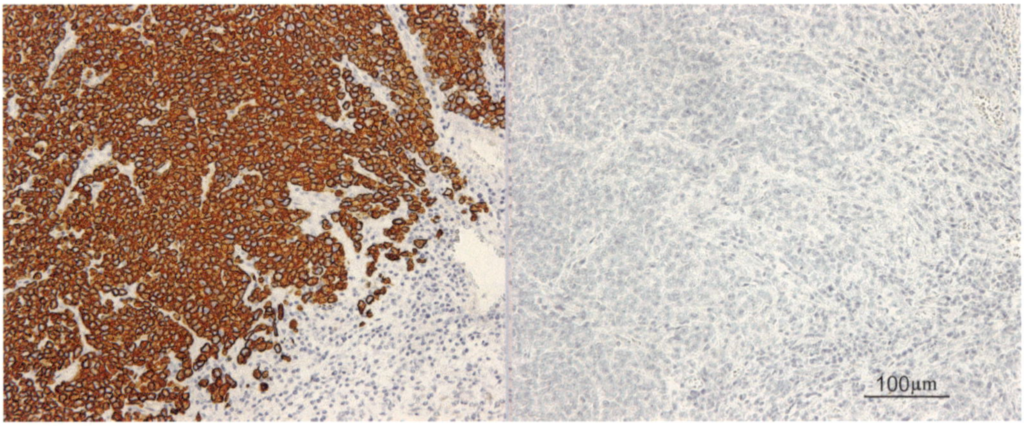

Fig. 7. Loss of E-cadherin expression in cohesive tumor. Left: cytokeratin staining. Right: same area, stained for E-cadherin (internal domain).

Tumors with preserved E-cadherin expression (both domains) trended to have smaller size (AreaV, R=0.37), with less mp portion (R=0.36). External domain of E-cadherin was stronger preserved in those advanced UGC with LS, which demonstrated minor tubular component

(R=0.73) (such as the case a#08, Fig. 3). Intriguingly, the tendency to lose internal domain was stronger in all tumors with more prominent cohesive component (R=0,41), all advanced UGC with total E-cadherin loss were mostly cohesive [Fig. 7 and Fig. 3, cases a#03, a#06, a#11, a#12, a#15].

Loss of external and internal E-cadherin domains correlated with each other (R=0.78), being more severe for external domain (Fig. 6).

3.3 Integrins expression and UGC histopathological features

Non-neoplastic (NN) pattern of integrin expression was described earlier (Yanchenko et al., 2009), briefly see Table 3.

	α6	a2	b1	b4	α3	a1	a5	aV	aVb5	aVb3	aVb6
NN	+++	+++	+++	G+	G+	–	–	+/–	+/–	–	–
Early UGC	0.85± 0.04	0.75± 0.03	0.87± 0.05	0.73± 0.05	0.83± 0.03	0.04± 0.01	0.12± 0.03	0.30± 0.06	0.11± 0.03	0.04± 0.02	0.10± 0.04
Advanced UGC	0.87± 0.02	0.72± 0.05	0.84± 0.03	0.65± 0.05	0.71± 0.06	0.19± 0.03	0.13± 0.02	0.47± 0.08	0.28± 0.06	0.07± 0.03	0.10± 0.03
T-test	NS	NS	NS	NS	NS	<0.01	NS	NS	<0.05	NS	NS

"+++" - expressed strongly in all epithelial cells, "G+" - expressed mostly in glandular portion, "–" - no expression, "+/–" - expressed in areas of plastic changes.

Table 3. Percentage of integrin positive cells

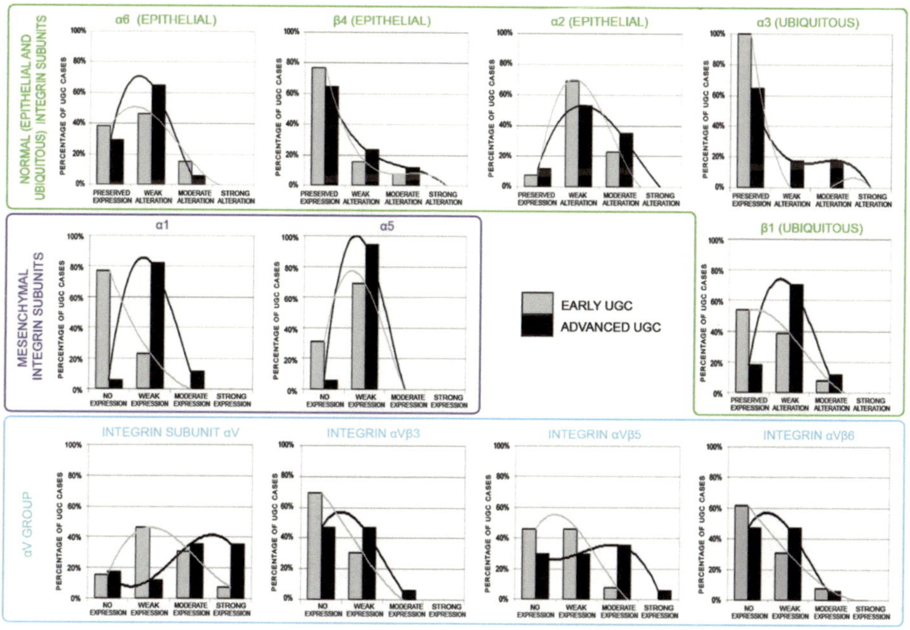

Fig. 8. UGC distribution according integrin expression pattern.

3.3.1 Epithelial integrins

All integrin subunits, common for normal stomach epithelium (α2, α3, α6, β1, β4) similar to internal domain of E-cadherin, demonstrated strong trend to be preserved both in early and advanced UGC (Table 3). However, unlike E-cadherin, none of the UGC cases demonstrated total loss of any normal integrins and most of cases showed normal or weakly depressed epithelial integrin expression (Fig. 8). Also, in contrast to E-cadherin, epithelial integrins did not demonstrate any tendency to be preserved more in tumors with weaker invasive potential. Strictly epithelial integrin subunits (α2, α6, β4) expression correlated with each other (R=0.48), i.e. they trended to be preserved better in the same tumors.

3.3.2 Mesenchymal integrins

α1 integrin (collagen receptor) expressed stronger in advanced carcinomas, whereas α5 (fibronectin receptor) did not reveal such tendency (Table 3). However, both subunits expressed rather weakly (Fig. 8). In the whole UGC pool, α1 correlated with such signs of higher local invasive potential as bigger tumor size (AreaV, R=0.51), prevalence of extramucosal over mucosal portion (R=0.50), as well as with bigger number of LN metastasis (R=0.39). α5 integrin subunit did not demonstrate such linkage with invasion features, correlating only with bigger tumor size (AreaH, R=0.57) in advanced UGC.

Regarding prevailed histotype (SIG or POR) α1 and α5 demonstrated different tendencies. α1 in all UGC pool trended to express in mostly poorly differentiated tumors with smaller SRC and LS component (R=0.53) (Fig. 9A, poorly differentiated tumor [left pair] is positive; SRC tumor [right pair] is negative) , whereas α5 in early UGC expressed stronger in SRC areas (Fig. 9B). In advanced UGC α5 demonstrated the same trend as α1, but it was non-significant. Both mesenchymal integrins expressed stronger in UGCs with prominent scirrhous component (α1 R= 0.50, α5 R=0.64) (Fig. 9C).

3.3.3 αV group

Like mesenchymal integrin subunit, percentage of cells, expressing each individual integrin of this group was low, being significantly higher in advanced UGC only for αVβ5 integrin (Table 3). αV subunit, which formed a part of all three integrins, as well as paired with two other β subunits (β1, β8), was expressed more often (Table 3). Tumors, expressing αVβ3 and αVβ6 integrins, expressed them in mostly in a weak manner (Fig. 8). Percentage of tumors with moderate or strong expression of αVβ5 integrins and αV subunit was higher (Fig. 8).

In a whole tumor group αV integrin subunit expression demonstrated linkage with such local invasive features as bigger tumor size (R=0.50), prevalence of extramucosal (especially, mp) growth (R=0.44), as well as with γ-INF (R=0.56) and veins invasion (R=0.37). αVβ5 integrin was also expressed more frequently if tumors with prevailed mp portion (R=0.42) and unclear invasion front (γ-INF, R=0.37). αV subunit was rarely seen in advanced cohesive UGC (R=0.74) (Fig. 10A) and advanced UGC with developed signet-ring cell (R=0.53) and mucinous component (R=0.57). Tubular component in advanced carcinomas was linked with stronger αVβ6 expression (R=0.51) (Fig. 10B: only tubular, but not poorly differentiated component of the tumor expresses αVβ6).

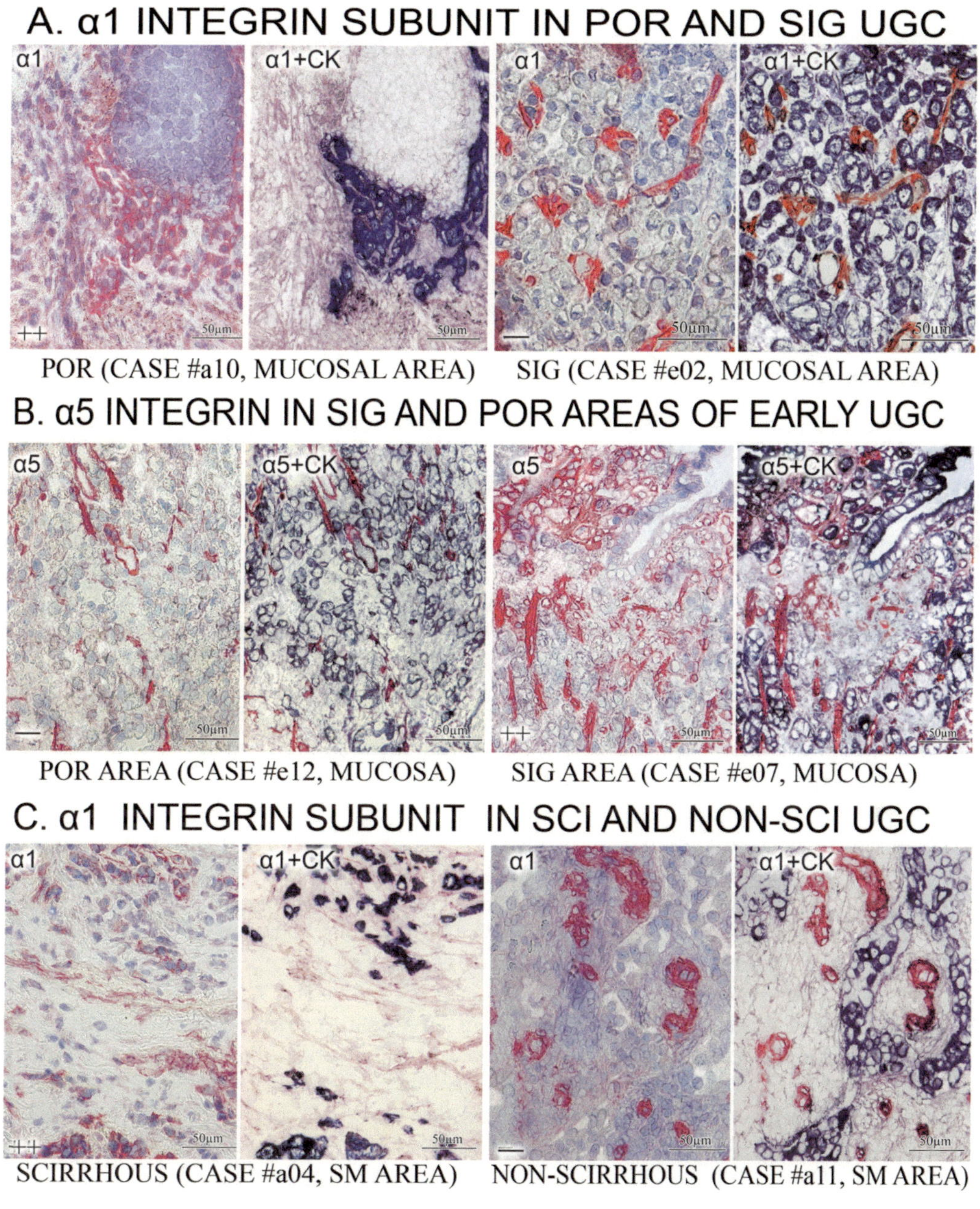

Fig. 9. Mesenchymal integrin expression. Microphotos of each area were taken twice: after staining for integrin (left photo in each pair; integrins are stained with magenta) and after staining for cytokeratins (2nd step of double staining, right photo, CK are stained with purple-blue). Double staining was performed for better quantitative assessment of integrin positive cells in frozen samples of UGC with poor morphological representation (for details see Yanchenko N. et al, 2009). Symbols in the bottom-left corner of each microphoto depict the intensity of integrin staining.

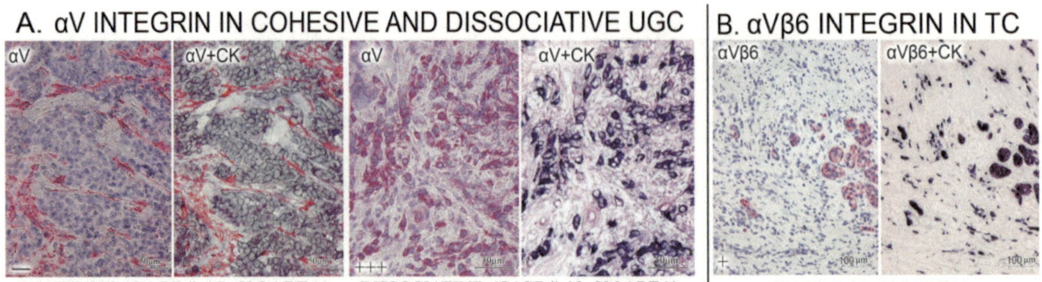

Fig. 10. aV-group integrin expression (for explanations see Fig. 9).

4. Discussion

4.1 Quantitative analysis proves loss of gastric differentiation and its impact into UGCs progression

Precise quantitative analysis provided plenty of data regarding UGCs structure and its impact into tumor progression. It quantitatively proved empirically observed tendency to lose gastric-cell differentiation while tumor invades in extramucosal areas, as we demonstrated substitution of relatively differentiated SRC component (in early carcinomas) by poorly differentiated component in advanced UGC.

Layered arrangement of SRC in mucosa, which reflects rudimentary gastric-mucosal differentiation (Natsagdorj et al., 2008; Sugihara et al., 1987) and is predominant in most early carcinomas, also demonstrated a tendency to be disorganised in advanced UGCs, and mucosal portions of those "primary" UGC which arose form LS-abundant early UGC almost totally lose this relatively ordered layered arrangement. Additionally, the more significantly advanced tumor loses LS, the more clearly it demonstrates the tendency for penetrative vs. spreading growth.

However, even those tiny remnants of LS are very important as they were shown to be necessary for prediction of the prognostic role of SRC component. We could conclude that the tendency for lymphatic (and venous) penetration, considered to be reason of poor prognosis in advanced SRC (Humar et al., 2007; Hyung et al., 2002; Kim et al., 1997; Li et al. 2007) is observed only in advanced "secondary" UGCs, arose form dedifferentiated tubular carcinomas, but not in advance "primary" UGCs.

On the other hand, from the position of local invasive features prominent SRC component, in both early and advanced UGCs could be considered as favourable prognostic feature, as SRC demonstrated a tendency to spread in connective tissue (lamina propria in early UGCs or submucosa in advanced UGCs), but not penetrate muscle layers. We could suppose that one of the probable reasons observed in this study is lack of abnormal mesenchymal (α1 and α5) and aV-integrins (shown to be essential for mp penetration) in SRC.

Diffuse α5 integrin subunit expression in SRC areas of early carcinomas, was not associated with local invasive features and probably reflected its role in reparative (Herard et al., 1996) and inflammatory (Liebert et al., 1994) processes rather in invasion, as its ligand fibronectin is topographically associated with the front of invasion of GC (David et al., 1993).

4.2 E-cadherin loss in cohesive component of UGC

As could be expected, UGCs we predominantly cohesive cell arrangement and clearly seen invasion front demonstrated less aggressive behaviour. Surprisingly they also demonstrated significantly higher tendency to lose E-cadherin expression than tumors with predominantly dissociative cell arrangement. This findings demonstrate that significance of solely E-cadherin down-regulation in cell dissociation could be rather questionable, especially in advanced UGC.

Simultaneously observed low expression of abnormal (mesenchymal and especially αV integrins) in highly cohesive tumors with compact, non-dissociative cell arrangement could mean that for dissociation and spreading UGC cells need not only to lose cell-cell adhesion but also to acquire abnormal cell-ECM contacts and motility mechanisms.

Previously, E-cadherin loss (extracellular domain was studied) was proved to be obligatory first step of carcinogenesis in hereditary diffuse GC, in sporadic early GC however such E-cadherin loss was considered as important, however optional event (Humar et al., 2007). Our data also proved that E-cadherin loss is not a critical requirement for tumor progression, as we demonstrated remarkable preservation of E-cadherin in both early and advanced sporadic UGC. Moreover, expression of E-cadherin in mucosal parts of advanced tumors with E-cadherin-negative extramucosal parts could mean that E-cadherin loss in such tumors is a secondary event, supporting the idea of gradual alteration of E-cadherin with UGC progression (Nakamura et al., 2005).

4.3 Scirrhous stromal component and mesenchymal integrin gain

Dissociative cell arrangement was clearly demonstrated to be not necessarily accompanied scirrhous stroma development, and even some cohesive tumors could develop areas of scirrhous stroma. However, in all cases scirrhous stroma prevalence contributed to local invasiveness. Possible reason of this findings is stronger expression of mesenchymal (α1, α5), but not epithelial (α2, αVβ6) collagen and fibronectin receptors in scirrhous areas. It could be supposed that stronger desmoplastic response recruits integrins responsible for mesenchymal fibroblast-like movements, albeit fibronectin production is not directly linked to desmoplastic response (David et al., 1993).

Epithelial fibronectin receptor αVβ6 in the whole tumor was not correlated with scirrhous stroma development, as its expression was shown to be confined to invasion front (Breuss et al., 1995). However, αVβ6 association with tubular component in advanced UGC supports the idea of the its predominant role for cohort migration, which was proved to depend on fibronectin (Shimao et al., 1999).

4.4 E-cadherin down-regulation is more important than epithelial integrin down-regulation

In all UGCs studied normal epithelial integrin phenotype seems to be more stable than E-cadherin expression and did not demonstrate linkage with tumor invasiveness. One of the possible reasons of the absence of significant relationship between expression of normal integrin and tumor behavior is impossibility to predict their role in tumor spreading. They are characterised by broad range of modulation of their functions by external and internal signals, e.g. α3β1 and α6β4 integrins could form both sedentary and moving contacts, enhancing both anti- and pro-invasive properties of cancer cells (Giannelli et al., 2002). Conversely, E-cadherin is responsible only for homophilic adhesion and acting only as invasion suppressor, and its significant alteration causes an increase of local invasive features of UGC. However, as was mentioned above, even total loss of cell-cell adhesiveness without abnormal integrin gain does not lead to highly invasive phenotype.

From the position of the whole integrin phenotype, gain of abnormal integrins seems to be more important for UGC growth and invasion, than normal epithelial integrins down-regulation. Even minute or moderate gain of both mesenchymal and αV group integrins is linked with local invasion features such as tendency to penetrate deeper in muscularis propria, accompanied by γ infiltration pattern, linked with more rapid growth in UGC (our data) and poor prognosis of ovarian tumors (Spannuth et. al., 2005).

5. Conclusion

Thorough quantitated analysis of UGC histology, supplemented by simultaneous analysis of the integrin and E-cadherin phenotype, pioneered in this study, revealed not only tight correlation between UGCs histological components (such as signet-ring cell component, layer structures, cohesive cell arrangement, and scirrhous stromal development) and tumor invasive features, but also proposed E-cadherin down-regulation and abnormal (mesenchymal and αV-group) integrin up-regulation as the possible reason of this correlation.

6. References

Breuss, JM., Gallo, J., DeLisser, HM., Klimanskaya, IV., Folkesson, HG., Pittet, JF., Nishimura, SL., Aldape, K., Landers, DV., Carpenter, W. et al. (1995). Expression of the beta 6 integrin subunit in development, neoplasia and tissue repair suggests a role in epithelial remodeling. J Cell Sci., Vol. 108, Pt. 6, (June 1995), pp. 2241-51

Choi, S., Lee, SA., Kwak, TK., Kim, HJ., Lee, MJ., Ye, SK., Kim, SH., Kim, S., Lee, JW. (2009). Cooperation between integrin alpha5 and tetraspan TM4SF5 regulates VEGF-mediated angiogenic activity. Blood, Vol. 113, No.8, (February 2009), pp. 19; 1845-55

Crew, KD., Neugut, AI. (2006). Epidemiology of gastric cancer. *World J Gastroenterol.*, Vol.12, No.3, (January 2006) pp. 354-62

David, L., Mandel, U., Clausen, H., Sobrinho-Simoes, M. (1993). Immunohistochemical expression of oncofetal fibronectin in benign and malignant lesions of the stomach. Eur J Cancer. Vol.29, No.14, (August 1993), pp. 2070-1

Friedl, P., Wolf, K. (2003). Tumour-cell invasion and migration: diversity and escape mechanisms. *Nat Rev Cancer*, Vol. 3, No.5, (May 2003), pp. 362-74

Giannelli, G., Astigiano, S., Antonaci, S., Morini, M., Barbieri, O., Noonan, DM., Albini, A. (2002). Role of the α3β1 and α6β4 integrins in tumor invasion. *Clin Exp Metastasis*, Vol.19, No.3, (March 2002), pp. 217-23

Guszczyn, T., Sobolewski, K. (2004). Deregulation of collagen metabolism in human stomach cancer. *Pathobiology*, Vol. 71, Iss. 6; (June 2004), p. 308

Hazan, RB., Qiao, R., Keren, R., Badano, I., Suyama, K. (2004). Cadherin switch in tumor progression. *Ann N Y Acad Sci.*, Vol. 1014, (April 2004), pp. 155-63

Herard, AL., Pierrot, D., Hinnrasky, J., Kaplan, H., Sheppard, D., Puchelle, E., Zahm, JM. (1996). Fibronectin and its α5β1-integrin receptor are involved in the wound-repair process of airway epithelium. *Am J Physiol.*, Vol.271, No.5, Pt.1, (November 1996 Nov), pp. L726-33

Humar, B., Fukuzawa, R., Blair, V., Dunbier, A., More, H., Charlton, A., Yang, HK., Kim, WH., Reeve, AE., Martin, I., Guilford, P. (2007). Destabilized adhesion in the gastric proliferative zone and c-Src kinase activation mark the development of early diffuse gastric cancer. Cancer Res., Vol.67, No.6, (March 2007), pp. 2480-9

Hyung, WJ., Noh, SH., Lee, JH., Huh, JJ., Lah, KH., Choi, SH., Min, JS. (2002). Early gastric carcinoma with signet ring cell histology. *Cancer*, Vol.94, No.1, (January 2002), pp. 78-83.

Stefansson, IM., Salvesen, HB., Akslen, LA. (2004). Prognostic Impact of Alterations in P-Cadherin Expression and Related Cell Adhesion Markers in Endometrial Cancer. *Journal of Clinical Oncology*, Vol 22, No 7 (April 2004), pp. 1242-1252

Japanese Gastric Cancer Association. (1998). Japanese Classification of Gastric Carcinoma - 2nd English Edition. Gastric Cancer. Vol.1, No.1, (December 1998), pp. 10-24

Kaneko, S., Yoshimura, T. (2001). Time trend analysis of gastric cancer incidence in Japan by histological types, 1975-1989. Br J Cancer., Vol.84, No.3, (February 2001), pp. 400-5

Kim, JP., Kim, SC., Yang, HK. (1994). Prognostic significance of signet ring cell carcinoma of the stomach. *Surg Oncol.*, Vol.3, No.4, (August 1994), pp. 221-7

Li, C., Kim, S., Lai, JF., Hyung, WJ., Choi, WH., Choi, SH., Noh, SH. (2007). Advanced gastric carcinoma with signet ring cell histology. *Oncology*, Vol. 72, No.1-2, (November 2007), pp. 64-68

Liebert, M., Washington, R., Stein, J., Wedemeyer, G., Grossman, HB. (1994). Expression of the VLA beta 1 integrin family in bladder cancer. *Am J Pathol.*, Vol. 144, No.5, (May 1994), pp. 1016-22

Nabeshima, K., Inoue, T., Shimao, Y., Kataoka, H., Koono., M. (1999). Cohort migration of carcinoma cells: differentiated colorectal carcinoma cells move as coherent cell clusters or sheets. Histol Histopathol., Vol.14, No.4, (October 1999), pp.1183-97

Nakamura, E., Sugihara, H., Bamba, M., Hattori, T. (2005). Dynamic alteration of the E-cadherin/catenin complex during cell differentiation and invasion of undifferentiated-type gastric carcinomas. *J Pathol.*, Vol.205, No.3, (February 2005), pp. 349-58

Natsagdorj, L., Sugihara, H., Bamba, M., Hattori, T. (2008). Intratumoural heterogeneity of intestinal expression reflects environmental induction and progression-related loss of induction in undifferentiated-type gastric carcinomas. *Histopathology*, Vol.53, No.6, (December 2008), pp. 685-97

Shimao, Y., Nabeshima, K., Inoue, T., Koono, M. (1999). Role of fibroblasts in HGF/SF-induced cohort migration of human colorectal carcinoma cells: fibroblasts stimulate migration associated with increased fibronectin production via upregulated TGF-beta1. Int J Cancer, Vol.82, No.3, (July 1999), pp. 449-58

Sidoni, A. Differential trends in the intestinal and diffuse types of gastric carcinoma. *Arch Pathol Lab Med.*, Vol.129, No.3, (March 2005), p. 290

Spannuth, WA., Rocconi, RP., Kirby, TO., Huh, WK., Conner, MG. (2005). Gamma mode of infiltration associated with poor prognosis in malignant teratoma of the ovary: A case report. *Gynecol Oncol.*, Vol.98, No.1, (July 2005), pp. 155-7

Sugihara, H., Hattori, T., Fukuda, M., Fujita, S. (1987). Cell proliferation and differentiation in intramucosal and advanced signet ring cell carcinomas of the human stomach. *Virchows Arch A Pathol Anat Histopathol*, Vol. 411, No.2, (1987), pp. 117-127

Yanchenko. N., Sugihara, H., Hattori, T. (2009). Application of a novel method of double APAAP staining with subsequent quantitative image analysis to the examination of integrin expression in undifferentiated-type gastric carcinomas. *J Histochem Cytochem.*, Vol.57, No.12, (December 2009), pp. 1183-93

Yang, Z., Zhang, X., Gang, H., Li, X., Li, Z., Wang, T., Han, J., Luo, T., Wen, F., Wu, X. Up-regulation of gastric cancer cell invasion by Twist is accompanied by N-cadherin and fibronectin expression. *Biochem Biophys Res Commun*. Vol.358, No.3, (July 2007) pp. 925-30

7

Exploring the Utility of Carbohydrate Associated Transferase Activities as Potential Tumor Markers for Human Gastric Cancer

E.V. Chandrasekaran and Khushi L. Matta
Department of Cancer Biology, Roswell Park Cancer Institute, Buffalo, NY USA

1. Introduction

Mucins are large, highly O-glycosylated proteins that are present at the surface of most epithelial cells and are involved in the protection and lubrication of the epithelium (Gendler and Spicer 1995). The expression of mucin genes is organ-and cell-type specific. The increased expression and altered glycosylation of mucins influence cellular growth, differentiation, transformation, adhesion and immune surveillance (Hollingworth and swanson 2004) and are associated with the development of cancer. Mucins have been implicated in the biologic behavior and progression of several cancers. During carcinogenesis, aberrant glycosylation leads to the development of tumor subpopulations with different adhesion properties (Taniguchi et al. 1996; Hiraiwa et al. 1996). Alterations of mucins during the pathogenesis of cancer have been well documented (Hakomori et al. 2002). The under glycosylation of mucins results in the creation of tumor associated cryptic carbohydrate core structures Tn, sialyl Tn and T (Taylor-Papadimitriou et al. 1999).

The Gram-negative bacterium Helicobacter pyroli infects over 50% of the world's population and causes various gastric diseases such as chronic gastritis, peptic ulcer and gastric cancer. Peripheral lymph node addressin (PNAd) containing 6-sulfo sialyl Lewis X-capped O-glycans on high endothelial venule (HEV)-like vessels are closely associated with pathogenesis of H pyroli-related diseases. The α1,4 GlcNAc-capped O-glycans expressed by gastric gland mucous cell-derived mucin prevents colonization of H pyroli. Thus, the differential expression of distinct O-glycans in stomach provides therapeutic potentialities based on specific carbohydrate modulation (Nakayama et al. 1999; Reis et al. 2000 and Kobayashi et al. 2009).

Werther et al. (1996) examined the frequency of sialyl Tn expression and its prognostic value in gastric cancer by immunohistochemical analysis of 340 gastric tumors and found that sialyl Tn expression is a marker of gastric cancer progression suggesting that cancer associated mucins play a role in the malignant behavior of the tumor. Santos-Silva et al. (2005) have reported that polymorphism in the MUC1 tandem repeat exerts influence on the expression of cryptic carbohydrate core structures in gastric cancer cells and the aggressive gastric tumors tend to express T antigen. Immunohistochemical study of Amado et al. (1998) for the expression of dimeric sialyl Lewis^x in 97 gastric carcinomas revealed a correlation between high expression of dimeric sialyl Lewis^x and venous invasion and poor outcome in gastric cancer patients. Petretti *et al* (1999) studied RNA expression of several glycosyltransferases in surgical specimens of gastric carcinomas and found significant enhancement in the expression of ST3Gal IV and FucT IV.

A comprehensive study by Carvalho et al. (1999) on mucin expression in a panel of gastric carcinoma cell lines found no apparent relationship between the mucin core proteins and the simple mucin type or Lewis^x carbohydrate antigens that are expressed in each cell line. Thus there exists a complexity in glycosyltransferase activities which lead to several tumor-associated carbohydrate structures in gastric carcinoma.

A comparative study of gene-expression profiles of adenocarcinoma metastases and primary adenocarcinomas (Ramaswamy et al. 2003) indicated that a subset of primary tumors resembled metastatic tumors with respect to a gene-expression signature and that solid tumors carrying this gene-expression signature were most likely to be associated with metastasis and poor clinical outcome. These results further suggested that the metastatic potential of human tumors is encoded in the bulk of a primary tumor and thus challenged the notion that metastases arise from rare cells within a primary tumor that have the ability to metastasize (Poste et al. 1980). Thus, it became obvious that a very consistent change of some biological events in a primary tumor as opposed to the normal tissue has the possibility of being related to the malignant potential of the tumor. Recently, we examined the patterns of glycosyl- and glycan-sulfotransferase activities in several cancer cell lines and the resulting data strongly suggested an association of unique carbohydrate structures with signature potential in individual cancers (Chandrasekaran et al. 2006). The present study was aimed to identify the glycosyl- or sulfotransferase which exhibits the most marked and consistent change of activity in gastric tumorigenesis, by comparing the pattern of various glycosyl and glycan: sulfotransferase activities in tumorous and normal gastric tissues of each patient in ten gastric carcinoma cases.

2. Materials and methods

2.1 Tissue specimens

Human gastric tumor specimens were obtained during surgical procedures at Roswell Park Cancer Institute and stored frozen within 1h at -70°C. We studied the gastric tumor as well as non-tumor stomach tissue specimens from the same patient in ten gastric carcinoma cases and, in addition, two gastric tumor specimens in which case normal stomach tissue specimens were unavailable. The Pathology report on the tumors is presented in Table 1 and Table 4.

When the samples were collected from Pathology, a portion of the sample adjacent to that used for enzyme assay was fixed in formalin and embedded in paraffin. Slides were prepared from the paraffin blocks, and stained with hematoxylin and eosin by standard procedures. A board-certified pathologist studied the slides to determine the distribution of cell types within the tumor tissue compared to the control tissue from the same case (although in three cases non-tumor tissue was not available). Due to the invasiveness of the gastric cancer in these cases, both the tumor and the non-tumor tissue samples generally contained smooth muscle. The smooth muscle component existed at roughly equivalent percentage in the tumor sample and non-tumor control on a case by case basis sometimes being a little larger in either tumor or non-tumor sample. The major difference between the normal and tumor sample in this study was that the tumor contained malignant epithelial cells, and the normal never did. With the exception of case 10, the amount of protein solubilized from the tumor and the corresponding non-tumor specimen by Triton X-100 did not vary much as evident from the values reported in **Table 1**. Thus, it becomes evident that a comparison of each glycosyltransferase and glycan:sulfotransferase activity per mg protein of the tissue extract between tumor and the corresponding non-tumor specimen is quite meaningful in understanding the quantitative change of each enzyme activity in tumorigenesis.

Gastric cancer cases	Tumor Site	STG	Smooth muscle (%) N	Smooth muscle (%) T	Specimen Wt. (g) N	Specimen Wt. (g) T	Protein (mg) in Triton X-100 solubilized extract / g tissue N	Protein (mg) in Triton X-100 solubilized extract / g tissue T
1	Overlapping lesion of stomach		30	40	3.5	1.9	52.8	67.4
2	Lesser curvature of stomach, NOS	3A	30	50	1.9	2.5	58.5	53.6
3	Lesser curvature of stomach, NOS	3A	20	30	4.2	1.9	54.6	42.2
4	Lesser curvature of stomach, NOS	2	N/A	70	6.0	1.0	60.0	41.0
5	Gastric antrum	3A	20	20	0.8	0.8	80.0	80.0
6	Gastric antrum	1B	20	30	0.8	0.6	60.4	67.5
7	Gastric antrum	2	10	0	1.7	0.5	52.4	82.8
8	Body of stomach	3A	10	10	0.6	2.1	68.9	80.2
9	Body of stomach	1B	20	10	0.6	2.0	52.9	86.9
10	Cardia, NOS	3A	40	30	1.9	2.3	112.0	23.5
11	Stomach, NOS	4	N/A	60	N/A	3.6		58.3
12	Lesser curvature of stomach, NOS		N/A	0	N/A	3.5		76.8

N; Non-tumor gastric tissue; T: Tumor gastric tissue N/A Not available

Table 1. The cancer site, stage and the details of the gastric tumor and non-tumor specimens from 12 patients

2.2 Acceptor compounds

The synthetic compounds used as acceptors in this study have already been used in our earlier studies (Chandrasekaran et al. 1995; 1996; 2001; 2004; 2005; 2006) and, thus, are well-documented acceptors for measuring the reported enzyme activities.

2.3 Processing of tissue specimens

The tissues were homogenized at 4°C with 4 volumes of 0.1 M Tris Maleate pH 7.2, 0.1% NaN_3 using kinematica. After adjusting the concentration of TritonX-100 to 2%, these homogenates were mixed in the cold room for 1h using Speci-Mix (Thermolyne) and then centrifuged at 20,000g for 1h at 4°C. The clear fat-free supernatant was stored frozen at -20°C until use. Aliquots of 10μL from this extract were used in assays run in duplicates.

2.4 Enzyme assays

Glycosyltransferase activity in tumor extract was determined by mixing the tumor extracts with acceptor and radiolabeled monosaccharide donor under the reaction conditions detailed below, followed by separation of unreacted donor from the radioactive product using anionic or hydrophobic chromatography. In all cases, the radioactive content of isolated products was determined by using 3a70 scintillation cocktail (research Products International, Mount Prospect, IL) and a Beckman LS9000 scintillation counter. Controls for each assay contained the reaction mixture with everything except the acceptor. Radioactivity of control was subtracted from that of product to obtain the results presented in the Tables. All assays were run in duplicate. Results from duplicate runs did not vary by more than 5%. The following are the conditions for individual enzymatic assays. Reaction temperature in all cases was 37°C.

2.5 Sialyltransferase

α2,3- and α2,6 sialyltransferase (ST) assay reactions proceeded for 2h in a mixture containing 100mM sodium cacodylate buffer (pH 6.0), 7.5mM acceptor, CMP-[9-^{3}H] NeuAc (typically 0.2μCi) and 10μl tumor extract in a total volume of 20μl (Chandrasekaran et al. 1995, 2005).

2.6 Gal/GalNAc transferases

βGlcNAc: β1,4Gal-T and αGalNAc:β1,3Gal-T assay mixtures in duplicate contained 0.1M Hepes-NaOH pH 7.0, 7mM ATP, 20mM Mn acetate, 1mM UDP-Gal. UDP [^{14}C] Gal (0.05μCi; 327mCi/mmol; Amersham), 0.5mM acceptor (unless otherwise stated) and 10μl tumor extract in a total volume of 20μL (Chandrasekaran et al. 2001). It was incubated for 4h; βGlcNAc:β1,4GalNAc-T assay mixtures in duplicate contained 0.1M Hepes-NaOH ph7.0, 7mM ATP, 20mM Mn acetate, UDP [^{3}H] GalNAc (0.20μCi; 7.8Ci/mmol: New England Nuclear Corp.) 7.5mM acceptor and incubated for 4h (Chandrasekaran et al. 2001).

2.7 Fucosyltransferases

α1,2, α1,3- , α1,4-fucosyltransferase and FT VI assay reactions were carried out for 2h in a reaction mixture containing 50mM Hepes buffer (pH 7.5), 5mM $MnC1_2$, 7mM ATP, 3mM NaN_3, 3mM synthetic acceptor, 0.05μCi GDP-[^{14}C]Fuc (290mCi/mmol) and 10μl tumor extract in a total volume of 20μl (Chandrasekaran et al. 1996).

2.8 Glycan: sulfotransferases

Sulfotransferase (Sulfo-T) assay reactions took 2h and required a mixture containing 100mM Tris-Maleate (pH 7.2), 5mM Mg Acetate, 5mM ATP, 10mM NaF, 10mM BAL, 7.5mM acceptor, 0.5μCi of [^{35}S]PAPS (specific activity 2.4Ci/mmol) and 10μl of tumor extract in a total volume of 30μl (Chandrasekaran et al. 2004).

2.9 Chromatographic methods

Dowex-1-Cl or Sep-Pak C18 cartridges were used to isolate radiolabeled product from the reaction mixture. For Gal-T, GalNAc-T and FT assays, the incubation mixture was diluted with 1ml water and passed through a 1ml bed volume of Dowex-1-Cl column (Chandrasekaran et al. 1996, 2001). The column was washed twice with 1ml water. The breakthrough and the water wash contained the [^{14}C]-galactosylated or [^{14}C]-fucosylated products formed with neutral acceptors. 3ml of 0.1M NaCl was used to obtain [^{14}C]-fucosylated products from sialylated acceptors after water elution. For sialyltransferase assays, the radioactive products from benzylglycosides were separated by hydrophobic chromatography on Sep-Pak C18 cartridge (Water, Milford, MA), and elution of the product was done with 3ml methanol (Chandrasekaran et al. 2005; Palcic et al. 1998). For sulfotransferase assays, elution of the [35S]-sulfated compound from Dowex-1-Cl column could be achieved by 3ml of 0.2M NaCl (Chandrasekaran et al. 2001).

2.10 Effect of divalent cations on gastric tumor Gal: 3-O-sulfotransferase activity

For seeing the effect of divalent cations on Gal: 3-O-sulfotransferase activity the incubation mixture contained varying concentration (1-50mM) of Mg acetate, Mn acetate or Ca acetate under the standard incubation conditions. Gal3Sulfo-T4 activity was assayed using 3-O-Me Galβ1, 4 GlcNAcβ1,6(Galβ1,3)GalNAcα-O-Bn as the acceptor. Gal3Sulfo-T2 activity was measured with the acceptor Galβ1, 4 GlcNAcβ1, 6(3-O-MeGalβ1, 3)GalNAcα-O-Bn.

2.11 N-Acetylglucosaminltransferase assay

The reaction mixture (30µl) contained 5mM acceptor, 70 mM Hepes-NaOH pH7.0, 7mM GlcNAc 1, 5 lactone, 14mM Mn acetate, 5mM ATP, 2mM NaN_3, 0.2µCi UDP-[6-^{3}H] GlcNAc (NEN-Dupont) and 15µl tumor extract and incubated for 4h at 37°C. The radioactive products from benzyl glycosides were separated by hydrophobic chromatography on Sep-Pak C18 cartridge and from allyl glycoside by Biogel P2 column chromatography as described above.

2.12 β N-acetylhexosaminidase treatment

10 µl of the [6-^{3}H] N-acetyl glucosamine containing products were incubated at 37°C for 20h with 0.1 unit of this enzyme as recommended by supplier (GLYKO) in a reaction volume of 20µl.

2.13 β1, 3Galactosidase (recombinant enzyme from calbiochem) treatment

10 µl of the [6-^{3}H] N-acetyl glucosamine containing product from Galβ1, 3 (GlcNAc β 1, 6) GalNAc α O-Al was mixed with 10µl of 0.1M citrate buffer-0.1% BSA pH 5.0 and 10µl (20 mU) recombinant enzyme and incubated at 37°C for 20h.

2.14 Lectin-agarose chromatography

PNA-agarose (Sigma), ConA-agarose (Sigma) and GSL II-agarose (Vector) columns of 5 ml bed volume were used under conditions as recommended by suppliers.

2.15 Thin layer chromatography

TLC was carried out on Silica gel GHLF (250 µm scored 20x20cm; Analtech, Newark DE). The solvent systems A [1 propanol/NH_4OH/H_2O (12/2/5 V/V)] and B [n-butanol/acetic acid/H_2O (3/2/1)] were used. The acceptor compounds were located on the plates by spraying with sulfuric acid in ethanol and heating at 100°C. The radioactive products were located by scraping 0.5cm width segments of silica gel and soaking them in 2 ml water in vials followed by liquid scintillation counting.

3. Results

3.1 Non-reducing terminal of complex carbohydrate chains

Several glycosyltransferases and glycan-sulfotransferases act on the non-reducing terminal of mucin Core2 tetra-and tri-saccharides and Globo backbone unit of gangliosides, core 1 disaccharide and Asparagine linked complex carbohydrate chains terminating in Gal residues, leading to a complexity of cancer-associated terminal glycan structures as shown in **Table 2.** Hence, we examined the levels of many of these enzyme activities in gastric tumor tissue as well as non-tumor gastric tissue of the same patient in ten gastric cancer cases for identifying any significant consistent change in any of these enzyme activities in gastric cancer. The specific acceptor compounds used in the present study for assaying the enzymes are reported in **Table 3.** The results on various enzyme levels are presented in **Tables 4** and **5.**

Carbohydrate chain terminal	Modifying glycosyl-and sulfo-transferases
1. *GlcNAcβ1,6(Galβ1,3)GalNAcα-O-Ser/Thr (mucin core2 trisaccharide)	β1,3Gal/GalNAcTs; FTVI; β1,4Gal/GalNAcTs; GlcNAc6SulfoT
2. a) *Galβ1,4GlcNAcβ1,6(Galβ1,3)GalNAcα-O-Ser/Thr (mucin core2 tetrasaccharide) b) Asparagine linked complex carbohydrate chains terminating in *Gal residues	Gal3SulfoT2; Gal3SulfoT3 ST3Gal III; ST3Gal IV α1,2-FT; α1,4-GlcNAcT β1,3-GlcNAcT
3. a) Galβ1,4GlcNAcβ1,6(*Galβ1,3)GalNAcα-O-Ser/Thr b) GlcNAcβ1,6(*Galβ1,3)GalNAcα-O-Ser/Thr c) *Galβ1,3 GalNAcα-O-Ser/Thr (mucin core1 disaccharide) d) *Galβ1,3 GalNAcβ 1,3 Galα-O-R (Globo unit of gangliosides)	Gal3SulfoT4; ST3Gal I ST3Gal II; α1,2-FT α1,4-GlcNAcT β1,3-GlcNAcT

* Denotes the terminal unit utilized by the enzyme to transfer monosaccharide or sulfate

Table 2. Glycosyl-and sulfo-transferases involved in carbohydride chain terminal modification

3.2 Fucosyltransferase activities in gastric carcinoma

α1,3-FT contributed the major FT activity in both normal and tumor specimens in all cases. In nine cases, the tumor specimens as compared to normal (with the exception case 10) contained lower α1,3-FT activity (a decrease of 10-60%). There was a marked reduction (40-90%) of α1, 2-FT activity in seven cancer cases (2, 3, 4, 5, 6, 7 and 9). Thus, it is interesting to note that a decrease of α 1, 3- and α 1, 2- FT activities occurred in the same specimens. On the other hand, α1,4-FT activity and FTVI activity were present in increased level in the same five cancer cases (1, 3, 4, 7 and 10) and in decreased level in the same five cases (2, 5, 6, 8 and 9). Four tumor specimens (cases 7, 4, 1 and 10) which include two Signet ring cell CA and two mucin producing adenocarcinoma exhibited high elevation of FTVI activity (8.9, 10.5, 51.4 and 199.5 fold respectively) as compared to the corresponding normal specimen. Further, a highly noteworthy finding is that the gastrointestinal stromal tumor specimen (case 12) was distinct in having a low level of α1, 3-FT activity and negligible amounts of α1, 4-FT, α1,2-FT and FTVI activities as compared to other tumor specimens.

Glycosyl- or Sulfo-transferases	Acceptors
Fucosyltransferases: α 1, 2-FT α 1, 3-FT α 1, 4-FT FTVI	 Gal β-O-Bn 2-O-Me Gal β 1, 4 GlcNAc 2-O-Me Gal β 1, 3 GlcNAc GlcNAc β 1, 4 GlcNAc β-O-Bn
Sialyltransferases: ST3(O) ST3(N) ST6(N)	3-O-Me Gal β 1, 4 GlcNAc β 1, 6 (Gal β 1, 3) GalNAc α-O-Bn 2-O-Me Gal β 1, 3 GlcNAc β-O-Bn Gal β 1, 4 GlcNAc β 1, 6 (3-O-Me Gal β 1, 3) GalNAc α-O-Bn [corrected for ST3(N) activity]
β Gal/GalNAc transferase: β 1, 4 Gal-T β 1, 4 GalNAc-T α GalNAc: β 1, 3 Gal-T	 3-O-Me Gal β 1, 3 (GlcNAc β 1, 6) GalNAc α-O-Bn 3-O-Me Gal β 1, 3 (GlcNAc β 1, 6) GalNAc α-O-Bn 4-Fluoro GlcNAc β 1, 6 GalNAc α-O-Bn
Glycan: Sulfotransferases Gal 3 Sulfo-T_2 Gal 3 Sulfo-T_4 GlcNAc 6 Sulfo-T	Gal β 1, 4 GlcNAc β 1, 6 (3-O-Me Gal β 1, 3) GalNAc α-O-Bn 3-O-Me Gal β 1, 4 GlcNAc β 1, 6 (Gal β 1, 3) GalNAc α-O-Bn GlcNAc β 1, 3 Gal β 1, 4 Glc

Table 3. Specific acceptors for measuring Glycosyl- and Sulfo- transferase activities in gastric tumor and non-tumor specimens

3.3 Sialyltransferase activities in gastric carcinoma

ST3 (O) activity, which forms 3'-sialyl T hapten (NeuAcα2, 3Galβ1, 3GalNAcα) was the predominant sialyltransferase activity in all gastric tissue specimens. This activity increased (1.7-172.0 fold) in six (cases 2, 3, 4, 6, 9 and 10) and decreased in four (cases 1, 5, 7 and 8) gastric tissue specimens. ST6(N) activity synthesizing 6'-LacNAc type 2 unit (NeuAcα2,6Galβ1,4GlcNAcβ-) ranged 4% - 78% of the ST3(O) activity in the tumor tissue specimens studied and ST3(N) activity forming 3'-sialyl LacNAc was even far less than ST6(N) activity. Three out of four tumor specimens from Signet ring cell carcinoma (cases 2, 3 and 4) and three out of five tumor specimens from adenocarcinoma (cases 6, 9 and 10) showed an increased level of ST3 (O) activity. Two cases of Signet ring cell CA (1 and 3) and three cases of adinocarcinoma (7, 8 and 9) showed significant ST6 (N) activity in the range 8.2 - 78.0% of ST3 (O) activity.

3.4 β-GlcNAc : β1,4-Gal/GalNAc and α-GalNAc : β1,3-Gal transferase activities in gastric carcinoma

Three tumor specimens (cases 3, 4 and 10) while exhibiting an increase in β1, 4Gal-T activity, other tumor specimens contained lower level of this activity than the corresponding normal specimens. Six tumor specimens (cases 3, 4, 5, 6, 8 and 10) showed an increased level of β1, 4GalNAc-T activity. It is remarkable that two tumor specimens (cases 5 and 6) from adenocarcinoma contained only 30% and 40% level of α-GalNAc: β1, 3Gal-T activity as compared to the normal specimens. On the contrary, the tumor specimen of case 10 as compared to other tumor specimens had a high level of this activity, which exceeded even the levels of its β1, 4Gal/GalNAc-T activities. The level of αGalNAc : β1,3Gal-T activity was also higher than β1,4Gal/GalNAc-T activity in Litinis Plastica specimen (case 11)

Enzyme Activity		Glycosyltransferase activities in Tissue specimens: Incorporation of [14C] or [3H] monosaccharides (CPMx10-3) into the enzyme specific acceptor catalyzed by 1mg protein of the tissue extract											
		1	2	3	4	5	6	7	8	9	10	11	12
Fucosyl-transferases													
α1,2-FT	N	127.2	146.8	76.8	62.9	197.2	109.4	70.9	102.7	108.9	19.9		
	T	111.2	83.3	49.0	35.0	16.5	22.0	132.1	34.4	62.5	131.9	88.5	2.5
		(0.9)	(0.6)	(0.6)	(0.6)	(0.1)	(0.2)	(1.9)	(0.3)	(0.6)	(6.6)		
α1,3-FT	N	449.6	494.1	533.2	422.2	448.8	428.4	526.3	367.8	483.5	166.4		
	T	390.5	382.6	448.3	184.0	180.2	198.2	352.8	278.9	328.7	655.0	452.2	107.0
		(0.9)	(0.8)	(0.8)	(0.4)	(0.4)	(0.5)	(0.7)	(0.8)	(0.7)	(3.9)		
α1,4-FT	N	68.3	9.1	268.3	71.5	12.3	405.2	189.5	173.6	417.0	18.4		
	T	193.9	2.3	322.6	201.3	0.0	211.3	325.6	91.2	294.5	671.6	193.4	0.9
		(2.8)	(0.3)	(1.2)	(2.8)	(0.0)	(0.5)	(1.7)	(0.5)	(0.7)	(36.5)		
FT-VI	N	3.1	138.6	42.7	1.5	16.7	137.9	13.6	5.4	227.0	0.8		
	T	159.2	60.6	51.7	15.8	1.2	2.7	121.0	3.8	181.7	159.6	90.5	0.8
		(51.4)	(0.4)	(1.2)	(10.5)	(0.1)	(0.0)	(8.9)	(0.7)	(0.8)	(199.5)		
Sialyl-transferases													
α2,3(O)ST	N	184.5	54.4	180.4	15.6	234.2	104.2	379.7	306.5	148.6	1.9		
	T	53.8	145.1	309.0	122.7	155.2	240.3	83.3	245.1	308.2	326.8	114.0	91.9
		(0.3)	(2.7)	(1.7)	(7.9)	(0.7)	(2.3)	(0.2)	(0.8)	(2.1)	(172.0)		
α2,3(N)ST	N	2.1	1.9	0.7	0.0	1.1	1.7	0.6	2.6	3.6	0.4		
	T	3.1	4.0	2.5	0.0	1.6	2.3	4.2	2.2	3.8	7.1	1.1	2.7
		(1.5)	(2.1)	(3.6)	(0.0)	(1.5)	(1.4)	(7.0)	(0.8)	(1.1)	(4.3)		
α2,6(N)ST	N	0.4	15.4	24.5	0.0	16.2	48.3	40.5	8.3	50.1	0.0		
	T	32.9	8.3	25.2	7.3	6.4	11.9	65.0	38.4	41.5	0.0	8.7	8.2
		(82.2)	(0.5)	(1.0)	(7.3)	(0.4)	(0.2)	(1.6)	(4.6)	(0.8)	(0.0)		
Gal/GalNAc transferases													
β1,3 Gal-T	N	36.6	34.8	67.2	25.6	70.2	102.0	88.1	98.9	110.6	39.7		
	T	43.3	44.1	65.9	31.6	19.4	36.3	138.1	83.0	166.4	244.9	103.3	23.8
		(1.2)	(1.3)	(1.0)	(1.2)	(0.3)	(0.4)	(1.6)	(0.8)	(1.5)	(6.2)		
β1,4 Gal-T	N	172.2	167.8	255.3	113.2	232.2	275.0	362.5	229.8	264.5	26.7		
	T	111.6	151.9	403.9	124.1	199.0	258.4	211.4	205.7	207.0	161.9	92.9	62.3
		(0.6)	(0.9)	(1.6)	(1.1)	(0.9)	(0.9)	(0.6)	(0.9)	(0.8)	(6.1)		
β1,4 GalNAc-T	N	51.7	44.3	36.0	12.2	36.8	38.5	39.7	37.9	74.8	15.3		
	T	27.2	38.1	50.5	25.8	44.0	43.9	32.4	40.3	28.7	61.0	28.9	10.1
		(0.5)	(0.9)	(1.4)	(2.1)	(1.2)	(1.1)	(0.8)	(1.1)	(0.4)	(4.0)		

N: Non-tumor gastric tissue; T: Tumor gastric tissueValues in parentheses indicate fold of enzyme activity in tumor with respect to the normal

Table 4. The levels of glycosyltransferase activities in human gastric non-tumor and tumor specimens

Gastric cancer cases	Tumor Histology	Differen-tiation		Sulfotransferase activities in tissue specimens: Incorporation of ^{35}S-sulfate (CPMx10^{-3}) into enzyme specific acceptors catalyzed by 1mg protein of the tissue extract		
				Gal3sulfo T2	Gal3sulfo T4	GlcNAc6 sulfo T
1	Signet ring cell CA Krukenberg Tumor	Poor	N T	0.8 60.7 (75.9)	3.4 49.1 (14.4)	33.8 43.8 (1.3)
2	Signet ring cell CA Krukenberg Tumor	Poor	N T	2.1 329.0 (156.7)	12.9 91.4 (7.1)	19.5 53.7 (2.8)
3	Signet ring cell CA, Krukenberg Tumor	Poor	N T	10.1 208.1 (20.6)	1.8 111.0 (61.7)	1.8 3.6 (2.0)
4	Signet ring cell CA, Krukenberg Tumor	Moderate	N T	0.1 2.6 (26.0)	0.1 0.5 (5.0)	0.1 0.7 (7.0)
5	Adenocarcinoma nos	Poor	N T	1.1 11.7 (10.6)	27.8 75.8 (2.7)	31.1 49.8 (1.6)
6	Adenocarcinoma nos	Poor	N T	1.4 2.6 (1.9)	6.7 34.3 (5.1)	6.0 3.3 (0.6)
7	Mucin producing adenocarcinoma	Poor	N T	0.3 2.1 (7.0)	0.4 59.6 (149.0)	1.9 5.2 (2.7)
8	Adenocarcinoma nos	Moderate	N T	1.3 2.7 (2.1)	0.7 2.3 (3.3)	2.9 4.1 (1.4)
9	Adenocarcinoma nos	Moderate	N T	0.4 3.3 (8.3)	7.1 19.8 (2.4)	1.9 15.3 (8.1)
10	Mucin producing adenocarcinoma	Poor	N T	0 1.4 (1.4)	0.2 12.3 (61.5)	2.3 86.3 (37.5)
11	Litinis Plastica	Poor	T	2.3	56.2	58.3
12	Gastrointestinal stromal sarcoma	Non-epithelial Poor	T	1.1	4.6	76.8

N: Non-tumor gasrteic tissue; T: Tumor gastric tissue Values in parentheses indicate fold of enzyme activity in tumor with respect to the normal

Table 5. The levels of sulfotransferase activities in human gastric non-tumor and tumor specimens

3.5 Glycan: Sulfotransferase activities in gastric carcinoma

Both Gal3Sulfo-T_4 activity specific for Galβ1, 3GalNAcα- and Gal3Sulfo-T_2 activity utilizing mainly Galβ1,4GlcNAcβ- were found, respectively, at 2.4→61.7 fold and 1.7→156.7 fold elevated level in all the gastric tumor specimens studied. On the other hand, an increased level of GlcNAc6-Sulfo-T activity was also evident but to a lesser extent in nine gastric tumor specimens. Five tumor specimens, all from adinocarcinoma (cases 5, 6 7, 9 and 10) contained predominantly Gal3Sulfo-T_4 while Gal3Sulfo-T_2 dominated in three specimens of Signet ring cell CA(cases 1, 2 and 3).

3.6 The identity of Gal: 3-O-Sulfo transferases in human gastric tumor specimens

Acceptor specificities: A consistent marked elevated Gal: 3-O-Sulfotransferase activities in gastric tumors prompted us to establish further the identity of these enzymes with the known cloned Gal3Sulfotransferases (Chandrasekaran et. al. 2004). We studied four tumor specimens (cases 2, 3, 6 and 7) for acceptor specificities and the results are presented in **Table 6.**

	Gal : 3-O-Sulfotransferase Activity %			
Acceptor	case 6	case 7	case 2	case 3
Galβ1,4GlcNAc	3.2	8.8	100.0 (2438)	100.0 (17550)
Galβ1,3GalNAcα-O-Al	100.0 (2679)	100.0 (3409)	22.7	16.5
3-O-MeGalβ1,4GlcNAcβ1,6(Galβ1,3)GalNAcα-O-Bn	230.2	326.8	48.4	42.9
Galβ1,4GlcNAcβ1,6(3-O-MeGalβ1,3)GalNAcα-O-Bn	11.1	16.7	80.1	73.2
Galβ1,3(GlcNAcβ1,6)GalNAcα-O-Al	489.4	657.3	112.8	90.2
Galβ1,3GalNAcβ1,3Galα-O-Me	222.8	304.2	210.7	178.0
Fetuin triantennary asialo glycopeptide	21.3	15.9	44.0	29.7

Table 6. Establishing the identity of Gal : 3-O-Sulfotransferases in Human Gastric Tumor Specimens

The values in parentheses are the actual CPM designated as 100% for the acceptor Galβ1, 3GalNAcα-O-Al in the cases 6 and 7 and for the acceptor Galβ1,4GlcNAc in the cases of 2 and 3

Gal3Sulfo-Ts of tumor specimens from cases 2 and 3 showed low activity towards Galβ1, 3GalNAcα-O-Al and that from cases 6 and 7 very low activity towards Galβ1, 4GlclNAc. Tumor specimens 6 and 7 contained mostly Gal3Sulfo-T_4 (Chandrasekaran et. al. 2004). Gal3Sulfo-Ts of tumor specimens 2 and 3 were found to be less active towards Fetuin triantennary asialo glycopeptides, which was established as the best acceptor in our earlier studies for Gal3Sulfo-T_3 (Chandrasekaran et. al. 2004). Further, the above enzymes were very active towards Galβ1, 3GalNAcβ1, 3Galα-O-Me whereas Gal3Sulfo-T_3 showed very low activity towards this acceptor. Gal3Sulfo-Ts of tumor specimens 2 and 3 were found to have the identity of cloned Gal3Sulfo-T_2 (Chandrasekaran et. al. 2004).

Influence of divalent metal ions (see **Fig 1**): None of the divalent metal ions Ca^{2+}, Mn^{2+} and Mg^{2+} had any significant stimulating effect on Gal3Sulfo-T of tumor specimen 7. In fact, a gradual decline in enzyme activity was noticed upon increasing the concentration of Mn^{2+} in the reaction mixture. Thus, this enzyme resembled Gal3Sulfotransferase from breast tumor (Chandrasekaran et. al. 1997) as well as the cloned Gal3Sulfo-T_4 (Chandrasekaran et. al. 2004). On the other hand, the metal ions Ca^{2+}, Mn^{2+} and Mg^{2+} stimulated the activity of tumor specimen 3. Mn^{2+} stimulated the activity between 5-20mM and then the activity decreased reaching the initial level at 50mM. This pattern of influence by Mn^{2+} on the activity was quite similar to that of Gal3Sulfotransferase from colon tissue (Chandrasekaran et. al. 1997) and cloned Gal3Sulfo-T_2 (Chandrasekaran et. al. 2004). On the contrary, the activity of cloned Gal3Sulfo-T_3 was stimulated by Mn^{2+} reaching the maximum at 40-50mM

(Chandrasekaran et. al. 2004). Thus, Gal3Sulfo-T of tumor specimen 7 was similar to GalSuflo-T_4 and that of tumor specimen 3 closely resembled Gal3Sulfo-T_2.

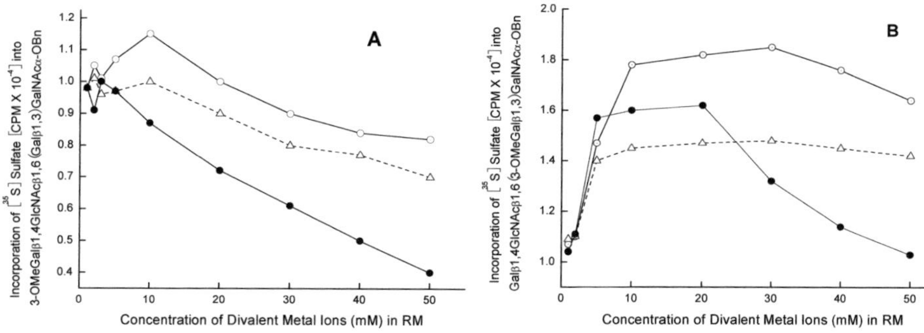

A. Case 7 tumor specimen; B. Case 3 tumor specimen • Mn;Δ Mg; ○ Ca

Fig. 1. Influence of divalent metal ions on gastric tumor Gal3 Sulfotransferase activities.

3.7 Identification of human gastric tissue α- GlcNAc transferase acting on terminal GlcNAc residue

The present investigation identified two N-acetylglucosaminyltransferase activities in gastric tissues using mucin core 2 tri- and tetra-saccharides as acceptors as reported in **Table 7**. An increased level (1.5-8.5 fold) of GlcNAc transferase activity on mucin core 2 tetrasaccharide was observed in three gastric tumor specimens as compared to that of the corresponding non-tumor specimens. Further, the level of this enzyme is about two-fold as compared to the corresponding activity of the other enzyme. The linkages of [6-³H] GlcNAc residues attached to mucin core 2 tri- and tetra-saccharides were further examined by utilizing TLC and lectin-agarose chromatography techniques (see sections 3.8 and 3.9).

Gastric cancer cases		Incorporation [6-³H] GlcNAc (CPM x 10^{-3}) catalyzed by 1 mg protein of the tissue extract	
		Gal β 1, 3 (GlcNAc β 1, 6) GalNAc α-O-Al	Gal β 1, 3 (Gal β 1, 4 GlcNAc β 1, 6) GalNAc α-O-Bn
1	N	5.9	9.8
	T	5.8	14.4
2	N	8.4	18.4
	T	6.8	24.5
5	N	15.7	27.2
	T	5.2	26.7
10	N	2.1	2.7
	T	15.0	23.0
11	T	7.0	16.4

Table 7. The levels of human gastric tissue N-Acetylglucosaminyltransferase activities towards mucin core 2 tri-and tetra-saccharides

3.8 TLC studies

Fig 2 A (lanes A, B, C and D respectively) shows the mobilities (solvent system A) of the acceptor 3-O-Me Gal β 1, 3 (GlcNAc β 1, 6) GalNAcα-O-Bn, the [6-^{3}H] GlcNAc containing product, [6-^{3}H] GlcNAc containing product incubated with and without β-N-acetyl hexosaminidase (Jack bean). Lanes B, C and D show that the radioactive products have the same mobility. It is evident from these results that β-N-acetyl hexosaminidase (Jack bean) was not able to hydrolyze the [6-^{3}H] GlcNAc containing product. Fig 2 B (lanes A and B)shows the mobilities (solvent system B) of 3-O-Me Gal β 1, 3 (GlcNAc β 1, 6) GalNAcα-O-Bn and 3-O-Me Gal β 1, 3 (Gal β 1, 4 GlcNAc β 1, 6) GalNAcα-O-Bn. Lane c shows the mobilities of 3-O-Sulfo Gal β 1, 3 (Gal β 1, 4 GlcNAc β 1, 6) GalNAcα-O-Bn and Std. GlcNAc. Lanes D, E and F show respectively the mobilities of [6-^{3}H] GlcNAc containing product from 3-O-Me Gal β 1, 3 (GlcNAc β 1, 6) GalNAcα-O-Bn, 3-O-Me Gal β 1, 3 (Gal β 1, 4, GlcNAc β 1, 6) GalNAcα-O-Bn and 3-O-Sulfo Gal β 1, 3 (Gal β 1, 4, GlcNAc β 1, 6) GalNAcα-O-Bn after treatment with β-N-acetyl hexosaminidase (Jack bean). It is clear that [6-^{3}H] GlcNAc was released only from the radioactive products arising from the last two acceptors (Lanes E and F) indicating that [6-^{3}H] GlcNAc is β linked to mucin core 2 tetrasaccharide . **Fig 2 C** lane A shows the mobilities (Solvent system B) of acceptor Gal β 1, 3 (GlcNAc β 1, 6) GalNAcα-O-Al and Std. GlcNAc. Treatment with recombinant β 1, 3 Galactosidase resulted in the removal of Gal as evident from the faster mobility of the radioactive product (lane C). β-N-Acetylhexosaminidase (Jack bean) did not act on the radioactive product (compare lanes E and F).

3.9 Lectin-agarose chromatography

The primary sugar specificity of PNA is Gal linked β 1, 3to GalNAc. ConA binds Man and Glc and GSL II binds terminal GlcNAc but these lectins have additional structural requirements for binding. **Fig 3** shows PNA-agarose affinity chromatography of [6-^{3}H] GlcNAc containing product from Gal β 1, 3 (GlcNAc β 1, 6) GalNAcα-O-Al. More than 90% of the product binds to this column as shown in Fig 3 A indicating that [6-^{3}H] GlcNAc is not transferred to the Gal terminal. The radioactive product after recombinant β 1, 3 Galactosidase treatment was subjected to PNA-agarose affinity chromatography and it showed > 90% non-binding to this column. On the contrary to these results, Nakayama et al. (1999) without showing data just mentioned in their paper that their cloned human α 1, 4 N-acetylglucosaminyltransferase acted only on the Gal moiety of mucin core 2 trisaccharide. We find that [6-^{3}H] GlcNAc linkage to β 1, 6 linked GlcNAc in mucin core 2 is completely resistant to Jack bean β-N-acetyl hexosaminidase which has a broad specificity cleaving non-reducing terminal β 1- 2, 3, 4 or 6 linked GlcNAc and GalNAc residues (Li and Li 1970). This enzyme was also able to cleave very efficiently GlcNAc linked β 1, 4 to GlcNAc (N, N'-Diacetylchitobiose) (Li and Li 1970). Thus GlcNAc transferred to β 1, 6 linked GlcNAc has been found to be in α-linkage. Nakayama et al. (1999) reported that α 1, 4 GlcNAc-T was responsible for the formation of GlcNAc α 1, 4 Gal β-R which in turn was responsible for class III mucin ConA reactivity. In this connection, it is noteworthy that the present study found that the radioactive compound [6-^{3}H] GlcNAc α GlcNAc β 1, 6 (Gal β 1, 3) GalNAc α-O-Al did not bind to ConA-agarose as well as GSL II-agarose (**Fig 4 A and B**). After the removal of Gal by recombinant β 1, 3 galactosidase treatment, the resulting radioactive compound still did not bind to GSL II-agarose (**Fig 4 C**).

A

	A	B	C	D
20		59	180	181
19		48	110	174
18		55	106	213
17		62	114	147
16		85	154	80
15		81	180	159
14		527	170	208
13		482	1861	1910
12		69	218	313
11		50	78	121
10		55	132	102
9		50	66	152
8		48	85	97
7		54	79	106
6		40	71	109
5		49	97	110
4		42	127	118
3		49	148	108
2		47	68	139
1		48	114	153

B

	A	B	C	D	E	F
20				80	135	104
19				67	115	78
18				46	125	81
17				72	806	433
16				63	2996	2503
15				55	1954	2238
14				63	303	414
13				67	108	79
12				54	75	51
11				48	107	52
10				74	92	99
9				85	134	136
8				435	288	240
7				512	109	98
6				58	93	52
5				44	108	51
4				58	97	62
3				47	89	47
2				42	79	62
1				50	115	66

C

	A	B	C	D	E
20		62	96	155	102
19		97	62	74	106
18		95	67	102	109
17		98	100	119	94
16		114	99	83	107
15		84	106	90	115
14		83	703	219	247
13		233	2942	158	265
12		142	249	123	100
11		95	97	114	136
10		109	125	233	86
9		816	400	3217	1404
8		3550	392	997	2988
7		287	84	109	136
6		150	62	116	127
5		113	84	124	137
4		130	84	98	102
3		94	69	102	98
2		108	63	137	104
1		85	72	128	121

Fig. 2. TLC Identification of βGlcNAc: αGlcNAc transferase activity in human gastric tumor

Fig. 2 A (solvent system A).
A: Acceptor compound 3-O-Me Gal β 1, 3 (GlcNAc β 1, 6) GalNAc α-O-Bn
B: [6-^{3}H] GlcNAc containing product resulting from A
C and D: B incubated with and without β N-acetylhexosaminidase (Jack bean)
Fig. 2. B (solvent system B).
A: 3-O-Me Gal β 1, 3 (GlcNAc β 1, 6) GalNAc α-O-Bn
B: 3-O-Me Gal β 1, 3 (Gal β 1, 4 GlcNAc β 1, 6) GalNAc α-O-Bn
C: 3-O-Sulfo Gal β 1, 3 (Gal β 1, 4 GlcNAc β 1, 6) GalNAc α-O-Bn and Std. GlcNAc
D, E and F: [6-^{3}H] GlcNAc containing products resulting from A, B and C respectively after β N- acetylhexosaminidase(Jack bean) treatment
Fig. 2. C (Solvent system B).
A: The acceptor Gal β 1, 3 (GlcNAc β 1, 6) GalNAc α-O-Al and Std. GlcNAc
B: [6-^{3}H] GlcNAc containing product resulting from the acceptor in A
C: B after β 1, 3 galactosidase (recombinant) treatment
D and E: B incubated with and without β N- acetylhexosaminidase (Jack bean)

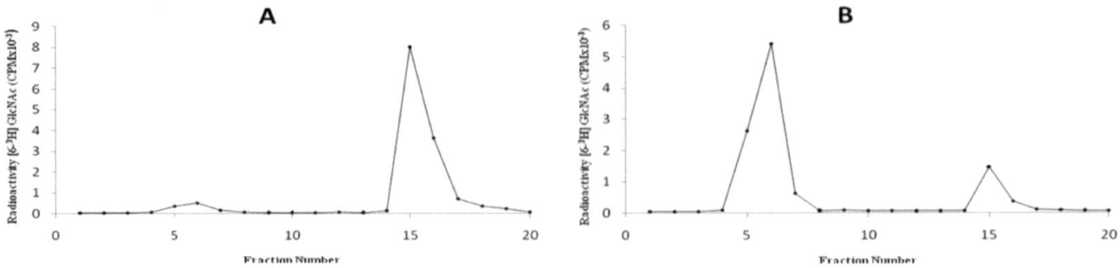

A: [6-³H] GlcNAc containing product resulting from the acceptor Gal β 1, 3 (GlcNAc β 1, 6) GalNAc α-O-Al

B: β 1, 3 galactosidase (recombinant) treated [6-³H] GlcNAc containing product

Fig. 3. PNA-agarose affinity chromatography of [6-³H] GlcNAc containing product

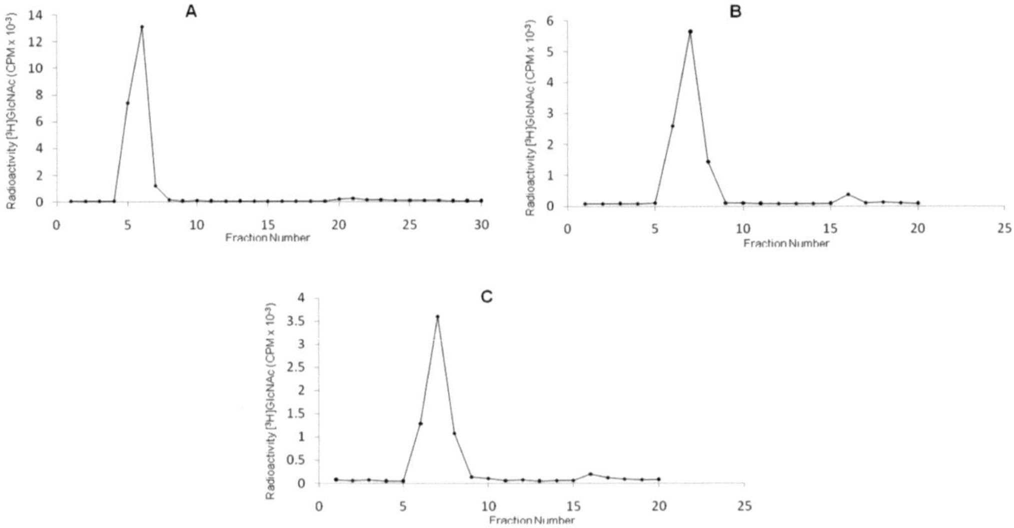

Affinity chromatography of [6-³H] GlcNAc containing product resulting from the acceptor Gal β 1, 3 (GlcNAc β 1, 6) GalNAc α-O-Al on A: Con A-agarose; B: GSL II-agarose; C: GSL II-agarose after β 1, 3 galactosidase (recombinant) treatment

Fig. 4. Chromatography on ConA-agarose and GSL II-agarose

4. Discussion

Many risk factors have been associated with the development of gastric cancer, and the pathogenesis is most likely multifactorial. One postulation on the development of this disease involves a succession of histologic changes that commence with atrophic gastritis, advance to mucosal metaplasia, and eventually result in a malignancy (Layke et al. 2004). Tumor development and growth can be viewed as uncontrolled tissue growth. Tumor growth relies on blood supply by the blood vessels (Kobayashi et al. 2003). It has been known that a growing tumor secretes factors that induce blood vessel growth (i.e., neovascularization) to support its own growth and survival (Folkman et al. 1995). A primary cell type of the blood vessels, especially microvessels in a tumor, is an endothelial cell. Therefore, focus has been to discover factors that specifically control endothelial cell proliferation (Davis et al. 2003). The roles of other factors are just beginning to be understood (Sogn et al. 2005). The tumor microenvironment needs to be completely characterized for understanding its role in tumor progression and metastasis (Sogn et al. 2005). Glycoproteins play a role in pathological processes due to immunological response to the altered oligosaccharides (Fukuda et al. 1996). They have roles in cell adhesion during inflammation and metastasis (Fukuda et al. 1996). Hence it is anticipated that glycoproteins may have a definite role in tumor microenvironment.

Recently an important role for galectins in cancer micrometastasis became evident from the report of Khaldoyandidi, et al. (2003) that interactions between T-antigen of breast cancer cells and galectin-3 mediate both homotypic and heterotypic intercellular adhesion of metastatic breast cancer cells under conditions of flow *in vitro* and *in vivo*. A substitution of sulfate at C-3 position of β-galactosyl residue in T-hapten enhanced its binding efficiency about 15 fold towards galectin-4 and 3 fold towards galectin-3 (Ideo et al. 2002). Similarly, the studies of our laboratory on galectin specificities showed that 3-O-Sulfo Galβ1, 4GlcNAc as compared to Galβ1, 4GlcNAc was 3 fold more efficient in binding to galectin-1 (Allen et al. 1998). Thus, the enhancement of the binding ability to galectins by 3-O-Sulfation of β-galactosyl residues appears to be a common characteristic of galectin family. In addition, 3'-sialylation Core1 in contrast to 3'-sulfated Core1 had very weak affinity for galectin-4 (Ideo et al. 2002). Hippo et al. (2001) analyzed six gastric cancer cell lines by Northern Blot and observed an up-regulation of galectin-4. Sulfatide was found as a major acidic glycolipid in human gastric mucosa (Natomi et al. 1993) and the expression of cerebroside sulfotransferase mRNA in endoscopic bioptic specimens of eleven gastric cancer cases was reported by Kobayashi et al. (1999). The present study finds several fold consistent increase in Gal3Sulfotransferase activity in gastric tumor. The resulting 3-O-Sulfogalactosyl residues in gastric tumor cell glycoproteins and glycolipids may facilitate the interaction of gastric tumor cells with galectin-4, resulting in intercellular homotypic and heterotypic adhesion of gastric cancer cells.

5. Conclusion

It becomes evident from the present study that among the various transferases, which can modify the terminal Gal residues in carbohydrate chains as shown in **Table 2**, only Gal3Sulfotransferases show a consistent several fold elevated activity in all gastric tumor specimens: Gal3-sulfo-T_4 (Gal3-sulfortransferase specific for Galβ1,3GalNAcα-O-Ser/Thr) and GlcNAc6-Sulfo-T are apparently associated with poorly differentiated gastric adenocarcinoma whereas poorly differentiated Signet ring cell gastric carcinoma expresses a high level of Gal3Sulfo-T_2, a Gal3Sulfotransferase acting on Galβ1,4GlcNAcβ- terminal unit. The most consistent change in glycosyltransferase activity could be found only with α1, 2-FT. A significant decrease in this activity was seen in the range 40 – 90% in seven gastric tumor specimens. Thus, the present study was able to show that down regulation of α1,2-FT activity accompanied by induction of Gal3-O-Sulfotransferase activities acting on Gal terminals could be involved in the facile sulfation of carbohydrate chains, which may contribute to the microenvironment suitable for interaction with galectin-4 in promoting tumor growth and metastasis. Furthermore, the sulfation of Gal terminal as well as GlcNAc residues would render the carbohydrate chains strong anionic charge, resistance to degradation by sialidases, galactosidases and hexosaminidases and this would increase their half-life in receptor-mediated glycoprotein clearance.

6. Acknowledgements

This research was supported by the NIH (USA) Grant CA35329 and Comprehensive Cancer Center Support Grant CA160561.

7. References

Allen HJ, Ahmed H, Matta KL (1998) Binding of synthetic sulfated ligands by human splenic galectin 1, a β-galactoside-binding lectin. Glycoconj J 15:691-695.

Amado M, Carneiro F, Seixas M, Clausen H, Sobrinho-Simoes M (1998) Dimeric sialyl-Le(x) expression in gastric carcinoma correlates with venous invasion and poor outcome. Gastroenterology 114:462-470.

Carvalho F, David L, Aubert JP, Lopez-Ferrer A, De Bolos C, Reis, CA, Gartner F, Peixoto A, Alves P, Sobrinho-Simoes M (1999) Mucins and mucin-associated carbohydrate antigens expression in gastric carcinoma cell lines. Virchows Arc 435:479-485.

Chandrasekaran EV, Jain RK, Larsen RD, Wlasichuk K, Matta KL (1995) Selectin-ligands and tumor associated carbohydrate structures: specificities of α2,3-sialyltransferases in the assembly of 3′-sialyl, 6-sulfo/sialyl Lewis a and x, 3′-sialyl, 6′-sulfo Lewis x and 3′-sialyl, 6-sialyl/sulfo blood group T-hapten. Biochemistry 34:2925-2936.

Chandrasekaran EV, Jain RK, Larsen RD, Wlasichuk K, DiCioccio RA, Matta KL (1996) Specificity analysis of three clonal and five non-clonal α1,3-L-fucosyltransferases with sulfated, sialylated, or fucosylated synthetic carbohydrates as acceptors in relation to the assembly of 3′-sialyl-6′-sulfo Lewis x (the L-selectin ligand) and related complex structures. Biochemistry 35:8925-8933.

Chandrasekaran EV, Jain RK, Vig R, Matta KL (1997) The enzymatic sulfation of glycoprotein carbohydrate units: blood group T-hapten specific and two other distinct Gal:3-O-sulfotransferases as evident from specificities and kinetics and the influence of sulfate and fucose residues occurring in the carbohydrate chain on C-3 sulfation of terminal Gal. Glycobiology 7:753-768.

Chandrasekaran EV, Chawda R, Piskorz C, Locke RD, Ta A, Sharad G, Odunsi K, Lele S, Matta KL (2001) Human ovarian cancer, lymphoma spleen, and bovine milk GlcNAc:β1,4Gal/GalNAc transferases: two molecular species in ovarian tumor and induction of GalNAcβ1,4Glc synthesis by α-lactalbumin. Carbohydr Res 334:105-118.

Chandrasekaran EV, Lakhaman SS, Chawda R, Piskorz CF, Neelamegham S, Matta KL (2004) Identification of physiologically relevant substrates for cloned Gal:3-O-sulfotransferases (Gal3STs): distinct high affinity of Gal3ST-2 and LS180 sulfotransferase for the Globo H backbone, Gal3ST-3 for N-glycan multiterminal Galβ1, 4GlcNAcβ- units and 6-sulfoGalβ1, 4GlcNAcβ-, and Gal3ST-4 for the mucin core-2 trisaccharide. J Biol Chem 279:10032-10041.

Chandrasekaran EV, Xue J, Xia J, Chawda R, Piskorz C, Locke RD, Neelamegham S, Matta KL (2005) Analysis of the specificity of sialyltransferases toward mucin Core2, Globo, and related structures. Identification of the sialylation sequence and the effects of sulfate, fucose, methyl and fluoro substituents of the carbohydrate chain in the biosynthesis of selectin and siglec ligands and novel sialylation by cloned α2,3(O)sialyltransferase. Biochemistry 44:15619-15635.

Chandrasekaran EV, Xue J, Neelamegham S, Matta KL (2006) The pattern of glycosyl- and sulfotransferase activities in cancer cell lines: a predictor of individual cancer-associated distinct carbohydrate structures for the structural identification of signature glycans. Carbohydr Res 341:983-994.

Folkman J (1995) Angiogenesis in cancer, vascular, rheumatoid and other disease. Nat Med 1:27-31.

Gendler S J, Spicer A P (1995) Epithelial mucin genes. Annu Rev. Physiol. 57:607-634

Hakomori S (2002) Glycosylation defining cancer malignancy: new wine in an old bottle. Proc Natl Acad Sci USA 99:10231-10233.

Hippo Y, Yashiro M, Ishii M, Taniguchi H, Tsutsumi S, Hirakawa K, Kodama T, Aburatani H (2001) Differential gene expression profiles of scirrhous gastric cancer cells with high metastatic potential to peritoneum or lymph nodes. Cancer Res 61:889-895.

Hiraiwa N, Dohi T, KawakamiKimura N, Yumen M, Ohmori K, Maeda M, Kannagi R (1996) Suppression of sialyl Lewis X expression and E-selectin-mediated cell adhesion in cultured human lymphoid cells by transfection of antisense cDNA of an alpha1→3 fucosyltransferase (Fuc-T VII). J Biol Chem 271:31556-31561.

Hollingsworth M A, Swanson B J (2004) Mucins in cancer: Protection and control of the cell surface. Nat. Rev. Cancer 4:45-60

Ideo H, Seko A, Ohkura T, Matta KL, Yamashita K (2002) High-affinity binding of recombinant human galectin-4 to SO_3-→3Galβ1→3GalNAc pyranoside. Glycobiology 12:199-208.

Khaldoyanidi SK, Glinsky VV, Sikora L, Glinskii AB, Mossine VV, Quinn TP, Glinsky GV, Sriramarao P (2003) MDA-MB-435 human breast carcinoma cell homo- and heterotypic adhesion under flow conditions is mediated in part by Thomsen-Friedenreich antigen -galecin-3 interactions. J Biol Chem 278:27-4134.

Kobayashi T, Honke K, Tsunematsu I, Kagaya H, Nishikawa S, Hokari K, Kato M, Takeda H, Sugiyama T, Higuchi A, Asaka M (1999) Detection of cerebroside sulfotransferase mRNA in human gastric mucosa and adenocarcinoma. Cancer Lett 138:45-51.

Kobayashi M, Lee H, Nakayama J, Fukuda M (2009) Roles of gastric mucin-type O-glycans in the pathogenesis of Helicobacter pylori infection. Glycobiol. 19:453-461

Layke JC, Lopez PP (2004) Gastric Cancer: Diagnosis and treatment options. Am Family Physician 69:1133-1140.

Li S-C, Li Y-T (1970) Studies on the glycosidases of Jack bean meal. III Crystallization and properties of β N-acetylhexosaminidase. J. Biol. Chem. 245:5153-5160

Nakayama J, Yeh J C, Misra A K, Ito S, Katsuyama T, Fukuda M (1999) Expression cloning of a human α1,4- N acetyl glucosaminyltransferase that forms GlcNAcα1, 4 Galβ-R, a glycan specifically expressed in the gastric gland mucous cell-type mucin. Proc. Natl. Acad. Sci. USA 96:8991-8996.

Natomi H, Saitoh T, Sugano K, Iwamori M, Fukayama M, Nagai Y (1993) Systemic analysis of glycosphingolipids in the human gastrointestinal tract: enrichment of sulfatides with hydroxylated longer-chain fatty acids in the gastric and duodenal mucosa. Lipids 28:737-742.

Palcic MM, Heerze LD, Pierce M, Hindsgaul O (1988) The use of hydrophobic synthetic glycosides as acceptors in glycosyltransferase assays. Glycoconj J 5:49-63.

Petretti T, Schulze B, Schlag PM, Kemmner W (1999) Altered mRNA expression of glycosyltransferases in human gastric carcinomas. Biochim Biophys Acta 1428:209-218.

Poste G, Fidler IJ (1980) The pathogenesis of cancer metastasis. Nature 283:139-146.

Ramaswamy S, Ross KN, Lander ES, Golub TR (2003) A molecular signature of metastasis in primary solid tumors. Nat Genet 33:49-54.

Reis CA, David L, Carvalho F, Mandel U, de Bolos C, Mirgorodskaya E, Clausen H, Sobrinho-Simoes M (2000) Immunohistochemical study of the expression of MUC6 mucin and co-expression of other secreted mucins (MUC5AC and MUC2) in human gastric carcinomas. J. Histochem. Cytochem. 48:377-388

Santos-Silva F, Fonseca A, Caffrey T, Carvalho F, Mesquita P, Reis C, Almeida R, David L, Hollingsworth MA (2005) Thomsen-Friedenreich antigen expression in gastric carcinomas is associated with MUC1 mucin VNTR polymorphism. Glycobiology 15:511-517.

Sogn JA, Anton-Culver H, Singer DS (2005) Meeting Reports: NCI Think Tanks in Cancer Biology. Cancer Res 65:9117-9120.

Taniguchi N, Yoshimura M, Miyoshi E, Ihara Y, Nishikawa A, Fuji S. (1996) Remodeling of cell surface glycoproteins by N-acetylglucosaminyltransferase III gene transfection: modulation of metastatic potentials and down regulation of hepatitis B virus replication. Glycobiology 6:691-694.

Taylor-Papadimitriou J, Burchell J, Miles DW, Dalziel M (1999) MUC1 and cancer. Biochim Biophys Acta 1455:301-313.

Werther JL, Tatematsu M, Klein R, Kurihara M, Kumagai K, Llorens P, Neto JG, Bodian C, Pertsemlidis D, Yamachika T, Kitou T, Zkowitz S (1996) Sialosyl-Tn antigen as a marker of gastric cancer progression: an international study. Int J Cancer 69:193-199.

8

Human Epidermal Growth Factor Receptor Family (HER) in Gastric Cancer

Jolanta Czyzewska
Department of Clinical Laboratory Diagnostics Medical University of Bialystok Poland

1. Introduction

The epidermal growth factor receptor family consists of four members with similar structures: HER1/erbB1, HER2/erbB2, HER3/erbB3 and HER4/erbB4. The genes encoded for Erb are proto-oncogenes, or precursor genes, which under normal conditions are present in all cells of an organism. Proto-oncogenes can be activated in several ways, most often it is through structural changes of the cell genome such as point mutation, translocation or amplification (Ghaderi, 2002).

These receptors play an important role in the processes of proliferation and differentiation of normal cells. Hence, any aberrations in their structure or function can be the cause of tumor development and progression. All members of the epidermal growth factor receptor family have a similar structure with an extracellular domain linking the ligand, transmembrane domain and intracytoplasmic domain of the tyrosine kinase. The binding of the ligand to these receptors causes the creation of homodimers and heterodimers as well as the activation of downstream signaling pathways (Ghaderi, 2002). The ligand by inducing extracellular homo and heterodimerization of the ErbB receptors undergoes auto-phosphorylation using intracellular tyrosine residues by arranging the tyrosine kinase domains next to each other. The phosphorylated tyrosine endings of the cytoplasmic receptor act as sites that bind different intracytoplasmic transduction particles, which participate in the cellular response depending on ErbB stimulation (Tvorogov 2009). For this reason the HER family can contribute to tumor progression. Most research has shown a high level expression of the HER family members in patients suffering from gastric cancers (Ghaderi, 2002).

Signaling through the HER pathway plays a fundamental role in the regulation of correct cell growth, proliferation, migration and takes part in such processes like the healing of wounds, cell repair and skin maintenance. However, it has been shown that signaling through the HER pathway plays a very important role in the growth process, replication, migration and survival of cancer cells. Since the HER signaling pathway cascades, causing the strengthening of the growth signal on progressing levels, small changes in the amount or activity of EGRF can significantly accelerate the development or progression of the tumor by facilitating cell replication and migration, and suppression of the apoptosis process (programmed cell death). What is more, many studies have shown that HER signaling, a fundamental factor in correct cell growth and repair, can be activated as a response to different therapies used to treat cancer, like chemotherapy or radiation therapy, and can

lead to cell and tissue damage. It has been suggested that HER pathway activation can contribute to the development of resistance to cancer therapies (Zhou, 1992; Liang, 2003).
Under normal conditions the activation of the EGFR family is controlled by spatial and periodic expression of its ligands, which belong to the EGF-related peptide growth family, such as EGF, heparin-binding EGF (HB-EGF), transforming growth factor alpha (TNF-α) and neuroregulin. These growth factors are synthesized as transmembrane precursors released from the cell surface by proteolytic cleavage and subsequently activate RTKs of the EGFR family in an autocrine or paracrine fashion. Despite the abundance of ligands identified for EGFR, ErbB3 and ErbB4, no direct ligand for HER2 has been discovered. Instead, HER2 functions as a homo or heterodimer with other members of the EGFR family through interaction with anonistic ligands, such as EGF, HB-EGF and TNF-α (Iwamoto, 2006).
Constant activation of receptor kinases leads to excessive activation of the signaling pathway. The causes of kinase over-expression can vary, mutations, autocrine kinase activation or amplification, for example. Elevated signal transfer activity can be connected to an increased risk of tumor development and malignancy (Walles, 1999).

2. HER 1/ EGFR/ HERA/c-erbB1

Epidermal growth factor receptor (EGFR) is one of four receptors in the pathway of epidermal growth factor transfer (HER, human epidermal growth factor receptor). It is a transmembrane glycoprotein consisting of 1186 amino acid residues. The gene encoding ErbB1 is located on chromosome 7 at p12.3-12.1. The emergence of mutation in this region leads to the appearance of mutated forms of EGFR. Three variants of these forms have been identified: I, II, III, with the mutation variant III (ΔEGFR) being most common. It involves the loss of the ligand binding site and leads to permanent spontaneous activation of the tyrosine kinase domain (Wojtukiewicz, 2010).
The EGFR has three domains: extracellular, transmembrane and intracellular. The extracellular domain contains relatively high levels of cysteine residue. It is a site of mitogen activator binding (ligands ErbB1) ex. epidermal growth factor (EGF), tumor necrosis factor α (TNF α), and heparin binding EGF - (HB-EGF). After the ligand attaches to the EGFR there is a change in the conformational isomerism of the receptor particle and dimerization takes place. This interaction allows for the greatest utilization of the characteristics of various combining receptors (Wojtukiewicz, 2010).

3. HER1/EGFR in gastric cancer

Experiments using monoclonal antibodies against c-erbB1 have been carried out during the treatment of different tumors. Among others, tumor fighting properties of the monoclonal human-mouse chimera antibody have been used to neutralize cancer cells in the large intestine both *in vitro* and *in vivo*. The antibody, in the second phase of the experiment, has been adapted for patients with head, neck and lung tumors (Ghaderi, 2002).
Meta-analysis showed the expression of c-erbB1 in gastric cancer in the range from 7.1% to as high as 80.0%. Positive correlation has been shown between the expression of this receptor and the diameter of the tumor, local invasion of the tumor and the spread of cancer cells to surrounding lymph nodes. Additionally, a relationship has been discovered between the stage of the tumor and the expression of c-erbB1. These results suggest c-erbB1

involvement in the progression of gastric cancer in patients from Iran and can be considered to be a prognosticating factor in these tumors. Similarly, high expression of c-erbB1 and its positive correlation with those prognosticating factors can become useful tools for diagnosing and prognosis in gastric patients from Iran. As a result it has been suggested that the expression of this receptor should be monitored as part of routine patient screening (Ghaderi, 2002).

4. c-erbB2, HER2/neu

HER2/neu is a proto-oncogene encoding transmembrane tyrosine kinase with a mass of 185 kDa. c-erbB-2 is encoded by a gene located on chromosome 17 (Ghaderi, 2002). Located on the cell membrane it binds with its extracellular growth factor ligands to HER-2 which leads to dimer formation with another HER-2 molecule or with HER-1, HER-3 or HER-4. Dimerization causes phosphorylation of tyrosine residue in the cytoplasmic domain of the receptor and a further activation of the intracellular transfer pathway, which regulates various biological reactions, including cell proliferation, differentiation, movement and survival. High expression of c-erbB-2 has been described in various types of tumors such as breast cancer, ovarian cancer, lung cancer, salivary gland cancer, cancer of the large intestine, prostate cancer and pancreatic cancer. It has also been suggested that this protein is an indicator of an unfavorable outcome (Satiroglu- Tufan, 2006).

ErbB2 does not have its own ligands and plays the role of a co-activator in relation to the other proteins of the ERBB family. Its basic signaling results from the ability to react with other ERBB receptors. The receptor can undergo stabilization as well as transactivation through the ligands specific to ERBB1 and ERBB3, which allows ERBB2 to take part in signal transfer. Heterodimers created by ERBB2 are considered to be particularly active (Citki, 2003; Lee, 2001).

Attachment of various ligands to the extracellular domain initiates the cascading of signal transduction. The ligand attaching to the EGFR induces homodimerization and heterodimerization with other types of HER proteins. HER2 does not attach to any known ligand but it is a preferred partner of heterodimerization for other members of the HER family. The HER2 gene, located adjacent to the topoisomerase IIa, is related to the oncogene v-erbB of the avian erythroblastosis virus. In tumors HER2 behaves like an oncogene, mainly because high level of gene amplification induces over-expression of the protein on the cell membrane and which then acquires characteristics typical to atypical cells (Gravalos, 2008).

In normal cell signal transduction Her2 plays a role of a growth factor and is connected with the regulation of cell growth, survival and differentiation. Its downstream signaling can be activated by point mutations, gene amplification or gene over-expression. There exists a hypothesis that high ERBB2 expression aids spontaneous dimerization which contributes to ERBB2 activation and downstream signaling (Arrington, 2009).

Amplification of the ERBB2 gene and/or the over-expression of its protein have been discovered in 20-30% of breast cancers. Over-expression of HER2, along with negative estrogen reception and early metastasis of these cancers, is treated as an independent factor predicting survivability and recurrence of the disease (Arrington, 2009).

5. HER2 in gastric cancer

HER2 expression in gastric cancer was described for the first time in 1986 (Gravalos, 2008). In breast tumors ERBB2 functions as an oncogene, with gene amplification and protein overexpression in the cell membrane. Not only is gene amplification an indicator of unfavorable prognosis it is also a predictive marker for therapies using the monoclonal antibody trastuzumab on patients with breast cancer with metastases. Amplification of ERBB2 has been found not only in breast cancers but in other malignant tumors such ovarian cancer, lung cancer, cancer of the large intestine and gastric cancer. With the use of immunohistochemistry, in gastric cancer the expression of ERBB2 has been shown in 5.2-22.6% of cases, while the percentage of ERBB2 amplification with the use of fluorescent in situ hybridization (FISH) was within the range of 3.8-12.2%. However, clinical significance of ERBB2 amplification/overexpression in gastric cancer patients is still unclear (Barros-Silva, 2009).

An anomaly most commonly found in tumors is gene amplification with an increase of HER2 protein expression. In people with gastric cancer HER2 over-expression/amplification is detected in 15-59% of advanced tumors. In gastric cancer the up-regulation of HER2 expression can control the cell cycle, cell movement and invasion through several intracellular paths. HER2 signaling plays a fundamental role in the development, progression and metastasis of gastric cancer (Lee, 2010).

When the HER2 signal spreads from the cell surface to the intracellular effectors it requires a signal transducer and activates Grb2 (growth factor receptor- bound 2). It is thought that Grb2, which facilitates HER2 signaling, plays a fundamental role in the development of breast cancer, its progression and metastasis. Janes et al. (1994) have shown that in breast cancer cells HER2 over-expression was connected with the Grb2-SOS1 complex, which activated the Raf/MEK/MAPK pathway through Ras. However, the role of Grb2 and its connection to HER2 were seldom described in gastric cancer. Yu et al. (2009) have shown that Grb2 overexpression in the main mass of the tumor as well as in metastasis occurs late in the process of gastric cancer development. Overexpression of Grb2, however, was connected with unfavorable prognosis for these patients. Researchers have also shown a significant correlation between Grb2 and HER2 in stomach tumors (Yu, 2009).

Bao et al. (2010) utilized RNA interference in gastric cancer from SGC-7901 and MNK-45 cultures to halt the activity of the HER2 oncogene. Through this work they have shown that HER2 is not only closely connected to tumor growth but also to its invasiveness. Even as Sarna-HER2 stopped the growth of gastric cancer cells, HER2 reduced the migration and invasiveness of cancer cells. By comparing the HER2- knockdown group with the control group the researchers discovered the presence of several markers of metastasis: COL1A1, ACTA2, E- katherine, MMP-2 and MMP-9. The knockdown of HER2 was accompanied by significant deregulation of MMP-1, despite unchanged levels of MMP-2 and MMP-9. They also demonstrated that HER2 can regulate MMP-1 expression at the transcription level. HER2 does not increase transcription activity through Myc, SRY, CREB or NF-κB attachment sites. This could be caused by downstream particles that have not been detected in bioinformatic analysis and which have the ability to attach to the MMP-1 promoter region and to regulate its transcription activity. Another interesting phenomenon was the fact that when MMP-1 was reduced the invasiveness of cells was nearly completely blocked. However, transcription of the MMP-1 expressing vector into shRNA-HER2 cells, which displayed a low ability for metastasis, resulted in only a partial restoration of the invasiveness of these cells. This data shows that MMP-1 is a downstream effector of HER2 and that HER2 can have an influence on other particles connected to metastasis, with the exception of MMP-1 (Bao, 2010).

6. HER3

The ERBB3 encoding gene is located on the 12 chromosome at q13. The proteins encoded by it show a low activity of tyrosine kinase. In comparison to ERBB2 and ERBB4, ERBB3 displays a much lower homologation of the endothelial and cytoplast domains with the ERBB1 receptor, (Kraus, 1989; Lebeau, 2001). In all probability the ERBB3 by itself does not function as an oncogene, but increase of its expression can strengthen the oncogenic effect caused by the over expression of the ERBB2 receptor (Alimandii, 1995).

7. HER3 in gastric cancer

The expression of the HER3 protein is very often observed in advanced gastric tumors. It has been shown that HER3 expression is connected with gastric cancer progression and prognoses, while the HER1 or HER2 expression did not show a similar relationship. In the conducted *in vitro* experiments, HER3 blocking caused the decrease of the downstream signals and the death of tumor cells. It would seem that HER3 could be potentially useful in clinical treatment of cancer patients, especially those with stomach tumors. HER3 is associated with the signals mediated from HER1 or HER2, and it may be also associated with the resistance to anti-HER1 or anti-HER2 therapies. High expression of the HER3 protein could be an indicator of an unfavorable prognosis for gastric cancer patients. Positive staining has been observed more often in advanced tumors with high malignancy when compared to early stage cancers, which can point to the involvement of this protein in the progression process of the disease. Co-expression of HER3 and HER2 has not been connected to gastric cancer prediction. The creation of a heterodimer of HER3/HER1 has been observed in gastric cancer cells. What is more, a relationship between the expression of HER3 and HER1 proteins has been observed. The expression of HER1 has been accepted as a prognosis indicator for patients with gastric cancer. The expression of HER3 protein had a stronger correlation with remote metastases and the survival time of gastric cancer patients then HER1 expression. The role of the HER4 protein expression in gastric cancer has not been determined. A positive immunohistochemical reaction to this protein has been equally often observed in early stage and in advanced gastric cancer. A recent study of gastric cancer cells show that the GER family kinases were targets of amplified fibroblast growth factor receptor 2, and the inhibition of HER3 which resulted in the loss of cell proliferation initiated by the fibroblast growth factor receptor 2. For this reason, therapies involving blocking of HER3 can become part of the new strategy in gastric cancer treatment, along with therapies using anti-HER1 and anti-HER2 treatments (Hayashi, 2008).
Kabayashi et al. (2003) demonstrated that activation of phosphoinositide-3-kinase (P13K)/Akt triggered by phosphorylation of HER3 was important for dedifferentiatiated phenotypes of gastric cancer cell cultures. They also showed that HER3 signal pathway contributed to the development of dedifferentiated carcinomas by promoting motility and invasion of adenocarcinoma cells. This evidence supports the possible involvement of HER3 in the dedifferentiation process of gastric cancer.

8. HER4

The gene encoding ERBB4 is located on chromosome 2 at q33.3-34 (Zimonjic, 1995). This gene is activated after combining with a neuroregulator, betacellulin and heparin-binding

EGF-like growth factor. Its activation leads to cell proliferation, chemotaxis or differentiation through the utilization of particular signal transferring proteins like P13K kinase and Shc (Carpentre, 2003). Even though the ERBB4 structure and function is similar to other members of the ERBB family it is still unclear what role, general or specific, ERBB4 plays in human tumor development. Protooncogenes, including EGFR and ERBB2, are most often evaluated in the light of mutation presence in tumors (Lynch, 2004; Peaz, 2004; Pao, 2004; Stephens, 2004; Shigama, 2005). For this reason it can be assumed that ERBB4 as a protooncogene is also subject to mutation in human tumors (Soung, 2006).

Tvorogov et al (2009) has shown that 2 of 10 mutations destroy the catalytic activity of ERBB4 tyrosine kinase. However, despite losing tyrosine kinase activity, two mutated receptors were still able to form a "working" heterodimer with ERBB2 and to activate mitogen-actived protein kinase Erk and phosphoinositide 3-kinase/Akt pathway. The mutant receptors were able to activate Erk and phosphoinositide 3-kinase/Akt signaling pathway to a similar extent as the wild-type ERBB4. ERBB4 kinase activity was required for NRG-induced activation of the signal transducer and activator of transcription 5 (STAT5), resulting in failure of ERBB4 mutants to activate STAT5 (Tvorogov, 2009). Whereas Erk and phosphoinositide 3-kinase/Akt pathway have been implicated in the survival and proliferation of cancer cells, the role of STAT5 signaling in cancer is not yet fully understood, however increased STAT5 signaling has been associated with transformation. (Yu, 2004).

9. HER4 in gastric cancer

The role of ERBB4 in the process of carcinogenesis has not been completely defined. YH Soung et al. (2006) described ERBB4 kinase domain mutation in gastric, breast, lung and large intestine tumors. It is the first report describing mutation of the ERBB4 kinase domain in human tumors. The location of the mutation in the kinase domain, a location very important for functioning, can suggest that the discovery of ERBB4 mutation could be a change in function. (Soung, 2006). Stephens et al. (2005) found ERBB4 mutation in 1 of 25 studied breast tumors and it was found outside the kinase domain. Soung et al. (2006) has shown a convergence in the presence of ERBB4 and K-RAS mutations in gastric cancer, which can occur and could play a role in the process of pathogenesis of gastric cancer. These observations are different from previous observations where the K-RAS mutation in patients with lung cancer was not connected to neither EGFR nor ERBB2 mutations (Kosaka, 2004). The presence of ERBB4 mutation in commonly appearing human tumors, can act as a green light to initiate research into introduction of therapies aimed at eliminating mutated ERBB4.

HER4 gene expression was higher in cancerous tissue in comparison to healthy tissue of a gastric tumor (Kataoka , 2008).

10. HER2 amplification

The amplification of the oncogene HER2 is an important biomarker in identification of patients who could react to HER2 therapy using the humanized monoclonal antibody transtuzumab (herceptin). Fluorescence *in situ* hybridization (FISH) or chromogenic *in situ* hybridization (CISH) can be used to assess weather tissue samples contain gene amplification. The FISH method is currently considered to be the "gold standard" in HER2 amplification detection. This method has a high sensitivity (96.5%) and specificity (100%)

(Pauletti, 1996). An additional advantage of this method is that it can be used on small samples and cuttings preserved in formaldehyde or paraffin. FISH facilitates the direct display of gene amplification in the cell nucleus and enables gene and chromosome count on a cell-by-cell basis (Park, 2006). CISH is an attractive alternative to FISH. Tissue preparation and the process of sample hybridization are the same for both methods. These techniques differ in the method of detection which in CISH involves the initiation of a reaction with peroxidase which can be seen with the help of an optical microscope and that allows for an easy assessment of tissues and amplification products. Additionally, CISH allows the creation of a permanent record and is much cheaper than FISH. Since CISH is a relatively new method, the comparison between CISH and FISH is still being made in the clinical setting (Park, 2006).

Wolf- Yadlin et al. (2006) made an attempt at explaining different effects of HER2 amplification in carcinomas with different growth patterns. These researches suggested that HER2 overexpression causes an increase in cell migration but has a minimal effect on proliferation of cells being stimulated by the epidermal growth factor (EGF) or heregulin. For this reason HER2 amplification can increase cell migration in expanding tumors, while infiltrative carcinomas, which posses high invasive potential, do not gain additional advantages with HER2 amplification.

Many researchers have shown that HER2 overexpression can be used as a prognostic factor for gastric cancer patients. The multi-variative analysis study performed by Brien et al. (1998) showed that the pathological stage and HER2 gene amplification are independent prognostic factors for survivability. Allgayer et al. (2000) confirmed the importance of HER2 status as a prognostic factor in a prospective study of gastric cancer. They have demonstrated a significant association between the level of HER2 expression and shorter recovery and overall survival.

11. Therapies using antibodies against the her family members

11.1 Trastuzumab (herceptin)

Trastuzumab (herceptin) is a recombined humanized monoclonal antibody anti-HER2mAb (rhuMAb HER2) with particle mass of 145531.5 g/mol. It was engineered from a cloned human IgG, with structure and antigen-binding residues of a potent murine mAb 4D5. Exact mechanics of how it behaves are not known, however it has been speculated that it plays a role in blocking the division of the HER2 receptor and dimerization; impedes the intracellular transference path P13K; has an anti-angiogenic effect by modulating the effects of pro and anti-angiogenic factors; or arresting cell proliferation in the G1 phase (Baselga, 2009;Valabrega, 2007; Hayashi, 2008).

Usually tastuzumab is well tolerated. When administered during therapy as the only medication side effects such as bone marrow suppression, nausea and vomiting or baldness are seldom observed (Hudis, 2007). However, trastuzumab therapy is connected with an increased risk of cardiotoxicity. This heart disorder is the most part reversible after discontinuation of the drug (Okines, 2010).

It has been shown that in patients with HER2 positive breast cancer, herceptin treatment does extend survival time. Among breast cancer patients with metastases, high HER2 expression and presence of amplification signified better effectiveness of trastuzumab therapy (Slamon, 2001).

HER2 status is usually determined by immunohistochemistry (IHC) and/or *in situ* hybridization. In IHC the four-tiered scoring system described originally for the Food and

Drug Administration (FDA), the HerceptTest, has been approved. Samples scored as 0 and 1+ are negative, 2+ as equivocal and 3+ as positive. However, the American Society of Clinical Oncology/College of American Pathologists (ASCO/CAP) guidelines require in-house validation of 1+ and 3+ samples with ISH before a certified laboratory can confine ISH retesting to 2+ samples (Batran, 2008). Recently, a modification of the HercepTest scoring system for gastric carcinomas was proposed (Table 1).

Intensity score	Staining pattern		HER2 expression
	surgical specimen	biopsy specimen	
0	no reactivity or membranous reactivity in <10% of tumor cells	no reactivity or membranous reactivity in any tumor cell	negative
+1	faint/barely perceptible membranous reactivity in ≥10% of tumor cells; cells are reactive only in part of their membrane	tumor cell clusters with faint/ barely perceptible membranous reactivity, regardless of percentage of tumor cells stained	negative
+2	weak-to-moderate complete, basolateral or lateral membranous reactivity in ≥10% of tumor cells	tumor cell clusters with weak-to-moderate complete, basolateral or lateral membranous reactivity, regardless of percentage of tumor cells stained	equivocal
+3	strong complete, basolateral or lateral membranous reactivity in ≥10% of tumor cells	tumor cell clusters with strong complete, basolateral or lateral membranous reactivity, regardless of percentage of tumor cells stained	positive

Table 1. Recommended scoring system to evaluate immunohistochemistry staining patterns in patients with advanced gastric cancer. (Yoon, 2011).

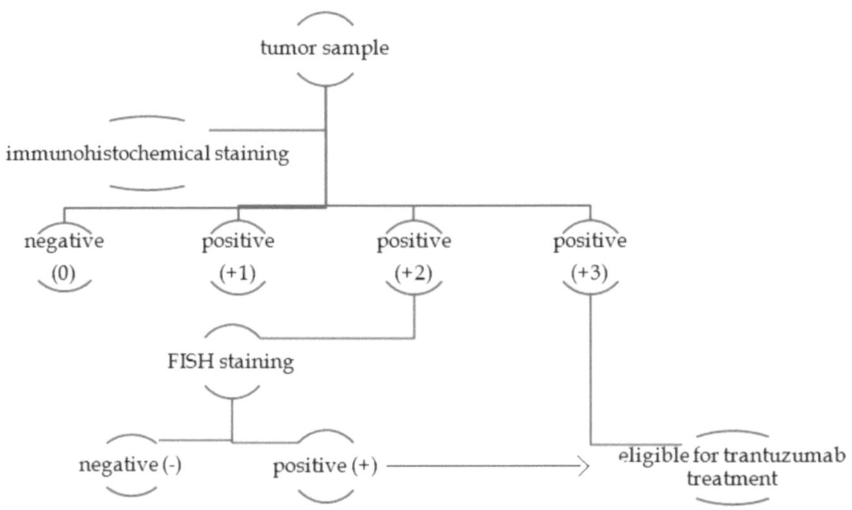

Fig. 1. HER2 testing algorithm in metastatic gastric and esophagogastric junction cancers. FISH: Fluorescence *in situ* hybridization; IHC: Immunohistochemistry (Yoon, 2011).

11.2 Cetuximab (anti-epidermal growth factor receptor monoclonal antibody)

Cetuximab is a class IgG1 monoclonal antibody designed to bind with the epidermal growth factor receptor (GFR) (Martinelli, 2009). Cetuximab binds to the extracellular domain of the EGFR in its non-active configuration and competes to bind with the receptor through sealing the ligand binding site. This interaction of the antibody and the receptor prevents dimerization of the receptor and so blocks the tyrosine kinase activation dependant on the EGFR ligand. Additionally cetuximab induces EGFR internalization, downregulation and degradation. By provoking an anti-cancer response dependant on the immune system, cetuximab represses the proliferation of cancer cells (stops the G1 phase), the production of vascular endothelial growth factor (VEGF), tumor dependant angiogenesis and the invasion of cancer cells (Ciardiello, 2008; Lordick, 2010).

The monoclonal antibody cetuximab has demonstrated antitumor efficacy both as a monotherapy and when combined with chemotherapy. (Lenz, 2006; Van Custen, 2007). Importantly, cetuximab treatment partially indicates that EGFR may improve resistance to irinotecan-based chemotherapy in a group of patients (Cuninghtam, 2004). Previous studies also reported that the EGFR TKI gefitinib worked well in combination with topo I inhibitors and platinum agents (Nagashima, 2006; Braun, 2005; Stewart, 2004; Van Schaeybroech, 2005).

Pinto et al. (2009) published the results of the II phase of a study concerned with the treatment of patients with advanced gastric cancer with the drug combination: cetuximab and cisplatin. The response to this combination of drugs, observed at 41%, was higher than treatment with cisplatin or docetaxel alone. These researches have also shown that the entire progression rate was approximately eight months and was longer than during treatment with irinotecan or %- fluorouracil. Similar results were obtained by Lordick et al. (2010), with an average disease progression rate of 7.6 months. A slightly shorter disease progression time (about 5.5 months) and a response to treatment with cetuximab at 50% were observed by Han et al. (2009) in their research.

11.3 Lapatinib

Lapatinib is a potent ATP - a competitive inhibitor that simultaneously inhibits both EGFR and HER2. In cell-free biochemical kinase assays, lapatinib inhibits the recombinant EGFR and HER2 tyrosine kinase by 50% at concentrations of 10.8 and 9.3 nmol/L, respectively. In cell-based assays, lapatinib inhibits the growth of HER2-overexpressing BT474 breast cancer cells at comparably low concentrations of 100 nmol/L (Konecny, 2006).

Lapatinib showed significant results when combined with trastuzumab in HER2- amplified gastric cancer cells. The combination of lapatinib and trastuzumab induces nearly complete tumor regression in all of the mice that have been treated. Those effects were much more pronounced than either lapatinib or trastuzumab alone (Wainberg, 2010). Although results of Wainberg et al. (2010) were only preliminary, they support the ongoing investigation of lapatinib in gastric cancer as well as its possible combination with trastuzumab in HER2-amplified disease. The addition of anti-HER2 therapy to standard chemotherapy could have direct clinical benefit and makes the investigation of additional anti-HER2 therapies in upper gastrointestinal cancers, very desirable (Wainberg, 2010).

HER2 amplification is an important prognosis factor for the growth inhibitory activity of lapatinib in gastric cancer. Kim et al. (2008) has shown that lapatinib inhibits the phosphorylation of EGFR and HER2, and through this also impedes signal transfer from Akt and Erk in the gastric cancer cells sensitive to lapatinib. Lapatinib halted the G1 phase of the cell cycle in cell cultures SNU-216, NCI-N87 and SNU-484, which displayed a growth inhibitory effect at higher concentrations. Furthermore, cMyc reduction and $p27^{kip1}$ induction were also observed after lapatinib treatment. Conversely, the induction of apoptosis by lapatinib is linked to the inhibition of the Akt pathway, rather than the Erk pathway (Kim, 2008). Lapatinib blocks Erk phosphorylation through the stimulation of the IGF-1 ligand. However, the inhibitory effects for IGF-1- stimulated phosphorylation of the IGF-1 receptor were not seen in SNU-484. It could be that lapatinib inhibits the downstream signaling of the phosphorylated IGF-1 receptor via EGFR, considering that it is a complex between the IGF-1 receptor and EGFR which activates the Erk pathway (Kim, 2008).

Lapatinib, in combination with 5-FU, is currently used as the prodrug capecitabine in treating patients with breast cancers with HER2 expression in a clinical investigation of solid tumors (Geyer, 2006). It has been shown that lapatinib exhibits a high anticancer effectiveness in cells with high EGFR or HER2 expression (Rusnak, 2007; Konecny, 2006). Overexpression and/or amplification of HER2 in patients with breast cancer have been determined to be important prognostic factors in treating with lapatinib (Konecny, 2006).

11.4 Gefitinib

Gefitinib is an orally active, quinazoline tyrosine kinase inhibitor, selective for EGFR. Its anticancer effectiveness has been shown in lung cancer treatment. Somatic mutations within the ATP- binding pocket of the tyrosine kinase domain of the EGFR, including small in-frame deletions and missense substitutions, are present in lung adenocarcinomas and confer responsiveness to gefitinib in lung cancer patients (Lynch, 2004; Paez, 2004). Yokoyama et al. (2006), have shown for the first time that cell cultures (GLM-1, GLM-2 i GLM-4, NCI-N87) of gastric cancers were more sensitive to gefitinib than traztuzumab. Gefitinib induced apoptosis in cells demonstrating HER2 overexpression, something that has not been observed in commonly used gastric cancer cell cultures without HER2 expression.

It still seems unclear why gefitinib, an EGFR inhibitor, displays anticancer properties with gastric cancer cells that are HER2 positive but not those that are EGFR positive. Anido et al. (2003) have put forward a hypothesis that gefitinib prevents the formation of HER2/HER3 heterodimers by taking part in the sequestration of HER2 and HER3 with inactive (nonphosphorylated) EGFR/HER2 and EGFR/HER3 heterodimers. Yokoyama et al. (2006) has shown that gefitinib can selectively arrest the phosphorylation of Akt only in cells with HER2 overexpression, although cells with low HER2 expression also displayed constitutive activation of P13K/Akt pathway. This suggests that gefitinib can selectively block activated P13K/Akt pathways only because it is simply driven by HER2 overexpression along with relatively high expression of HER3, which permits the formation of the HER2/HER3 heterodimer (Yokoyama, 2006). The other interesting discovery made by these researchers has been the claim that gastric cancer cell cultures with HER2 overexpression become resistant to gefitinib. Gefitinib resistant cells of the GLM-1R culture have displayed an increase of EGFR expression and a more differentiated morphology in comparison to parental cells of the GLM-1 culture. The Shs and Erk1/2, upstream and downstream signaling molecules of the MAPK pathway, were also upregulated in GLM-1R cells. Additionally, the inhibition of the phosphorylation of Akt in GLM-1 parental cells in response to gefitinib treatment was weakened when the path Ras/MAPK was highly stimulated by higher concentrations of EGF. These observations can suggest that the pathway EGFR-Ras-MAPK is really (but in moderation) activated in compensation for the blockage of the HER2-P13K-Akt pathway in GML-1R cells, which results in persistent growth when gefitinib is present and the build up of resistance (Yokoyama, 2006).

12. Immunohistochemical evaluation expression of her2 and her1/egfr

Many investigators subsequently evaluated HER2 status in gastric cancer cells by IHC (immunohistochemistry). The frequency of HER2 overexpression was varied widely from 8 to 31 %. The consensus of almost all reports is that the majority of positive cases are the intestinal type histologically. Methods of IHC which evaluate for HER2 status in gastric cancer have not been standardized and that is a wide range in the frequency of overexpression, furthermore, there have been few reports claiming to have demonstrated HER2 gene amplification in gastric cancer (Sato, 1997; Takehana, 2002).

There are conflicting results in studies of HER2 with regard to its relationship to prognosis in gastric cancer patients. Some studies have reported that HER2 overexpression is a poor prognostic factor for gastric cancer (Uchino, 1993; Chariyalertsah, 1994; Mizutani, 1993). DI Park 2006 demonstrated that HER2 is an prognostic parameter in gastric cancer. Similar finding demonstrated Yonemura et al. (1991, 1991). They showed that immunoreactivity to HER2 can be an independent prognostic value in gastric cancer. Mizutani et al. (1993) reported significantly poorer prognoses for patients suffering from early gastric cancer who were HER2 positive in IHC. However, other studies have failed to fund any association with prognosis whatsoever (Hilton, 1992; Kołodziejczyk, 1994; Tateishi, 1992; Sasano, 1993). Orita et al. (1997) elucidated prognostic significance of the expression of c-erbB-2 oncogene in gastric cancer patients. They found out that c-erbB-2 protein expression was associated with considerably shorter postoperative survival time. In patients with positive and negative c-erbB-2 expression, a 5-year survival reached 29% and 47%, respectively. Similar results have been reported by some other authors (Tsugawa, 1998; Nakajima, 1999; Pinto-de-Sousa, 2002). These data suggest that c-erbB-2 expression can be a prognostic factor for gastric cancer patients. However, according to other studies, c-erbB-2 does not exert a significant effect on the overall survival time of gastric cancer patients (Gurel, 1999; Polakowski, 1999).

The first preliminary data concerning the level of EGFR in the gastric wall were described by Yasiu et al. (1988), indicating an increase in the level of EGFR in neoplastic tissue compared to normal mucus. Similar observations have been reported by other authors (Kopp, 2002; Coyle, 1999). Kopp et al. (2002) suggested that in case of chronic inflammation or tissue damage the physiological effect of the ligand for the EGF-receptor pathway, associated with the regulation of regeneration and healing in the gastric mucus, may additionally stimulate the process of neoplastic transformation in the gastric mucus and tumor progression. We observed EGFR expression in 50% of the evaluated cases of gastric cancer. High expression was observed mainly in the intestinal type and poorly differentiated cancers, as well as in those infiltrating the whole gastric wall or at least into the muscular layer. However, we found no statistical significance. As reported by Gamboza-Dominguez et al. (2004), lack or low expression of EGFR protein was significantly correlated with prolonged postoperative survival time, as compared to the moderate and strong expression.

13. Conclusion

Signaling through the HER pathway plays a fundamental role in the regulation of cell growth, proliferation, migration and survival of neoplastic cells. Moreover, HER signaling can be activated as a response to different therapies used to treat cancer, like chemotherapy or radiation therapy, and can lead to cell and tissue damage. Elevated signal transfer activity can be connected to an increased risk of tumor development and malignancy. Positive correlation has been shown between the expression of these receptors and the local invasion of the tumor, lymph nodes metastases and stage of gastric cancer. .Overexpression of these factors may be a prognosticating factor in these tumors. As a result it has been suggested that the expression of HER family receptors should be monitored as part of routine patient screening. It was suggested, that blocking of the action of GER family receptors can be used in the treatment of gastric cancer. These agents, combined with chemiotherapy and other targeted can be used in the future as a oncological therapy.

14. Referenses

Ghaderi, A; Vasei, M; Maleck-Hosseini, SA; Gharesi- Fard, B; Khodami, M; Dorouchi, M; Modjtahedi, H. (2002). The expression of c-erbB-1 and cerbB-2 in Iranian patients with gastric carcinoma. *Pathology Oncology Research*, Vol.8, No.4, pp252-256.

Zhau, HE; Wan, DS; Zhou, J; Miller, GJ; von Eschenbach, AC. (1992). Expression of c-erbB-2/neu proto- oncogene in human prostate cancer tissues and cell lines. *Mol Carcinog*, 5, pp320-327.

Liang, K; Ang, KK; Milas, L; Hunter, N; Fan, Z. (2003). The epidermal growth factor receptor mediates radioresistance. *Int J Radiat Oncol Biol Phys*, 57, pp246-245

Iwamoto, R; Mekada, E. (2006). ErbB and HG-EGF signaling in heart development and function. *Cell Struct Funct*, 31, pp1-14.

Walles, A. (1999). EGF receptor. *Int J Biochem Cell Biol*, 31, pp637.

Wojtukiewicz, MZ; Sierko, E; Szambora, P. (2010). Patofizjologiczne podstawy terapii ukierunkowanej na zahamowanie funkcji receptora czynnika wzrostu naskórka (EGFR). *Onkol Prak Klin*, Vol.6, No.5, pp217-227.

Satiroglu- Tufan, NL; Bir, F; Calli-Demirkan, N. (2006). Investigation of HER-2 codon 655 single nucleotide polymorphism frequency and c-ErbB-2 protein expression alterations in gastric cancer patients. *World J Gastroenterol*, Vol.12, No.20, pp3283-3287, ISSN 1007- 9327.

Citki, A; Kochuperakkal, BS; Yarden, Y. (2003). The deaf and dumb: the biology of ErbB-2 and ErbB-3. *Exp Cell Res*, 284, pp54.

Lee, H; Akita, RW; Sliwkowski, MX; Maihle, NJ. (2001). A naturally occurring secreted human ErbB-2, ErbB-3, and ErbB- 4. *Cancer Res*, pp4467.

Gravalos, C; Jimeno, A. (2008). HER2 in gastric cancer: a new prognostic factor and a novel therapeutic target. *Annals of Oncology*, 19, pp1523-1529.

Arrington, AK; Dahlerg PS; Davydova, J; Veckers, SM; Yamamoto, M. (2009). ERBB2 suppression decreases cell growth via apoptosis in gastrointestinal adenocarcinomas. *Surgery*, 146, pp213-219.

Barros-Silva, JD;Leitão, D; Afonso, L; Vieira, J; Dinis- Riberio, M; Fragoso, M; Bento, MJ; Santos, L; Ferreira, P; Rêgo, S; Brandão,C; Carneiro, F; Lopes, C; Schmitt, F; Teixeira, MR. (2009). Association of ERBB2 gene status with histopathological parameters and disease- specific survival in gastric carcinoma patients. *British Journal of Cancer*, 100, pp487-493.

Lee, MS; Cha, EY; Thuong, PT; Kim, JY; Ahn, MS; Sul, JY. (2010). Down-regulation of human epidermal growth factor receptor 2/neu oncogene by corosolic acid induces cell cycle arrest and apoptosis in NCI-N87 human gastric cancer cells. *Biol Pharm Bull*, 33, pp931-937.

Janes, PW; Daly, RJ; DeFazio, A; Sutherland, RL. (1994). Activation of the Ras signaling pathway in human breast cancer overexpressing erbB-2. *Oncogene*, 9, pp3601-3608.

Yu, GZ; Chen, Y; Wang, JJ. (2009). Overexpression of Grb2/HER2 signaling in Chinese gastric cancer: their relationship with clinicopathological parameters and prognostic significance. *J Cancer Res Clin Oncol*, 135, pp1331-1339.

Bao, W; Fu, HJ; Jia, LT; Zhang, Y; Li, W; Jin, BQ; Yao, LB; Chen, SY; Yang, AG. (2010). HER2-mediated upregulation of MMP-1 is involved in gastric cancer cell invasion. *Archives of Biochemistry and Biophysics*, 499, pp49-55.

Kraus, MH; Issing, W; Miki, T; Popescu, NC; Aaronson, SA (1989). Isolation and characterisation of c-erbB3, a third member of the erbB-epidermal growth factor receptor family; evidence of overexpression in a subset of human mammary tumours. *Proc Natl Acad Sci, USA*, 86, pp9193- 9197.

Lebeau, A; Deimling, D; Kaltz, C; Sendelhofert, A; Iff, A; Luthardt, B; Untch, M; Löhrs U. (2001). HER-2/neu analysis in archival tissue samples of human breast cancer: comparision of immunohistochemistry and fluorescence in situ hybridization. *J Clin Oncol*, 19, pp354- 363.

Alimandii, M; Romano, A; Curia, MC, Muraro, R; Fedi, P; Aaronson, SA; Di Fiore, PP; Kraus, MH. (1995). Cooperative signaling of ERB-3 and ERB-2 in neoplastic transformation and human mammary carcinomas. *Oncogene*, 10, pp1813.

Hayashi, M; Inokuchi, M; Takagi, Y; Yamada, H; Kojima, K; Kumagai, J; Kawano, T; Sugihara, K. (2008). High expression of HER3 is associated with decreased survival in gastric cancer. *Clin Cancer Res*, 14,pp7843-7849.

Kabayashi, M; Iwamatsu, A; Shinohara-Kanda, A; Ihara, S; Fukui, Y. (2003). Activation of ErbB3-P13-kinase pathway is correlated with malignant phenotypes of adenocarcinomas. *Oncogene*, 22, pp1294-1301.

Zimonjic, DB; Alimandii, M; Miki, T; Popescu, NC; Kraus, MH. (1995). Localization of the human HER4/ERBB-4 gene to chromosome 2. *Oncogene*, 10, pp1235- 1237.

Carpentre, G. (2003). ErbB-4: mechanism of action and biology. *Exp Cell Res*, 284, p66-77.

Lynch, TJ; Bell, DW; Sordella, R; Gurubhagavatula, S; Okimoto, RA; Brannigan, BW; Harris, PL; Haserlat, SM; Supko, JG; Haluska, FG; Louis, DN; Christiani, DC; Settleman, J; Haber, DA. (2004). Activating mutations in the epidermal growth factor receptor underlaying responsiveness of non-small-cell lung cancer to gefitinib. *N Engl J Med*, 350, pp2129- 39.

Peaz, JG; Janne, PA, Lee, JC; Tracy, S; Greulich, H; Gabriel, S; Herman, P; Kaye, FJ; Lindeman, N; Boggon, TJ; Naoki, K; Sasaki, H; Fujii, A; Eck, MJ; Sellers, WR; Johnson, BE; Meyerson, M. (2004). EGFR mutations in lung cancer: correlation with clinical response to gefitinib therapy. *Science*, 304,pp1497-500.

Pao, W; Miller, V; ZAkowski, M; Doherty, J; Politi, K; Sarkaria, I; Singh, B; Heelan, R; Rusch, V; Fulton, L; Mardis, E; Kupfer, D; Wilson, R; Kris, M; Varmus, H. (2004). EGF receptor gene mutations are common on lung cancer from "never smokers" and are associated with sensitivity of tumors to gefitinib and erlotinib. *Proc Natl Acad Sci USA*, 101, pp13306-13311.

Stephens, P; Hunter, C; Bignell, G; Edkins, S; Davies, H; Teague, J; Stevens, C; O'Meara, S; Smith, R; Parker, A; Barthorpe, A; Blow, M; Brackenbury, L; Butler, A; Clarke, O; Cole, J; Dicks, E; Dike, A; Drozd, A; Edwards, K; Forbes, S; Foster, R; Gray, K; Greenman, C; Halliday, K; Hills, K; Kosmidou, V; Lugg, R; Menzies, A; Perry, J; Petty, R; Raine, K; Ratford, L; Stepherd, R; Small, A; Stephens, Y; Tofts, C; Varian, J; West, S; Widaa, S; Yates, A; Brassuer, S; Cooper, CS; Flanagan, AM; Knowles, M; Leung, SY; Louis, DN; Looijenga, LH; Malkowicz, B; Pierotti, MA; Teh, B; Chenevix-Trench, G; Weber, BL; Yuen, ST; Harris, G; Goldstraw, P; Nicholson, AG;

Futreal, PA; Wooster, R; Stratton, MR. (2004). Lung cancer: intragenic ERBB2 kinase mutations in tumours. *Nature*, 431, pp525-526.

Shigematsu, H; Takahashi, T; Nomura, M; Majmudar, K; Suzuki, M; Lee, H; Witsuba, II; Fong, KM; Toyooka, S; Shimizu, N; Fujisawa, T; Minna, JD; Gazdar, AF. (2005). Somatic mutations of the HER2 kinase domain in lung adenorarcinomas. *Cancer Res*, 65, pp1642-1646.

Soung, YH; Lee, JW; Kim, SY; Wang, YP;Jo, KH; Moon, SW; Park, WS; Nam, SW; Lee, JY; Yoo, NJ; Lee, SH. (2006). Somatic mutations of the ERBB4 kinase domain in human cancers. *Int J Cancer*, 118, pp1426-1429.

Tvorogov, D; Sundvall, M; Kurppa, K; Hollmén, M; Repo, S; Johnson, MS; Elenius, K. (2009). Somatic mutations of ErbB4- selective loss-of-function phenotype affecting signal transduction pathways in cancer. *J Biol Chem*, 284, pp5582-5591.

Yu, H; Jove, R. (2004). The STATs of cancer--new molecular targets come of age. *Nat Rev Cancer*, 4, pp97-105. Stephens, P; Edkins, S; Davies, H; Greenman, C, Cox C; Hunter, C; Bignell, G; Teague, J; Smith, R; Stevens, C; O'Meara, S; Parker, A; Tarpey, P; Avis, T; Barthorpe, A; Brackenbury, L; Buck, G; Butler, A; Clements, J; Cole, J; Dicks, E; Edwards, K; Forbes, S; Gorton, m; Gray, K; Halliday, K; Harrison, R; Hills, K; Hinton, J; Jones, D; Kosmidou, V; Laman, R; Lugg, R; Menzies, A; Perry, J; Petty, R; Raine, K; Shepherd, R; Small, A; Solomon, H; Stephens, J; Tofts, C; Varian, J; Webb, A; West, S; Widaa, S; Yates, A; Brasseur, F; Cooper, CS; Flanagan, AM; Green, A; Knowles, M; Leung, SY; Looijenga, LH; Malkowicz, B; Pierotti, AM; Teh, B; Yuen, ST; Nicholson, AG; Lakhani, S; Easton, DF; Weber, BL; Stratton, MR; Futreal, PA; Wooster, R. (2005). A screen of the complete protein kinase gene family identifies diverse patterns of somatic mutations in human breast cancer. *Nat Genet*, 37, pp590-592.

Kosaka, T; Yatabe, Y; Endoh, H; Kuwano, H; Takahashi, T; Mitsudomi, T. (2004). Mutations of the epidermal growth factor receptor gene in lung cancer: biological and clinical implications. *Cancer Res*, 64, pp8919-8923.

Kataoka,H; John, T; Kasugasi, K; Okayama, N; Moriyama, A; Asai, K; Kato, T. (2008). Expression of mRNA for heregulin and its receptor, ErbB-3 and ErbB-4, in human upper gastrointestinal mucosa. *Life Sci*, 63, pp553-564.

Pauletti, G; Godophin, W; Press, MF, Salomon, DJ. (1996). Detection and quantitation of HER-2/neu gene amplification in human breast cancer archival material using fluorescence in situ hybridization. *Oncogene*, 13, pp63-72.

Park, DIL; Yun, JW.; Park, JH; Oh, SJ, Kim, HJ; Cho, YK; Sohn, CIL; Jeon, WK; Kim, BI; Yoo, CH; So, BH; Cho, EY; Chae, SW; Kim, EJ; Sohn, JH; Ryu, SH; Sepulveda, AR. (2006). HER-2/neu amplification is an independent prognostic factor in gastric cancer. *Dig Dis Sci*, 51, pp1371-1379.

Wolf-Yadlin, A; Kumar, N; Zhang, Y; Hautaniemi, S; Zaman, M; Kim, HD; Grantcharova, V; Lauffenburger, DA; White, FM. (2006). Effects of HER2 overexpression on cell signaling networks governing proliferation and migration. *Mol Syst Biol*, 2,pp1-15.

Brien, TP; Depowski, PL; Sheehan, CE; Ross, JS; McKenna, BJ. (1998). Prognostic factors in gastric cancer. *Mod Pathol*, 11, pp870-877.

Allgayer, H; Babic, R; Gruetzner, KU; Tarabichi, A; Schiidberg, FW; Heiss, MM. (2000). c-erb-B2 is on independent prognostic relevance in gastric cancer and is associated with the expression of tumor- associated protease system. *J Clin Oncol*, 18, pp2201-2209.

Baselga, J; Swain, SM. (2009). Novel anticancer targets: revisting ERBB2 and discovering ERBB3. *Nat Rev Cancer*, 9, pp463-475.

Valabrega, G; Montemurro, F; Aglitta, M. (2007). Transtuzumab:mechanism of action, resistance and future perspectives in HER2-overexpressing breast cancer. *Ann Oncol*, 18, pp977-984.

Hudis, CA. (2007). Transtuzumab- mechanism of action and use in clinical practice. *N Engl J Med*, 357, pp39-51.

Okines, AFC; Cunningham, D. (2010). Transtuzumab in gastric cancer. *European Jurnal of Cancer*, 46, pp1949-1959.

Slamon, DJ; Leyland-Jones, B; Shak,S Fuchs, H; Paton, V; Bajamonde, A; Fleming, T; Eiermann, W; Wolter, J; Pegram, M; Baselga, J; Norton, L. (2001). Use of chemotherapy plus a monoclonal antibody against HER2. *N Engl J Med*, 344, pp783-792.

Batran, AL; Hartmann, JT; Probst, S; Schmalenberg, H; Hollerbach, S; Hofheinz, R; Rethwisch, V; Seipelt, G; Homann, N; Wilhelm, G; Schuch, G; Stoehlmacher, J; Derigs, HG; Hegewisch-Becker, S; Grossmann, J; Pauligk, C; Atmaca, A; Bokemeyer, C; Knuth, A; Jäger, E. (2008). Phase III trial in metastatic gastroesophagel adenocarcinoma with fluorouracil, leucovorin plus either oxaplatin or cisplatin: a study of the Arbeitsgemeinschaft Internistiche Onkologie. *J Clin Oncol*, 26, pp1435-1442.

Yoon, H; Kang, YK. (2011). Recommended scoring system to evaluate immunohistochemistry staining patterns in patients with advanced gastric cancer. Results and implications of the Trastuzumab for Gastric Cancer (ToGA) trial. *Clinical Investigation* 1(1), pp87-95.

Mortinelli, E; De Palma, R; Orditura, M; De Vita, F; Ciardiello, F. (2009). Anti-epidermal growth factor receptor monoclonal antobodies in cancer therapy. *Clin Exp Immunol*, 158,pp1-9.

Ciardiello, F; Tortora, G. (2008). EGFR antagonists in cancer treatment. *N Ehngl J Med*, 358, pp1160-1174.

Lordick, F; Luber, B; Lorenzen, S; Hegewisch-Becker, S; Folprecht, G; Wöll, E; Decker, E; Endlicher, E; Röthling, N; Schuster, T;Keller, G; Fend, F; Peschel, C. (2010). Cetuximab plus oxaliplatin/leucovorin/5-fluorouracil in first-line metastatic gastric cancer: a phase II study of the Arbeitsgemeinschaft Internistiche Onkologie (AIO). *British Journal of Cancer*, 102, pp500-505.

Lenz, HJ; Van Custem, E; Khambata-Ford, S; Mayer, RJ; Gold, P; Stella P; Mirtsching, B; Cohn, AL; Pippas, AW; Azarnia, N; Tsuchihashi, Z; Mauro, DJ; Rowinsky, EK. (2006). Multicenter phase II and Translational study of cetuximab in metastatic colorectal carcinoma refractory to irinotecan, oxaliplatin, and fluoropyrimidines. *J Clin Oncol*, 24, pp4914-4921.

Van Cutsem, E; Nowacki, MP; Lang, I; Cascinu, S; Shcheptin, I; Maurel, J; Rougier, P; Cunningham, D; Nippen, J; Kohne, C. (2007). Randomized phase III study of irinotecan and 5-FU/FA with or without cetuximab in the first-line treatment of patients with metastatic colorectalcancer (mCRC): the CRYSTAL trial. *J Clin Oncol*, 25, abstract 4000.

Cunningham, D; Humblet, Y; Siena, S; Khayat, D; Bleiberg, H; Santoro, A; Bets, D; Mueser, M; Harstrick, A;

Verslype, C; Chau, I, Van Cutsem, E. (2004). Cetuximab monotherapy and cetuximab plus irinotecan in irinotecan-refractory metastatic colorectal cancer. *N Engl J Med*, 351, pp337-345.

Nagashima, S; Soda, H; Oka, M; Kitazaki, T; Shiozawa, K; Nakamura, Y; Takemura, M; Yabuuchi, H; Fukuda, M; Tsukamoto, K; Kohno, S. (2006). BCRP/ABCG2 levels account for the resistance to topoisomerase I inhibitors and reversal effects by gefitinib in non-small cell lung cancer. *Cancer Chemiother Pharmacol*, 58,pp594-600.

Braun, AH; Stark, K; Dirsch, O; Hilger, RA; Seeber, S; Vanhoefer, U. (2005). The epidermal growth factor receptor tyrosine kinase inhibitor gefitinib sensitizes colon cancer cells to irinotecan. *Anticancer Drungs*, 16, pp1099-1108.

Steward, CF; Leggas, M; Schuetz, JD; Panetta, JC; Cheshire, PJ; Peterson, J; Daw, N; Jenkins, JJ; Gilberson, R;

Germain, GS; Harwood, Fc; Houghton, PJ. (2004). Gefitinib enhances the antitumor activity and oral bioavailability of irinotecan in mice. *Cancer Res*, 64, pp7491-7499.

Van Schaeybroeck, S; Karaiskou-McCaul, A; Kelly, D; Longley, D; Galligan, L; Van Cutsem, E; Johnson, P. (2005). Epidermal growth factor receptor activity determines response of colorectal cancer cells to gefitinib alone and in combination with chemiotherapy. *Clin Camcer Res*, 11, pp7480-7489.

Pinto, C; Di Fabio, F; Siena, S; Cascinu, S; Llimpe, FL; Ceccarelli, C; Mutri, V; Giannetta, L; Giaquinta, S; Funaioli, C; Berardi, R; Longobardi, C; Piana, E; Martoni, AA. (2007). Phase II study of cetuximab in combination with FOLFIRI in patients with untreated advanced gastric or gastroesophageal junction adenocarcinoma (FOLCETUX study). *Ann Oncol*, 18, pp510-517.

Han, SW; Oh, DY; Im, SA; Lee, KW; Song, HS; Lee, NS; Lee, KH; Choi, IS; Lee, MH; Kim, MA; Kim, WH; Bang, YJ; Kim, TY. (2009). Phase II study and biomarker analisis of cetuximab combined with modifiedFOLFOX6in advanced gastric cancer. *Br J Cancer*, 100, pp298-304.

Konecny, GE; Pegram, MD, Venkatesan, N; Finn, R; Yang, G; Rahmeh, M; Untch, M; Rusnak, DW; Spehar, G; Mullin, RJ; Keith, BR; Gilmer, TM; Berger, M; Podratz, KC; Slamon, DJ. (2006). Activity of the dual kinase inhibitor lapatinib (GW572016) against HER-2- overexpression and transtuzumab- treated brest cancer cells. *Cancer Res*, 66, pp1630-1639.

Wainberg, ZA; Anghel, A; Desai, AJ; Ayala, R; Luo, T; Safran, B; Fejzo, MS; Hecht, JR; Slamon, DJ; Finn, RS. (2010). Lapatinib, a dual EGFR and HER2 kinase inhibitor, selectively inhibits HER2- amplified human gastic cancer cells and is synergistic with Trastuzumab *in vitro* and *in vivo. Clin Cancer Res*,16, pp1509-1519.

Kim, JW.; Kim, HP; Im, SA; Kang, S; Hur, HS; Yoon, YK; Oh, DY; Kim, JH; Lee, DS.; Kim, TY; Bang, YJ. (2008). The growth inhibity effect of lapatinib, a dual inhibitor of EGFR and HER2 tyrosine kinase, in gastric cancer cell lines. *Cancer Letters*, 272, pp296-306.

Geyer, CE; Forster, J; Lindquist, D; Chan, S; Romie, CG; Pienkowski, T; Jagiello- Gruszweld, A; Crown, J; Chan, A; Kauffman, B; Skarlos, D; Campone, M; Davidson, N; Berger, M; Oliva, C; Rubin, SD; Stein, S; Cameron, D. (2006). Lipatinib plus capecitabine for HER2-positive advanced breast cancer. *N Engel J Med.*, 355, pp2733-2743.

Rusnak, DW; Alligood, KJ; Mullin, RJ; Spahar, GM; Arenas-Elliott, C; Martin, AM; Degenhardt, Y; Rudolph, SK; Haws, TF; Hudson-Curtis, BL; Gilmer, TM. (2007). Assessment of epidermal growth factor receptor (EGFR, ErbB1) and HER2 (ErbB2) protein expression levels and response to lapatinib (Tykerb, GW572016) in an expanded panel of human normal and tumor cell lines. *Cell Prolif*, 40, pp580-594.

Yokoyama, H; Ikehara, Y; Kodera, Y; Ikehara, S; Yatabe, Y; Mochizuki, Y; Koine, M; Fujiwara, M; Nakao, A; Tatematsu, M; Nakanishi, H. (2006). Molecular basis for sensitivity and acquired resistance to gefitinib in HER2-overexpressing human gastric cancer cell lines derived from liver metastasis. *British J Cancer*, 95, pp1504-1513.

Anido, J; Matar, P; Albanell, J; Guzman, M; Rojo, F; Arribas, J; Averbuch, S; Baselga, J. (2003). ZD1839, a specific epidermal growth factor receptor (EGFR) tyrosine kinase inhibitor, induces the formation of inactive EGFR/HER2 and EGFR/HER3 heterodimers and prevents heregulin signaling in HER2-overexpressing breast cancer cells. *Clin Cancer Res*, 9, pp1274-1283.

Sato, T; Abe, K; Kurose, A; Uesugi, N; Todokori, T; Sasaki, K. (1997). Ampification of the c-erbB-2 gene detected by FISH in gastric cancers. *Pathol Int*, 47, pp179-182.

Takehana, T; Kunitomo, K; Kono, K; Kitahara, F; Iizuka, H; Matsumoto, Y; Fujino, AF; Ooi, A. (2002). Status of c-erbB-2 in gastric adenocarcinoma: a comparative study o immunohistochemistry, fluorescencje *in situ* hybrydyzation and enzyme-linked immunosorbent assai. *Int J Cancer*, 98, pp833-837.

Uchino, S; Truda, H; Marayama, K; Kinoshita, T; Sasako, M; Saito, T; Kobayashi, M; Hirohashi, S. (1993). Overexpression of c-erb-B2 protein in gastric cancer. Its correlation with long term survival of patients. *Cancer*, 72, pp3179-3184.

Chariyalertsak, S; Sugano, K; Ohkura, H; Mori, Y. (1994). Comparison of c-erb-B2 oncoprotein expression in tissue and serum of patients with stomach cancer. *Tumor Biol*, 15, pp294-303.

Mizutani, T; Onda, M; Tokunaga, A; Yamanaka, N; Sugisaki, Y. (1993). Relationship of c-erb- B2 protein expression and gene amplification to invasion and metastasis in human gastric cancer. *Cancer*, 72, pp2083-2038.

Yonemura, Y; Ninomiya, I; Ohoyama S; Kimura, H; Yamaguhi, A; Fushida, S; Kosaka, T; Miwa, K; Miyazaki, I; Endou, Y; at al.(1991). Expression of c-erbB-2 oncoprotein in gastric carcinoma. Immunoractivity for c-erbB-2 protein is an indicator of poor short- term prognosis in patients with gastric carcinoma. *Cancer*, 67, pp2914-2918.

Yonemura, Y; Ninomiya, I; Yamaguchi, A; Fushida, S; Kimura, H; Ohoyama, S; Miyazaki, I; Endou, Y; Tanaka, M; Sasaki, T. (1991). Evaluation expressionof immunoractivity for erbB-2 protein as a marker of poor short term prognosis in gastric cancer. *Cancer Res*,51;pp1034-1038.

Hilton, DA; West, KP. (1992). c-erb-B2 oncogene product expression and prognosis in gastric carcinoma. *J Clin Pathol*, 45, pp454-456.

Kolodziejczyk, P; Yao, T; Oya, M; Nakamura, S; Utsunomiya, T; Ishikawa, T; Tsuneyoshi, M. (1994). Long- term follow-up study of patients with gastric adenomas with malignant transformation. An immunohistochemical and histochemical analysis. *Cancer*, 74, pp2896-2907.

Tateishi, M; Toda, T; Minamisono, Y; Nagasaki, S. (1992). Clinicopathological significance of c-erb-B2 protein expression in human gastric carcinoma. *J SurgOncol*, 49, pp209-212.

Sasano, H; Date, F; Imatani, A; Asaki, S; Nagura, H. (1993). Double immunostaining for c-ereb-B2 and p53 in human stomach cancer cells. *Hum Pathol*, 24, pp584-589.

Orita, H; Maehara, Y; Emi, Y; Kakeji, Y; Baba, H; Korenaga, D; Sugimachi, K. (1997). c- erbB-2 expression is predictive for lymphatic spread of clinical gastric carcinoma. *Hepato-Gastroenterology*, 44, pp 294-298.

Tsugawa, K; Yonemura, Y; Hirono, Y; Fushida, S; Kaji, M; Miwa, K; Miyazaki, I; Yamamoto, H. (1998). Amplification of the c-met, c-erbB-2 and epidermal growth factor receptor gene in human gastric cancers: correlation to clinical features. *Oncology*, 55, pp475- 481.

Nakajima, M; Sawada, H; Yamada, Y; Watanabe, A; Tatsumi, M; Yamashita, J; Matsuda, M; Sakaguchi, T; Hirao, T; Nakano, H. (1999). The prognostic significance of amplification and overexpression of c-met and c-erbB-2 in human gastric carcinomas. *Cancer*, 85, pp1894- 1902.

Pinto-de-Sousa, J; David, L; Almeida, R; Leitão, D; Preto, JR; Seixas, M; Pimenta, A. (2002). c-erbB-2 expression is associated with tumor location and venous invasion and influences survival of patients with gastric carcinoma. *Int J Surg Pathol*, 10, pp247-256.

Gurel, S; Dolar, E; Yerci, O; Samli, B; Ozturk, H; Nak, SG; Gulten, M; Memik, F. (1999). The relationship between c-erbB-2 oncogene expression and clinicopathological factors in gastric cancer. *J Int Med Res*, 27, pp74- 78.

Polkowski, W; van Sandick, JW; Offerhaus, GJ; ten Kate, FJ; Mulder, J; Obertop, H; van Lanschot, JJ. (1999). Prognostic value of Lauren classification and c-erbB-2 oncogene overexpression in adenocarcinoma of the esophagus and gastroesophageal junction. *Ann Surg Oncol*, 6, pp290- 297.

Yasui, W; Sumiyoshi, H; Hata, J; Kameda, T; Ochiai, A; Ito, H; Tahara, E. (1988). Expression of epidermal growth factor in human gastric and colonic carcinomas. *Cancer Res*, 48, pp137- 141.

Kopp, R; Ruge, M; Rothbauer, E; Cramer, C; Kraemling, HJ; Wiebeck, B; Schildberg, FW; Pfeiffer, A. (2002). Impact of epidermal growth factor (EGF) radioreceptor analysis on long-term survival of gastric cancer patients. *Anticancer Res*, 22, pp1161-1167.

Coyle, WJ; Sedlack, RE; Nemec, R; Peterson, R; Duntemann, T; Murphy, M; Lawson, J. (1999). Eradication of *Helicobacter pylori* normalizes elevated mucosal levels of epidermal growth factor and its receptor. *Am J Gastroenterol*, 94, pp2885- 2889.

Gamboza- Dominguez, A; Dominguez- Fonseca, C; Quintanilla- Martinez, L; Reyes-Gutierrez, E; Green, D; Angles- Angles, A; Busch, R; Hermannstadter, C; Nahrig, J; Becker, KF; Becker, I; Hofler, H; Fend, F; Luber, B. (2004). Epidermal growth factor receptor expression correlates with poor survival in gastric adenocarcinoma from Mexican patients: a multivariate analysis using a standardized immunohistochemical detection system. *Mod Pathol*, 17, pp579-587.

9

Free Radicals and Gastric Cancer

Mahmoud Lotfy[1] and Yousery E. Sherif[2]
[1]*Associate Professor of Molecular Cell Biology & Immunology, Molecular and Cellular Biology Department, Genetic Engineering and Biotechnology Research Institute, Minufiya University, Sadat City, Minufiya, Egypt and Department of Applied Medical Sciences, Jouf University, Qurayat,*
[2]*Clinical Pharmacology Department, Faculty of Medicine, Mansoura University, Mansoura, Egypt and Department of Chemistry, Faculty of Science and Arts, Olla, Taibah University, Saudi Arabia*

1. Introduction

The inflammation is linked to tumorigenesis by a variety of molecules. The prostaglandins, cytokines, nuclear factor-kappa B (NF-kappa B), chemokines, angiogenic growth factors, and free radicals, are key factors involved in that process. Reactive oxygen and nitrogen species play a crucial role in the progression from normal gastric mucosa to cancer. Oxidative stress is associated with gastric disorders such as chronic gastritis, peptic ulcers, gastric cancer and mucosa-associated lymphoid tissue (MALT) lymphoma. During malignant transformation, the increased oxygen radicals generation initiates lipid peroxidation and DNA and proteins oxidation processes causing DNA and proteins structural and functional damages that lead finally to the loss of cell integrity. The major interest in elucidating the role of oxidative stress in a range of diseases has focused attention on drugs that can prevent the generation of reactive oxygen species or enhance their metabolism. The response to such interventions can give insight into the underlying role of reactive oxygen species in the pathophysiology and may point to future therapeutic targets. In this chapter, we present the most updated knowledge on free radicals and antioxidants in gastric cancer.

2. Free radicals

Free radicals are molecules containing unpaired electrons such as $O_2•$, •OH, ROO•, and RO• (Figure 1). They are unstable and highly reactive components. Proteins, lipids, and nucleic acids are subject to oxidation by reactive oxygen species (ROS) generated during normal metabolism and even more so under conditions of oxidative stress. The intracellular levels of oxidized proteins have been shown to increase during aging and in the development of many age-related diseases, including Alzheimer's disease, rheumatoid arthritis, atherosclerosis, and Parkinson's disease (Khan et al, 2004) (Table 1). Moreover, an increase in intracellular ROS leads to initiation of various types of cell death (Yuyama et al., 2003).

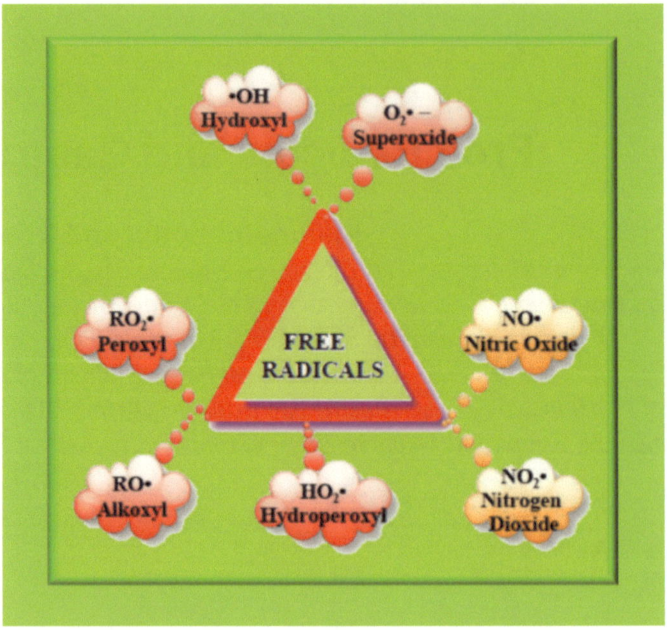

Fig. 1. Reactive oxygen species (ROS) and reactive nitrogen species (RNS).

Generation of oxygen as superoxide, hydrogen peroxide and hydroxyl radicals are involved in killing microorganisms by leukocytes. However, these same reactive oxygen species may damage cells (Babior et al, 1973). To counteract these oxidants, cells have several antioxidant enzymes including superoxide dismutase (SOD; EC 1.15.1.I), glutathione peroxidase (GSH-PX) and catalase. Eukaryotic cells have two forms of SOD; one found in the mitochondrial matrix, the manganese SOD (Mn-SOD), and another found predominantly in the cytosol, the copper-zinc SOD (Cu/Zn-SOD). Prokaryotes have another, iron SOD (Marklund, 1984). These enzymes dismutate superoxide to H_2O_2, which is then converted to water by either catalase or GHX-PX. The GSH-PX uses the reduced glutathione to convert H_2O_2 to water as well as to convert lipid peroxide to lipid metabolites and eicosenoids. A delicate balance exists between expression of each SOD and GHX-PX to provide cellular resistance to oxidative stress (Kelner & Bagnell, 1990). It has been shown that in some cancers, reduced expression of Mn-SOD is due to mutations in the promoter of the gene, while in other types of cancer, reduced levels of Mn-SOD are due to abnormal methylation, loss of heterozygosity or mutation in the coding sequence (Hernandez-Saavedra & McCord, 2003). These different mechanisms cause the chaotic results about SOD in malignant tumors including gastric cancer, colorectal cancer and other gastrointestinal tumors (Hwang et al, 2007; Skrzydlewska et al, 2003; Tandon et al, 2004).

Proteins are ubiquitous in all cells and tissues, constituting more than 50% of the dry weight of cells, and are susceptible to oxidative/nitrosative modifications. When reactive oxygen species (ROS) and reactive nitrogen species (RNS) levels exceed the cellular antioxidant capacity, a deleterious condition known as oxidative/nitrosative stress occurs (Figures 2 & 3). It describes a status in which cellular antioxidant defenses are insufficient to keep the levels of ROS/RNS below a toxic threshold. This may be either due to excessive production of ROS/RNS, loss of antioxidant defenses or both. Unchecked, excessive ROS/RNS generation can lead to the destruction of cellular components including proteins, and ultimately cell death via apoptosis or necrosis (Giustarini et al, 2004).

Condition	Reference
Cancer	Hofseth, (2008).
Cigarette Smoking	Pasupathi et al, (2009) & El-Zayadi, (2006).
Aging	Adiga & Adiga, (2009).
Atherosclerosis	Shaikh & Suryakar, (2009) & Sumathi et al, (2010).
Rheumatoid Arthritis	Shinde et al, (2010) & Ahmed, (2005).
Diabetes	Kundu et al, (2011).
Infertility	Duru et al, (2001).
Asthma	Fabian et al, (2011).
COPD	Hakhamaneshi et al, (2007).
Neurodegeneration	Abraham et al, (2005).
Acute Ischaemic Stroke	Aygul et al, (2006).
Epilepsy	Hamed & Abdellah, (2004).
Skin disease	Aly & Shahin (2010).
Schistosomiasis Infection	Rizk et al, (2006).
Alcoholic Liver Disease	Maithreyi et al, (2010).
Esophagitis	Jiménez et al, (2005).

Table 1. Some clinical situations that are associated with altered oxidative/antioxidative balance as evidenced in the mentioned studies.

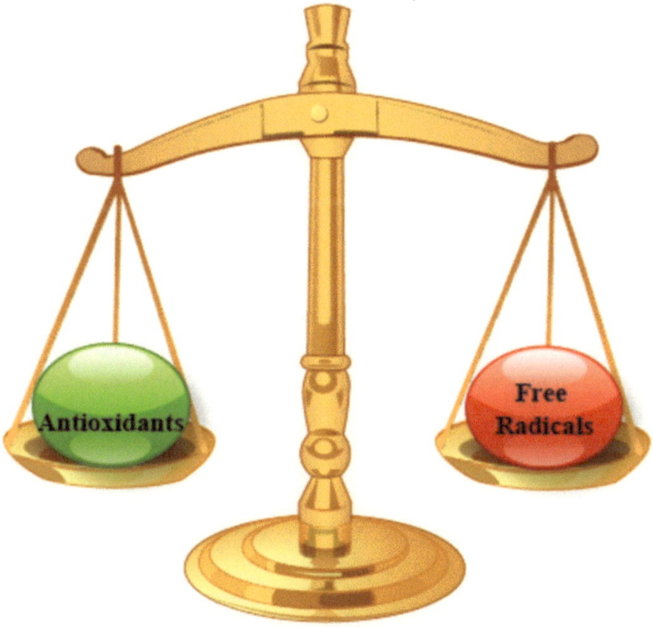

Fig. 2. The balance between free radicals levels and antioxidant defense system is favoring the health. On the contrary, the imbalance between them is leading to the oxidative stress and hence to the damage of cellular compartments and consequently to the disease.

3. Cancer and free radicals

Malignancy comprises a diverse set of diseases that not only originate from almost every tissue but also display remarkable heterogeneity in presentation and prognosis. Despite this immense range of clinical characteristics, all human tumors share a limited set of behaviors that define the malignant state (Hanahan &Weinberg, 2000). Among these hallmarks, unlimited replicative potential and widespread genomic disarray are among the most common characteristics exhibited by human cancer cells. Although numerous distinct molecular pathways regulate specific aspects of each of these phenotypes, emerging evidence now implicates that the oxidative stress and the programmed cell death are essential determinant s of the cell life span.
A role of free radicals has been proposed in the pathogenesis of numerous diseases as indicating above including cancer of different organs such as breast, gastric, colon, multiple myeloma, ovarian, renal, skin, leukemia, biliary, thyroid, and lung cancer (Table 2 & Figure 3).

Cancer	Reference
Prostate Cancer	Pace et al, (2010).
Renal Cell Carcinoma	Soini et al, (2006).
Breast Cancer	Yeon et al, (2011).
Biliary Epithelial Cancer	Elsing et al, (2011).
Colon Cancer	Sangeetha et al, (2010).
Gastric Carcinoma	Tandon et al, (2004).
Hepatocellular Carcinoma	Gayathri et al, (2009).
Esophageal Carcinoma	Lee et al, (2001).
Thyroid Cancer	Koduru et al, (2010).
Lung Cancer	Gupta et al, (2010).
Cervical Cancer	Beevi et al, (2007).
Head and Neck Squamous Cell Carcinoma	Bentz, (2007).
Skin Cancer	Cooke et al, (2007).
Laryngeal Carcinoma	Dwivedi et al, (2008).
Leukemia	Kato et al, (2003).

Table 2. Oxidative stress as a result of altered oxidative/antioxidative balance is proposed as key factor in the pathogenesis of different tumors as shown above.

4. Gastric cancer

4.1 Epidemiology

Gastric carcinoma was the major cancer burden worldwide in the twentieth century. Its etiology and pathogenesis were obscure. Several events have changed that outlook, and currently, it ranks in the second place of mortality from cancer, after lung cancer. In the United States, the number of cases has remained around 20,000 for several years. The geographic distribution of gastric cancer is spotty. Areas of highest risk have traditionally been Japan, Korea, China, Eastern Europe, and the Andean regions of the Americas. In contrast, Australia, Africa, the coastal regions of the Americas, and Southern Asia have

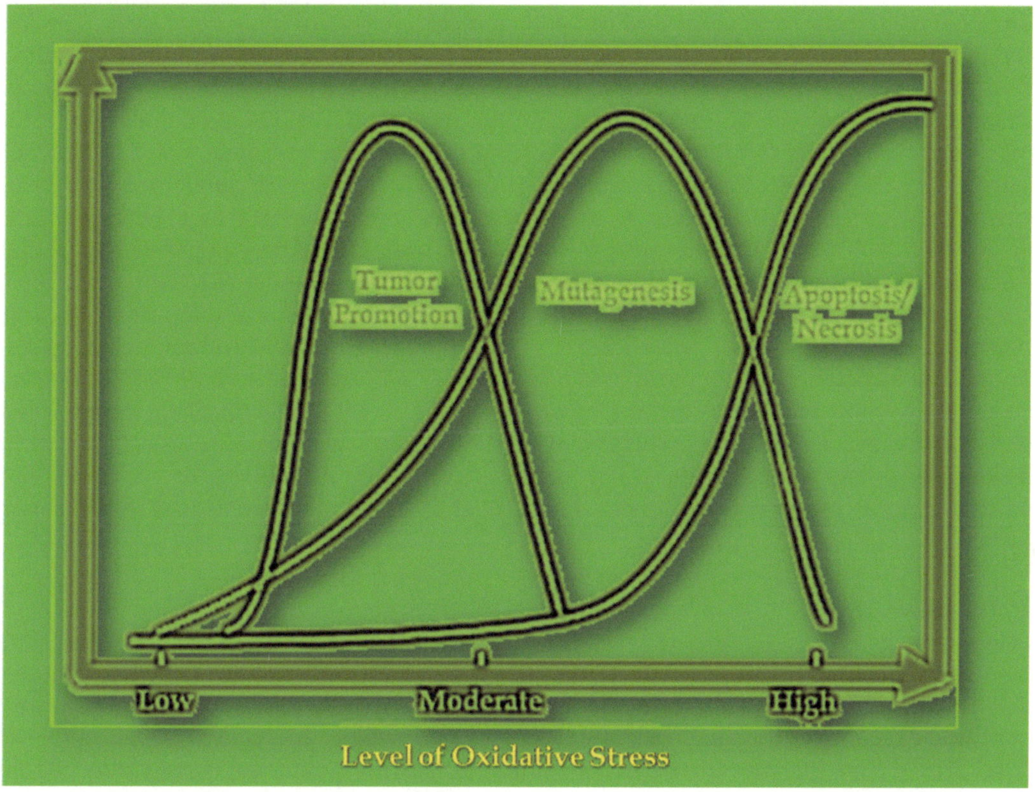

Fig. 3. The link between the dose of oxidative stress and the dependant effect on tumor promotion, mutagenesis and the apoptosis/necrosis (modified from Valko et al, 2007).

traditionally been areas of low risk. Western Europe and North America, with considerably higher risk several decades ago, have experienced a marked decrease since then, and at the present time are considered areas of low risk (reviewed in Correa et al, (2009).

4.2 Risk and protective factors

As reported earlier (Karagianni & Triantafillidis, 2010), the available evidence is indicating a probable protective role of vegetables, especially allium vegetables, fish, and fruit consumption against gastric cancer risk. It also seems probable that high salt intake increases gastric cancer risk. Furthermore, the available evidence is suggestive of a protective role of pulses and foods containing selenium. Limited, but still suggestive evidence exists concerning an inverse association between chilli, processed meat, smoked foods and grilled or barbecued animal foods with gastric cancer risk. Moreover, it has also been proposed that reducing the prevalence of smoking, obesity and gastroesophageal reflux could decrease the incidence of gastric cancer (Engel et al, 2003). Recently, it was reported that the salt intake is an important dietary risk factor for gastric cancer regardless of *H. pylori* infection and virulence, smoking, tumor site and histological type (Peleteiro et al, 2011).

Meta-analysis is a statistical methodology that can combine the results from multiple studies that investigating the same rationale. The utility of the meta-analysis is to conclude a clear statement from these conflicting studies. Meta-analysis consists of three basic steps. The first step is the systematic search of the literature to identify the studies according to certain criteria. The second one to extract the numerical data from each study for the experimental versus control subjects in randomized clinical trials, on various outcomes and their difference. Finally, the third step is carried out to calculate the parameters and reflect their statistical confidence. Recently, numerous meta-analysis studies were publicized concerning with gastric cancer investigation. A recent meta-analysis showed that a high intake of pickled vegetables may increase gastric cancer risk and their data suggested that a high consumption of fresh vegetables is important to reduce gastric cancer risk (Kim et al, 2010). It was evidenced recently in this type of studies that nonsteroidal anti-inflammatory drugs (NSAIDs), including aspirin is associated with a decrease in the development of gastric cancer. The associations were more obvious after they adjusted for several risk factors that are known to contribute to the development of gastric cancer (Tian et al, 2010). Reduced risk of noncardia gastric cancer is associated with the regular use of aspirin especially among Caucasians (Yang et al., 2010). Dairy product consumption (Huang et al, 2009), and *Helicobacter pylori* eradication treatment (Fuccio et al, 2009), might decrease the risk of gastric cancer.

4.3 Oxidative stress

Reactive oxygen species are closely associated with the intracellular signal cascade, thus strongly implicating involvement in tumor progression. The antioxidant enzymes activities such as GSH-PX, SOD, G6PD (glucose-6-phosphate dehydrogenase), MDA and GR were found to be related with malignant phenotype in gastric cancer and colorectal cancer (Kekec et al, 2009). The increase in oxidative stress in gastric carcinoma was evidenced by significant rise in plasma lipid peroxidation marker MDA measured as TBARS. There was a significant fall in serum albumin level in patients due to its protective effect against deleterious oxidative damage (Reddy et al, 2009). The source of cellular ROS production includes activated phagocytes for examples neutrophils and macrophages. The level of myeloperoxidase (MPO) (enzyme of granulocyte) and TAS (total antioxidant status) was evaluated in the plasma of gastric carcinoma patients. MPO is a measurement of neutrophils activation and synthesis of ROS. In gastric carcinoma patients before and after operation (1 and 10 day) MPO concentration was 3 times higher in comparison to the control group, but TAS level was decreased. These results suggest the presence of prolonged oxidative stress in malignant disease but it requires long time observation after surgery (Czygier et al, 2010). It was indicated that gastric cancer patients were characterized by increased the advanced oxidation protein products (AOPP) levels (Noyan et al, 2009).

Increased level of lipid peroxidation and significant differences in glutathione level and glutathione peroxidase, glutathione -S-transferase and glutathione reductase activities were observed in serum taken before and after surgery from patients with gastrointestinal tract tumors compared to those in control serum of healthy blood donors. Increase of lipid peroxidation and changes in GSH level and related enzyme activities, suggest oxidative stress in patients with gastrointestinal tract tumors. These alterations reflect the presence of functional defense mechanism against oxidative stress related firmly to the glutathione metabolism. The impaired antioxidant system may favor accumulation of free radicals (Ścibior et al, 2008). It has been found that low levels of essential antioxidants in the circulation are associated with an increased risk of cancer (Diplock, 1991). Persistent generation of reactive oxygen species such as superoxide, H_2O_2, and hydroxyl radicals is an

inevitable consequence of mitochondrial respiration in aerobic organisms, whose ATP requirements are correlated with the level of metabolic activity. Several potential mechanisms are thought to contribute to the increased ROS in cancer cells. First, oncogenic signals have been shown to cause increased ROS generation. The oncogene c-myc, for example, increases ROS generation, induces DNA damage, and mitigates p53 function.
Another possible mechanism by which cancer cells generate increased amounts of ROS may involve malfunction of the mitochondrial respiratory chain. Since the mitochondrial DNA (mtDNA) codes for 13 components of the respiration complexes and contains no introns, mutations of mtDNA are likely to affect the function of its encoded proteins and lead to malfunction of the mitochondrial respiratory chain. It is also known that mtDNA is more vulnerable to damage than nuclear DNA, and mtDNA mutations are frequently detected in cancer cells (reviewed in Pelicano et al, 2004).

4.3.1 Helicobacter pylori

Helicobacter pylori (H. pylori) infection (Figures 4 & 5), the main cause of chronic gastritis, increases gastric cancer risk. It was reported that *H. pylori* is implicated in many diseases in addition to the gastric cancer (Abdel-Hady et al, 2007; El-Masry et al, 2010; El-Shahat et al, 2005).The infection causes inflammatory cells to produce reactive oxygen metabolites that may damage DNA and promote carcinogenesis. It was showed that *H. pylori* water extract induces tumor formation via reactive oxygen species production (Ishikawa et al, 2006). Successful eradication treatment of *H. pylori* prevents the production of reactive oxygen metabolites (Farkas et al, 2005; Mashimo et al, 2006). In a recent study, a close relationship was demonstrated between the plasma malondialdehyde and nitric oxide levels, gastric histopathology and genotypes of *H. pylori* (Tiwari et al, 2010). In patients with *H. pylori* infection, NO metabolites concentration was increase demonstrating a positive correlation with grade of inflammatory lesions in gastric mucosa. The effective antibacterial therapy causes the decrease of NO metabolites concentration in gastric juice, especially in patients with chronic active gastritis. Eradication decreases the grade of lesions in gastric mucosa just in 12 months after effective antibacterial therapy (Walecka-Kapica et al, 2008).
8-Hydroxy-2'-deoxyguanosine (8-oxo-dG) levels in the gastric mucosa were increased in carriers of *H. pylori*, and were further increased in subjects infected with strains positive for the cagA gene, encoding the cytotoxin-associated protein, cagA. Oxidative DNA damage was more pronounced in males, in older subjects, and in *H. pylori*-positive subjects suffering from gastric dysplasia. Moreover, 8-oxo-dG levels were significantly higher in a small subset of subjects having a homozygous variant allele of the 8-oxoguanosine-glycosylase 1 (OGG1) gene, encoding the enzyme removing 8-oxo-dG from DNA. Conversely, they were not significantly elevated in glutathione S-transferase M1 (GSTM1)-null subjects. Thus, both bacterial and host gene polymorphisms affect oxidative stress and DNA damage, which is believed to represent a key mechanism in the pathogenesis of gastric cancer. The interplay between bacterial and host gene polymorphisms may explain why gastric cancer only occurs in a small fraction of *H. pylori*-infected individuals (Izzotti et al, 2007).
The mRNA of inflammatory markers and oxidant and antioxidant enzymes was investigated in gastritis, gastric ulcer and gastric cancer in gastric biopsy of patients infected with *H. pylori* and the results showed that the oxidant status in gastritis is different in the three lesions slightly. In gastritis, a significant expression of TNF-α (tumor necrosis factor-α), IL-8 (interleukin-8), IL-12, Nox1 (NADH oxidase 1) and iNOS (pathogen-inducible nitric oxide synthase) was detected. In gastric ulcer, a significant expression for TNF-α, IL-8, IL-12

and Nox1 was observed, while in gastric cancer a significant expression for TNF-α, IL-8, IL-1β, IL-10, IL-12, iNOS and Nox1 was evidenced. The oxidant status in gastritis was the only condition where TNF-α and IL-8 expression was associated to *H. pylori* virulence suggesting that they are the main oxidant stress markers responsible to trigger an increase in ROS levels that contributes to decrease the expression of the MnSOD and GSH-PX in gastritis (Augusto et al, 2007)(see Figure 6).

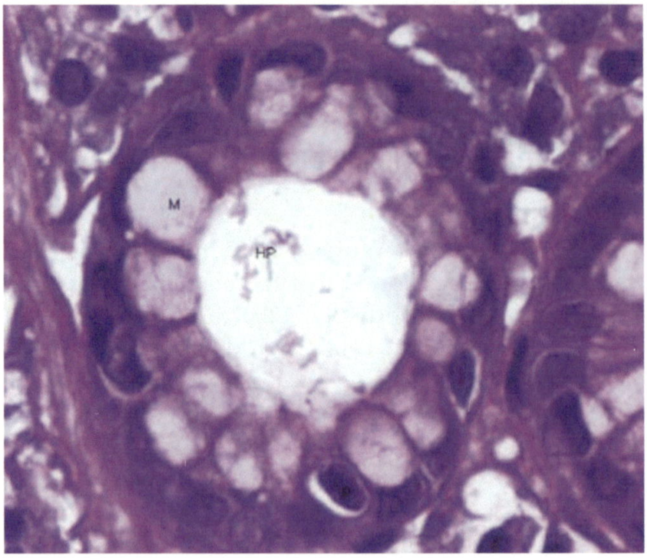

Fig. 4. Presence of *H. pylori* in corpus section stained with hematoxylin and eosin. M; Mucus secreting cells & HP; *H. pylori* (from Abusini et al, 2009).

There are three possible mechanisms by which *H. pylori* infection leads to loss of genomic integrity and promote carcinogenesis (Figure 7). The first is the increase in DNA damage and decrease in repair activity. The second is the mutations in mtDNA. The last is the induction of a transient mutator phenotype resulting in mutations in the DNA upon infection with *H. pylori*. Due to *H. pylori* infection and to inflammatory response, increased amounts of ROS are generated in the gastric epithelial cells that induce oxidative damage in the DNA. *H. pylori* infection also leads to methylation of gene promoters, causing gene silencing and is associated with several other DNA alterations such as chromosomal instability, p53 mutations, influence on the expression of p53 and c-Myc, as well as MSI. At the same time, infection leads to a deficiency in the activity of major repair pathways. The increase in DNA damage coupled to the decrease in repair activity may be two of the key factors involved in the induction of a transient mutator phenotype that could contribute to nuclear and mtDNA mutations. The appearance of mtDNA mutations after *H. pylori* infection might be partly due the down-regulation of BER. BER is one of the best characterized DNA repair pathways in the mitochondria. Several proteins involved in BER have been described in mitochondria, such as DNA glycosylases, APE1, polymerase γ and DNA ligase III . It was observed that APE1 expression is down-regulated in gastric cells infected with *H. pylori*, suggesting an imbalance between generation and repair of AP sites. This could be one the mechanisms behind the induction of mtDNA mutations, which may lead to the impairment of oxidative phosphorylation, cell damage, and disease (reviewed in Machado et al, 2010).

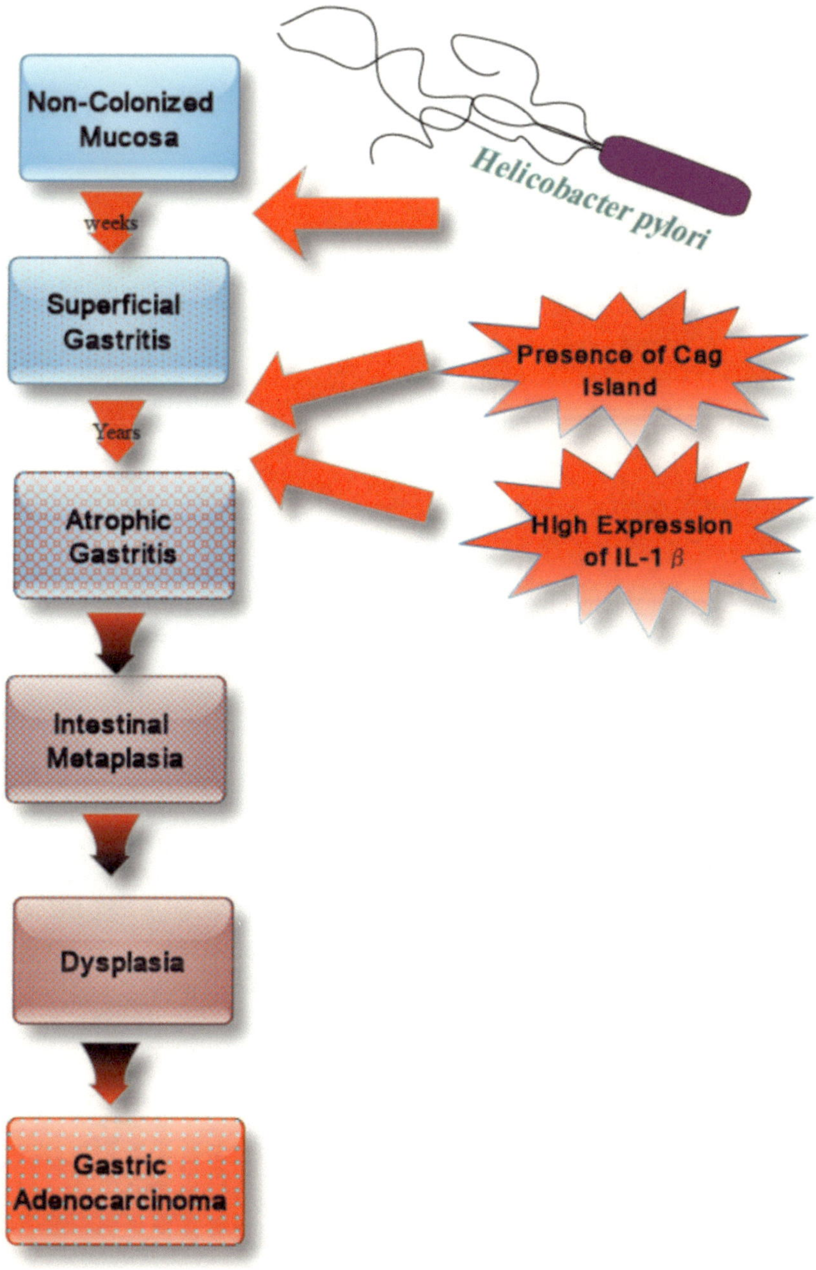

Fig. 5. Multi-step development of intestinal-type gastric adenocarcinoma. *Helicobacter pylori* cag pathogenicity island within *H. pylori* strains and host polymorphisms that promote high expression levels of the cytokine interleukin-lβ augment the risk for gastric adenocarcinoma (adapted from Israel & Peek, 2006). It is well known that gastric cancer is associated with alterations of oncogenes and tumor suppressor genes. Furthermore, prostaglandins, cytokines, nuclear factor-kappa B, chemokines, angiogenic growth factors, and free radicals are involved in GC pathogenesis.

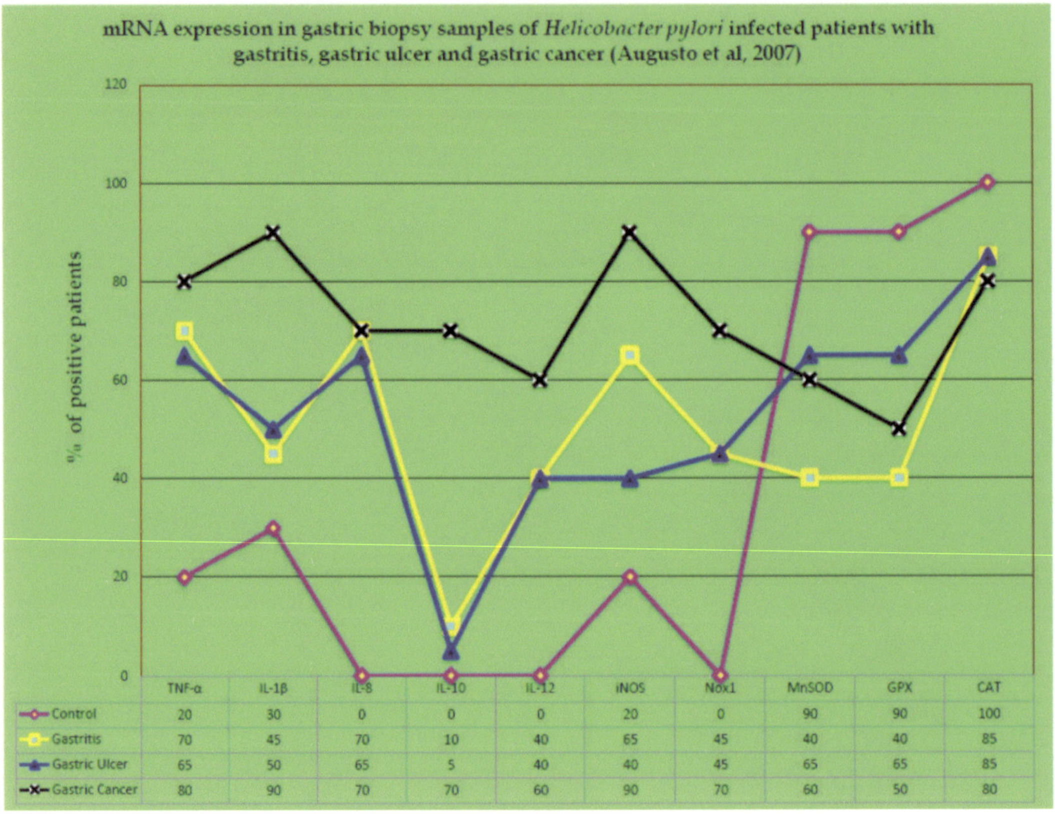

Fig. 6. mRNA expression of inflammatory markers and both oxidant and antioxidant enzymes in gastric biopsy samples of *Helicobacter pylori* infected patients with gastritis, gastric ulcer and gastric cancer. This figure was produced based on the data presented in table 2 of Augusto et al, (2007) publication with permission of Rightslink, Copyright Clearance Center (CCC), and Elsevier.

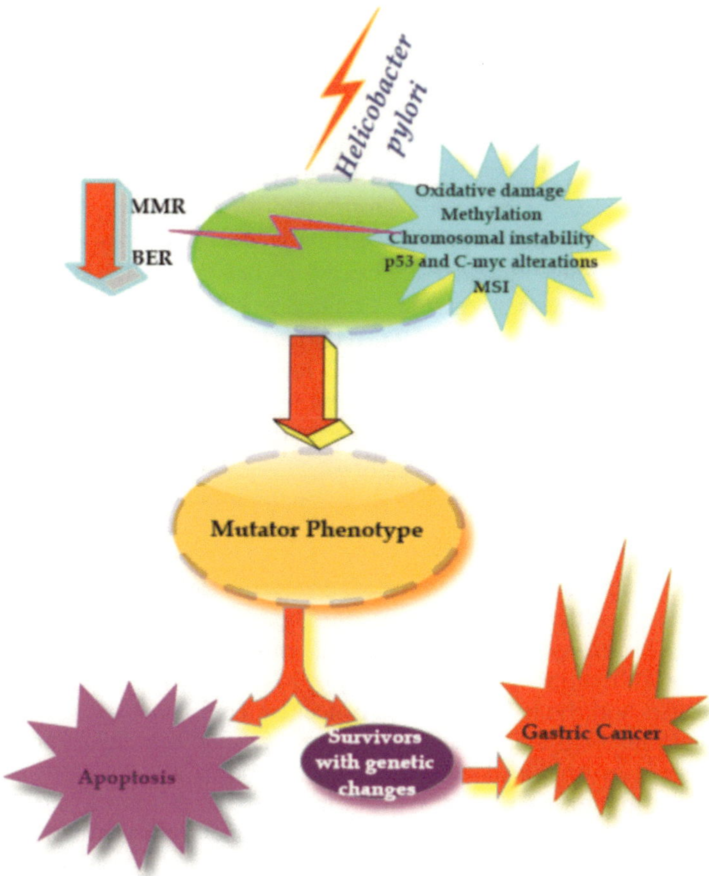

Fig. 7. Proposed model for the development of gastric cancer (adapted from Machado et al, 2010). Microsatellite instability (MSI) is simple repetitive sequences or microsatellites may undergo length alterations. MMR is the DNA mismatch repair pathway. MSI can lead to deficiency of MMR. *H. pylori* gastritis might lead to a deficiency of MMR in gastric epithelium that may increase the risk of mutation accumulation in the gastric mucosa cells during chronic *H. pylori* infection. Base excision repair (BER) is another major repair pathway critical for the maintenance of genome stability as it repairs a number of endogenously generated DNA lesions. Therefore, it is possible that this repair pathway plays an important role ensuring genetic stability in gastric cells. BER removes various forms of base damage such as oxidation, methylation, deamination, depurination and hydroxylation. BER is initiated by DNA glycosylases that recognize and cleave the damaged bases, creating abasic (AP) sites. The AP sites created are cytotoxic and mutagenic and are, therefore, further processed by DNA glycosylases with AP-lyase activity or by APE1. The single nucleotide gap is filled and the nick sealed to complete the repair reaction. It was suggested that increased levels of cellular damage and death due to reactive oxygen species would lead to increased inflammation and consequently to the production of more ROS and tumor-promoting cytokines. It also strongly indicates that one mechanism underlying genetic instability caused by *H. pylori* infection is deregulation of central DNA repair pathways (see Machado et al, 2010).

4.3.2 Smoking

Tobacco smoke contains many toxic, carcinogenic and mutagenic chemicals, as well as stable and unstable free radicals and reactive oxygen species (ROS) in the particulate and the gas phase with the potential for biological oxidative damage. Epidemiological evidence established that smoking is one of the most important extrinsic factor of premature morbidity and mortality (Valavanidis et al, 2009). It was estimated that the number of gastric cancer cases attributable to tobacco smoking occurring worldwide, in total, over 80,000 cases of gastric cancer (11% of all estimated cases) may be attributed to tobacco smoking each year. The majority of published studies reported a positive association between gastric cancer and cigarette smoking. Meta-analysis suggested a risk of stomach cancer among smokers of the order of 1.5–1.6 as compared to non-smokers (Trédaniel et al, 1997).

Thiobarbituric acid reactive substances (TBARS) level was found higher in smokers than non-smoking gastric cancer patients. The activities of superoxide dismutase, catalase, glutathione peroxidase, glutathione-S-transferase, reduced glutathione, and vitamins A, E and C were decreased in gastric cancer patients who were smokers as compared to other groups ($p < 0.001$). The lipid peroxidation and possible breakdown of antioxidant status in the cigarette smoking may increase the risk of gastric cancer. Thus, chronic smoking enhances erythrocyte lipid peroxidation in gastric carcinoma patients with concomitant failure of both plasma and erythrocyte antioxidant defense mechanisms. The low antioxidant status of healthy smokers may predispose them to oxidant-mediated tissue damage, which may increase the risk of gastric cancer (Pasupathi et al, (2009). It was concluded that the TNF-alpha-857 C/T polymorphism may play an independent role in gastric carcinogenesis and the risk for gastric cancer by TNF genetic effect is pronounced by cigarette smoking (Yang et al, 2009). Recently, it was detected that the cigarette smoking was associated with risk of oesophageal squamous cell carcinoma, oesophageal adenocarcinoma, gastric cardia adenocarcinoma and gastric non-cardia adenocarcinoma (Steevens et al, 2010). Plasma levels of MDA were significantly increased but melatonin content of the blood was significantly decreased in smokers as compared to nonsmokers. It seems that melatonin can reduce free radical damage to the respiratory system induced by cigarette smoke (Ozguner et al, 2005). A significant decrease in free malondialdehyde levels in light smokers after one month phytonutrient supplementation was achieved (Bamonti et al, 2006). The effect of the consumption of a pear, an apple and 200 ml orange juice, during 26 days, on total plasma antioxidant capacity and lipid profile of chronic smokers and non-smoking healthy adults was analyzed. Fruit consumption increased total plasma antioxidant capacity in non-smokers, but not in smokers. In non-smokers, total cholesterol, high-density lipoprotein-cholesterol, and low-density lipoprotein-cholesterol increased significantly; while in smokers, total cholesterol and low-density lipoprotein-cholesterol decreased (Alvarez-Parrilla et al, 2010). Antioxidant-rich food was found to modulate positively the cellular stress defense of smokers (Bohn et al, 2010).

5. Antioxidants

ROS are generated during normal aerobic metabolism and increased levels are present during oxidative stress. It has been proposed that ROS is necessary for life and essential for the regulation of essential physiologic functions. However, at high concentrations, ROS are cytotoxic. ROS are important in cell differentiation, apoptosis, and cell proliferation. These functions are regulated by redox-sensitive signal transduction pathways. The amount of antioxidants in the cells is high and so cells prevent or repair the damages caused by

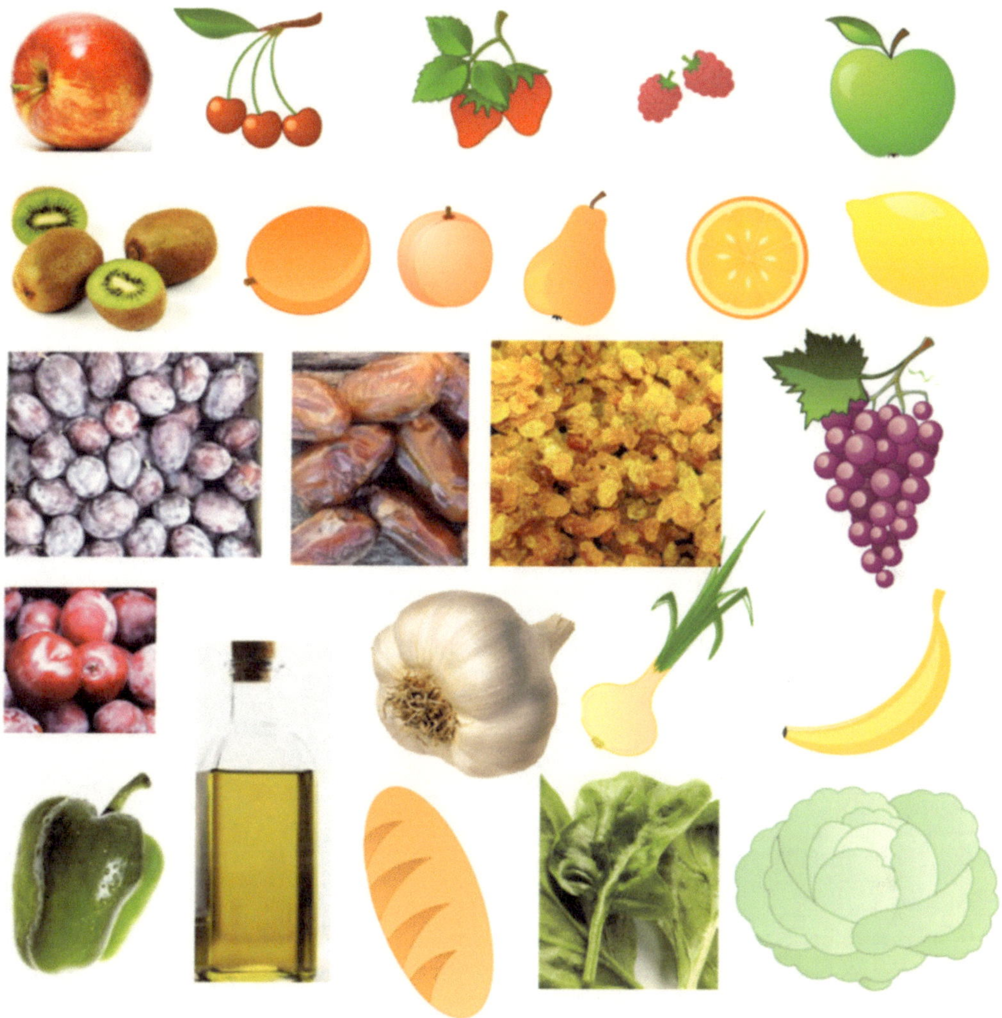

Fig. 8. The antioxidant content is different from food to another. Dried fruits (dates, raisins, and prunes), vegetables (red cabbages, spinach, and garlic), fruits (red grape, different types of berries, red apple, and red plum) and juices such as orange juices are among the foods with highest antioxidant content. Furthermore, drinks such as espresso coffee and oils such as soybean and virgin olive oil are rich sources of antioxidants. On the other hand, the most powerful natural foods to scavenge the oxygen free radicals and to inhibit the lipid peroxidation are blackberry, orange, lemon, strawberry, kiwi, garlic, green pepper, and cabbages (Miller et al, 2000; Pellegrini et al, 2003).

ROS. ROS-induced damage can result in cell death, mutations, chromosomal aberrations and also carcinogenesis (Cerutti, 1985). The antioxidants are antioxidant enzymes and some vitamins (Figures 8-12). There are three major types of antioxidant enzymes in mammalian cells: superoxide dismutase, catalase, and peroxidase, of which glutathione peroxidase is the most important component of these (Hurt et al, 2007) (Figure 12). Both endogenous and exogenous antioxidants play an important and interdependent role in preventing cancer.

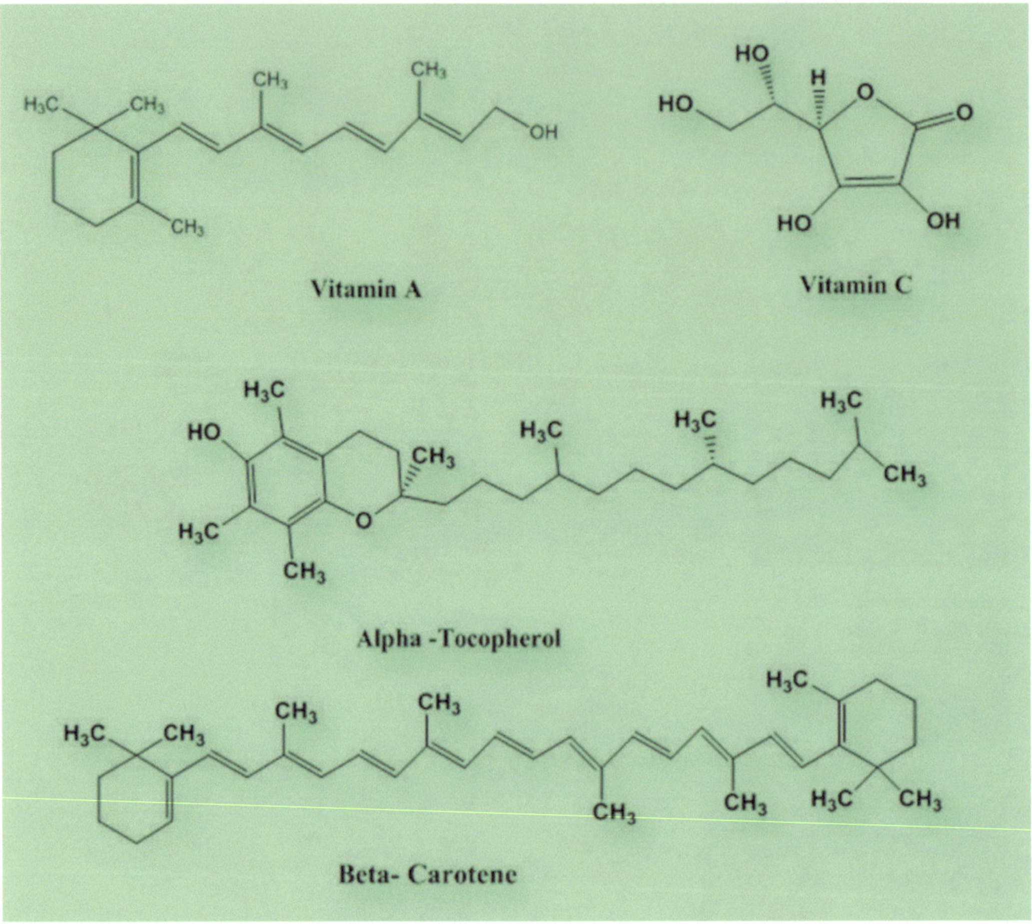

Fig. 9. Antioxidant vitamins include vitamin A, E, and C. The ascorbic acid is the only one feature of the ROS scavenging capacity of fresh fruit and vegetable juices. Other free radical scavengers present in fruits and vegetables are flavonoids, carotenoids, organic acids (cinnamic acid and gallic acid), vitamin E, and sulfhydryl compounds. A well balanced diet of fruit and vegetables may enhance the antioxidant defenses against ROS induced injuries to cells and tissues (Leonard et al, 2002).

It was evidenced that the MnSOD Val-9Ala polymorphism may contribute to cancer development through a disturbed antioxidant balance, where the decreased consumption level of dietary antioxidant s is an essential contributing factor (Li et al, 2005 & Wang et al, 2009). It was showed that ascorbic acid protects against gastric cancer by scavenging reactive radical species which would otherwise react with DNA, with resultant genetic damage (Drake et al, 1996). Vitamin C-releasing acetylsalicylic acid in comparison with plain acetylsalicylic acid induces less gastric mucosal damage and this protective effect is probably due to the attenuation of oxidative stress in gastric mucosa (Konturek et al, 2004). High dietary antioxidant quercetin intake is inversely related to the risk of noncardia gastric adenocarcinoma, and the protection appears to be particularly strong for women exposed to oxidative stress, such as tobacco smoking (Ekstrom et al, 2011). Treatment with Allopurinol (inhibits the enzyme xanthine oxidase which is responsible for the formation of superoxide radicals and scavenges hydroxyl radicals) and dimethyl sulphoxide (DMSO; scavenges hydroxyl radicals) was found to provide gastric cancer patients with a survival advantage (Salim, 1992). In was observed upon following up 29,133 male smokers that the higher dietary intake of retinol was protective, but dietary intake of α-tocopherol and γ-tocopherol increased risk of gastric cardia cancer. Higher intakes of fruits, vitamin C, tocopherols, and lycopene were protective against gastric noncardia cancer (Nouraie et al, 2005).

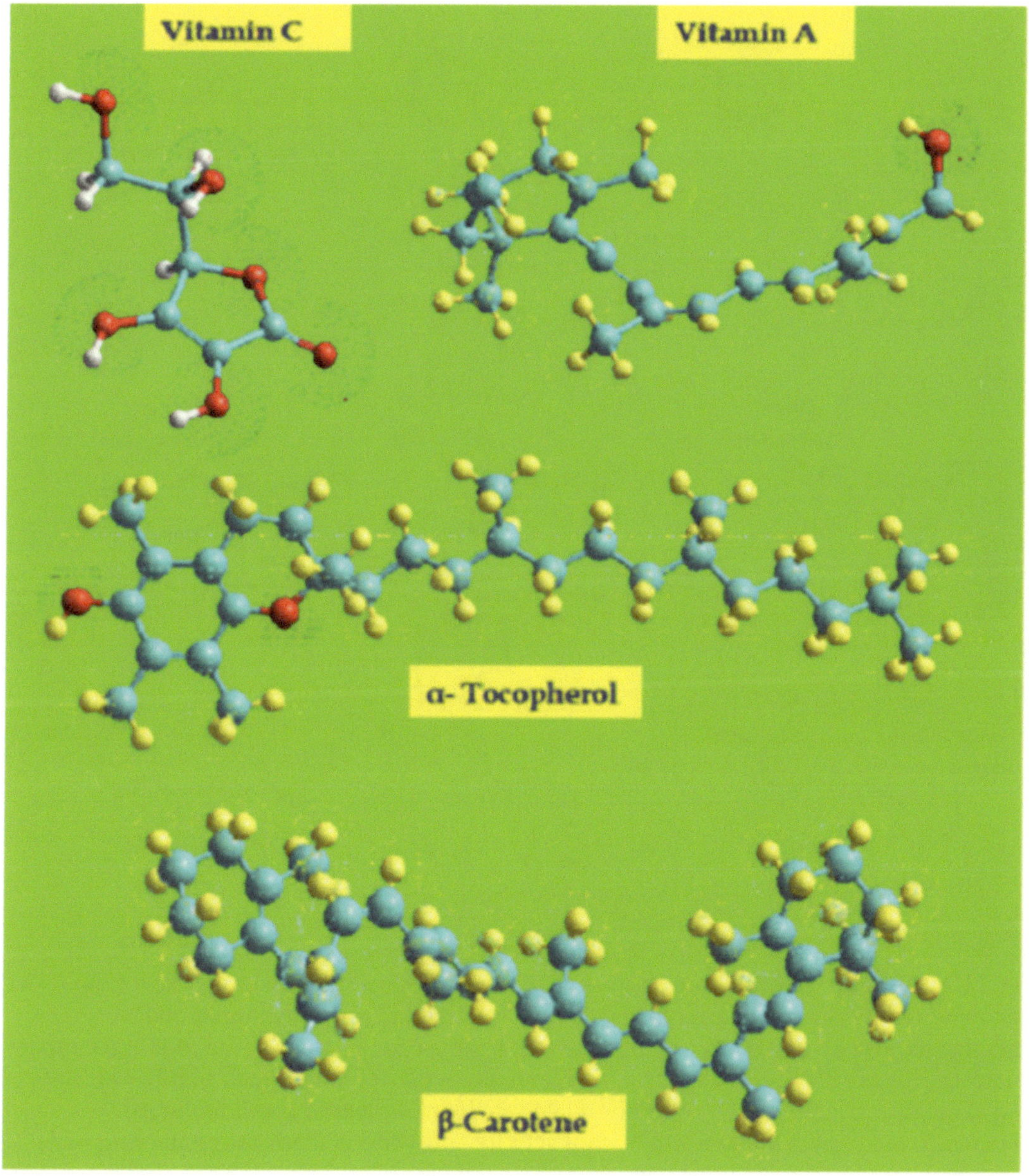

Fig. 10. Vitamins with antioxidant activity in three dimensional structures.

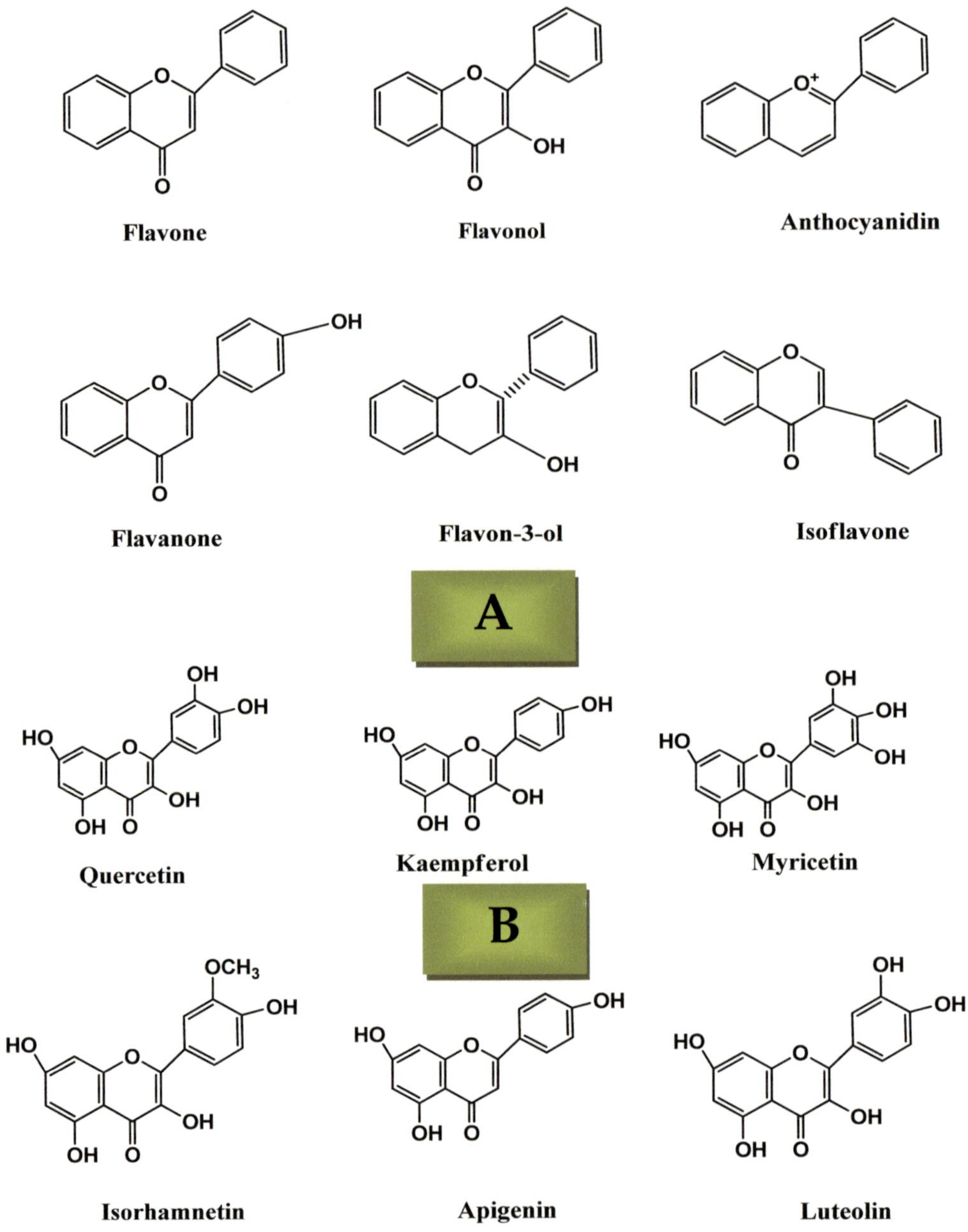

Fig. 11. Fruits and vegetables are sources of polyphenolic compounds called flavonoids. The flavonoid family is flavonols, flavones, flavan-3-ols, isoflavones, flavanones and anthocyanidins (A). Flavonols and flavones are synthesized in plant tissues and it comprises quercetin, myricetin, kaempferol and isorhamnetin, while a more limited number of fruits and vegetables contain the structurally-related flavones, apigenin and luteolin (B). Flavonoids are known to have antioxidant activity and various foods are containing such components as blueberry, onion, lettuce, tomato, and tea (Crozier et al, 2000). Tea is a good scavenger of free radicals as indicated previously (El-Sayed et al, 2006; Oyama et al, 2010).

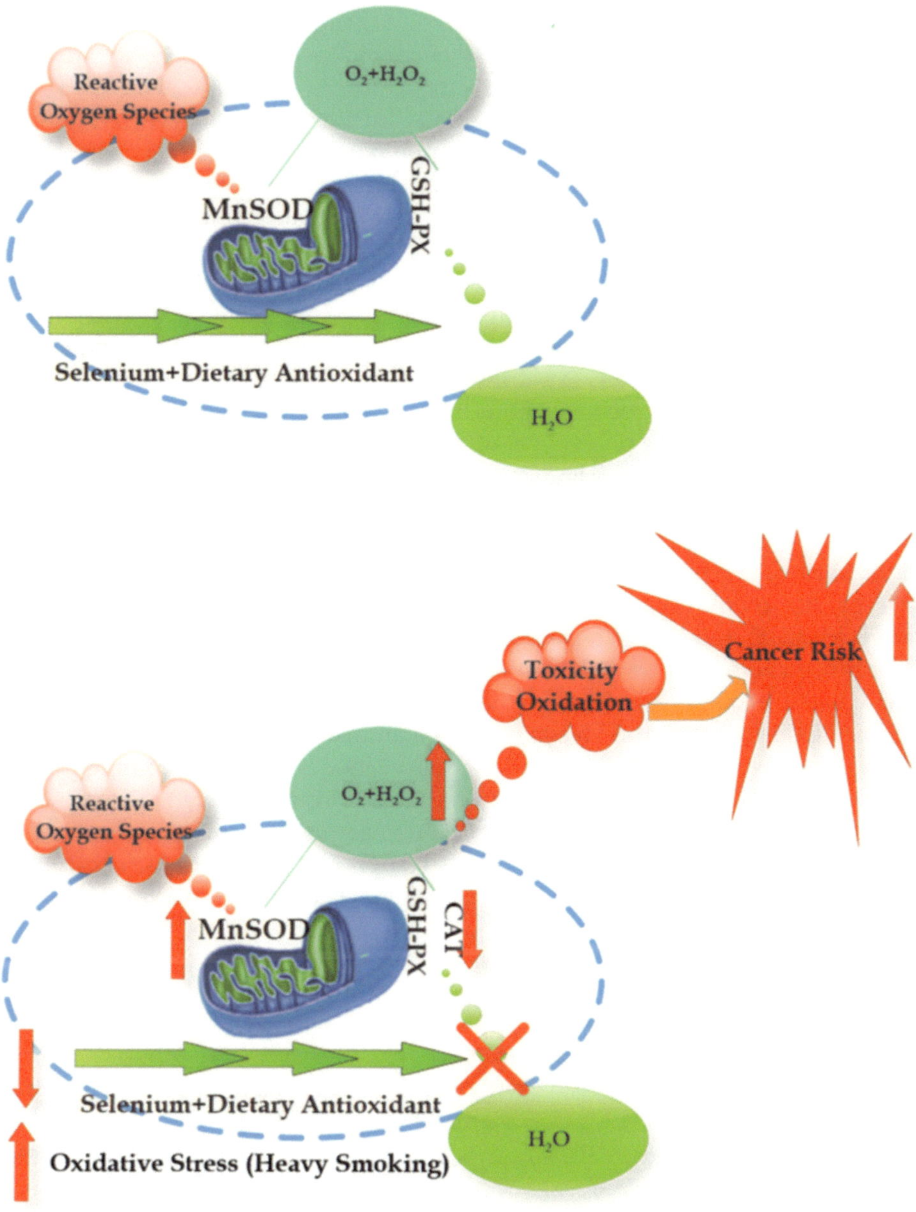

Fig. 12. Potential mechanism for the interaction between MnSOD and antioxidant status in cancer development (modified from Li et al, 2005 & Wang et al, 2009). In mitochondria, the ROS is dismutated by MnSOD into oxygen and hydrogen peroxide (H_2O_2), which is further detoxified to water (H_2O) by mitochondrial glutathione peroxidase (GSH-PX) (an enzyme requiring selenium) and catalase (CAT). High levels of MnSOD expression may lead to increased O_2 and H_2O_2, and induce toxicity if glutathione peroxidase activity is low due to inadequate selenium or dietary antioxidant intake. The normal pathway is shown above and the altered one is shown below.

6. Conclusions

Gastric cancer ranks the second leading cause of cancer-specific mortality worldwide. It has a poor prognosis; 5-year survival rate of gastric cancer is less than 20%-25% in the USA, Europe, and China (Hartgrink et al, 2009). Cells in tissues and organs are continuously subjected to oxidative stress and free radicals on a daily basis. This free radical attack has exogenous or endogenous (intracellular) origin. The cells withstand and counteract this occurrence by the use of several and different defense mechanisms ranging from free radical scavengers like glutathione (GSH), vitamins C and E and antioxidant enzymes like catalase, superoxide dismutase and various peroxidases to sophisticated and elaborate DNA repair mechanisms (Kryston et al, 2011). Reactive oxygen species along with reactive nitrogen species are well recognized for playing a dual role as both deleterious and beneficial species. The "two-faced" character of ROS is substantiated by growing body of evidence that ROS within cells act as secondary messengers in intracellular signalling cascades, which induce and maintain the oncogenic phenotype of cancer cells, however, ROS can also induce cellular senescence and apoptosis and can therefore function as anti-tumourigenic species. The cumulative production is common for many types of cancer cell that are linked with altered redox regulation of cellular signalling pathways. Oxidative stress induces a cellular redox imbalance which has been found to be present in various cancer cells compared with normal cells; the redox imbalance thus may be related to oncogenic stimulation. DNA mutation is a critical step in carcinogenesis and elevated levels of oxidative DNA lesions (8-OH-G) have been noted in various tumors, strongly implicating such damage in the etiology of cancer (Valko et al, 2006). Finally, the eradication treatment for *H. pylori*, smoking quitting, eating of fresh and dried fruits with high antioxidant content such as dates, raisins, and prunes, and avoiding the salts and pickled vegetables, all are seemingly justifiable means for reduction the gastric cancer prevalence and for general health. Further studies are warranted to explore the effect of different combinations of antioxidants on the healthy heavy smokers to find out if these compounds can protect them or lessen both the gastric cancer incidence and the other debilitating diseases associated with smoking.

7. References

Abdel-Hady H., Zaki, A., Badra, G., Lotfy, M., Selmi, C., Giorgini, A., El-Sayed, M., Badr, R. (2007). *Helicobacter pylori* infection in hepatic encephalopathy: Relationship to plasma endotoxins and blood ammonia. *Hepatology Research*, Vol. 37, pp. 1026-1033.

Abraham, S., Soundararajan, C.C., Vivekanandhan, S. & Behari, M. (2005). Erythrocyte antioxidant enzymes in Parkinson's disease. *Indian Journal Medical Research*, Vol. 121, pp. 111-115.

Abusini, H., Abuelteen, K., Elkarmi, A., Alenzi, F.Q., Lotfy, M. (2009). Investigation of *Helicobacter pylori* infection in Jordanian patients using six enzyme immunoassays for immunoglobulin G (IGG) and IGA testing. *Roumanian Archives of Microbiology and Immunology*, Vol. 68, pp. 240-245.

Adiga, U., Adiga, S. (2009). Total antioxidant activity in old age. *Biomedical Research,* Vol. 19, pp.185-186.

Ahmed, R. G. (2005). The physiological and biochemical effects of diabetes on the balance between oxidative stress and antioxidant defense system (Review Article). *Medical Journal of Islamic World Academy of Sciences* Vol. 15, pp. 31-42.

Alvarez-Parrilla, E., De La Rosa, L.A., Legarreta, P., Saenz, L., Rodrigo-Garcia, J., Gonzalez-Aguilar, G.A. (2010). Daily consumption of apple, pear and orange juice differently affects plasma lipids and antioxidant capacity of smoking and non-smoking adults. *International Journal of Food Sciences & Nutrition*, 61, 369-380.

Aly, D.G. & Shahin, R.S. (2010). Oxidative stress in *lichen planus*. *Acta Dermatovenerologica Alpina, Pannonica et Adriatica*, Vol. 19, pp. 3-11.

Augusto, A.C., Miguel, F., Mendonça, S., Pedrazzoli, J., Jr., Gurgueira, S.A. (2007). Oxidative stress expression status associated to *Helicobacter pylori* virulence in gastric diseases. *Clinical Biochemistry*, Vol. 40, pp. 615–622.

Aygul, R., Kotan, D, Demirbas, F., Ulvi, H, & Deniz, O. (2006). Plasma oxidants and antioxidants in acute ischaemic stroke. *The Journal of International Medical Research*, Vol. 34, pp. 413 - 418.

Babior, B.M., Kipnes, R.S., Curnutte, J.T. (1973). Biological defense mechanism. The production by leukocytes of superoxide, a potential bactericidal agent. *Journal of Clinical Investigation*, Vol. 52, pp.741.

Bamonti, F., Novembrino, C., Ippolito, S., Soresi, E., Ciani, A., Lonati, S., Scurati-Manzoni, E., Cighetti, G. (2006). Increased free malondialdehyde concentrations in smokers normalise with a mixed fruit and vegetable juice concentrate: a pilot study. *Clinical Chemistry & Laboratory Medicine*, Vol. 44, pp. 391-395.

Beevi, S.S., Rasheed, M.H. , Geetha, A. (2007). Evidence of oxidative and nitrosative stress in patients with cervical squamous cell carcinoma. *Clinica Chimica Acta*, Vol. 375, pp. 119-123.

Bentz, B. (2007). Head and neck squamous cell carcinoma as a model of oxidative-stress and cancer. *Journal of Surgical Oncology*, Vol. 96, pp. 190-191.

Bohn, S.K., Myhrstad, M.C., Thoresen, M., Holden, M., Karlsen, A., Tunheim, S.H., Erlund, I., Svendsen, M., Seljeflot, I., Moskaug, J.O., Duttaroy, A.K., Laake, P., Arnesen, H., Tonstad, S., Collins, A., Drevon, C.A., Blomhoff, R. (2010). Blood cell gene expression associated with cellular stress defense is modulated by antioxidant-rich food in a randomised controlled clinical trial of male smokers. *BMC Medicine*, Vol. 8, pp. 54.

Cerutti, P.A. (1985). Prooxidant states and cancer. *Science*, Vol. 227, pp. 375–381.

Cooke, M.S., Osborne, J.E., Singh, R., Mistry, V., Farmer, P.B., Evans, M.D. , Hutchinson, P.E. (2007). Evidence that oxidative stress is a risk factor for the development of squamous cell carcinoma in renal transplant patients. *Free Radical Biology & Medicine*, Vol. 43, pp. 1328-1334.

Correa, P., Camargo, M.C., & Piazuelo, M.B. (2009). Overview and pathology of gastric cancer, In: *The biology of gastric cancers*, Wang TC., Fox, J.G.& Giraud, A.S. (eds.), pp. 1-24, Springer Science + Business Media, ISBN: 978-0-387-69181-7, USA.

Crozier, A., Burns, J., Aziz, A.A., Stewart, A.J., Rabiasz, H.S., Jenkins, G.I., Edwards, C.A., Lean, M.E. (2000). Antioxidant flavonols from fruits, vegetables and beverages: measurements and bioavailability. *Biological Research*, vol. 33, pp. 79-88.

Czygier, M., Kamocki, Z., Lawicki, S., Szmitkowski, M. (2010). The plasma level of myeloperoxidase (MPO) and total antioxidant status (TAS) in gastric cancer patients after surgery. *Przeglad lekarski*, 67, 443-445.

Diplock, A.T. (1991). Antioxidant nutrients and disease prevention: an over-view. *American Journal of Clinical Nutrition*, Vol. 53, pp. 189–193.

Drake, I.M., Davies, M.J., Mapstone, N.P., Dixon, M.F., Schorah, C. J., White, K.L.M., Chalmers, D.M., Axon, A.T.R. (1996). Ascorbic acid may protect against human gastric cancer by scavenging mucosal oxygen radicals. *Carcinogenesis*, vol.17, pp. 559-562.

Duru, N., Morshedi, M., & Oehninger, S. (2001). Effects of hydrogen peroxide on DNA and plasma membrane integrity of human spermatozoa. *Fertility & Sterility*, Vol. 74, pp. 1200-1207.

Dwivedi, R., Raturi, D., Kandpal, N., Singh, R., Puri, V. (2008). Oxidative stress in patients with laryngeal carcinoma. *Indian Journal Cancer*, Vol. 45, pp. 97-99.

Ekstrom, A.M., Serafini, M., Nyren, O., Wolk, A., Bosetti, C. , Bellocco, R. (2011). Dietary quercetin intake and risk of gastric cancer: results from a population-based study in Sweden. *Annals of Oncology*, 22, 438-443.

El-Masry, S., El-Shahat, M., Badra, G., Aboel-Nour, M.F., Lotfy, M. (2010). *Helicobacter pylori* and hepatitis C virus coinfection in Egyptian patients. *Journal of Global Infectious Diseases*, Vol. 2, pp. 4-9.

El-Sayed, I.H., Lotfy, M., El-Khawaga, O.A., Nasif, W.A. , El-Shahat, M. (2006). Prominent free radicals scavenging activity of tannic acid in lead-induced oxidative stress in experimental mice. *Toxicology and Industrial Health*, 22, 157-163.

El-Shahat, M., El-Masry, S., Lotfy, M., El-Kenawy, A.M., Nasif, W.A. (2005). Relationship of *Helicobacter pylori* to Bcl-2 family expression, DNA content and pathological characteristics of gastric cancer. *International Journal of Gastrointestinal Cancer*, Vol. 36, pp. 61-68.

Elsing, C., Voss, A., Herrmann, T., Kaiser, I., Huebner, C.A., Schlenker, T. (2011). Oxidative stress reduces Na+/H+ exchange (NHE) activity in a biliary epithelial cancer cell line (Mz-Cha-1). *Anticancer Research*, Vol.31, pp. 459-465.

El-Zayadi, A.R. (2006). Heavy smoking and liver. *World Journal Gastroenterology*, Vol. 12, pp. 6098-6101.

Engel, L.S., Chow, W., Vaughan, T.L., Gammon, M.D., Risch, H.A., Stanford, J.L., et al. (2003). Population attributable risks of esophageal and gastric cancers. *Journal National Cancer Institute*, Vol. 95, pp.1404-1413.

Fabian, E., Pölöskey, P., Kósa, L., Elmadfa, I., Réthy, L.A. (2011). Activities of antioxidant enzymes in relation to oxidative and nitrosative challenges in childhood Asthma. *Journal of Asthma*, (In Press).

Farkas, R., Pronofai, L., Tulassay, Z., Selmeci, L. (2005). Relationship between eradication of *Helicobacter pylori* and gastric mucosal superoxide dismutase activity. *Anticancer Research*, Vol. 25(6C), pp. 4763-4767.

Fuccio, L., Zagari, R.M., Eusebi, L.H., Laterza, L., Cennamo, V., Ceroni, L., Grilli, D., Bazzoli, F. (2009). Meta-analysis: can *Helicobacter pylori* eradication treatment reduce the risk for gastric cancer? *Annals of Internal Medicine*, Vol.151, pp. 121-128.

Gayathri, R., Priya, D.K., Gunassekaran, G.R., Sakthisekaran, D. (2009). Ursolic acid attenuates oxidative stress-mediated hepatocellular carcinoma induction by diethylnitrosamine in male Wistar rats. *Asian Pacific Journal of Cancer Prevention*, Vol. 10, pp. 933-938.

Giustarini, D., Rossi, R., Milzani, A., Colombo, R., Dalle-Donne, I. (2004). S-Glutathionylation: From redox regulation of protein functions to human diseases. *Journal of Cellular and Molecular Medicine* 2004; 8 (2): 201-212.

Gupta, A., Srivastava, S., Prasad, R., Natu, S.M., Mittal, B., Negi, M.P., Srivastava, A.N. (2010). Oxidative stress in non-small cell lung cancer patients after chemotherapy: association with treatment response. *Respirology*, Vol. 15, pp. 349-356.

Hakhamaneshi M. S., Mesbah-Namin S. A., Houshmand M., Lotfi A. S. (2007). Alteration in antioxidant capacity in patients with chronic obstructive pulmonary disease. *Tanaffos*, Vol.6, pp. 13-17.

Hamed S.A., & Abdellah, M.M. (2004).Trace elements and electrolytes homeostasis and their relation to antioxidant enzyme activity in brain hyperexcitability of epileptic patients (Critical Review). *Journal of Pharmacological Sciences*, Vol. 96, pp. 349 - 359.

Hanahan, D., Weinberg, R.A. (2000). The hallmarks of cancer. *Cell*, Vol.100, pp. 57-70.

Hartgrink, H.H., Jansen, E.P., van Grieken, N.C., van de Velde, C.J. (2009). Gastric cancer. *Lancet*, Vol. 374, pp. 477- 490.

Hernandez-Saavedra, D., McCord, J.M. (2003). Paradoxical effects of thiol reagents on Jurkat cells and a new thiol-sensitive mutant form of human mitochondrial superoxide dismutase. *Cancer Research*, Vol.63, pp.159–163.

Hofseth, L.J. (2008). Nitric oxide as a target of complementary and alternative medicines to prevent and treat inflammation and cancer (Mini-review). *Cancer Letters*, Vol. 268, pp. 10–30.

Huang, Y.X., Qin, L.Q., Wang, P.Y. (2009). Meta-analysis of the relationship between dairy product consumption and gastric cancer. *Zhonghua Yu Fang Yi Xue Za Zhi* (*Chinese Journal of Preventive Medicine*), Vol.43, pp.193-196.

Hurt, E.M., Thomas, S.B., Peng, B., Farrar, W.L. (2007). Integrated molecular profiling of SOD2 expression in multiple myeloma. *Blood*, Vol.109, pp.3953–3962.

Hwang, T.S., Choi, T.K., Han, H.S. (2007). Differential expression of manganese superoxide dismutase, copper/zinc superoxide dismutase and catalase in gastric adenocarcinoma and normal gastric mucosa. *European Journal of Surgical Oncology*, Vol. 33, pp. 474–479.

Ishikawa, T., Yoshida, N., Tokuda, H., Kokura, S., Nakabe, N., Kuchide, M., Ichiishi, E., Imaeda, A., Ichikawa, H, Naito, Y, Okanoue, T, Yoshikawa, T. (2006). Role of oxygen-derived free radicals in *Helicobacter pylori* water extract-induced mouse skin carcinogenesis. *Biofactors*, Vol. 28, pp.1-7.

Israel, D.A. & Peek, R.M., Jr.(2006). Mechanisms of *Helicobacter pylori*-induced gastric inflammation. In: *Physiology of the Gastrointestinal Tract,* (4th edition), Johnson, L.R., pp. 1091-1114, Academic Press, USA.

Izzotti, A., De Flora, S., Cartiglia, C., Are, B.M., Longobardi, M., Camoirano, A., Mura, I., Dore, M.P., Scanu, A.M., Rocca, P.C., Maida, A., Piana, A. (2007). Interplay between

Helicobacter pylori and host gene polymorphisms in inducing oxidative DNA damage in the gastric mucosa. Carcinogenesis, Vol. 28, pp. 892-898.

Jiménez, P., Piazuelo, E., Sánchez, M.T., Ortego, J., Soteras, F., Lanas, A. (2005). Free radicals and antioxidant systems in reflux esophagitis and Barrett's esophagus. *World Journal of Gastroenterology,* Vol. 11, pp. 2697-2703.

Karagianni, V., Triantafillidis, J.K. (2010). Prevention of gastric cancer: diet modifications. *Annals of Gastroenterology,* Vol. 23, pp. 237-242.

Kato, M., Minakami, H., Kuroiwa, M., Kobayashi, Y., Oshima, S., Kozawa, K., Morikawa, A., Kimura, H. (2003). Superoxide radical generation and Mn- and Cu-Zn superoxide dismutases activities in human leukemic cells. *Hematol Oncol,* Vol. 21, pp.11-16.

Kekec, Y., Paydas, S., Tuli, A., Zorludemir, S., Sakman, G., Seydaoglu, G. (2009). Antioxidant enzyme levels in cases with gastrointesinal cancer. *European Journal of Internal Medicine,* Vol. 20, pp.403-406.

Kelner, M.J., & Bagnell. R. (1990). Alteration of endogenous glutathione peroxidase, manganese superoxide dismutase, and glutathione transferase activity in cells transfected with a copper-zinc superoxide dismutase expression vector. *Journal of Biological Chemistry,* Vol. 265, pp. 10872.

Khan, M.A.S., Oubrahim, H., Stadtman, E.R. (2004). Inhibition of apoptosis in acute promyelocytic leukemia cells leads to increases in levels of oxidized protein and LMP2 immunoproteasome. *PNAS,* Vol. 101, pp.11560–11565.

Kim, H.J., Lim, S.Y., Lee, J.S., Park, S., Shin, A., Choi, B.Y., Shimazu, T., Inoue, M., Tsugane, S., Kim, J. (2010). Fresh and pickled vegetable consumption and gastric cancer in Japanese and Korean populations: a meta-analysis of observational studies. *Cancer Science,* Vol. 101, pp. 508-516.

Koduru, B., Tejaswini, A., Thakur, A., Kamath, S.U., Shenoy, K.R., Kamath, U ., Reshma, K. (2010). Indicators of oxidative stress in thyroid cancer. *Indian Journal of Biochemistry & Biophysics,* Vol. 47, pp. 121-123.

Konturek, P.C., Kania, J., Gessner, U., Konturek, S. J., Hahn, E.G., Konturek, J.W. (2004). Effect of vitamin C-releasing acetylsalicylic acid on gastric mucosal damage before and after *Helicobacter pylori* eradication therapy. *European Journal of Pharmacology,* Vol. 506, pp. 169– 177.

Kryston, T.B., Georgiev, A.B., Pissis, P., Georgakilas, A.G. (2011). Role of oxidative stress and DNA damage in human carcinogenesis. *Mutation Research/ Fundamental and Molecular Mechanisms of Mutagenesis,* doi:10.1016/j.mrfmmm.2010.12.016 (In press).

Kundu, S., Bala, A., Ghosh, P., Mukhopadhyay, D., Mitra, A., Sarkar, A., Bauri, A.K., Ghosh, A., Chattopadhyay, S., Chatterjee, M. (2011). Attenuation of oxidative stress by allylpyrocatechol in synovial cellular infiltrate of patients with rheumatoid arthritis. *Free Radicals Research,* Vol.45, pp. 518-526.

Lee, J.S., Oh, T.Y., Ahn, B.O., Cho, H., Kim, W.B., Kim, Y.B., Surh, Y.J., Kim, H.J., Hahm, K.B. (2001). Involvement of oxidative stress in experimentally induced reflux esophagitis and Barrett's esophagus: clue for the chemoprevention of esophageal carcinoma by antioxidants. *Mutation Research,* Vol. 480-481, pp.189-200.

Leonard, S.S., Cutler, D., Ding, M., Vallyathan, V., Castranova V, Shi, X. (2002). Antioxidant properties of fruit and vegetable juices: more to the story than ascorbic acid. *Annals of Clinical & Laboratory Science*, Vol. 32, pp. 193-200.

Li, H., Kantoff, P.W., Giovannucci, E., et al. (2005). Manganese superoxide dismutase polymorphism, prediagnostic antioxidant status, and risk of clinical significant prostate cancer. *Cancer Research*, Vol. 65, pp. 2498–2504.

Machado, A.M.D., Figueiredo, C., Seruca, R., Rasmussen, L.J. (2010). *Helicobacter pylori* infection generates genetic instability in gastric cells (Review). *Biochimica et Biophysica Acta*, Vol.180, pp.658–665.

Maithreyi, R., Janani, A.V., Krishna, R., Shweta, A., Edwin, R.R., Mohan, S. K. (2010). Erythrocyte lipid peroxidation and antioxidants in chronic alcoholics with alcoholic liver disease. *Asian Journal of Pharmaceutical and Clinical Research*, Vol. 3, pp. 183-185.

Marklund, S.L. (1984). Extracellular superoxide dismutase and other superoxide dismutase isozymes in tissue from nine mammalian species. *Biochemistry J*, Vol. 222, pp. 649.

Mashimo, M., Nishikawa, M., Higuchi, K., Hirose, M., Wei, Q., Haque, A., Sasaki, E., Shiba, M., Tominaga, K., Watanabe, T., Fujiwara, Y., Arakawa, T., Inoue, M. (2006). Production of reactive oxygen species in peripheral blood is increased in individuals with *Helicobacter pylori* infection and decreased after its eradication. *Helicobacter*, Vol. 11, pp. 266-271.

Miller, H.E., Rigelhof, F., Marquart, L., Prakash, A., Kanter, M. (2000). Antioxidant content of whole grain breakfast cereals, fruits and vegetables. *Journal of the American College of Nutrition*, Vol. 19, pp. 312S–319S.

Nouraie, M., Pietinen, P., Kamangar, F., Dawsey, S.M., Abnet, C.C., Albanes, D., Virtamo, J., Taylor, P.R. (2005). Fruits, vegetables, and antioxidants and risk of gastric cancer among male smokers. *Cancer Epidemiology, Biomarkers & Prevention*, Vol. 14, pp. 2087-2092.

Noyan, T., Guducuoglu, H. , Ilhan, M. (2009). A study of oxidative stress parameters in anti-*helicobacter pylorus* immunoglobulin g positive and negative gastric cancer patients. *Yonsei Medical Journal*, 50, 677-682.

Oyama, J., Maeda, T., Sasaki, M., Kozuma, K., Ochiai, R., Tokimitsu, I., Taguchi, S., Higuchi, Y. , Makino, N. (2010). Green tea catechins improve human forearm vascular function and have potent anti-inflammatory and anti-apoptotic effects in smokers. *Internal Medicine*, 49, 2553-2559.

Ozguner, F., Koyu, A. , Cesur, G. (2005). Active smoking causes oxidative stress and decreases blood melatonin levels. *Toxicology and Industrial Health*, Vol. 21, pp. 21-26.

Pace, G., Di Massimo, C., De Amicis, D., Corbacelli, C., Di Renzo, L., Vicentini, C., Miano, L., Tozzi Ciancarelli, M.G. (2010). Oxidative stress in benign prostatic hyperplasia and prostate cancer. *Urologia Internationalis*, Vol. 85, pp. 328-333.

Pasupathi, P., Saravanan, G., Chinnaswamy, P., Bakthavathsalam, G. (2009). Effect of chronic smoking on lipid peroxidation and antioxidant status in gastric carcinoma patients. *Indian Journal of Gastroenterology*, Vol. 28, pp. 65–67.

Peleteiro, B., Lopes, C., Figueiredo, C., Lunet, N. (2011). Salt intake and gastric cancer risk according to *Helicobacter pylori* infection, smoking, tumour site and histological type. *British Journal of Cancer*, Vol.104, pp. 198-207.

Pelicano, H., Carney, D., Huanga, P. (2004). ROS stress in cancer cells and therapeutic implications. *Drug Resistance Updates*, Vol. 7, pp. 97–110.

Pellegrini, N., Serafini,M., Colombi, B., Del Rio, D., Salvatore, S., Bianchi, M., Brighenti, F. (2003).Total antioxidant capacity of plant foods, beverages and oils consumed in Italy assessed by three different *in vitro* assays. *The Journal of Nutrition*, Vol. 133, pp. 2812–2819.

Reddy, E.P., Reddy, V.S., Mouli, C. K., Rao, P.S. (2009). Physiological antioxidant system and oxidative stress in stomach cancer patients with normal renal and hepatic function. *Online Journal of Health Allied Sciences*, Vol.8, pp.9.

Rizk, M., Fayed, T.A., Badawy, M., Sabaa El-Regal, N. (2006). Effect of different durations of *Schistosoma mansoni* infection on the levels of some antioxidants in mice. *Medical Journal of Islamic World Academy of Sciences*, Vol.16, pp. 25-34.

Salim, A. S. (1992). Oxygen-derived free-radical scavengers prolong survival in gastric cancer. *Chemotherapy*, Vol. 38, 135-144.

Sangeetha, N., Aranganathan, S., Nalini, N. (2010). Silibinin ameliorates oxidative stress induced aberrant crypt foci and lipid peroxidation in 1, 2 dimethylhydrazine induced rat colon cancer. *Investigational New Drugs*, Vol. 28, pp. 225-233.

Ścibior, D., Skrzycki, M., Podsiad, M., Czeczot, H. (2008). Glutathione level and glutathione-dependent enzyme activities in blood serum of patients with gastrointestinal tract tumors. *Clinical Biochemistry*, Vol.41, pp. 852–858.

Shaikh, A.K., Suryakar, A.N. (2009). Oxidative stress and antioxidant status before and after supplementation of A-Z anti-oxidant tablets in coronary artery disease. *Biomedical Research*, Vol. 20, pp.136-140.

Shinde S. A., Suryakar, A.N., Sontakke A.N., & More U.K. (2010). Effect of antioxidant vitamin supplementation on erythrocyte membrane composition in type I diabetes mellitus in context of oxidative stress. *Biomedical Research*, Vol. 21, pp. 156-160.

Skrzydlewska, E., Kozuszko, B., Sulkowska, M., Bogdan, Z., Kozlowski, M., Snarska, J., et al. (2003). Antioxidant potential in esophageal, stomach and colorectal cancers. *Hepatogastroenterology*, Vol. 50, pp. 126–131.

Soini, Y., Kallio, J.P., Hirvikoski, P., Helin, H., Kellokumpu-Lehtinen, P., Kang, S.W., Tammela, T.L., Peltoniemi, M., Martikainen, P.M. , Kinnula, V.L. (2006). Oxidative/nitrosative stress and peroxiredoxin 2 are associated with grade and prognosis of human renal carcinoma. *Acta Pathologica, Microbiologica, et Immunologica Scandinavica*, Vol. 114, pp. 329-337.

Steevens, J., Schouten, L.J., Goldbohm, R.A., van den Brandt, P.A. (2010). Alcohol consumption, cigarette smoking and risk of subtypes of oesophageal and gastric cancer: a prospective cohort study. *Gut*, Vol.59, pp. 39-48.

Sumathi, M.E., Tembad M.M., Jayaprakash Murthy D.S., Preethi, B.P. (2010). Study of lipid profile and oxidative stress in chronic renal failure. *Biomedical Research*, Vol. 21, pp. 451- 456.

Tandon, R., Khanna, H.D., Dorababu, M., Goel, R.K. (2004). Oxidative stress and antioxidants status in peptic ulcer and gastric carcinoma. *Indian Journal of Physiology and Pharmacology*, Vol. 48, pp. 115-118.

Tian, W., Zhao, Y., Liu, S ., Li, X. (2010). Meta-analysis on the relationship between nonsteroidal anti-inflammatory drug use and gastric cancer. *European Journal of Cancer Prevention*, Vol.19, pp. 288-298.

Tiwari, S.K., Manoj, G., Sharma, V., Sivaram, G., Saikant, R., Bardia, A., Sharma, V.K., Abid, Z., Khan, A.A., Habeeb, M.A., Habibullah, C.M., Kumar, B.S., Nandan, A. (2010). Relevance of *Helicobacter pylori* genotypes in gastric pathology and its association with plasma malondialdehyde and nitric oxide levels. *Inflammopharmacology*. Vol. 18, pp. 59-64.

Trédaniel, J., Boffetta, P., Buiatti, E., Saracci, R., Hirsch, A. (1997). Tobacco smoking and gastric cancer: review and meta-analysis. *International Journal of Cancer*, Vol. 72, pp. 565-573.

Valavanidis, A., Vlachogianni, T., Fiotakis, K. (2009). Tobacco smoke: involvement of reactive oxygen species and stable free radicals in mechanisms of oxidative damage, carcinogenesis and synergistic effects with other respirable particles. *International Journal of Environmental Research and Public Health*, Vol. 6, pp. 445-462.

Valko, M., Leibfritz, D., Moncol, J., Cronin, M.T.D., Mazur, M., Telser, J. (2007). Free radicals and antioxidants in normal physiological functions and human disease (Review). *The International Journal of Biochemistry & Cell Biology*, Vol. 39, pp. 44–84.

Valko, M., Rhodes, C.J., Moncol, J., Izakovic, M., Mazur, M. (2006). Free radicals, metals and antioxidants in oxidative stress-induced cancer (Mini-review). *Chemico-Biological Interactions*, Vol. 160, pp. 1–40.

Walecka-Kapica, E., Knopik-Dabrowicz, A., Klupińska, G., Chojnacki, J. (2008). The assessment of nitric oxide metabolites in gastric juice in *Helicobacter pylori* infected subjects in compliance with grade of inflammatory lesions in gastric mucosa. *Pol Merkur Lekarski*, Vol.24, pp.95-100.

Wang, S., Wang, F., Shi, X., Dai, J., Peng, Y., Guo, X., Wang, X., Shen, H., Hu, Z. (2009). Association between manganese superoxide dismutase (MnSOD) Val-9Ala polymorphism and cancer risk - A meta-analysis. *European Journal of Cancer*, Vol. 45, pp. 2874 -2881.

Yang, J.J., Ko, K.P., Cho, L.Y., Shin, A., Gwack, J., Chang, S.H., Shin, H.R., Yoo, K.Y., Kang, D., Park, S.K. (2009). The role of TNF genetic variants and the interaction with cigarette smoking for gastric cancer risk: a nested case-control study. *BMC Cancer*, Vol. 9, pp. 238.

Yang, P., Zhou, Y., Chen, B., Wan, H.W., Jia, G.Q., Bai, H.L., Wu, X.T. (2010). Aspirin use and the risk of gastric cancer: a meta-analysis. *Digestive Diseases & Sciences*. Vol. 55, pp. 1533-1539.

Yeon, J.Y., Suh, Y.J., Kim, S.W., Baik, H.W., Sung, C.J., Kim, H.S., Sung, M.K. (2011). Evaluation of dietary factors in relation to the biomarkers of oxidative stress and inflammation in breast cancer risk. *Nutrition* (In Press). DOI: S0899-9007(10)00353-9 [pii]10.1016/j.nut.2010.10.012

Yuyama, K., Yamamoto, H., Nishizaki, I., Kato, T., Sora, I., Yamamoto, T. (2003). Caspase-independent cell death by low concentrations of nitric oxide in PC12 cells: involvement of cytochrome C oxidase inhibition and the production of reactive oxygen species in mitochondria. *Journal of Neuroscience Research*, Vol. 73, pp.351–363.

Part 2

Immunology and Immunohistomorphology

10

Immune Cell Responses in Gastric Carcinoma: An Analysis Based on Histopathology

Haruo Ohtani
Department of Pathology, Mito Medical Center, National Hospital Organization, 280 Sakurano-sato, Ibarak, Ibaraki 311-3193, Japan

1. Introduction

Recent advances in tumor immunology have established the concept of tumor immunosurveillance, and cancers are considered to have developed after overcoming these host immunosurveillance mechanisms. As a result, established cancers are in an immunosuppressive microenvironment (Dunn et al. 2004; Finn 2008).

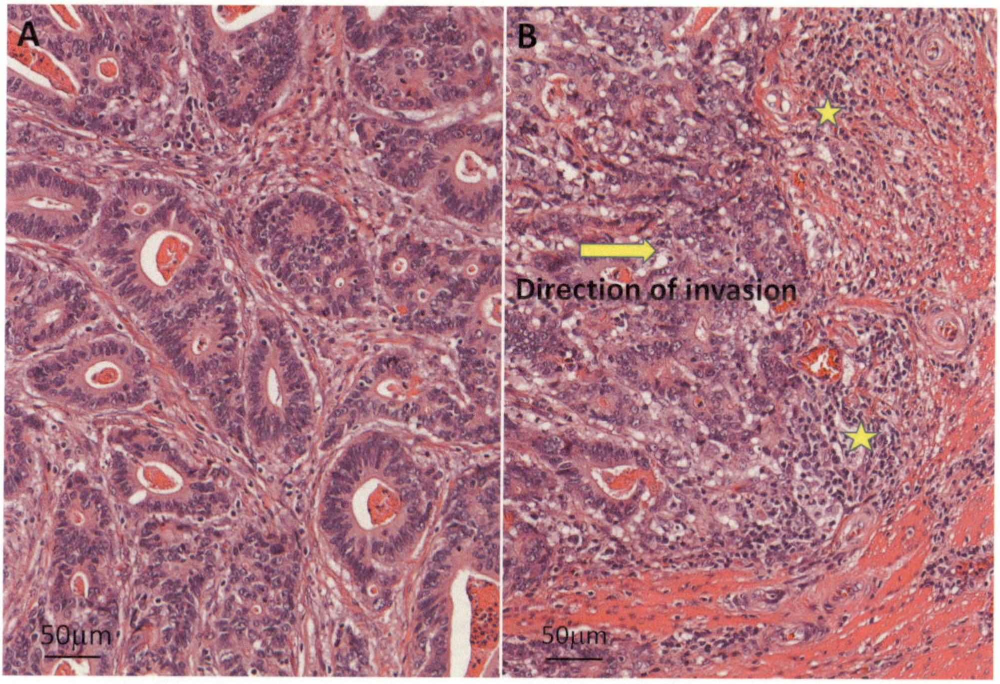

Fig. 1. Histology of conventional gastric cancer. **A)** Area inside conventional gastric cancer (well differentiated tubular adenocarcinoma). The stromal area is infiltrated by scanty tumor-infiltrating lymphocytes, a basic feature of cancer. **B)** Area of invasive margin in the same case. Note the presence of tumor-infiltrating lymphocytes along the invasive margin (asterisks). An arrow indicates the direction of invasion.

This concept implies that established tumors are either devoid of immune cell infiltrate (Fig. 1A) or, if present, the immune cell infiltrate is suppressed. Routine histopathological examination reveals that human cancer tissues are infiltrated to varying degrees by tumor-infiltrating lymphocytes, which if present, usually accumulate along the invasive margin (tumor-host interface) (Fig. 1B). In contrast, the stroma inside tumors tends to be devoid of tumor-infiltrating lymphocytes (Fig. 1A). Unraveling the biological significance of tumor-infiltrating lymphocytes is not straightforward because of the complexity of the cellular compositions of tumor-infiltrating lymphocytes themselves (Yu and Fu 2006). In several cancers, it is known that higher levels of tumor-infiltrating lymphocytes are prognostic of longer survival rates in patients (Naito et al. 1998; Sato et al. 2005; Galon et al. 2006; Sharma et al. 2007). Thus it appears likely that tumor-infiltrating lymphocytes may possess anti-tumor activity that alleviates cancer aggressiveness.

2. Gastric cancers with lymphoid stroma

Cancers with prominent tumor-infiltrating lymphocytic responses exist as extreme variants in tumor pathology; medullary carcinoma of the breast and nasopharyngeal carcinoma ("lymphoepithelial carcinoma") are two such examples. In gastric cancer, such variants are designated "gastric cancers with lymphoid stroma" or "lymphoepithelioma-like cancer".Such cancers are characterized by poorly differentiated cancer cells with a syncytial

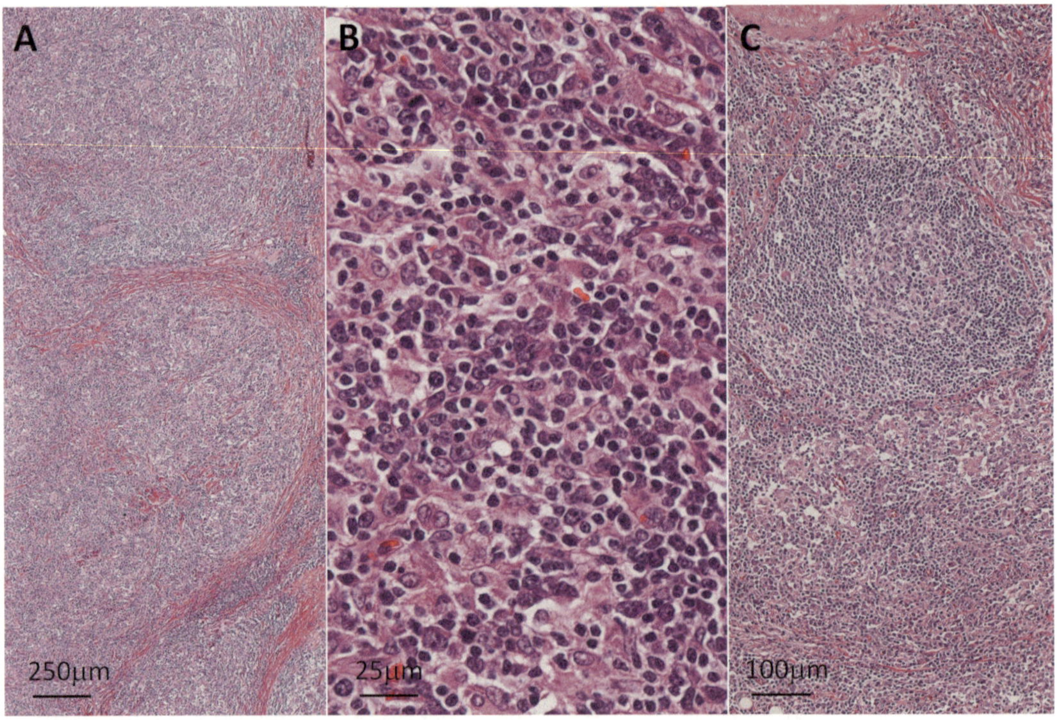

Fig. 2. A-C. **A, B**) Histology of lymphocyte-rich gastric cancer (typical case of lymphoepithelioma-like cancer). Low (A) and high power magnification (B). Note massive infiltration by lymphocytes, and poorly differentiated cancer cells. **C**) Occasionally formed lymph follicle with a germinal center.

appearance and massive lymphoid infiltrate (Fig. 2A, B). Formation of lymph follicles containing a germinal center is usually observed (Fig. 2C). The prognosis for typical cases is better than that for conventional gastric cancer cases (Watanabe et al. 1976; Minamoto et al. 1990). This suggests that the lymphoid stroma may produce an antitumor immune response. Most gastric cancers with lymphoid stroma are associated with Epstein-Barr virus (EB virus) (Tokunaga et al. 1993; Fukayama et al. 2010). It should be noted, however, that not all Epstein-Barr virus-associated gastric cancers have lymphoid stroma. In this chapter, attention is focused on how lymphoid infiltrate occurs in gastric cancers.

3. Cellular composition of the lymphocyte-rich stroma

The term "lymphocyte-rich gastric cancers" used here includes typical gastric cancers with lymphoid stroma (Fig. 2 A-C) and other types of gastric cancers associated with tumor-infiltrating lymphocytic responses in nearly whole stroma. The lymphocyte-rich gastric cancers are consistently infiltrated by $CD3^+$ T cells (Fig. 3A), among which both $CD8^+$ and $CD4^+$ T cells are present. Key antigen presenting cells, the $CD83^+$ myeloid-derived dendritic cells (Heath and Carbone 2009) are also distributed in the T cell-rich stroma of the lymphocyte-rich gastric cancers (Fig. 3B). B-lymphocytes are not generally abundant in the tissue (Fig. 3C), except in areas containing lymphoid follicles where abundant B-cell populations are observed. Saiki et al.'s (1996) finding that approximately 13% of $CD8^+$ T cells exhibited Ki-67 immunoreactivity implies that active immune responses with lymphocyte proliferative activity take place in lymphocyte-rich gastric cancers.

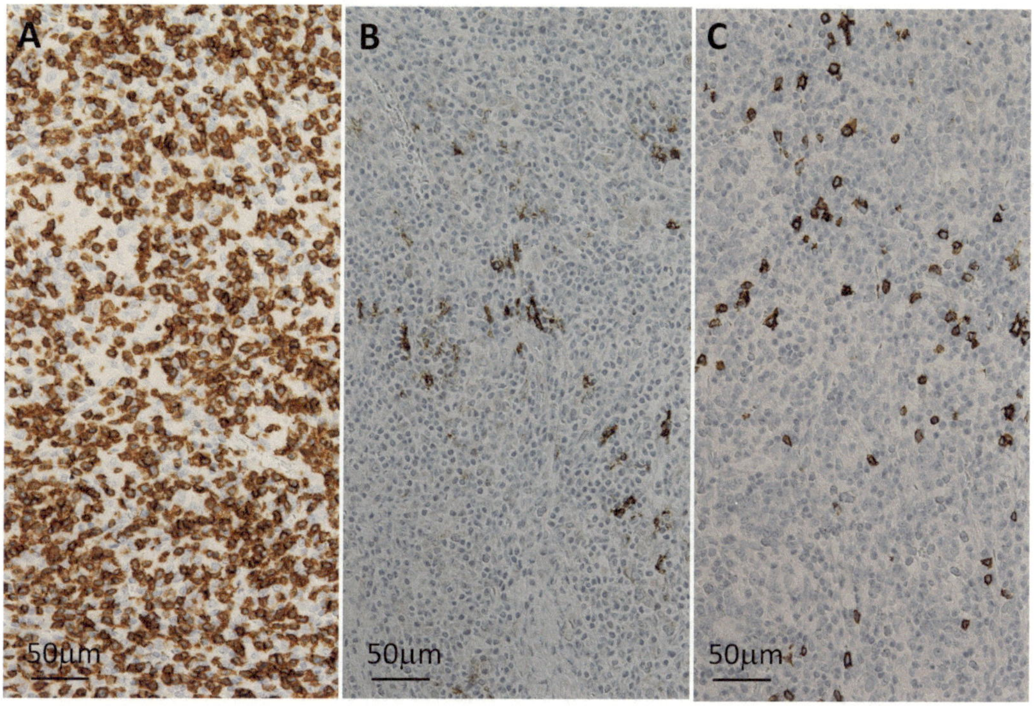

Fig. 3. Single immunohistochemistry of lymphocyte-rich gastric cancers for CD3 (**A**), CD83 (**B**), and CD20 (**C**) (signals shown with brown, hematoxylin-nuclear counterstaining). Note abundance of T-lymphocytes with mature dendritic cells. B-lymphocytes are not abundant.

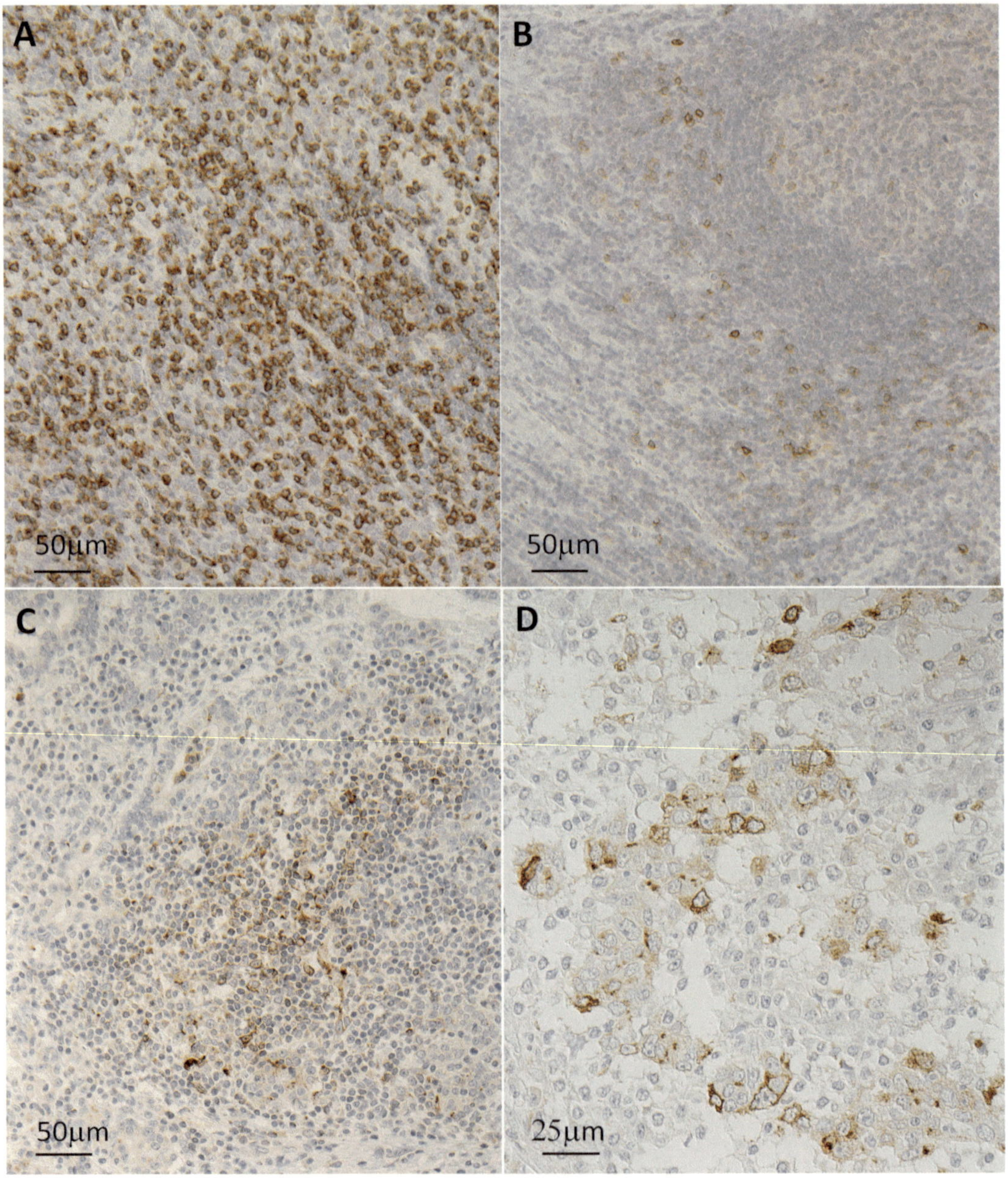

Fig. 4. A-D. Single immunohistochemistry of lymphocyte-rich gastric cancers for CXCR3 (**A**), CCR4 (**B**), and CXCL9 (**C** and **D**) (signals shown with brown, hematoxylin-nuclear counterstaining). **A**) Note abundance of CXCR3-positive lymphocytes. **B**) Expression of chemokine receptor CCR4 is sparse, which is mainly expressed by Th2 cell and regulatory T cells **C**) CXCL9 is mainly localized in stromal cells in lymphocyte-rich stroma. **D**) Only a part of cancer cells expresses CXCL9.

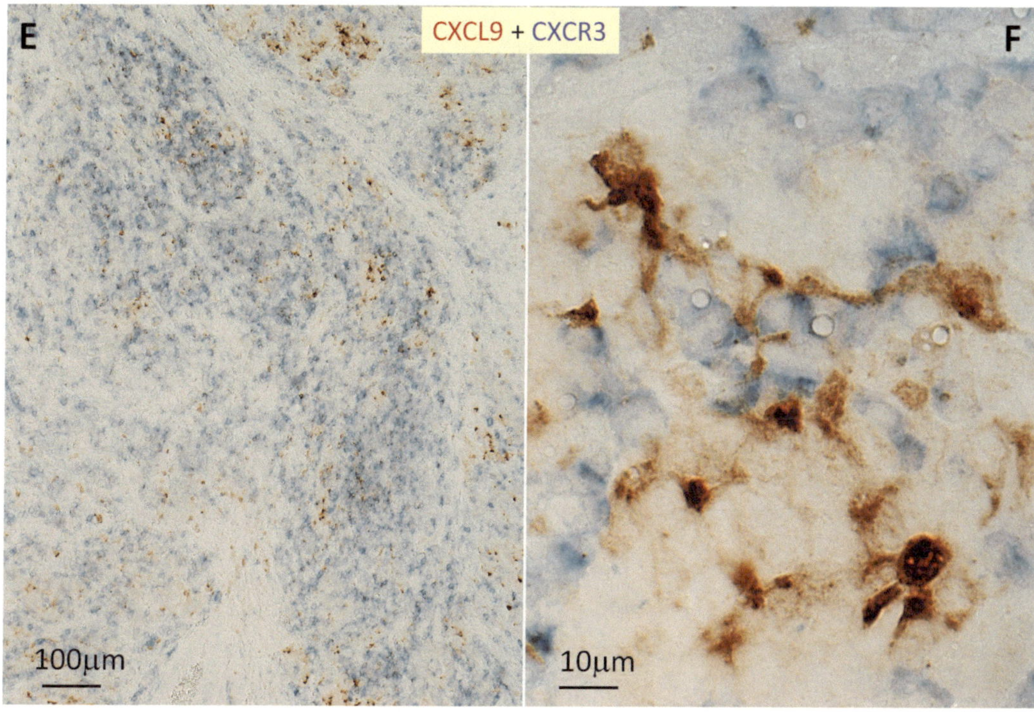

Fig. 4. E, F. Double staining of lymphocyte-rich gastric cancer for CXCL9 (brown) and CXCR3 (blue). Low power (**E**) and high power magnification (**F**) reveals that CXCL3+ stromal cells are in close contact with CXCR3+ lymphocytes; this is reminiscent of a dendritic cell-T cell distribution in the secondary lymphoid tissues such as lymph nodes.

4. Expression of chemokine CXCL9 and receptor CXCR3 in lymphocyte-rich gastric cancers

Chemokines are chemotactic cytokines, which cause migration of leukocytes and other cells that express cognate chemokine receptors (Zlotnik and Yoshie 2000; Murphy et al. 2000; Allen et al. 2007). Chemokines and their receptors play important roles in inflammation, lymphoid organogenesis and cancer cell invasion and/or metastasis. The chemokine receptor CXCR3 and two of its cognate ligands, CXCL9 (MIG) and CXCL10 (IP10) are described here because CXCR3 is widely expressed by T helper type 1 (Th1) cells and CD8+ T cells (Zlotnik and Yoshie, 2000; Ohtani et al. 2009).

By immunohistochemistry, CXCR3+ lymphocytes are abundant in the lymphoid stroma of lymphocyte-rich gastric cancers (Fig. 4A), which contrasts markedly with the sparse distribution of CCR4+ cells (Fig. 4B). This suggests a predominance of Th1 cells over Th2 cells in this tissue. CXCR3+ cells are sparse in the lymphoid follicles (B-cell zone). The CXCR3-ligands, CXCL9 and CXCL10, are mainly expressed by dendritic-shaped "stromal cells" that were distributed in CXCR3+ cell-rich lymphoid stroma (Fig. 4C). CXCL9 and CXCL10 are also expressed in only a small portion of cancer cells (Fig. 4D). Of the two, CXCL9 is more frequently observed in stromal cells of lymphocyte-rich gastric cancers than CXCL10. The author has designated this type of distribution "CXCR3+ T cell-CXCL9+ stromal cell clustering", which is clearly observed by double staining (Fig. 4E) (Ohtani et al.

2009, 2010). At higher magnification, a close cell-to-cell contact between CXCL9+ stromal cells and CXCR3+ cells is revealed (Fig. 2F). This clustering, reminiscent of T cell-dendritic cell clustering in the secondary lymphoid tissues, is confined to lymphocyte-rich gastric cancers, but not conventional gastric cancers. Hence, the results thus far suggest that the Th1 response is dominant and that CXCL9+ stromal cells are important for large-scale infiltration by CXCR3+ T cells.

5. Cell identification of CXCL9+ stromal cells

The shape of CXCL9+ stromal cells suggests that they may be dendritic cells. CD83+ mature, myeloid-derived dendritic cells are in fact found to be distributed in lymphocyte-rich gastric cancers (Fig. 3B). However, double immunohistochemistry reveals that only 10-20% of CXCL9+ stromal cells co-express CD83 (Fig. 5A), and half of CXCL9+ stromal cells co-expresses fascin (a wide marker of dendritic cells) (Fig. 5B). DC-Lamp, another marker of mature dendritic cells, is expressed also in a part of CXCL9+ stromal cells (Fig. 5C). A half of CXCL9+ stromal cells expresses CD68, a marker of macrophages including immature dendritic cells.

These data suggest that only a minor part of CXCL9+ stromal cell populations comprises mature, myeloid-derived dendritic cells, but more than half are stromal cells (probably myeloid-derived cells) that cannot be classified precisely at present.

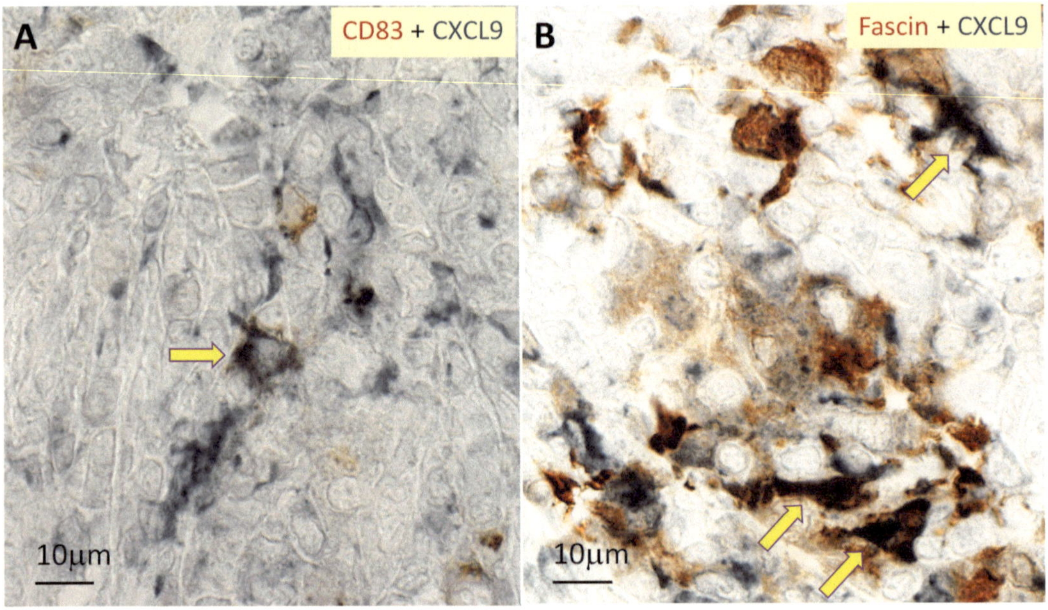

Fig. 5. A and B. **A)** Double staining for CD83 and CXCL9. An arrow indicates CD83+ (brown) mature dendritic cells also expressing CXCL9 (blue). **B)** Double staining for fascin (brown) and CXCL9 (blue). Arrows indicate fascin+ dendritic cells co-expressing CXCL9. These data suggest that a part of CXCL9-positive stromal cells are dendritic cells.

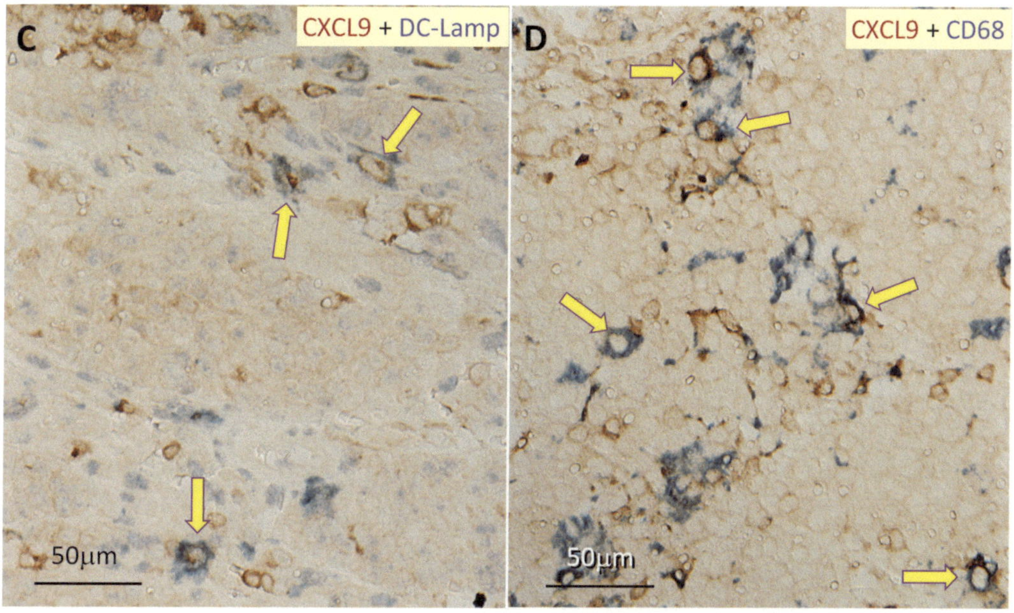

Fig. 5. C and D. **C**) Double staining for CXCL9 and DC-lamp (using frozen section). Arrows indicateDC-Lamp+ mature dendritic cells (blue) also expressing CXCL9 (brown) Double staining for CXCL9 (brown) and CD68 (blue). Arrows indicate double positive cells. These cells may be macrophages or immature dendritic cells.

6. Proliferative activity of T cells in close contact with CXCL9+ stromal cells

The proliferative activity of T cells in the histopathological samples can be assessed using Ki-67 immunohistochemistry. As shown in Fig. 6A, double staining reveals that CD45RO+ T cells (red) and CXCL9+ stromal cells (dark blue) exhibit close cell-to-cell contact (similar to Fig. 2B). Fig. 6B has Ki-67 immunostaining (brown) added to the double staining. This triple staining shows that CD45RO+(red)Ki-67+(brown) cells exist in close contact to CXCL9+ stromal cells (dark blue) (Fig. 6B, arrows). Approximately 10% of CD45RO+ cells co-express Ki-67. This indicates that CD45RO+ T cells in close contact with CXCL9+ stromal cells have proliferative activity. Taking account of the well-characterized T-cell and dendritic cell interactions, the data here imply that when CXCR3+ T cells are in close contact with CXCL9+ stromal cells, they may receive proliferative stimuli. Therefore, the lymphoid stroma is not a mere aggregation of lymphocytes, but a place where significant T cell–stromal cell interactions can occur.

7. Similarity to the regional lymph nodes

Given that peripheral tissue (with inflammatory changes) has a close connection with regional lymph nodes, it is important to compare potential changes occurring between gastric cancers and regional lymph nodes. As shown in figure 7A, CXCL9+ stromal cells are abundantly distributed in the T-cell zone in the regional lymph nodes of lymphocyte-rich gastric cancers. In contrast, regional lymph nodes in conventional gastric cancers show only sporadic expression of CXCL9+ cells (Fig. 7B). Hence, histopathological identification of CXCL9+ cells in both primary tumor and regional lymph nodes suggests that a functional relationship exists between them.

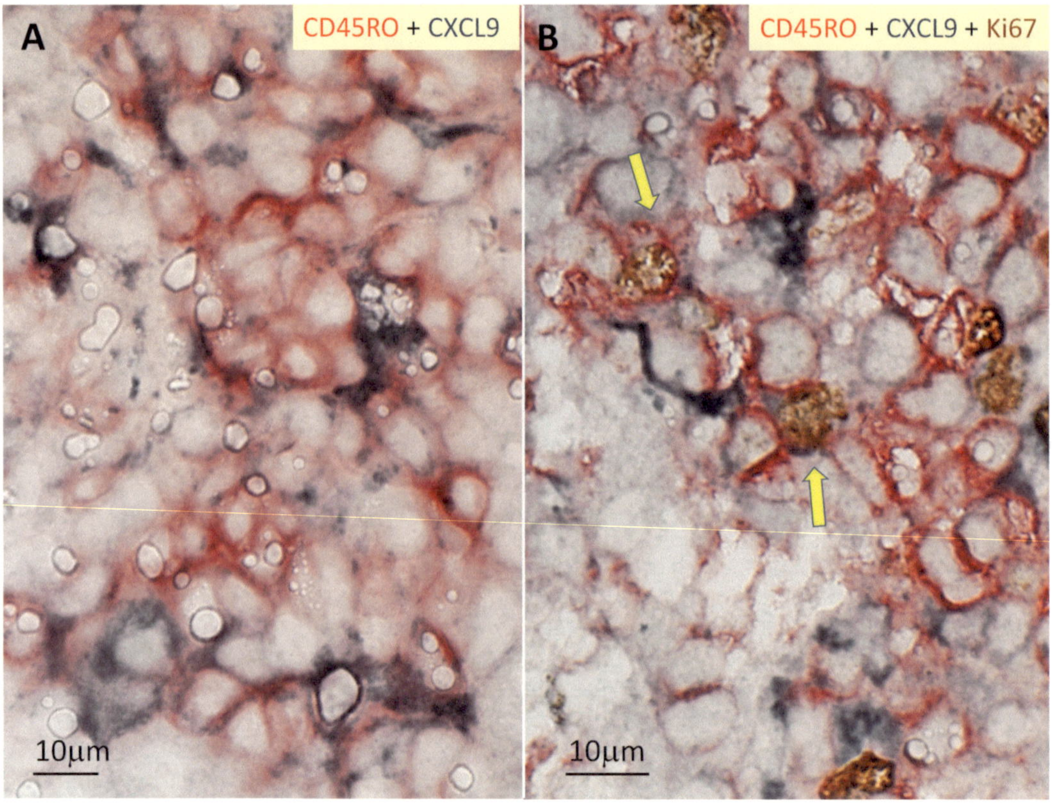

Fig. 6. Immunohistochemical analyses for proliferative activity of T cells in lymphocyte-rich gastric cancer. **A**) Double staining for CD45RO (red) and CXCL9 (dark blue), revealing that CXCL9+ stromal cells are in close contact with CD45RO+ T cells (similar to the results shown in Fig. 2B). **B)** Triple staining for CD45RO (red) + CXCL9 (dark blue) + Ki-67 (brown). Arrows indicate Ki-67+ T cells (brown and red) that are in close contact with CXCL9+ stromal cells (dark blue). This suggests that T cells in close contact with CXCL9+ cells are proliferating in lymphocyte-rich gastric cancers.

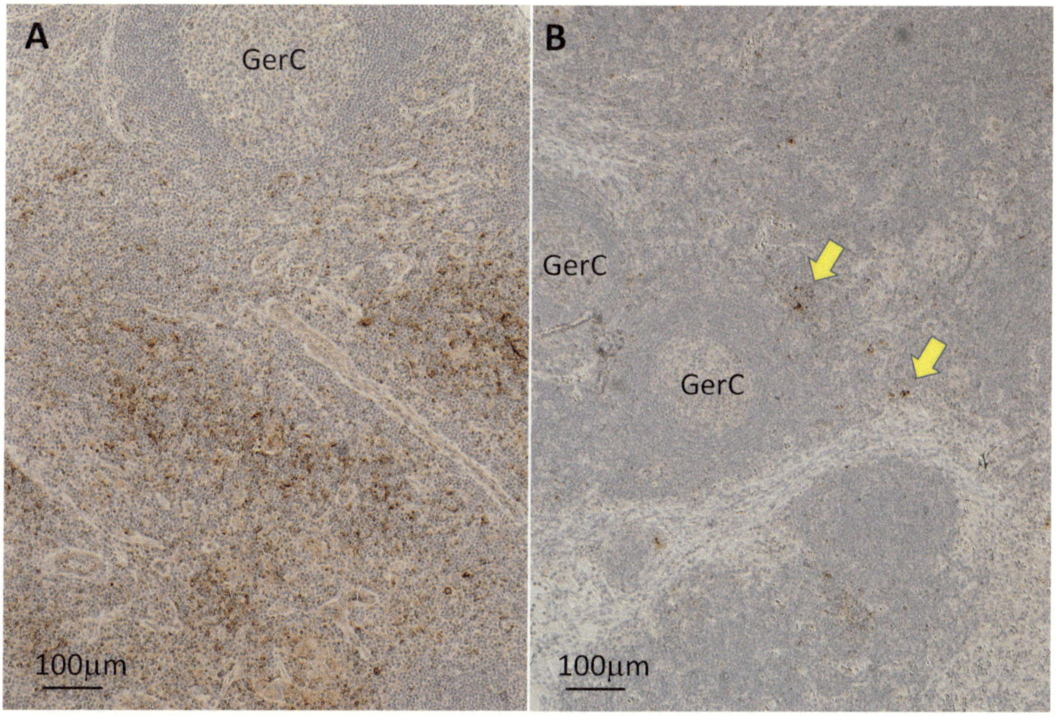

Fig. 7. Immunohistochemistry for CXCL9 in regional lymph nodes in lymphocyte-rich- (**A**) and conventional (**B**) gastric cancers. Note the abundance of CXCL9+ stromal cells in regional lymph nodes in lymphocyte-rich gastric cancers (A), contrasted by sparse distribution of CXCL9+ stromal cells (arrows) in regional lymph node of conventional gastric cancer (B). GerC in (B) and (C) represents germinal centers.

8. Regulatory T cells

The data thus far suggests the presence of pro-immune responses in lymphocyte-rich gastric cancers. However, current opinion on tumor immune evasion mechanisms maintains that immunosuppressive factors play a major role. Regulatory T-cells are one type of cell that exerts a suppressive function, and forkhead box protein-3 (Foxp3) is a reliable marker of the cells (Zou 2006). In gastric cancer, diffuse distribution of regulatory T cells is associated with a poorer prognosis of patients (Mizukami et al. 2008a,b). Fig. 8A shows the distribution of Foxp3+ regulatory T-cell in lymphocyte-rich gastric cancer. Using Foxp3 as a marker, quantitative immunohistochemistry shows a small increase in the number of regulatory T-cells in lymphocyte-rich gastric cancers, compared with conventional gastric cancers (Fig. 8B). This sharply contrasts with a marked increase in CXCR3+ lymphocytes observed in lymphocyte-rich gastric cancers compared with conventional gastric cancers (Fig. 8C). Hence, the ratio of CXCR3+ lymphocytes/regulatory T-cells is higher in lymphocyte-rich gastric cancers than in conventional gastric cancers. Overall, this suggests that the lymphoid stroma in lymphocyte-rich gastric cancers is shifted towards a pro-immune status compared with conventional gastric cancers. And, it is clear that immunosuppressive aspects of lymphoid stroma cannot be explained by a mere increase in regulatory T-cells alone.

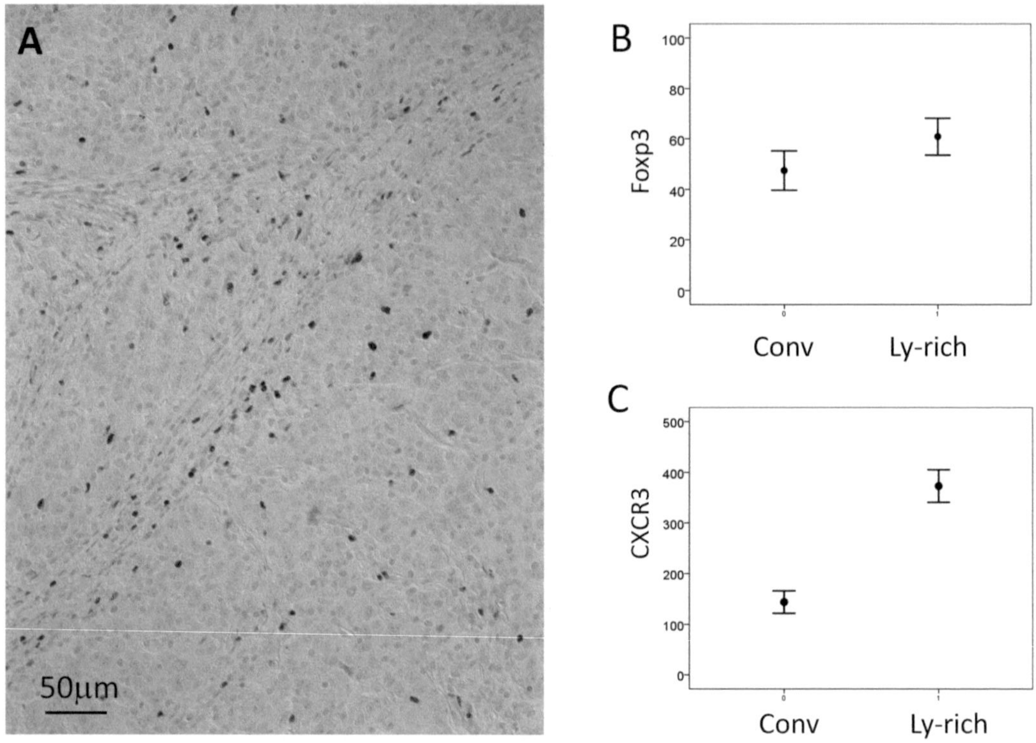

Fig. 8. Analysis on regulatory T cells. **A**) Immunohistochemitry for Foxp3 reveals that regulatory T-cells are also distributed in lymphocyte-rich gastric cancer. **B**) However, regulatory T-cells are mildly elevated in lymphocyte-rich gastric cancers than in conventional gastric cancer. (**C**) There are a sharp increase in the number of $CXCR3^{+}$ cells in lymphocyte-rich gastric cancers as compared with conventional gastric cancer (error bars for panels B and C are the mean ± standard error). Methods of B) and C). Immunohistochemistry for Foxp3 was performed on routine histopathological slides. The numbers of $Foxp3^{+}$ cells per unit area (0.0625 mm^2) were counted manually suing a 40x objective lens. At least three areas were counted. In lymphocyte-rich gastric cancer, areas with average infiltration were counted. In conventional gastric cancers, the most densely infiltrated areas were counted. Conv, conventional gastric cancer. Ly-rich, lymphocyter-rich gastric cancer. Verticals bar in B) and C) represent number of cells per unit area (0.0625 mm^2).

Next the immunohistochemical distribution of chemokine CCL22 (MDC) is described. CCL22 is one of the cognate ligands of CCR4 which is frequently expressed by regulatory T-cells and Th2 cells. CCL22 is focally expressed by mature dendritic cells in lymphocyte-rich gastric cancers, but not in conventional gastric cancers (Ohtani et al. 2010). It is generally believed that tumor-derived CCL22 promotes accumulation of CCR4⁺ regulatory T-cells, which subverts immune responses in cancer (Menetrier-Caux et al. 2009). Tan et al. (2011) suggested that regulatory T-cells can promote tumor metastasis through RANKL, a mechanism distinct from an immunoregulatory one. Therefore, it is conceivable that dendritic cells in lymphocyte-rich gastric cancers may have both tumor-inhibitory and tumor-promoting properties

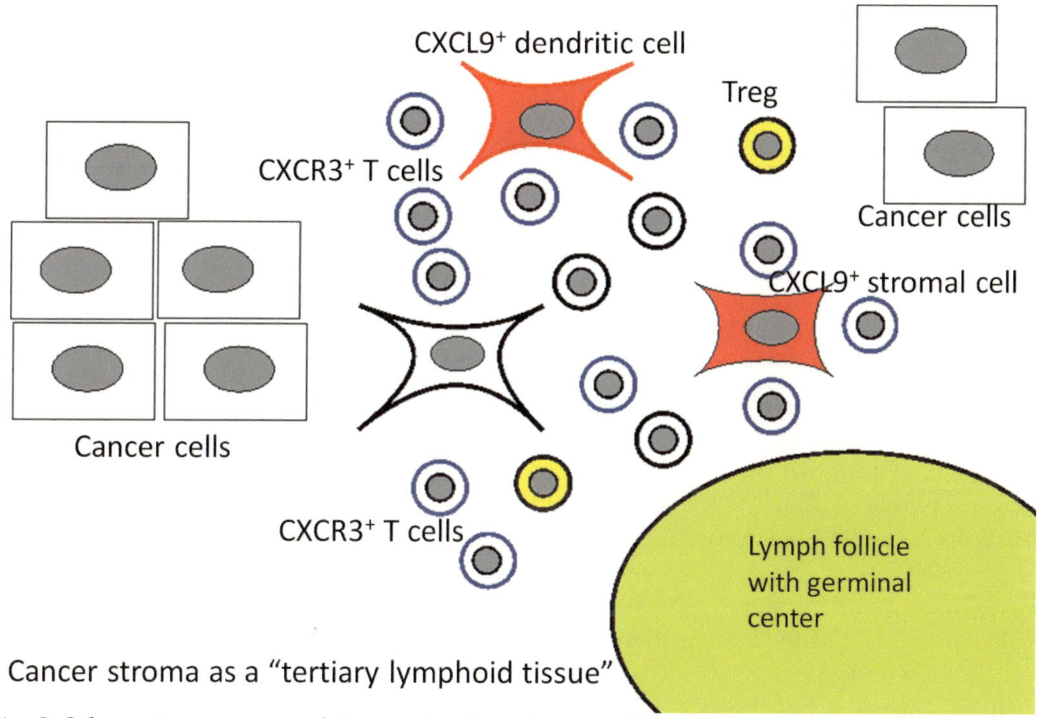

Fig. 9. Schematic summary of the results. Lymphocyte-rich gastric cancers are characterized by an abundance of CXCR3⁺ T cells with CXCL9⁺ stromal cells (CXCR3⁺ T cell-CXCL9⁺ stromal cell clustering). Dendritic cells are also distributed in the section. Together with the formation of lymphoid follicles with germinal centers, these data suggest that the stroma of lymphocyte-rich gastric cancer is a tertiary lymphoid tissue.

9. Conclusions

Fig. 9 is a schematic summary of this chapter. This depicts stromal elements of lymphocyte-rich gastric cancers. T cells are predominant in this lymphoid stroma, where chemokine CXCL9 and chemokine receptor CXCR3 are expressed by stromal cells and T cells, respectively, to form CXCL9⁺ stromal cell-CXCR3⁺ T cell clustering. Mature, myeloid-derived dendritic cells are also distributed in the tissue. A part of CXCL9⁺ cells corresponds to these mature dendritic cells. However, a large part of CXCL9⁺ stromal cells remains unclassified.

Regulatory T-cells are also present, but their relative density is lower in lymphocyte-rich gastric cancers than in conventional gastric cancers. Together with the occasional formation of lymph follicles with a germinal center, the lymphoid stroma in lymphocyte-rich gastric cancer is judged to be similar to the secondary lymphoid tissue (i.e., lymph nodes or Peyer patches). Lymphoid tissues newly formed in the peripheral tissues during chronic inflammation are designated "tertiary lymphoid tissues" (Aloisi et al. 2006). The author proposes, therefore, that lymphoid stroma in lymphocyte-rich gastric cancer can be regarded as tertiary lymphoid tissue (Ohtani et al. 2009). Hence, immunostimulatory aspects of lymphocyte-rich gastric cancers have been clarified in this chapter. A mere increase of regulatory T-cells is not observed in lymphocyte-rich gastric cancer. Further analyses of the immunoregulatory aspects of lymphoid stroma are now required because immunosubversion is considered to be a major obstacle to successful immunotherapy of cancer.

10. Acknowledgments

The author is grateful to Drs. Osamu Yoshie, Masaaki Miyazawa, Takashi Nakayama, Fuminori Katou, Eiichi Sato, Noriko Kimura, Hiroshi Naganuma, and Yuriko Saiki for their cooperation. Clerical assistance by Ms. Fumiko Date is also greatly appreciated.

11. References

Allen SJ, Crown SE, Handel TM. (2007) Chemokine: receptor structure, interactions, and antagonism. Annu Rev Immunol 25:787-820.

Aloisi F, Pujol-Borrell R. (2006) Lymphoid neogenesis in chronic inflammatory diseases. Nat Rev Immunol 6:205-217.

Dunn GP, Old LJ, Schreiber RD. (2004) The three Es of cancer immunoediting. Annu Rev Immunol 22:329-360.

Yu P, Fu YX. (2006) Tumor-infiltrating T lymphocytes: friends or foes? Lab Invest. 86:231-245.

Finn OJ. Cancer immunology. (2008) N Engl J Med. 358(25):2704-2715.

Fukayama M. (2010) Epstein-Barr virus and gastric carcinoma. Pathol Int. 60(5): 337-350.

Galon J, Costes A, Sanchez-Cabo F, Kirilovsky A, Mlecnik B, Lagorce-Pagès C, Tosolini M, Camus M, Berger A, Wind P, Zinzindohoué F, Bruneval P, Cugnenc PH, Trajanoski Z, Fridman WH, Pagès F. (2006) Type, density, and location of immune cells within human colorectal tumors predict clinical outcome. Science 313(5795):1960-1964.

Heath WR, Carbone FR. Dendritic cell subsets in primary and secondary T cell responses at body surfaces. (2009) Nat Immunol. 10:1237-1244.

Ménétrier-Caux C, Gobert M, Caux C. (2009) Differences in tumor regulatory T-cell localization and activation status impact patient outcome. Cancer Res. 69(20):7895-7898.

Minamoto T, Mai M, Watanabe K, Ooi A, Kitamura T, Takahashi Y, Ueda H, Ogino T, Nakanishi I. (1990) Medullary carcinoma with lymphocytic infiltration of the stomach. Clinicopathologic study of 27 cases and immunohistochemical analysis of the subpopulations of infiltrating lymphocytes in the tumor. Cancer 66:945-952.

Mizukami Y, Kono K, Kawaguchi Y, Akaike H, Kamimura K, Sugai H, Fujii H. (2008) Localization pattern of Foxp3+ regulatory T cells is associated with clinical behaviour in gastric cancer. Br J Cancer. 98:148-153.

Mizukami Y, Kono K, Kawaguchi Y, Akaike H, Kamimura K, Sugai H, Fujii H. (2008) CCL17 and CCL22 chemokines within tumor microenvironment are related to accumulation of Foxp3+ regulatory T cells in gastric cancer. Int J Cancer. 122:2286-2293.

Murphy PM, Baggiolini M, Charo IF, Hébert CA, Horuk R, Matsushima K, Miller LH, Oppenheim JJ, Power CA. (2000) International union of pharmacology. XXII. Nomenclature for chemokine receptors. Pharmacol Rev. 52(1):145-76.

Naito Y, Saito K, Shiiba K, Ohuchi A, Saigenji K, Nagura H, Ohtani H. (1998) CD8+ T-cells infiltrated within cancer cell nests as a prognostic factor in human colorectal cancer. Cancer Res 58:3491-3494.

Ohtani H, Jin Z, Takegawa S, Nakayama T, Yoshie O. (2009) Abundant expression of CXCL9 (MIG) by stromal cells that include dendritic cells and accumulation of CXCR3+ T cells in lymphocyte-rich gastric carcinoma. *J Pathol* 217:21-31.

Ohtani H and Yoshie O. (2010) Morphometric analysis of the balance between CXCR3+ T cells and FOXP3+ regulatory T cells in lymphocyte-rich and conventional gastric cancers. *Virchows Arch* 456:615-623.

Saiki Y, Ohtani H, Naito Y, Miyazawa M, Nagura H. (1996) Immunophenotypical characterization of Epstein-Barr virus-associated gastric carcinoma: Massive infiltration by proliferating CD8+ T-lymphocytes. Lab Invest 75: 67-76.

Sato E, Olson SH, Ahn J, Bundy B, Nishikawa H, Qian F, Jungbluth AA, Frosina D, Gnjatic S, Ambrosone C, Kepner J, Odunsi T, Ritter G, Lele S, Chen YT, Ohtani H, Old LJ, Odunsi K. (2005) Intraepithelial CD8+ tumor-infiltrating lymphocytes and a high CD8+/regulatory T cell ratio are associated with favorable prognosis in ovarian cancer. Proc Natl Acad Sci USA 102:18538-18543.

Sharma P, Shen Y, Wen S, Yamada S, Jungbluth AA, Gnjatic S, Bajorin DF, Reuter VE, Herr H, Old LJ, Sato E. (2007) CD8 tumor-infiltrating lymphocytes are predictive of survival in muscle-invasive urothelial carcinoma. Proc Natl Acad Sci USA. 104:3967-3972.

Tan W, Zhang W, Strasner A, Grivennikov S, Cheng JQ, Hoffman RM, Karin M.(2011) Tumour-infiltrating regulatory T cells stimulate mammary cancer metastasis through RANKL-RANK signaling. Nature 470:548-553.

Tokunaga M, Land CE, Uemura Y, Tokudome T, Tanaka S, Sato E. (1993) Epstein-Barr virus in gastric carcinoma. Am J Pathol. 143:1250-1254.

Watanabe H, Enjoji M, Imai T. (1976) Gastric carcinoma with lymphoid stroma. Its morphologic characteristics and prognostic correlations. Cancer 38: 232-243.

Zlotnik A, Yoshie O. (2000) Chemokines: a new classification system and their role in immunity. Immunity. 12(2):121-7.

Zou W. (2006) Regulatory T cells, tumour immunity and immunotherapy. Nat Rev Immunol 6:295-307.

11

Immunohistochemical Profile of Mucins in Gastric Carcinoma

Daniela Lazăr[1], Sorina Tăban[2] and Sorin Ursoniu[3]
[1]*Department of Gastroenterology,*
[2]*Department of Pathology,*
[3]*Department of Public Health. University of Medicine and Pharmacy*
„Victor Babeş" Timişoara
Romania

1. Introduction

Gastric cancer represents the second leading cause of cancer related death (after lung cancer) despite a global decline in both its incidence and mortality since the late half of the 20th century (Kelley & Duggan, 2003; Zheng et al., 2008). This type of cancer continues nowadays to be a major health problem due to the slow decrease in incidence in Asia and its high mortality in the western countries (Roukos et al., 2002). The overall prognosis is reserved, depending on the TNM stage in the moment of diagnosis and somewhat on its histological type (Lauren, 1965).

Based on morphological characteristics focused on gland formation and histogenetic background, gastric adenocarcinomas are divided into intestinal and diffuse types using the Lauren classification system (Lauren, 1965), or as differentiated and undifferentiated using the Nakamura classification system (Nakamura et al., 1968). Intestinal-type adenocarcinoma is considered to be equivalent to differentiated adenocarcinoma and the diffuse-type to the undifferentiated adenocarcinoma.

These different types of gastric carcinomas express particular biological behaviours. Helicobacter pylori infection leads to the development of chronic atrophic gastritis and intestinal metaplasia (Byrd et al., 1997). Usually the intestinal-type gastric carcinoma arises on the background of intestinal metaplasia (Stemmermann, 1994; Tahara, 1993), and, by contrary, the diffuse-type on the background of gastric mucosa without intestinal metaplasia (Nakamura et al., 1968). The diffuse-type, as classified according to the Lauren system (non-solid type of poorly differentiated adenocarcinoma and the signet-ring cell carcinoma according to a Japanese classification system) (Japanese Gastric Cancer Association, 1996), do not show glandular formation, can be further divided into two subtypes. In the first one, the tumor is predominantly composed of signet-ring cells (>50%) (signet-ring cell carcinomas) and in the other one, the adenocarcinoma contains few signet-ring cells (<50%) (non-signet ring cell carcinomas). Although these histological types can usually be distinguished using standard stainings, new advances in histochemical and immunohistochemical reactions using gastric and small intestinal cell markers determined emerging of gastric cancer classification into different phenotypes, according to mucin expression (Tatematsu et al., 1990).

Much effort is being carried out to identify markers with biological and therapeutical significance in gastric cancer. Mucins are expressed by various epithelial cell types, both normal and malignant. Mucins, high-weight glycoproteins, represent major components of the mucus layer which protects the gastric epithelium against chemical and mechanical aggressions (Corfiefd et al., 2000; Moniaux et al., 2001). In humans, at least 14 genes were identified, coding proteins of mucins, called MUC1, MUC2, MUC3, MUC4, MUC5AC, MUC5B, MUC6, MUC7, MUC8, MUC9, MUC11, MUC12, MUC13 and MUC16 (Pinto-de-Sousa et al., 2002; Silva et al., 2002). They are classified into two groups: membrane bound including MUC1, MUC3A, MUC3B, MUC4, MUC12, MUC13 and MUC 17, and secreted or gel forming including MUC2, MUC5AC, MUC5B and MUC6 (Fowler et al., 2001). All these mucins present common structural characteristics, but are distinct in their tandem repeat peptides. Abnormal expression of mucins has been reported to accompany cancer development, influence cellular growth, differentiation, transformation, adhesion, invasion and immune surveillance (De Bolos et al., 1995).

MUC1 is involved with cell signaling, immuno-regulation and inhibition of cell-cell and cell-matrix adhesion (Rakha et al., 2005; Wesseling et al., 1996). MUC1 cytoplasmic domain has been observed to interact with β-catenin through a similar mode found in E-cadherin, by this way inhibiting the formation of E-cadherin- β-catenin complex (Yamamoto et al., 1997). By this action, MUC1 may participate in tumor cell detachment, invasion and metastases, being associated with aggressive tumor behavior and poor prognosis. There have been reported interactions between MUC1 and members of EGFR family (Rahn et al., 2001). The cytoplasmic domain has a role of signaling mediator of tyrosine kinase receptors (phosphorylated MUC1-Grb2/SOS complex) (Schroeder et al., 2001). MUC1 is present on the apical surface of secretory epithelia, but in the malignant tissues is variable in amount and cellular localization (Pandey et al., 1995). The high aberrant MUC1 expression in tumors leads to antigenically recognizable epitopes on the MUC1 molecules and stimulation of the immune response, making MUC1 a potential immunotherapeutic target (Gendler, 2001).

MUC2 and MUC5AC are important proteins for producing the mucus that protects and lubricates epithelial surfaces. MUC2 is the major secretory glycoprotein expressed abundantly by intestinal and airway epithelium (Gum et al., 1994). Its expression is a common feature of all mucinous carcinomas derived from different organs, including stomach, colon, breast and prostate, acting as a potential prognostic marker (Utsunomiya et al., 1998; Yamashita et al., 1993; Zhang et al., 1998).

MUC5AC is found mainly in the mucosal layer of the cardia, fundus and antrum of the stomach, with the role of epithelia protection (Ho et al., 1995). Tumor phenotypes are classified on the basis of the expression of various markers, such as CD10 as a marker for the brush border on the luminal surface of enterocytes, mucin 2 (MUC2) as a marker of intestinal goblet cells, MUC5AC or human gastric mucin (HGM) as a marker of surface gastric epithelium (foveolar cells) and MUC6 as a marker for pyloric glands (Namikawa & Hanazaki, 2010).

CD10 and MUC2 are considered diagnostic markers of the intestinal phenotype and MUC5AC, HGM and MUC6 are markers of the gastric phenotype. Gastric cancer phenotypes can be classified into four groups, depending on the combination of mucin expression: intestinal type, gastric type, combined type and unclassified type (Shiroshita et al., 2004).

Intestinal metaplasia can be divided into incomplete (precancerous lesion), consisted by the presence of goblet cells in the gastric gland, and complete (not a precancerous lesion), consisted by the presence of both enterocytes and goblet cells (Kawachi et al., 1974; Segura & Montero, 1983; Tosi et al., 1993). Based on the type of intestinal metaplasia, there are four phenotypes of gastric cancer: complete intestinal type, incomplete intestinal type, gastric type and unclassified type. The complete intestinal type is positive for CD10 and MUC2, and negative for MUC5AC. The incomplete intestinal phenotype is positive for CD10 and MUC5AC, or positive for MUC2 alone. The gastric type is positive for MUC5AC, and negative for CD10 and MUC2. Unclassified phenotypes are negative for CD10, MUC2, MUC5AC and MUC6. This classification based on mucin phenotype is important for assessing the biological behavior of gastric carcinomas and different therapeutic options (Namikawa & Hanazaki, 2010).

Gastric-type mucins are mucins specific to the gastric mucosa, although differentiated gastric adenocarcinomas change their mucin phenotype as they grow and invade deeper into the gastric wall. Recent reports reveal an incidence of 7.9-23.9% for the gastric-type differentiated adenocarcinomas among early gastric cancers (Kabashima et al., 2002; Koseki et al., 2000; Matsuoka et al., 2003). This type of early cancer tends to form larger tumors and exhibit higher rates of submucosal invasion in comparison with the intestinal-type (Matsuoka et al., 2003).

Gastric- and intestinal-types of differentiated gastric adenocarcinoma present differences in terms of their biological behavior. Usually, gastric-type tumors show scirrhous infiltration and intestinal-type carcinomas show a solid growth inside the wall (Oda et al., 2003; Shimoda et al., 1991). Some authors reported a significantly poorer prognosis in patients with advanced gastric cancer presenting gastric-type tumors vs. intestinal-type carcinomas, associated with increased malignant potential in the early phase of invasion and metastasis (Tajima et al., 2001). Koseki et al. (2000) have reported a significantly higher incidence of lymphatic invasion, venous invasion, and lymph node metastasis in the gastric-type. For these reasons, even in the early phase of the gastric-type, the decision to perform endoscopic mucosal/submucosal resection or minimal surgical procedures as a curative treatment should be carefully taken (Namikawa & Hanazaki, 2010).

The undifferentiated gastric adenocarcinoma show no clinicopathological differences between gastric and intestinal phenotypes. However, gastric-types present different growth patterns compared with intestinal-type tumors (Kabashima et al., 2005), showing a tendency to spread through the middle layer of the mucosa.

Recent studies have reported a different genetic background of patients with differentiated gastric adenocarcinomas for gastric-type compared to intestinal-type (Endoh et al., 2000; Fiocca et al., 2001; Matsuoka et al., 2003; Sugai et al., 2004). Overexpression of p53 protein is a common feature in differentiated adenocarcinoma (in both gastric- and intestinal phenotypes), but is rare in undifferentiated carcinoma (Matsuoka et al., 2003; Sugai et al., 2004). Data suggest that differentiation to gastric gland cells is related to the presence of microsatellite instability (MSI), whereas differentiation to intestinal epithelial cells is related to mutations in APC gene (Endoh et al., 2000; Tajima et al., 2006; Yamazaki et al., 2006).

Usually, the phenotype of gastric cancer tends to imitate the surrounding mucosa, with gastric-type cancers arising in areas expressing gastric-type or mixed-type mucins (Kabashima et al., 2000). Intestinal metaplasia surrounding gastric-phenotype of differentiated adenocarcinoma seems to be immature or incomplete, compared with gastric-intestinal or intestinal phenotype (Egashira et al., 1999).

Pinto-de-Sousa et al (2002) showed that the mucin phenotype is associated with the tumor site. In the study of Toki et al (2010), the signet ring cell carcinomas and non-signet ring cell carcinomas were most frequently encountered in the upper or middle segments of the stomach. Over 95% of the advanced gastric cancers had either a G or GI phenotype. Pinto-de-Sousa et al (2002) studied the mucin phenotypes of 23 diffuse-type adenocarcinomas and showed that the MUC5AC expression rate in these tumors was significantly higher than that in the unclassified and expansive adenocarcinomas. Reis et al (1997), studying the expression of MUC5AC in early gastric cancers, demonstrate at least some G phenotype cells in the initial stages of the tumors.

Some studies show that the expression rates of the GI and I phenotypes in the cases of undifferentiated advanced gastric cancers were encountered in over half of the cases (Baresi et al., 2006; Tajima et al., 2001; Toki et al., 2010). Studies reported that the progression of the signet ring cell carcinomas was associated with a phenotype shift from the G-type to the I-type in order to progress to the deep layer (Bamba et al., 2001; Tian et al., 2007; Yamachika et al., 1997; Yamagishi et al., 2004). It is also suggested that the morphological features of the signet ring cells change and are subsequently classified as non-signet ring cell carcinomas during tumor progression (Toki et al., 2010).

In the present research we aimed to assess the profile of mucins in gastric carcinomas through immunohistochemical reactions using anti- MUC1, MUC2, and MUC5AC monoclonal antibodies. The purpose of this study is to compare the expression of mucins with clinicopathological factors and outcome of patients.

2. Material and method

From the total of 256 patients (186 males and 79 females), diagnosed clinically and histopathologically with gastric cancer in the period 1998-2002 that underwent surgical interventions in the Departments of Surgery of the Emergency County Clinical Hospital Timisoara, there were 67 patients selected. A prospective study was performed on this group, regarding the evolution and aggressiveness of gastric cancer, on a period of 5 years. Surgical interventions, performed with curative or palliative intention, were not preceded by chemotherapy or radiotherapy. The patients or their relatives were contacted periodically, on the phone or by medical letter, at 6-month intervals, survival being monitored on a variable period, between one month and 68 months. Patients who died postoperatively through various complications, or due to other conditions, were excluded from the study. Clinical and morphological (macroscopic and microscopic) data were collected for each case. Gastric carcinomas were classified and interpreted according to the evaluation protocol recommended by the American Joint Committee on Cancer (AJCC) and International Union against Cancer (UICC).

Survival time was calculated from the month of surgery until the month of death or confirmation of survival, and survival rate was represented by the percentage of survivals at the end of the interval monitored (in years and months). Out of the total of cases included in the prospective study, 6 patients died at variable intervals, between 7 and 26 months, due to other medical causes, being excluded from the study.

Immediately after excision, specimens were fixed in 10% neutral buffered formalin, embedded in paraffin wax, cut into 3 µm paraffin sections and stained with haematoxylin and eosin (HE) for routine light microscopy. For immunohistochemical staining, additional 3 µm thick sections were cut from paraffin-embedded tissue and placed on poly-L-lysine-coated glass slides. For the determination of mucin phenotypes, immunostaining was done for MUC 1 (monoclonal antibody Ab-5, MH1, Thermo Scientific), MUC2 (monoclonal antibody Ab-2, M53, Thermo Scientific) and MUC5AC (monoclonal antibody Ab-1, 45M1, Thermo Scientific). Immunohistochemistry used the UltraVision Detection System, HRP/DAB (Ready-To-Use). The nuclear counterstaining was accomplished using Mayer's hematoxylin. According to their immunoreactivity, the cases were classified in 2 categories:

- negative cases (negative or positive immunoreactions in less than 5% of cells examined);
- positive cases (positive immunoreactions in more than 5% of cells examined).

Statistical analysis was performed using STATA 9.2 software (Statacorp, Texas, USA). Frequencies and percentages are shown for categorical data. Chi-square test was used to compare categorical data. Survival time was calculated as the time from cancer diagnosis to death, censoring at the date of last contact. The Kaplan-Meier method was used to compute 5-year survival rates and disease-specific survival curves were drawn. Differences between survival curves were determined by log-rank test. Survival analysis was performed using a Cox proportional hazards model. A *P*-value <0.05 was considered statistically significant, and hazard ratios (HR) with their respective 95% confidence interval (CI) were calculated.

3. Results

The final group consisted of 61 patients (43 males and 18 females) who presented ages between 30 and 80 (average age = 59.34 years). The main clinicopathological features of cases of gastric cancer investigated are presented in Table 1. In the peritumoral mucosa, MUC1 reactivity was detected in specialized glands of the gastric body (Fig. 1), in the pyloric glands (Fig. 2), and at the level of the antrum, in surface mucous cells and mucous neck cells.

Clinicopathological factors		No. of cases
Males		43
Females		18
Average age (min-max) years		59.34 (30-80)
Location	Antrum	31
	Body	15
	Pangastric	10
	Eso-cardial	2
	Gastric stump	3
Early carcinoma		5
Advanced carcinoma		56
Borrmann	I	5
	II	20
	III	22
	IV	9
pTis/T1/T2/T3/T4		4/6/7/21/23
pN0/N1/N2/N3		18/16/23/4
pM0/M1		47/14

Table 1. Clinicopathological characteristics of gastric cancers studied

MUC5AC is expressed strongly in the foveolar epithelium of gastric antrum and body (Fig. 3 and Fig. 4). MUC2, an intestinal-type mucin, was identified only on foci of intestinal metaplasia of gastric mucosa (in goblet cells - Fig. 5).

The expression of mucins in gastric carcinomas studied is heterogeneous and includes mucins synthesized normally by the gastric mucosa, as well as intestinal mucins expressed "de novo". We identified 41 cases with positive immune reactions for MUC1 (67.2%), 25 cases with positive reactions for MUC2 (40%), and 43 cases for MUC5AC (70.5%) (Graphic 1).

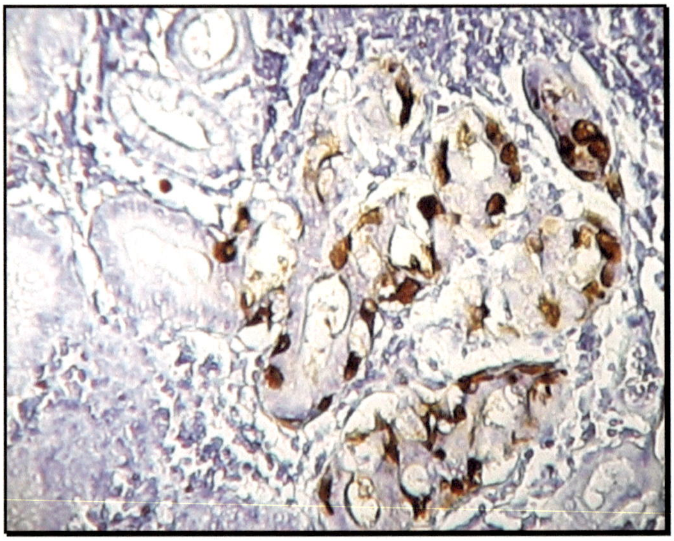

Fig. 1. MUC1-positive immunoreaction in specialized glands of the gastric body. DABx200.

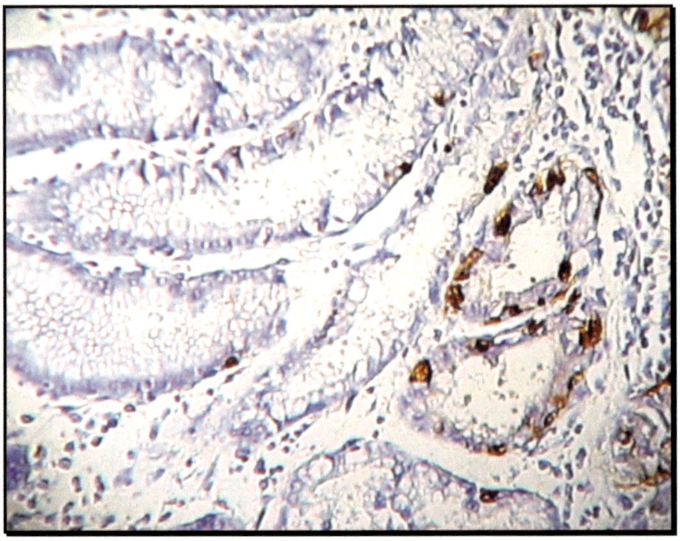

Fig. 2. MUC1 positive immunoreaction in pyloric glands. DABx200.

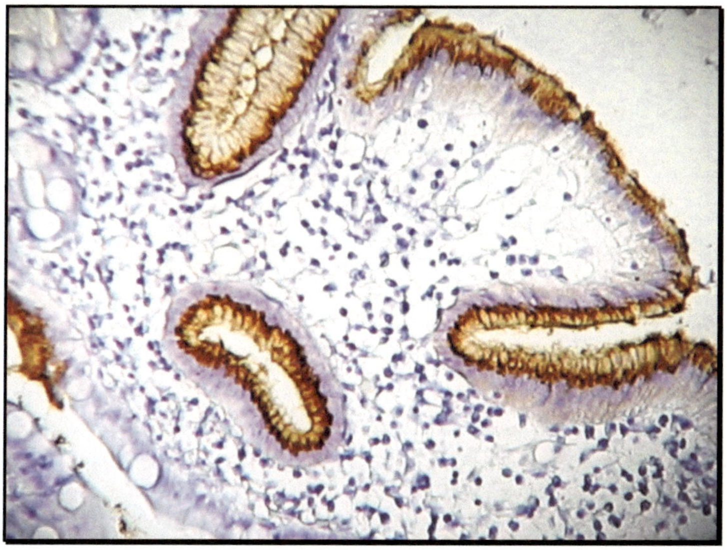

Fig. 3. MUC5AC-intensely positive immunoreaction in the gastric foveolar epithelium. DABx200.

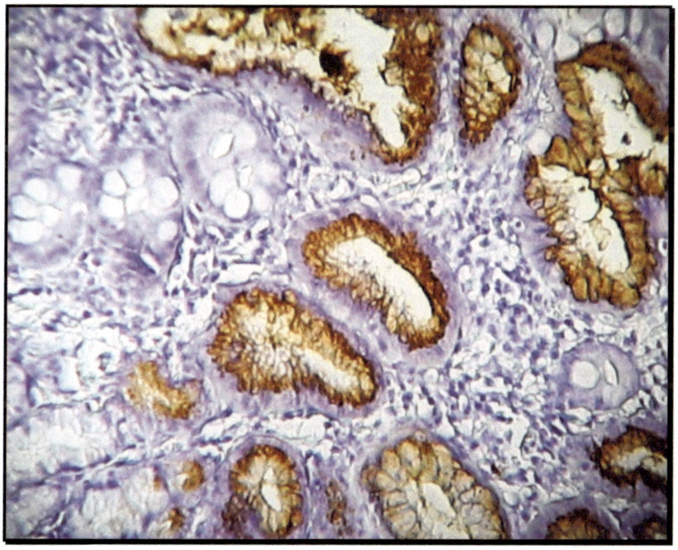

Fig. 4. MUC1-positive secretion in gastric glands; negative metaplastic foci. MUC1 immunoreaction, DABx200.

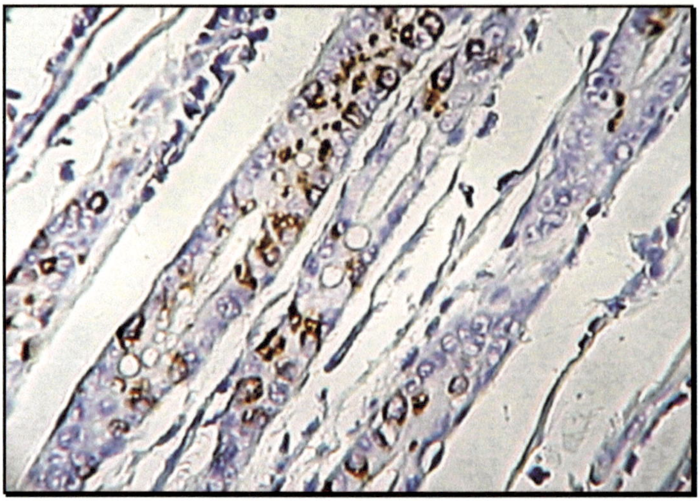

Fig. 5. MUC2-positive immunoreaction on foci of intestinal metaplasia. DABx200.

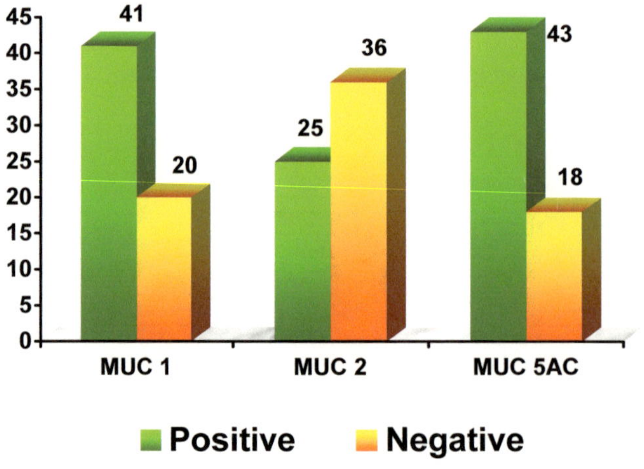

Graphic 1. Expression of mucins in gastric carcinomas

3.1 Immunohistochemical expression of MUC1 in gastric carcinomas

MUC1 antigen is expressed in most cases at the apical pole of cells and intraluminally (Fig. 6), and occasionally diffusely intracytoplasmatic (Fig. 7).

Our results do not show a relationship between the expression of MUC1 and gender of patients, but reveal greater immunopositive results in patients with ages over 61 (78.1%) in comparison with patients under 60 (55.2%) (P=0.057 borderline statistical significance) (Table 2). According to the location of tumors, we noted MUC1 positive immunoreactions in 64.5% of antral carcinomas, in 73.3% of body carcinomas, in 70% of carcinomas extended in the entire stomach, in 66.7% of carcinomas developed on the gastric stump and in 50% of carcinomas of the cardia.

Clinicopathological factors		MUC1 - n=20	MUC1 + (%) n=41	P
Gender	Males	13	30 (69.8%)	0.511
	Females	7	11 (61.1%)	
Age	≤ 60 years	13	16 (55.2%)	0.057
	≥ 61 years	7	25 (78.1%)	
Location	Antrum	11	20 (64.5%)	0.956
	Body	4	11 (73.3%)	
	Pangastric	3	7 (70%)	
	Cardia	1	1 (50%)	
	Gastric stump	1	2 (66.7%)	

Table 2. Relationship between gender of patients, age of patients and MUC1 expression

Classifying the tumors studied according to Lauren, we observed the greater frequency of MUC1-positive immune reactions (without reaching statistical significance) in carcinomas with glandular differentiation (73.7% - Fig. 8) (Table 3). The diffuse type of carcinoma became positive in 53% of cases (Fig. 9), and for the mixed type we obtained an intermediate value (66.7%).

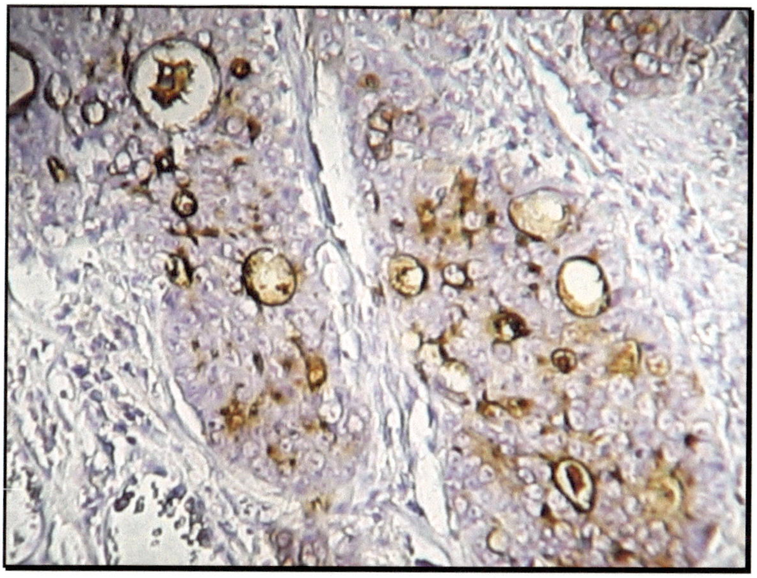

Fig. 6. MUC1-positive immunoreaction intra luminally and at the apical pole of malignant cells. DABx200.

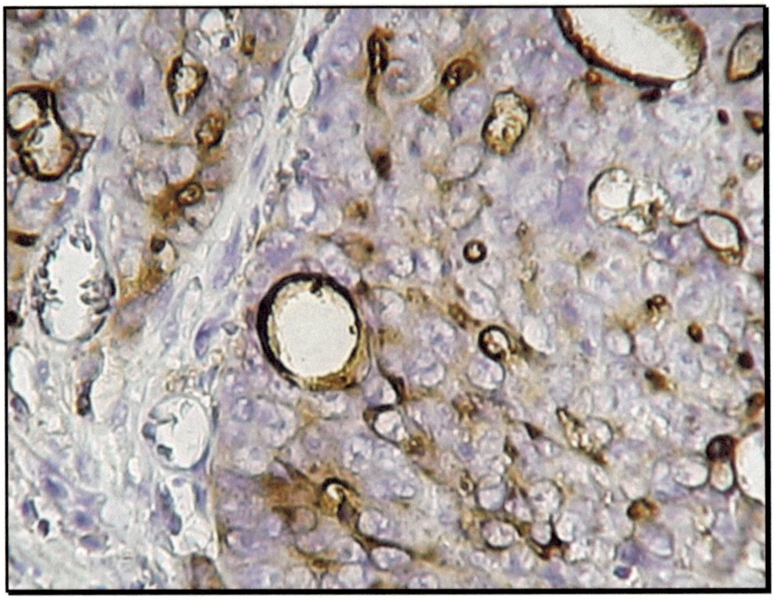

Fig. 7. MUC1 synthesis at the apical pole and intracitoplasmatical. MUC1 immunoreaction, DABx400.

Classifying the tumors studied according to Lauren, we observed the greater frequency of MUC1-positive immune reactions (without reaching statistical significance) in carcinomas with glandular differentiation (73.7% - Fig. 8) (Table 3). The diffuse type of carcinoma became positive in 53% of cases (Fig. 9), and for the mixed type we obtained an intermediate value (66.7%).

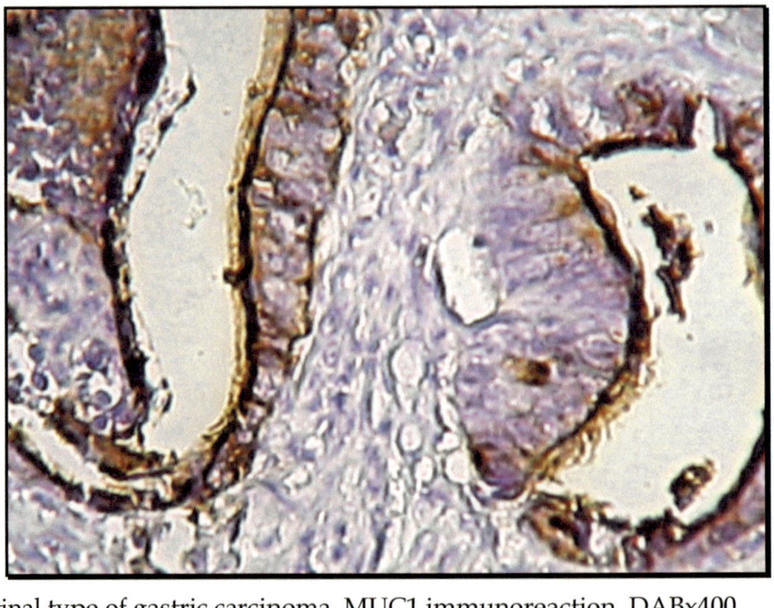

Fig. 8. Intestinal type of gastric carcinoma. MUC1 immunoreaction, DABx400.

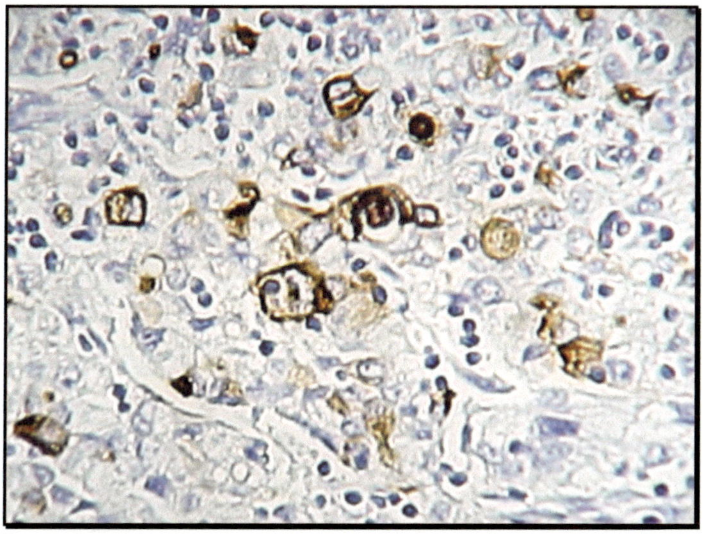

Fig. 9. Diffuse type of gastric carcinoma. MUC1 immunoreaction, DABx400.

From the histological forms, tubular and papillary adenocarcinomas (Fig. 10) became positive in a great number of cases (78.6% and 80%). For the mucinous adenocarcinoma we encountered 62.5% positive cases. The poorly differentiated forms, such as signet-ring cell carcinoma and anaplastic carcinoma (Fig. 11 and 12), expressed MUC1 in 53% and 33.3% of cases. In our study, the differences in MUC1 expression between various histological types were not statistically significant.

Clinicopathological factors		MUC1		P
		- n=20	+ (%) n=41	
Lauren classification	Intestinal type	10	28 (73.7%)	0.318
	Diffuse type	8	9 (53%)	
	Mixed type	2	4 (66.7%)	
Histological type	TA	6	22 (78.6%)	0.265
	PA	1	4 (80%)	
	MA	3	5 (62.5%)	
	SRCC	8	9 (53%)	
	AC	2	1 (33.3%)	
Tumor grade	G1	0	2 (100%)	0.468
	G2	8	12 (60%)	
	G3	12	27 (69.2%)	
Lymphovascular invasion	Present	13	25 (65.8%)	0.761
	Absent	7	16 (69.6%)	

TA-tubular adenocarcinoma; PA-papillary adenocarcinoma; MA-mucinous adenocarcinoma; SRCC-signet-ring cell carcinoma; AC- anaplastic carcinoma

Table 3. Relationship between the histological type, tumor grade, lymphovascular invasion and expression of MUC1

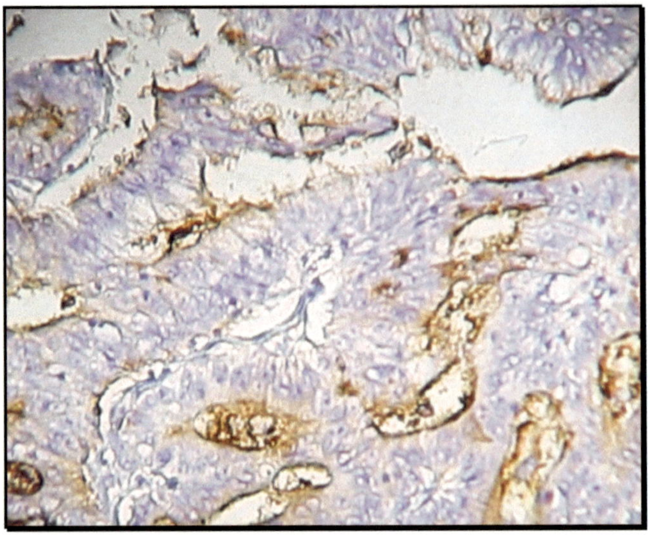

Fig. 10. Papillary adenocarcinoma. MUC1 immunoreaction, DABx200.

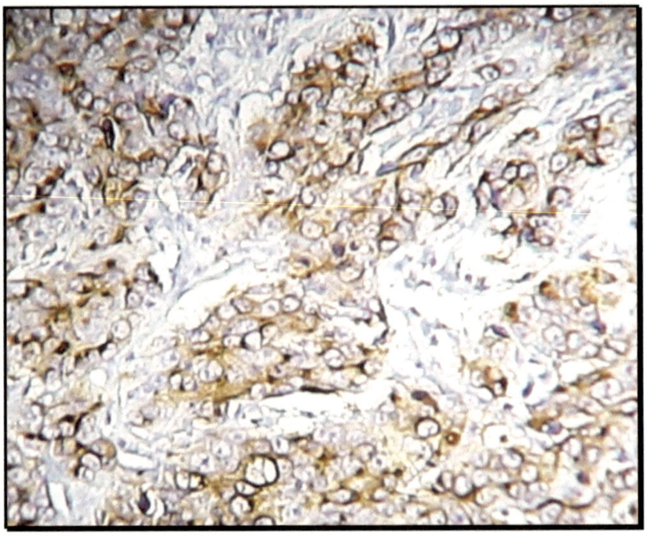

Fig. 11. Anaplastic carcinoma. MUC1 immunoreaction, DABx200.

The immunohistochemical expression of MUC1 is not correlated with the tumor histological grade and lymphovascular invasion. G1 carcinomas became positive for MUC1 in 100% of cases, but the result obtained could be influenced by the small number of cases included in this category.

From our data does not result a correlation between the MUC1 positive immune reaction and the level of tumor invasion (pT stage), the presence of distance metastases (pM stage) and pTNM staging (Table 4). However, we noted a largerer number of positive immunoreactions in cases with lymph node metastases (31 carcinomas - 72.1%) in comparison with tumors without metastases (10 cases - 55.6%), although not reaching statistical significance.

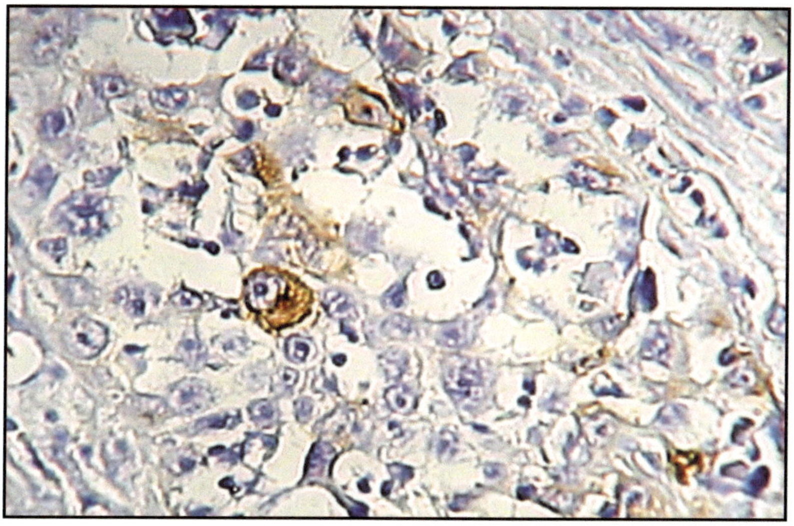

Fig. 12. Anaplastic carcinoma. MUC1 immunoreaction, DABx400.

Our results regarding survival of patients at 5 years demonstrate the role of MUC1 overexpression as a prognosis factor in gastric carcinomas. Patients with carcinomas which became positive for MUC1 survived significantly less than patients with MUC1 negative carcinomas (12.2% vs. 25% at 5 years) (P=0.0047) as shown in Graphic 2.

Clinicopathological factors		MUC1 - n=20	MUC1 + (%) n=41	P
pT	Tis	0	1 (100%)	0.870
	T1	1	3 (75%)	
	T2	3	6 (66.7%)	
	T3	7	10 (58.8%)	
	T4	9	21 (70%)	
pN	N0	8	10 (55.6%)	0.636
	N1	5	11 (68.7%)	
	N2	6	17 (74%)	
	N3	1	3 (75%)	
pM	M0	16	31 (66%)	0.702
	M1	4	10 (71.4%)	
pTNM	0	0	1 (100%)	0.884
	IA	1	2 (66.7%)	
	IB	1	4 (80%)	
	II	2	5 (71.4%)	
	IIIA	3	8 (72.7%)	
	IIIB	2	6 (75%)	
	IV	11	15 (57.7%)	

Table 4. Relationship between TNM staging and expression of MUC1

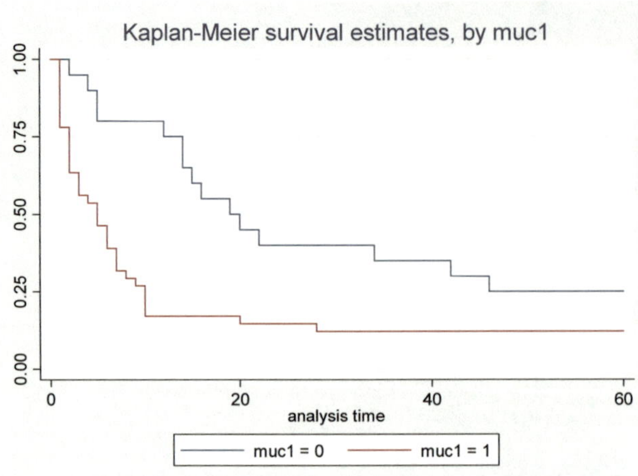

Mucl = 0 (negative expression); Mucl = 1 (positive expression)

Graphic 2. Survival at 5 years according to the MUC1 expression

A significant difference was also obtained by calculating the average survival in months, in the postoperative period, between the two types of patients (Graphic 3):

- for patients with MUC1-positive carcinomas: 12 months;
- for patients with MUC1-negative carcinomas: 28.5 months.

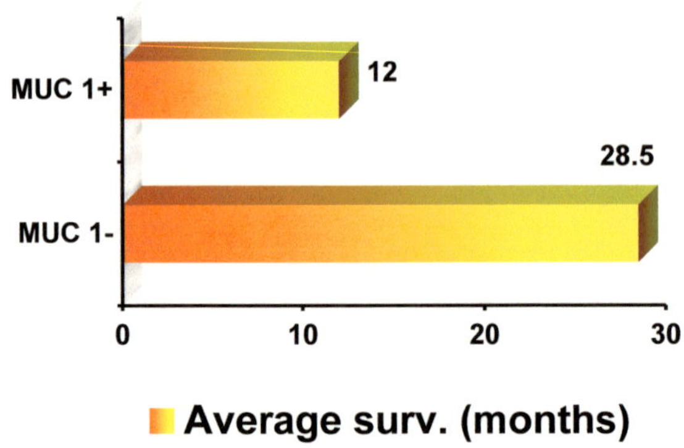

Graphic 3. Average survival of patients according to the MUC1 expression

Patients with MUC1 positive carcinomas were about two times more likely to die than those with MUC1 negative carcinomas (HR=2.30; 95%CI: 1.24-4.26; *P*=0.008).

3.2 Immunohistochemical expression of MUC2 in gastric carcinomas

Positive immunoreaction for MUC2 was observed only in malignant cells (intracytoplasmic) and in goblet cells from foci of intestinal metaplasia of gastric peritumoral mucosa (Fig. 13). We did not note the synthesis of MUC2 in epithelial cells of the normal gastric mucosa.

From the results obtained we conclude the absence of a relationship between the age and gender of patients and the immunohistochemical expression of MUC2 (Table 5).

According to the tumor location we noted MUC2 positive immunoreactions in 41.9% of antral carcinomas, 40% of gastric body carcinomas, 30% of pangastric carcinomas, and 25% of carcinomas developed on the gastric stump. We noted the tumors developed at the level of the cardia which expressed MUC2 in 100% of cases, suggesting the existence of a possible correlation between the overexpression of MUC2 and the cardial location of gastric carcinomas, but these data needs further confirmation by a larger number of cases.

Clinicopathological factors		MUC2		P
		- n=36	+ (%) n=25	
Gender	Males	25	18 (41.9%)	0.830
	Females	11	7 (38.9%)	
Age	≤ 60 years	18	11 (37.9%)	0.644
	≥ 61 years	18	14 (43.7%)	
Location	Antrum	18	13 (41.9%)	0.483
	Body	9	6 (40%)	
	Pangastric	7	3 (30%)	
	Cardia	0	2 (100%)	
	Gastric stump	2	1 (25%)	

Table 5. MUC2 expression and clinicopathological factors in gastric cancer

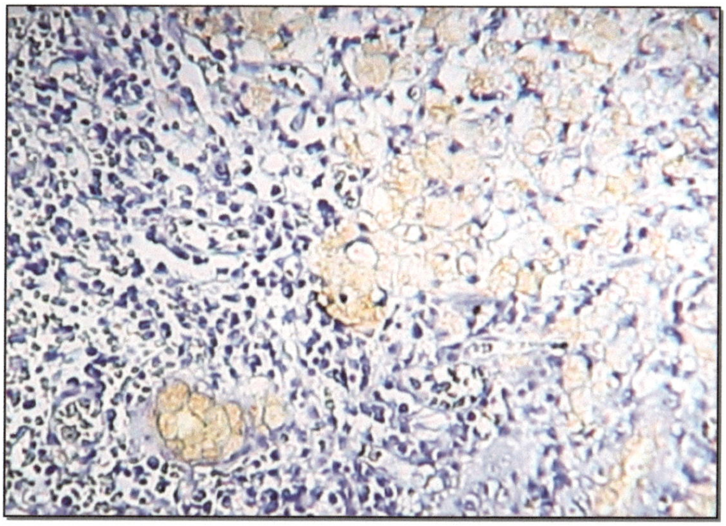

Fig. 13. Intracytoplasmic synthesis of MUC2 in tumoral cells and metaplastic foci. MUC2 immunoreaction, DABx100.

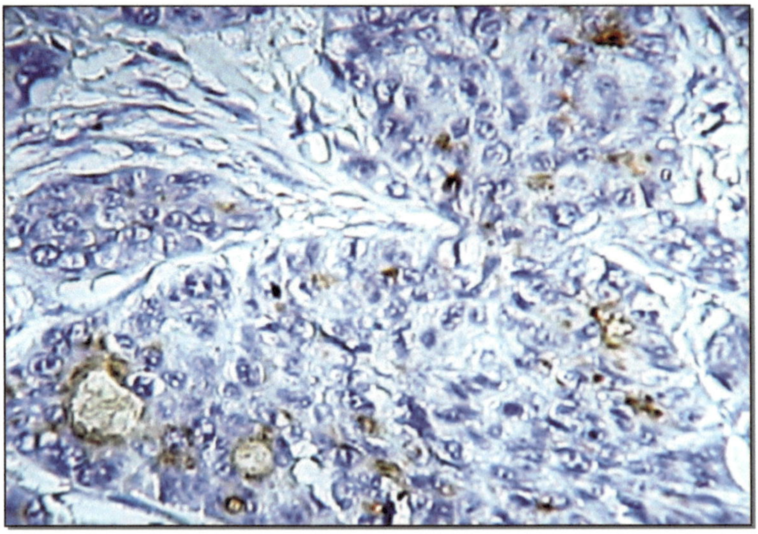

Fig. 14. Intestinal-type of gastric carcinoma. MUC2 immunoreaction, DABx100.

According to the Lauren classification, we noticed a greater immune positivity in intestinal-type carcinomas (47.4% - Fig. 14) and in mixed-type carcinomas (50%), in comparison with diffuse-type carcinomas (23.5% - Fig. 15) (Table 6), but without reaching statistical significance.

Clinicopathological factors		MUC2 - n=36	MUC2 + (%) n=25	P
Lauren classification	Intestinal type	20	18 (47.4%)	0.225
	Diffuse type	13	4 (23.5%)	
	Mixed type	3	3 (50%)	
Histological type	TA	17	11 (39.3%)	0.052
	PA	3	2 (40%)	
	MA	1	7 (87.5%)	
	SRCC	13	4 (23.5%)	
	AC	2	1 (33.3%)	
Tumor grade	G1	1	1 (50%)	0.859
	G2	11	9 (45%)	
	G3	24	15 (38.5%)	
Lymphovascular invasion	Present	22	16 (42.1%)	0.819
	Absent	14	9 (39.1%)	

TA-tubular adenocarcinoma; PA-papillary adenocarcinoma; MA-mucinous adenocarcinoma; SRCC-signet-ring cell carcinoma; AC- anaplastic carcinoma

Table 6. MUC2 expression and clinicopathological factors in gastric cancer

Overexpression of MUC2 is correlated (P=0.052 borderline statistical significance) with mucinous adenocarcinoma as histological form, being identified in 87.5% of cases (Fig. 16). From histological forms that are associated most rarely with the secretion of MUC2, we should mention the signet-ring cell carcinoma (23.5%). The data obtained are not suggestive for a relationship between the tumor histological grade or lymphovascular invasion and the immunohistochemical expression of MUC2.

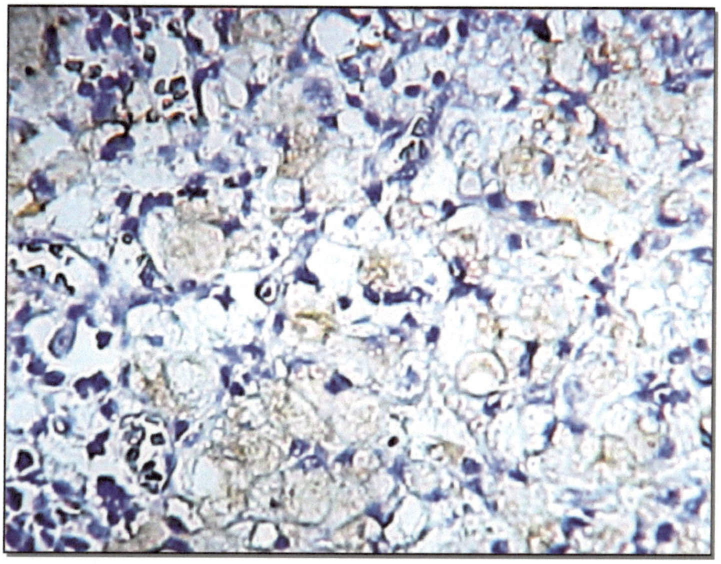

Fig. 15. Diffuse type of gastric carcinoma. MUC2 immunoreaction, DABx200.

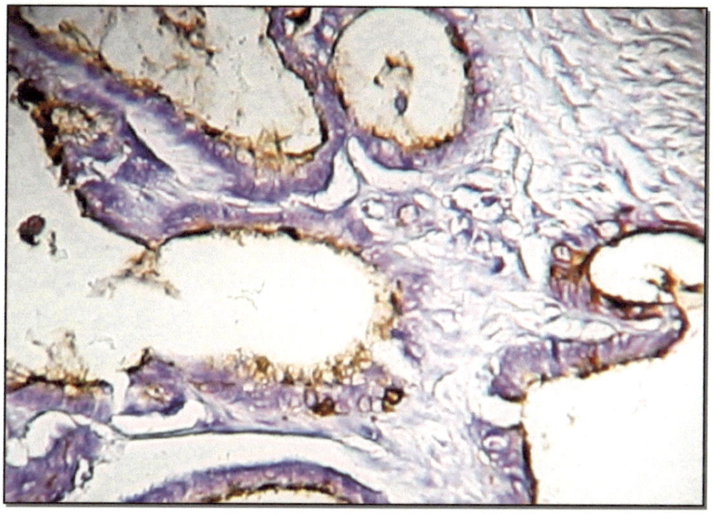

Fig. 16. Mucinous adenocarcinoma. MUC2 intensely positive immunoreaction, DABx200.

Based on the results obtained, we cannot point to the existence of a relationship between the pT, pN, pM, and pTNM factors, and the MUC2 immunoreaction in the gastric carcinomas examined (Table 7).

The immunohistochemical expression of MUC2 does not influence survival at 5 years of patients (16% for MUC2 positive patients vs. 16.7% for MUC2 negative patients) (P = 0.7568) (Graphic 4).

Clinicopathological factors		MUC2 - n=36	MUC2 + (%) n=25	P
pT	Tis	1	0 (0%)	0.927
	T1	2	2 (50%)	
	T2	5	4 (44.4%)	
	T3	10	7 (41.2%)	
	T4	18	12(40%)	
pN	N0	10	8 (44.4%)	0.953
	N1	10	6 (37.5%)	
	N2	14	9 (39.1%)	
	N3	2	2 (50%)	
pM	M0	28	19 (40.4%)	0.871
	M1	8	6 (42.9%)	
pTNM	0	1	0 (0%)	0.988
	IA	2	1 (33.3%)	
	IB	3	2 (40%)	
	II	4	3 (42.9%)	
	IIIA	6	5 (45.4%)	
	IIIB	5	3 (60%)	
	IV	16	10 (38.5%)	

Table 7. Expression of MUC2 and clinicopathological factors in gastric cancer

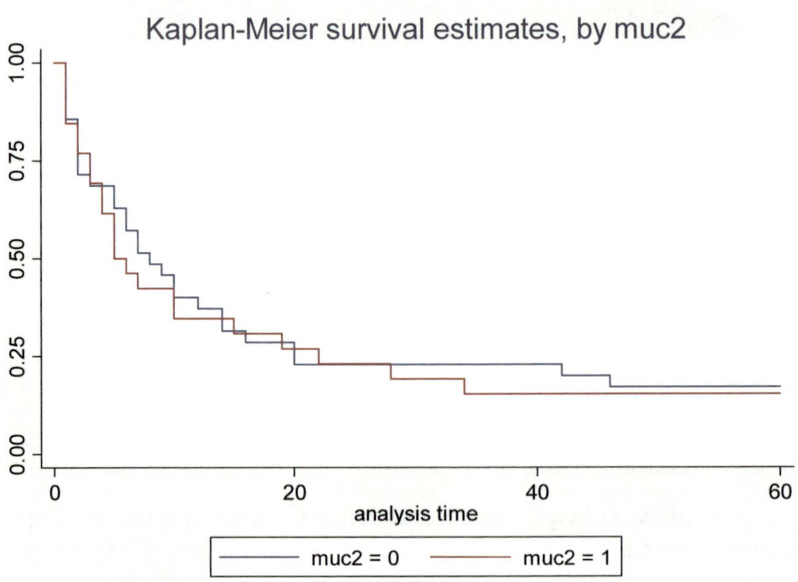

Muc2 = 0 (negative expression); Muc2 = 1 (positive expression)

Graphic 4. Survival at 5 years according to expression of MUC2

Average survivals calculated in months show the lack of correlation between the prognosis of patients and the immunohistochemical expression of MUC2 (16 months for patients with MUC2-positive carcinomas, and 18,4 months for patients with MUC2-negative carcinomas) (Graphic 5).

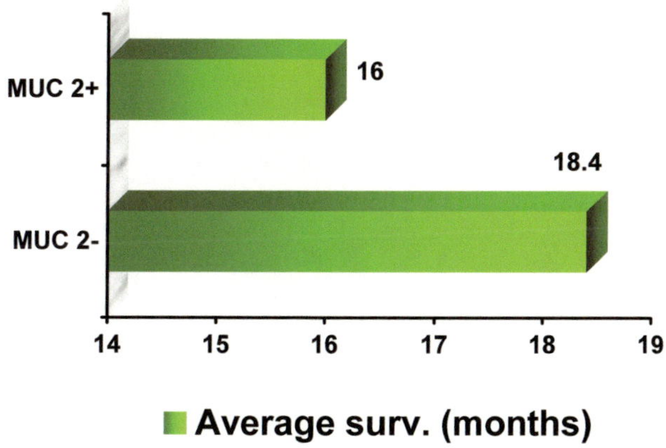

Graphic 5. Average survival of patients according to expression of MUC2

3.3 Immunohistochemical expression of MUC5AC in gastric carcinomas

Immunohistochemical reactions performed with the anti-MUC5AC antibody have demonstrated the strong expression of the foveolar epithelium of the gastric antrum and body (Fig. 17), as well as in the cytoplasms of malignant cells from 43 gastric carcinomas (70.5% - Fig. 18).

The results obtained do not show a relationship between the age or gender of patients and the expression of MUC5AC (Table 8).

Clinicopathological factors		MUC5AC		P
		- n=18	+ (%) n=43	
Gender	Males	12	31 (72.1%)	0.672
	Females	6	12 (66.7%)	
Age	≤ 60 years	9	20 (69%)	0.804
	≥ 61 years	9	23 (71.9%)	
Location	Antrum	6	25 (80.6%)	0.137
	Body	5	10 (66.7%)	
	Pangastric	4	6 (60%)	
	Cardia	2	0 (0%)	
	Gastric stump	1	2 (66.7%)	

Table 8. Expression of MUC5AC and clinicopathological factors in gastric cancer

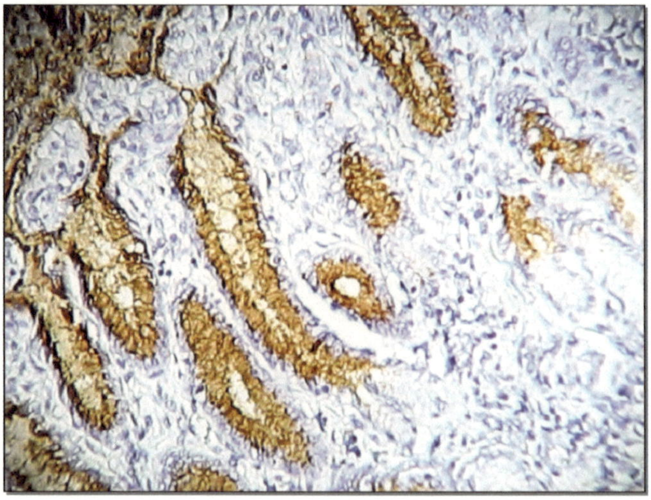

Fig. 17. MUC5AC intensely positive immunoreaction in the gastric foveolar epithelium. DABx100.

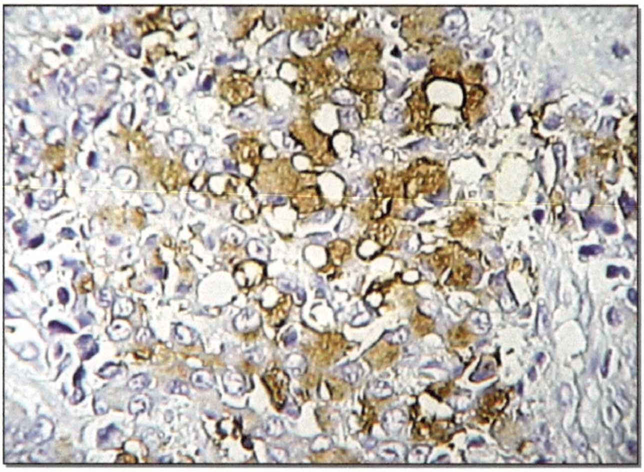

Fig. 18. MUC5AC immune reactivity in the cytoplasm of malignant cells. DABx200.

Analysis of MUC5AC according to location of tumors demonstrated the most frequent immunoreactivity of the antibody in antral carcinomas (80.6%) (without statistical significance). We identified positive immunoreactions in 66.7% of gastric body carcinomas, 60% of pangastric carcinomas and 66.7% of carcinomas developed on the gastric stump. Cardial tumors did not express the MUC5AC antigen.

The diffuse type of gastric carcinoma, as well as the signet-ring cell carcinoma, presented in a very high percentage (88.2%) MUC5AC positive immunoreactions (Tab. 9 - Fig. 19). Our results seem to show that MUC5AC is expressed mostly in the signet-ring cell carcinoma, but the differences between the histological subtypes did not reach statistical significance. According to the tumor histological grade, we noted 50% positive reactions in well-differentiated carcinomas, 70% positive reactions in moderately differentiated carcinomas and 71.8% in poorly differentiated carcinomas. We noted no relationship between the lymphovascular invasion and the expression of MUC5AC.

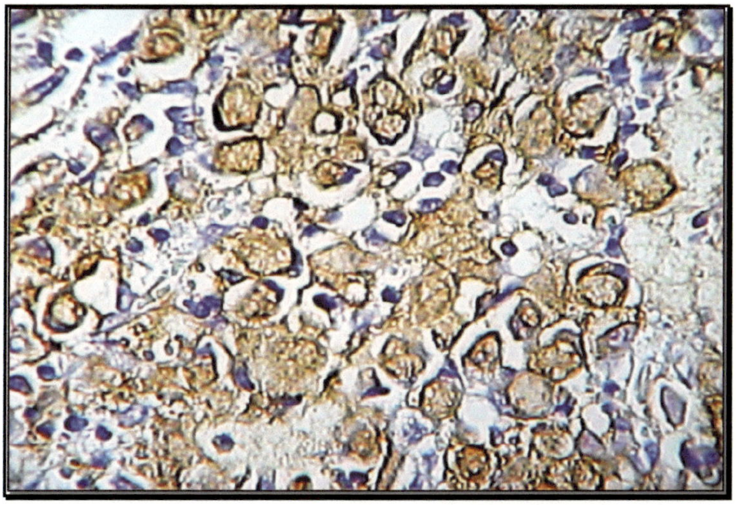

Fig. 19. Gastric signet-ring cell carcinoma. MUC5AC immunoreaction, DABx400.

Clinicopathological factors		MUC5AC		P
		- n=18	+ (%) n=43	
Lauren classification	Intestinal type	14	24(63.2%)	0.165
	Diffuse type	2	15 (88.2%)	
	Mixed type	2	4 (66.7%)	
Histological type	TA	20	18 (64.3%)	0.082
	PA	2	3 (60%)	
	MA	3	5 (62.5%)	
	SRCC	2	15 (88.2%)	
	AC	1	2 (66.7%)	
Tumor grade	G1	1	1 (50%)	0.958
	G2	6	14 (70%)	
	G3	11	28 (71.8%)	
Lymphovascular invasion	Present	12	26 (68.4%)	0.649
	Absent	6	17 (73.9%)	

TA-tubular adenocarcinoma; PA-papillary adenocarcinoma; MA-mucinous adenocarcinoma; SRCC-signet-ring cell carcinoma; AC- anaplastic carcinoma

Table 9. Expression of MUC5AC and clinicopathological factors in gastric cancer

Our results, similar with those obtained in analyzing MUC2, did not show the existence of a correlation between the level of tumor invasion, the presence of lymph node or distant metastases, the pTNM stage and the immunohistochemical expression of MUC5AC (Table 10).

Clinicopathological factors		MUC5AC - n=18	MUC5AC + (%) n=43	P
pT	Tis	0	1 (100%)	0.489
	T1	1	3 (75%)	
	T2	2	7 (77.8%)	
	T3	3	14 (82.4%)	
	T4	12	18 (60%)	
pN	N0	5	13 (72.2%)	0.992
	N1	5	11 (68.8%)	
	N2	7	16 (69.6%)	
	N3	1	3 (75%)	
pM	M0	14	33 (70.2%)	0.930
	M1	4	10 (71.4%)	
pTNM	0	0	1 (100%)	0.985
	IA	1	2 (66.7%)	
	IB	1	4 (80%)	
	II	2	5 (71.4%)	
	IIIA	4	7 (63.6%)	
	IIIB	2	6 (75%)	
	IV	8	18 (69.2%)	

Table 10. Expression of MUC5AC and clinicopathological factors in gastric cancer

The expression of MUC5AC does not constitute a prognostic factor in our study, the survival rate at 5 years being 16.3% for MUC5AC positive patients vs. 16.7% for MUC5AC negative patients (P = 0.5334; Graphic 6)

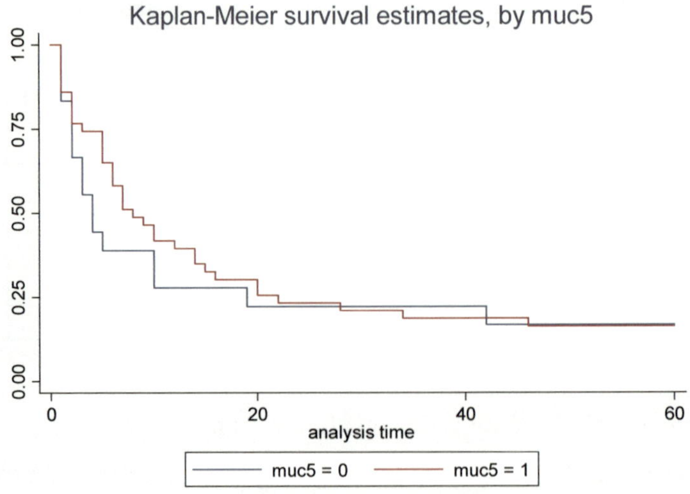

Muc5AC = 0 (negative expression); Muc5AC = 1 (positive expression)

Graphic 6. Survival at 5 years according to the expression of MUC5AC

The average survival rates, calculated in months, were of 18 months for patients with MUC5AC-positive carcinomas and 16.05 months for patients with MUC5AC-negative carcinomas, the two values being relatively close (Graphic 7).

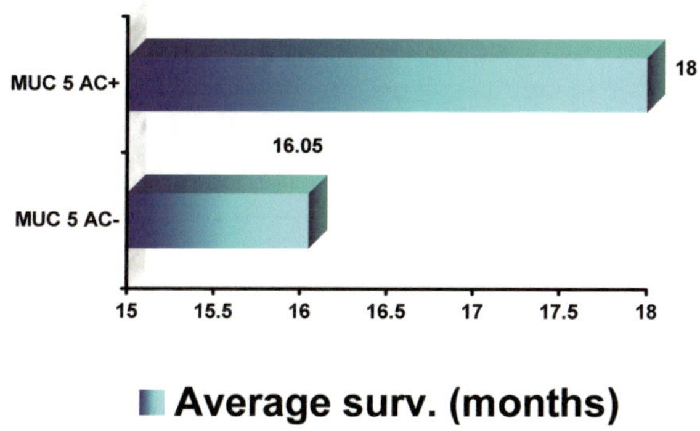

Graphic 7. Average survival rate (in months) according to the expression of MUC5AC

4. Discussions

The genes of mucins are expressed in normal cells and tissues. The stomach offers a very good example of expressing mucins. MUC1 can be identified in mucous cells of the surface epithelium and neck of glands at the level of the antrum, but also in the pyloric and oxyntic glands in the gastric body (Ho et al., 1995; Pinto-De-Sousa, 2002). The MUC5AC mucin is expressed strongly in the foveolar epithelium of the antrum and body and MUC5AC is limited to mucous neck cells of gastric body glands and pyloric glands of the antrum (Ho et al., 1995; Pinto-De-Sousa, 2002; Silva et al., 2002). The expression of mucins in gastric carcinomas is heterogeneous, including mucins synthesized normally by the gastric mucosa (MUC1, MUC5AC and MUC6), as well as intestinal mucins synthesized de novo (MUC2) (Baldus et al., 1998; Ho et al., 1993; Reis, 1997, 1998). Some authors suggested that the heterogeneous pattern of expression would offer information regarding the evolution of various forms of gastric cancer.

The progression of tumorigenesis involves abnormalities in the expressions of cyclins and other cell-cycle related genes (Ioachim, 2008). Abnormalities have been found for cyclins D1, A, E and their co-operating partners (cyclin-dependent kinase), that promote cell cycle progression (Handa et al., 1999; Ioachim, 2008). These progressive factors can be inhibited by blockers, such as p21, p27 and p57, p16, p15 and p18. Key regulators of progression through the G1 phase of the cell cycle are cyclin D1, cyclin E, p53, p21 and p27 (Gamboa-Dominguez et al., 2007; Mrena et al., 2006). Sugai et al. (2010), analyzing 190 gastric intramucosal differentiated-type cancers have suggested that the cellular mucin phenotypes are dependent on distinct cell cycle-related alteration. It was proposed a novel carcinogenesis model that relies on the mucin phenotype. Based on abnormalities of cell-cycle related proteins, overexpressions of p53 and cyclin A characterize gastric phenotype cancers, whereas overexpression of p27 is associated with the development of intestinal-phenotype cancers and overexpression of cyclin A with the mixt phenotype cancers.

Mucin and mucin O-glycosylation have attracted attention for their role in the adhesion of bacteria, cell-cell adhesion, and cancer cell metastization (Hollingsworth & Swanson, 2004).

The expression of mucins is often altered in cancer, with frequent aberrant glycosylation, resulting immature structures and exposure of the peptide backbone (Ferreira et al., ;Reis et al., 1998). These structures are useful markers of premalignant and malignant cells. Gomez et al (Gomes et al., 2009) have studied the pattern of expression of UDP-N-acetyl-D-galactosamine: polypeptide N-acetylgalactosaminyltransferase-6 (ppGal NAc-T6) in gastric mucosa, intestinal metaplasia and gastric carcinoma. ppGal NAc-T6 was expressed in normal mucosa (both antrum and body region), in 52% of the cases with intestinal metaplasia and had a heterogeneous expression in gastric carcinomas, being present in 79% of case. Its expression in gastric carcinomas was associated with venous invasion.

In our study we aimed to evaluate the profile of mucins in gastric carcinomas in the study group, through immunohistochemical reactions, using monoclonal anti-MUC1, MUC2, and MUC5AC antibodies. The purpose of the study is to compare the expression of mucins with clinicopathological factors and with the outcome of patients. In accordance with other works (Pinto-De-Sousa, 2002), the data obtained show that the immunohistochemical expression of mucins is associated with some characteristics of differentiation in gastric carcinomas. We noted the alteration of the profile of normal gastric mucins and the overexpression of intestinal mucin in the various forms of cancer.

In the peritumoral mucosa, the MUC1 immunoreactivity was detected in the specialized glands of the gastric body, in the pyloric glands, and at the level of the antrum (in surface mucous cells and neck mucous cells). Amongst the carcinomas studied we identified 41 cases with positive immunoreactions for MUC1, representing 67.2%. Using two specific monoclonal antibodies, Pinto-de-Sousa (2002) obtained positive reactions in 89% of cases with HFMG1 antibody and 50 of cases with SM3 antibody (which recognizes only the non-glycosylated forms of MUC1). Generally, the immunoreactivity for MUC1 varies in different studies between 24.3% and 100% (Gürbüz et al., 2002). The MUC1 antigen was expressed in most cases at the apical pole of cells and intraluminally, and occasionally diffusely intracytoplasmatic. Our results do not show a relationship between the expression of MUC1 and the gender of patients or the location of tumors, but reveal a greater immune positivity in patients with ages over 61 (78.1%), in comparison with patients under 60 years of age (55.2%) (borderline statistical significance).

Classifying the tumors studied, according to Lauren, we noticed a greater frequency of MUC1 positive immunoreactions in carcinomas with glandular differentiation (73.7%), although without reaching statistical significance. Concordant results were obtained by Gürbüz Y et al. (2002), Lee HS et al. (2001), Machado JC et al. (2000), Reis CA et al. (1998), Utsunomiya T et al. (1998). The diffuse type of carcinoma became positive in 53% of cases, and for the non-classifiable type we obtained an intermediate value (66.7%). Reis CA et al. (1998) note the significant association between the immune reactivity of SM3 and the non-classifiable gastric carcinoma.

In our study, the differences in MUC1 expression between various histological types were not statistically significant. Also, in the study of Pinto-De-Sousa et al (2002), the expression of HMFG1 and SM3 antibodies was not correlated with histological forms of gastric cancer.

The immunohistochemical expression of MUC1 is not correlated with the tumor histological grade and lymphovascular invasion. The G1 carcinomas became positive for MUC1 in 100% of cases, but the result obtained could be influenced by the small number of cases included in this category.

No correlation results from our study between the MUC1 immunoreaction and the level of tumor invasion (pT stage), the presence of distance metastases (pM stage) and pTNM staging. We noted, however, a greater number of positive immune reactions in cases with lymph node metastases (31 carcinomas - 72.1%), in comparison with tumors without lymph node metastases (10 cases - 55.6%), but without statistical significance. The correlation between MUC1 positivity and the presence of lymph node metastasis was observed by Zhang HK et al. (2004), together with the association between MUC1 and the advanced age of patients with gastric tumors of large dimensions.

In epithelial cancer cells, MUC1 is over-expressed, aberrantly glycosylated with short oligosaccharides and also loses its apical polarization and becomes expressed over the entire cell surface (Hilkens et al., 1992; Kim & Gum, 1996; Lloyd et al., 1996; Wesseling et al., 1996). MUC1 is an endogenous ligand of galectin-3 (an apoptosis inhibitor) in cancer cells (colon cancer), the interaction occurring via binding the galectin-3 to the oncofetal Thomsen-Friedenreich carbohydrate (TF) antigen on MUC1 (Yu et al., 2007). The increased expression of MUC1 and TF antigen are both associated with high metastatic potential of the cancer cell and poor prognosis (Nakamori et al., 1994). Over-expression of MUC1 promotes tumor cell release from primary tumor sites by inhibiting E-cadherin-mediated cell-cell and integrin-mediated cancer extracellular matrix interactions (Kondo et al., 1998). Thus, MUC1 may promote the formation of cancer cell aggregates/emboli and prolong the survival of disseminated cells in the circulation and contributes to cancer cell haematogenous dissemination (Zhao et al., 2010).

The role of MUC1 in invasion and metastasis has been shown in different models. The cytoplasmic tail of MUC1 was reported to enhance the invasion in breast cancer cells expressing wild-type GSK-3β and β-catenin (Lillehoj et al, 2003), suggesting possible interactions between these proteins. MUC1 expression is associated with increased steady-state levels of β-catenin in the cytoplasm and nucleus of breast carcinoma cells by blocking the GSK-3β-mediated phosphorylation of β-catenin, and preventing proteosomal degradation (Schroeder et al., 2003). It is possible that the cytoplasmic tail of MUC1 enables interaction between different regulators or alternatively might compete for or sequester β-catenin. In some cell types, the MUC1 cytoplasmic tail is also involved in the transcriptional activation of β-catenin-TCF-binding sites and transcriptional activation of cyclin D1 (Huang et al., 2005). MUC1 may play an antiapoptotic role in response to cellular stresses by stimulating Akt and the antiapoptotic protein Bcl-X to attenuate genotoxin-induced apoptosis (Raina et al., 2004). Recent reports suggest that this MUC1-mediated carcinogenesis is likely through the TGF-α signaling pathway (Pochampalli et al., 2007).

MUC1 is immunogenic in its hypoglycosylated form expressed on tumors, and the tumor-bearing patients generate both cellular and humoral immune responses to this antigen (Coronella-Wood & Hersh, 2003; Vlad et al., 2004). High levels of anti-MUC1 antibodies are associated with a better prognosis in some adenocarcinomas (Kurtenkov et al., 2007; Silk & Finn, 2007), an observation that has made MUC1 an attractive candidate for vaccines against these malignancies. Prophylactic vaccination is the most desirable strategy to prevent malignant diseases. Several vaccine trials involving MUC1 have been conducted, but none have resulted in therapeutically beneficial immune responses (Silk & Finn, 2007). Identification and understanding of the host factors that influence naturally occurring immune responses is an important prerequisite to successfully designing a vaccine that would induce therapeutic responses.

For MUC1 there are significant interindividual differences in naturally occurring antibody responses (Cramer et al., 2005). Recent studies in humans have shown that immune responsiveness to a variety of antigens- infectious agents, vaccines, autoantigens, including some tumor-associated antigens- are associated with particular GM and KM allotypes, hereditary antigenic determinants of γ and κ chains, respectively (Kameda et al., 1998; Pandey, 2001; Pertovaara et al., 2004). Pandey et al. (2008) have studied 169 Caucasian subjects with gastric cancer that were allotyped for several GM and KM markers. Their results have revealed that GM 3 23 5,13 phenotype is highly significantly associated with MUC1 IgG levels; subjects with this phenotype had lower antibody levels compared with those having other phenotypes. This phenotype had an interactive effect with KM phenotypes on the levels of IgG antibodies to this antigen. Association of non- GM 3 23 5,13 phenotypes with high responsiveness to MUC1 could aid in identifying subjects who are more likely to benefit from MUC1-based vaccines. For individuals with the low responder phenotype, MUC1 could be fused with appropriate adjuvants, such as heat shock proteins, in order to conceive a vaccine that could potentially generate high antibody responses in the majority of population (Li et al., 2006; Pandey et al., 2004).

In accordance with Reis CA et al (1998) and Baldus SE at al (1998), our results regarding the survival of patients at 5 years prove the association between the overexpression of MUC1 and the worse prognosis. Patients with carcinomas which became positive for MUC1 survived at 5 years significantly less (12.2%) than patients with MUC1-negative carcinomas (25%). A significant difference was also obtained by calculating, in months, the average survival in the postoperative period: for patients with MUC1-positive carcinomas - 12 months; for patients with MUC1-negative carcinomas – 28.5 months.

The results regarding the prognostic role for the immunohistochemical expression of MUC1 are contradictory. Studying a group of 94 gastric carcinomas, Pinto-De-Sousa et al. (2002) did not observe a relationship between MUC1 and the prognosis of patients.

The immunohistochemical reactions performed with the anti-MUC5AC antibody demonstrated a strong expression in the foveolar epithelium of the antrum and gastric body, as well as in the cytoplasms of malignant cells in 43 gastric carcinomas (70.5%).

The results obtained do not show a relationship between the age or gender of patients and the expression of MUC5AC. The analysis of MUC5AC according to the location of tumors demonstrated a frequent immunoreactivity of the antibody in antral carcinomas (80.6%), but without reaching statistical significance. Cardial tumors did not express the MUC5AC antigen.

The diffuse type of gastric carcinoma, as well as "signet-ring" cell carcinoma, presented in a very high percentage (88.2%) MUC5AC-positive immune reactions. Our results seem to show that MUC5AC is expressed mostly in the signet-ring cell carcinoma, but the differences between the histological subtypes did not reach statistical significance. The association between the expression of MUC5AC and the diffuse type carcinoma is mentioned also by other authors (Pinto-De-Sousa et al., 2002), suggesting keeping certain features of tumor differentiation in the gastric mucosa. Some studies signal the strong correlation between the immunoreactivity of MUC5AC and the tumors with infiltrative growth pattern (Gürbüz et al., 2002). This association reflects the modality of growth and invasion in diffuse type carcinomas.

We did not note a relationship between the tumor histological grade, the lymphovascular invasion and the expression of MUC5AC. Our results did not show the existence of a correlation between the level of tumor invasion, the presence of lymph node or distance metastases, the pTNM stage, and the immunohistochemical expression of MUC5AC.

In accordance with Pinto-De-Sousa`s results (2002), the expression of MUC5AC in our study does not constitute a prognostic factor, survival rates at 5 years being of 16.3% for patients with MUC5AC-positive carcinomas, and 16.7% for patients with MUC5AC-negative carcinomas. In the studies of Reis CA et al. (1998) and Hatori & Kushima (2002), the expression of MUC5AC was much frequently observed in incipient gastric carcinomas (100%) in comparison with advanced carcinomas (58.6%). The authors conclude that all gastric carcinomas are characterized by a "gastric" phenotype in the first stages of tumorigenesis. The average survival rates, calculated in months, were of 18 months for patients with MUC5AC-positive carcinomas, and 16.05 months for patients with MUC5AC-negative carcinomas, the two values being relatively close.

Several papers have described the relationship between mucin and pancreatic cancer, de novo expression of MUC5AC frequently occurring in intraductal papillary mucinous tumors and pancreatic adenocarcinoma (Kanno et al., 2006; Kim et al., 2002), while Takikita et al. (2009) reported that borderline statistically significant associations are seen between MUC5AC positivity and shorter survival time in patients with pancreatic cancer. Yamazoe S et al. (2010) demonstrated that suppression of MUC5AC reduced adhesive, invasive and metastatic potential of pancreatic cancer cell lines. MUC5AC might contribute to the progression of pancreatic cancer by inducing adhesiveness and invasiveness in extracellular matrix via VEGF overexpression.

Immune positivation for MUC2 was observed in our study only in malignant cells (intracytoplasmic) and in goblet cells in foci of intestinal metaplasia of peritumoral gastric mucosa. We did not note the MUC2 synthesis in epithelial cells of the normal gastric mucosa. Our results show that MUC2 intestinal mucine is expressed aberrantly in 25 gastric carcinomas (40% of cases).

Tumors developed at the level of the cardia expressed MUC2 in 100% of cases, suggesting the existence of a possible correlation between the overexpression of MUC2 and the cardial location of gastric carcinomas, but these data needs further confirmation by a larger number of cases.

According to the Lauren classification, we noted a greater immune positivation in intestinal-type carcinomas and mixed-type in comparison with diffuse-type carcinomas, but without reaching statistical significance.

In accordance with results of other studies (Pinto-De-Sousa et al., 2002; Reis et al., 2000), overexpression of MUC2 is correlated significantly (borderline statistical significance) with mucinous adenocarcinoma, being identified in 87.5% of cases. Overexpression of MUC2 was also described in colonic, pancreatic, mammary and ovarian mucinous carcinomas (Hanski et al., 1997). Immunoreactivity of MUC2 is tightly correlated with the presence of goblet cells. This fact suggests that the predominant cellular population in mucinous carcinoma consists of goblet cells.

Choi JS et al (2009) have studied human mucin gene expression and mucin phenotypes in mucinous and non-mucinous gastric carcinomas. Mucin gene expression profiles differed in nucinous vs. non-mucinous tumors. MUC2 was related distinctively to mucinous carcinomas and was expressed in 95.5% of these tumors, whereas it was observed in only 33.4% of non-mucinous carcinomas, suggesting that MUC2 is closely related to the mucinous histology and that it may play a role in the histogenesis of mucinous gastric carcinomas. MUC2 is expressed in normal colonic and small intestinal mucosa, but is not expressed in normal gastric mucosa. When intestinal metaplasia occurs in the stomach, MUC 2 is expressed in the goblet cells. In this study, mucinous gastric carcinomas were characterized by MUC1 negativity, MUC2 positivity, MUC5AC negativity, and MUC6 negativity compared with non-mucinous tumors. Mucinous carcinomas were categorized as intestinal mucin phenotype in 60.9%, mixed phenotype in 34.6%, and gastric phenotype in 2.3%. Patients who had the gastric or mixed phenotype had a shorter median survival than patients who had the intestinal phenotype, although the survival curves were not significantly different.

Data obtained in our study are not suggestive for a relationship between the tumor histological grade or lymphovascular invasion and the immunohistochemical expression of MUC2. Based on the results obtained, we cannot state the existence of a relationship between the pT, pN, pM, pTNM factors and the MUC2 immunoreaction in the gastric carcinomas examined.

The immunohistochemical expression of MUC2 does not influence survival at 5 years of patients, survival rates at 5 years being of 16% for patients with MUC2-positive carcinomas and 16.7% for patients with MUC2-negative carcinomas. Average survivals calculated in months show the lack of correlation between the prognosis of patients and the immunohistochemical expression of MUC2 (16 months for patients with MUC2-positive carcinomas and 18.4 months for patients with MUC2-negative carcinomas).

Immunohistochemical evaluation of the pattern of mucins can be considered an important method of interpretation and understanding of various clinical and pathological entities of gastric cancer. The expression of the intestinal mucin MUC2 was shown much more frequently in carcinomas located at the level of the cardia (100%), in comparison with antral tumors (41.9%), gastric body tumors (40%), pangastric tumors (30%), or tumors developed at the level of the gastric blunt (25%). This result suggests that cardial tumors are diagnosed and resected in advanced pTNM stages. In accordance with Ho and colab. (28), the data obtained in our study confirm the hypothesis according to which the heterogeneous expression of mucins and the "de novo" synthesis of non-gastric mucins correspond to advanced stages of gastric cancer.

Gastric carcinomas located at the level of the antrum express MUC5AC in a significantly greater proportion (80.6%) in comparison with tumors of the gastric body (66.7%), pangastric (60%) or cardial (0%). This high percentage could be due either to the slightly more advanced tumor stage in comparison with proximal carcinomas, either to the high frequency of diffuse-type carcinomas, located in the distal stomach.

5. Conclusions

The immunohistochemical evaluation of the pattern of mucines can be considered as an important method of interpreting and understanding the various clinical and pathological entities of gastric cancer.

The immunohistochemical expression of mucines is correlated with the histological type of gastric carcinoma (MUC1 with carcinomas with glandular differentiation, MUC2 with the mucinous carcinoma, and MUC5AC with the diffuse type of gastric carcinoma and the ring cell carcinoma). Our results suggest the different carcinogenesis of these histological types.

In our study, the immunohistochemical expression of MUC1 constitutes an important prognostic factor, survival at 5 years of patients with MUC1-positive carcinomas being significantly lower than survival at 5 years of patients with MUC1-negative carcinomas. Patients with MUC1 positive carcinomas were about two times more likely to die than those with MUC1 negative carcinomas.

The results obtained show that the immunohistochemical expressions of MUC2 and MUC5AC do not constitute prognostic factors in assessing the patients with gastric cancers.

According to the immunoreactivity of MUC2, the gastric mucinous carcinoma develops from a cellular population consisting predominantly of goblet cells.
The data obtained in our study confirms the hypothesis according to which the heterogeneous expression of mucines and the "de novo" synthesis of non-gastric mucines correspond to advanced stages of gastric cancer.

6. References

Baldus, SE.; Zirbes, TK.; Engel S., et al. (1998). Correlation of the immunohistochemical reactivity of mucins cores MUC1 and MUC2 with histopathological subtypes and prognosis of gastric carcinomas. Int J Cancer, 1998; 79: 133-138, ISSN 1097-0215

Bamba, M.; Sugihara, H.; Kushima, R., et al (2001). Time-dependent expression of intestinal phenotype in signet ring cell carcinomas of the human stomach. Virchows Arch. 2001; 438:49-56, ISSN 0945-6317

Barresi, V.; Vitarelli, E.; Grosso, M., et al (2006). Relationship between immunoexpression of mucin peptide cores MUC1 and MUC2 and Lauren`s histologic subtypes of gastric carcinomas. Eur J Histochem 2006; 50:301-309, eISSN 2038-8306

Byrd, JC.; Yan, P. ; Sternberg, L., et al (1997). Aberrant expression of gland-type gastric mucin in the surface epithelium of Helicobacter pylori-infected patients. Gastroenterology 1997; 113:455-464, ISSN 0016-5085

Choi, JS.; Kim, MA.; Lee, HE., et al (2009). Mucinous gastric carcinomas: clinicopathologic and molecular analyses. Cancer 2009; 3581-3590, ISSN 1097-0142

Corfiefd, AP.; Myerscough, N.; Longman R., et al (2000). Mucins and mucosal protection in the gastrointestinal tract: new prospects for mucins in the pathology of the gastrointestinal disease. Gut, 2000; 47: 589-594, ISSN 0017-5749

Coronella-Wood, JA. & Hersh, EM. (2003). Naturally occurring B-cell responses to breast cancer. Cancer Immunol Immunother 2003; 52:715–38, ISSN 0340-7004.

Cramer, DW.; Titus-Ernstoff, L.; Mc Kolanis, JR., et al (2005). Conditions associated with antibodies against the tumor-associated antigen MUC1 and their relationship to risk for ovarian cancer. Cancer Epidemiol Biomarkers Prev 2005; 14:1125–31, ISSN 1055-9965

De Bolos, C,; Garrido, M. & Real, FX. (1995). MUC6 apomucin shows a distinct normal tissue distribution that correlated with Lewis antigen expression in the human stomach. Gastroenterology 1995; 109:723-734, ISSN 0016-5085

Egashira, Y.; Shimoda, T. & Ikegami, M. (1999). Mucin histochemical analysis of minute gastric differentiated adenocarcinoma. Pathol Int 1999; 49: 55-61, ISSN 1440-1827

Endoh, Y.; Sakata, K.; Tamura, G., et al (2000). Cellular phenotypes of differentiated-type adenocarcinomas and precancerous lesions of the stomach are dependent on the genetic pathways. J Pathol 2000; 191: 257-263, ISSN 1096-9896

Ferreira, B.; Marcos, NT.; David, L., et al. Terminal alpha 1,4-linked N-acetyl glucosamine in Helicobacter pylori-associated intestinal metaplasia of the human stomach and gastric carcinoma cell lines. J Histochem Cytochem 54:585–591, ISSN 0022-1554

Fiocca, R.; Luinetti, O.; Villani, L., et al (2001). Molecular mechanisms involved in the pathogenesis of gastric carcinoma: interactions between genetic alterations, cellular phenotype and cancer histotype. Hepatogastroenterology 2001; 48: 1523-1530, ISSN 0172-6390

Fowler, J.; Vinall, L. & Swallow, D. (2001). Polymorphism of the human muc genes. Front Biosci 2001; 6:D1207-D1215, ISSN 1093-9946

Gamboa-Dominguez, A.; Seidl, S. ; Reyes-Gutierrez, E., et al (2007). Prognostic significance of p21WAF1/CIP1, p27Kip1, p53 and E-cadherin expression in gastric cancer. J Clin Pathol 2007, 60:756-761, ISSN 0021-9746

Gendler, SJ (2001). MUC1, the renaissance molecule. J Mammary Gland Biol Neoplasia 2001; 6:339-353, ISSN 1573-7039

Gomes, J. ; Marcos, NT.; Berois, N., et al (2009). Expression of UDP-N-acetyl-D-galactosamine: Polypeptide N-acetyl galactosaminyl transferase-6 in Gastric Mucosa, Intestinal Metaplasia, and Gastric Carcinoma. Journal of Histochemistry & Cytochemistry 2009, Volume 57(1):79–86, ISSN 0022-1554

Gum Jr, JR.; Hicks, JW.; Toribara, NW., et al (1994). Molecular cloning of human intestinal mucin (MUC2) cDNA. Identification of the amino terminus and overall sequence similarity to prepro-von Willebrand factor. J Biol Chem 1994; 269: 2440-2446, ISSN 0021-9258

Gürbüz, Y.; Kahlke, V. & Klöper G (2002). How do gastric carcinoma classification systems relate to mucin expression patterns? An immunohistochemical analysis in a series of advanced gastric carcinomas. Virchows Arch, 2002; 440: 505-511, ISSN 0945-6317

Handa, K.; Yamakawa, M.; Takeda, H., et al (1999). Expression of cell cycle markers in colorectal carcinoma superiority of cyclin A as an indicator of poor prognosis. Int J Cancer 1999, 84:225-233, ISSN 0020-7136

Hanski, C.; Hofmeier, M.; Schmitt-Graff, A., et al (1997). Overexpression or ectopic expression of MUC2 is the common property of mucinous carcinomas of the colon, pancres, breast and ovary. J Pathol, 1997; 182: 385-391, ISSN 1096-9896

Hattori, T. & Kushima, R (2001). Gastric differentiated stomach adenocarcinoma. Pathology, 2001; 22: 97-104, ISSN 1440-1827

Hilkens, J. ; Ligtenberg, MJ.; Vos, HL., et al (1992). Cell membrane-associated mucins and their adhesion-modulating property. Trends Biochem Sci 1992, 17:359-63, ISSN 0968-0004

Ho, SB.; Niehans, GA.; Lyftong, C., et al (1993). Heterogeneity of mucin gene expression in normal, preneoplastic and neoplastic human gastric epithelium. Cancer Res, 1993; 53: 641-651, ISSN 0008-5472

Ho, SB.; Shekels, LL.; Toribara, NW., et al (1995). Mucin gene expression in normal, preneoplastic, and neoplastic human gastric epithelium. Cancer Res 1995; 55:2681-2690, ISSN 0008-5472

Hollingsworth, MA. & Swanson, BJ (2004). Mucins in cancer: protection and control of the cell surface. Nat Rev Cancer 2004; 4:45–60, ISSN 1474-175X

Huang, L.; Chen, D.; Liu, D., et al (2005). MUC1 oncoprotein blocks glycogen synthase kinase 3beta-mediated phosphorylation and degradation of beta-catenin. Cancer Res 2005; 65:10413–22, ISSN 0008-5472

Ioachim, E (2008). Expression patterns of cyclins D1, E and cyclin-dependent kinase inhibitors p21waf1/cip1, p27kip1 in colorectal carcinoma: correlation with other cell cycle regulators (pRb, p53 and Ki-67 and PCNA) and clinicopathological features. Int J Clin Pract 2008, 62:1736-1743, ISSN 1368-5031

Japanese Gastric Cancer Association (1996). Japanese Classification of Gastric Carcinoma. 13th ed. Tokio: Kanahara Inc; 1996. p26

Kabashima, A. ; Yao, T. ; Sugimachi, K., et al (2000). Gastric or intestinal phenotypic expression in the carcinomas and background mucosa of multiple early gastric carcinomas. Histopathology 2000; 37: 513-522, ISSN 0309-0167

Kabashima, A.; Yao, T.; Sugimachi, K., et al. (2002) Relationship between biologic behaviour and phenotypic expression in intramucosal gastric carcinomas. Hum Pathol. 2002; 33:80-86, ISSN 0046-8177

Kabashima, A. ; Yao, T. ; Maehara, Y., et al (2005). Relationship between biological behavior and phenotypic expression in undifferentiated-type gastric carcinomas. Gastric Cancer 2005; 8: 220-227, ISSN 1436-3291

Kameda, H.; Pandey, JP.; Kaburaki, J., et al (1998). Immunoglobulin allotype gene polymorphisms in systemic sclerosis: interactive effect of MHC class II and Km genes on anticentromere antibody production. Ann Rheum Dis 1998; 57:366–70, ISSN 0003-4967

Kanno, A.; Satoh, K.; Kimura, K., et al (2006). The expression of MUC4 and MUC5AC is related to the biologic malignancy of intraductal papillary mucinous neoplasms of the pancreas. Pancreas 2006, 33(4):391-396, ISSN 0885-3177

Kawachi, T.; Kogure, K.; Tanaka, N., et al (1974). Studies of intestinal metaplasia in the gastric mucosa by detection of disaccharidases with "Tes-Tape". J Natl Cancer Inst 1974; 53:19-30, ISSN 0027-8874

Kelley, JR. & Duggan, JM. (2003). Gastric cancer epidemiology and risk factors. J Clin Epidemiol 2003; 56:1-9, ISSN 0895-4356

Kim, GE.; Bae, HI.; Park, HU., et al (2002). Aberrant expression of MUC5AC and MUC6 gastric mucins and sialyl Tn antigen in intraepithelial neoplasms of the pancreas. Gastroenterology 2002, 123(4):1052-1060, ISSN 0016-5085

Kim, YS. & Gum, Jr. (1996). Brockhausen I. Mucin glycoproteins in neoplasia. Glycoconj J 1996, 13:693-707, ISSN 0282-0080

Kondo, K.; Kohno, N.; Yokoyama, A., et al (1998). Decreased MUC1 expression induces E-cadherin-mediated cell adhesion of breast cancer cell lines. Cancer Res 1998, 58:2014-9, ISSN 0008-5472

Koseki, K. ; Takizawa, T. ; Koike, M., et al (2000). Distinction of differentiated type early gastric carcinoma with gastric type mucin expression. Cancer 2000; 89:724-732, ISSN 1097-0142

Kurtenkov, O.; Klaamas, K.; Mensdorff-Pouilly, S., et al (2007). Humoral immune response to MUC1 and to the Thomsen-Friedenreich (TF) glycotope in patients with gastric cancer: relation to survival. Acta Oncol 2007; 46:316–23, ISSN 0284-186X

Lauren, P. (1965). The two histological main types of gastric carcinoma: diffuse and so-called intestinal-type carcinoma. An attempt at a histo-clinical classification. Acta Pathol Microbiol Scand 1965; 64:31-49, ISSN:0108-0164

Lee, HS.; Lee, HK.; Kim, HS., et al (2001). MUC1, MUC2, MUC5AC and MUC6 expressions in gastric carcinomas. Their roles as prognostic indicators. Cancer, 2001; 92: 1427-1434, ISSN 1097-0142

Li, D.; Li, H.; Zhang, P., et al (2006). Heat shock fusion protein induces both specific and nonspecific anti-tumor immunity. Eur J Immunol 2006; 36:1324–36, ISSN 0014-2980

Lillehoj, EP.; Han, F. & Kim, KC (2003). Mutagenesis of a Gly-Ser cleavage site in MUC1 inhibits ectodomain shedding. Biochem Biophys Res Commun 2003; 307:743–9, ISSN 0006-291X

Lloyd, KO.; Burchell, J.; Kudryashov, V., et al (1996). Comparison of O-linked carbohydrate chains in MUC-1 mucin from normal breast epithelial cell lines and breast carcinoma cell lines: Demonstration of simpler and fewer glycan chains in tumor cells. J Biol Chem 1996, 271:33325-34, ISSN 0021-9258

Machado, JC.; Nogueira, AM.; Carneiro, F., et al (2000). Gastric carcinoma exhibits distinct types of cell differentiation: an immunohistochemical study of trefoil peptides (TFF1 and TFF2) and mucins (MUC1, MUC2, MUC5AC and MUC6). J Pathol, 2000; 190: 437-443, ISSN 0022-3417

Matsuoka, M. ; Aizawa, Y.; Nagamata, H., et al (2003). Significance of the mucin phenotype of early gastric cancer. Jikeikai Med J. 2003; 50:29-36, ISSN 0149-5992

Moniaux, N.; Escande, F.; Porchet, N., et al (2001). Structural organization and classification of the human mucin genes. Front Biosci, 2001; 6: D1192-1206, ISSN 1093-9946

Mrena, J.; Wiksten, JP.; Kokkola, A.; et al (2006). Prognostic significance of cyclin A in gastric cancer. Int J Cancer 2006, 119:1897-1901, ISSN 0020-7136

Nakamori, S.; Ota, DM.; Cleary, KR., et al (1994). MUC1 mucin expression as a marker of progression and metastasis of human colorectal carcinoma. Gastroenterology 1994, 106:353-61, ISSN 0016-5085

Nakamura, K.; Sugano, H. & Takagi, K. (1968). Carcinoma of the stomach in incipient phase: its histogenesis and histological appearances. Gann. 1968; 59:251-258, ISSN 0910-5050

Namikawa, T. & Hanazaki, K. (2010). Mucin phenotype of gastric cancer and clinicopathology of gastric-type differentiated adenocarcinoma. World J Gastroenterol 2010; 16(37):4634-4639, ISSN 1007-9327

Oda, I. ; Gotoda, T. ; Hasuike, N., et al (2003). Endoscopic features of differentiated-type early gastric carcinoma with gastric mucin phenotype. Stomach and Intestine 2003, 38: 684-692, ISSN 0536-2180

Pandey, JP.; Nietert, PJ.; von Mensdorff-Pouilly S., et al (2008). Immunoglobulin allotypes influence antibody responses to mucin 1 in patients with gastric cancer. Cancer Res 2008; 68:4 35, ISSN 0008-5472

Pandey, JP.; Prohászka, Z. ; Veres, A., et al (2004). Epistatic effects of genes encoding immunoglobulin GM allotypes and interleukin-6 on the production of autoantibodies to 60-and 65-kDa heat-shock proteins. Genes Immun 2004; 5:68–71.442-4446, ISSN 1466-4879

Pandey, JP. (2001). Immunoglobulin GM and KM allotypes and vaccine immunity. Vaccine 2001; 19:613–7, ISSN 0264-410X

Pandey, P.; Kharbanda, S. & Kufe, D. (1995). Association of the DF3/MUC1 breast cancer antigen with Grb2 and the Sos/Ras exchange protein. Cancer Res 1995; 55:4000-4003, ISSN 0008-5472

Pertovaara, M.; Hurme, M.; Antonen, J., et al (2004). Immunoglobulin KM and GM gene polymorphisms modify the clinical presentation of primary Sjögren's syndrome. J Rheumatol 2004; 31:2175–80, ISSN 0315-162X

Pinto-De-Sousa, J.; David, L.; Reis, A., et al (2002). Mucins MUC1, MUC2, MUC5AC and MUC6 expression in the evaluation of differentiation and clinico-biological behavior of gastric carcinoma. Virchows Arch, 2002; 440: 304-310, ISSN 0945-6317

Pochampalli, MR.; Bitler, BG. & Schroeder, JA. (2007). Transforming growth factor alpha dependent cancer progression is modulated by Muc1. Cancer Res 2007; 67:6591–8, ISSN 0008-5472

Rahn, JJ.; Dabbagh, L. ; Pasdar, M., et al (2001). The importance of MUC1 cellular localisation in patients with breast carcinoma: an immunohistologic study of 71 patients an review of the literature. Cancer 2001; 91:1973-1982, ISSN 1097-0142

Raina, D.; Kharbanda, S. & Kufe, D. (2004). The MUC1 oncoprotein activates the anti-apoptotic phosphoinositide 3-kinase/Akt and Bcl-xL pathways in rat 3Y1 fibroblasts. J Biol Chem 2004; 279:20607–12, ISSN 0021-9258

Rakha, EA.; Boyce, RW.; Rehim, DA., et al (2005). Expresion of mucins (MUC1, MUC2, MUC3, MUC4, MUC5AC and MUC6) and their prognostic significance in human breast cancer. Modern Pathology 2005; 18:1295-1304, ISSN 0893-3952

Reis, CA.; David, L.; Carvalho, F., et al (2000). Immunohistochemical study of the expression of MUC6 mucin and co-expression of other secreted mucins (MUC5AC and MUC2) in human gastric carcinomas. J Histochem Cytochem, 2000; 48: 377-388, ISSN 0022-1554

Reis, CA.; David, L.; Nielsen, PA., et al (1997). Immunohistochemical study of MUC5AC expression in human gastric carcinomas using a novel monoclonal antibody. Int J Cancer, 1997 74: 112-121, ISSN 0020-7136

Reis, CA.; David, L. ; Seixas, M., et al (1998). Expression of fully and under-glycosylated forms of MUC1. Mucin in gastric carcinoma. Int J Cancer, 1998; 79: 402-410, ISSN 0020-7136

Roukos, DH.; Agnantis, NJ.; Fatouros, M., et al (2002). Gastric cancer: introduction, pathology, epidemiology. Gastric & Breast Cancer 2002; 1:1-3, ISSN 1109 - 7655

Schroeder, JA.; Adriance, MC.; Thompson, MC., et al (2003). MUC1 alters beta-catenin-dependent tumor formation and promotes cellular invasion. Oncogene 2003; 22:1324–32, ISSN 0950-9232

Schroeder, JA.; Thompson, MC.; Gardner, MM., et al (2001). Transgenic MUC1 interacts with epidermal growth factor receptor and correlates with mitogen-activated protein kinase activation in the mouse mammary gland. J Biol Chem 2001; 276:13057-13064, ISSN 0021-9258

Segura, DI. & Montero, C. (1983). Histochemical characterisation of different types of intestinal metaplasia in gastric mucosa. Cancer 1983; 52: 498-503, ISSN 1097-0142

Shimoda, T.; Fujisaki, J.; Kashimura, H., et al (1991). Histological type of gastric carcinoma in relation to the mode of intramural spreading of cancer cells. Stomach and Intestine 1991; 26:1125-1134, ISSN 0536-2180

Shiroshita, H.; Watanabe, H.; Ajioka, Y., et al (2004). Re-evaluation of mucin phenotypes of gastric minute well-differentiated type adenocarcinomas using a series of HGM MUC5AC, MUC6, M-GGMC, MUC2 and CD10 stains. Pathol Int 2004;54:311-321, ISSN 1440-1827

Silk, AW. & Finn, OJ. (2007). Cancer vaccines: a promising cancer therapy against all odds. Future Oncol 2007; 3:299–306, ISSN 1479-6694

Silva, E.; Teixeira, A.; David, L., et al (2002). Mucins as key molecules for the classification of intestinal metaplasia of the stomach. Virchows Arch, 2002; 440: 311-317, ISSN 0945-6317

Stemmermann, GN. (1994). Intestinal metaplasia of the stomach. A status report. Cancer 1994; 74:556-564, ISSN 1097-0142

Sugai, T. ; Habano, W. ; Uesugi, N., et al (2004). Three independent genetic profiles based on mucin expression in early differentiated-type gastric cancers--a new concept of genetic carcinogenesis of early differentiated-type adenocarcinomas. Mod Pathol 2004; 17: 1223-1234, ISSN 0893-3952

Sugai, T.; Tsukahara, M.; Endoh, M., et al (2010). Analysis of cell cycle-related proteins in gastric intramucosal differentiated-type cancers based on mucin phenotypes: a novel hypothesis of early gastric carcinogenesis based on mucin phenotype. BMC Gastroenterology 2010, 10:55, ISSN 1471-230X

Tahara, E. (1993). Molecular mechanism of stomach carcinogenesis. J Cancer Res Clin Oncol 1993; 119:265-272, ISSN 0171-5216

Tajima, Y.; Shimoda, T. & Nakanishi, Y. (2001). Gastric and intestinal phenotypic marker expression in gastric carcinomas and its prognostic significance: immunohistochemical analysis of 136 lesions. Oncology. 2001; 61(3):212-20, ISSN 0030-2414

Tajima Y, Yamazaki K, Makino R, et al. (2006) . Gastric and intestinal phenotypic marker expression in early differentiated-type tumors of the stomach: clinicopathologic significance and genetic background. Clin Cancer Res 2006; 12: 6469-6479, ISSN 1078-0432

Takikita M, Altekruse S, Lynch CF, et al. (2009). Associations between selected biomarkers and prognosis in a population-based pancreatic cancer tissue microarray. Cancer Res 2009, 69(7): 2950-2955, ISSN 0008-5472

Tatematsu M, Ichinose M, Miki K, et al. (1990). Gastric and intestinal phenotypic expression of human stomach cancers as revealed by pepsinogen immunohistochemistry and mucin histochemistry. Acta Pathol Jpn 1990; 40: 494-504, ISSN 0001-6632

Tian MM, Zhao AL, Li ZW, et al. (2007). Phenotypic classification of gastric signet ring cell carcinoma and its relationship with clinicopathologic parameters and prognosis. World J Gastroenterol. 2007; 13:3189-3198, ISSN 1007-9327

Toki F, Takahashi A, Aihara R. (2010). Relationship between clinicopathological features and mucin phenotypes of advanced gastric adenocarcinoma. World J Gastroenterol. 2010 June 14; 16(22): 2764-2770, ISSN 1007-9327

Tosi P, Filipe MI, Luzi P, et al. (1993). Gastric intestinal metaplasia type III cases are classified as low-grade dysplasia on the basis of morphometry. J Pathol 1993; 169:73-78, ISSN 0022-3417

Utsunomiya T, Yonezawa S, Sakamoto H, et al. (1998). Expression of MUC1 and MUC2 mucins in gastric carcinomas: its relationship with the prognosis of the patients. Clin Cancer Res 1998; 4:2605-2614, ISSN 1078-0432

Vlad AM, Kettel JC, Alajez NM, et al. (2004). MUC1 immunobiology: from discovery to clinical applications. Adv Immunol 2004; 82:249–93, ISSN 0065-2776

Wesseling J, van der Valk SW, Hilkens J. (1996). A mechanism for inhibition of E-cadherin-mediated cell-cell adhesion by the membrane-associated mucin episialin/MUC1. Mol Biol Cell 1996; 7:565-577, ISSN 1059-1524

Yamachika T, Inada K, Fujimitsu Y, et al. (1997). Intestinalization of gastric signet ring cell carcinomas with progression. Virchows Arch. 1997; 431:103-110, ISSN 0945-6317

Yamagishi M, Noda M, Tatsumi Y, et al. (2004). Correlation between cyclooxygenase-2, proliferative activity, and mucin phenotype in human advanced gastric cancer. J Gastroenterol. 2004; 39:1143-1149, ISSN 0944-1174

Yamamoto M, Bharti A, Li Y, et al. (1997). Interaction of the DF3/MUC1 breast carcinoma-associated antigen and beta-catenin in cell adhesion. J Biol Chem 1997; 272: 12492-12494, ISSN 0021-9258

Yamashita K, Yonezawa S, Tanaka S, et al. (1993). Immunohistochemical study of mucin carbohydrates and core proteins in hepatolithiasis and cholangiocarcinoma. Int J Cancer 1993; 55:82-91, ISSN 0020-7136

Yamazaki K, Tajima Y, Makino R, et al. (2006). Tumor differentiation phenotype in gastric differentiated-type tumors and its relation to tumor invasion and genetic alterations. World J Gastroenterol 2006; 12: 3803-3809, ISSN 1007-9327

Yamazoe S, Tanaka H, Sawada T, et al. (2010). RNA interference suppression of mucin 5AC (MUC5AC) reduces the adhesive and invasive capacity of human pancreatic cancer cells. Journal of Experimental & Clinical Cancer Research 2010, 29:53, ISSN 0392-9078

Yu LG, Andrews N, Zhao Q, et al.(2007). Galectin-3 interaction with Thomsen-Friedenreich disaccharide on cancer-associated MUC1 causes increased cancer cell endothelial adhesion. J Biol Chem 2007, 282:773-781, ISSN 0021-9258

Zhang HK, Zhang QM, Zhao TH et al. (2004). Expression of mucins and E-cadherin in gastric carcinoma and their clinical significance. W J Gastroenterol, 2004; 10 (20): 3044-3047, ISSN 1007-9327

Zhang S, Zhang HS, Cordon-Cardo C, et al. (1998). Selection of tumor antigens as targets for immune attack using immunohistochemistry:protein antigens. Clin Cancer Res 1998; 4:2669-2676, ISSN 1078-0432

Zhao Q, Barclay M, Hilkens J, et al. (2010). Research interaction between circulating galectin-3 and cancer-associated MUC1 enhances tumour cell homotypic aggregation and prevents anoikis. Molecular Cancer 2010, 9:154, ISSN 1476-4598

Zheng HC, Li XH, Hara T, et al. (2008). Mixed-type gastric carcinomas exhibit more aggressive features and indicate the histogenesis of carcinomas. Virchow Arch 2008; 452:525-534, ISSN 0945-6317

Part 3

Microbial Infections and Their Implications

12

Genetic Factors Involved in the Genesis of Helicobacter Pylori-Induced Gastric Cancer

Asahi Hishida
Nagoya University Graduate School of Medicine
Japan

1. Introduction

Gastric cancer is the second most frequent cause of cancer-related mortality in the world, and is the most common malignancy of the gastrointestinal tract in East Asian populations (Parkin et al., 1997; Parkin et al. 1999). *Helicobacter pylori* (*H. pylori*) is an established risk factor for developing gastric cancer and its precancerous lesions, which was evidenced by numerous epidemiological studies (Hamilton & Aaltonen, 2000; Tsuji et al., 2006). More than 50% of the world's population is estimated to be infected with this bacterium (Danesh, 1999). It is demonstrated that the risk of the subjects with *H. pylori* infection is from 2- to 6-fold (Eslick et al., 1999). In addition, some trials on *H. pylori* eradication revealed that cure of its infection reduces the gastric cancer development in high-risk populations (Fukase et al., 2008; Wong et al., 2004).

2. Genetic factors involved in the genesis of *Helicobacter pylori*-induced gastric cancer

Accumulated evidence has shown that there are three steps in gastric carcinogenesis: *H. pylori* infection, development of gastric precancerous lesions, and gastric carcinogenesis (Hamajima et al., 2006). For each of these three steps there are specific genetic traits that influence the process interacting with lifestyle factors (Figure 1).

2.1 Genetic traits for the persistence of *Helicobacter pylori* infection

H. pylori is transmitted from person to person through the oral-oral or fecal-oral route mainly during the childhood.

Such factors as will directly affect the *H. pylori* transmission like sewage systems are also essential determinants of the infection. Although there is limited supporting biological evidence, some lifestyle factors such as salty food intake, low fruits intake, or smoking might play a role in persistent *H. pylori* infection.

Genetic traits could influence persistent *H. pylori* infection interacting with lifestyle factors.

2.1.1 Genetic polymorphisms of the molecules associated with gastric acid secretion

Gastric acid is secreted from parietal cells, and regulated by histamine, gastrin, and acetyl choline. It is known that IL-1β and TNF-α, proinflammatory cytokines, inhibit gastric acid

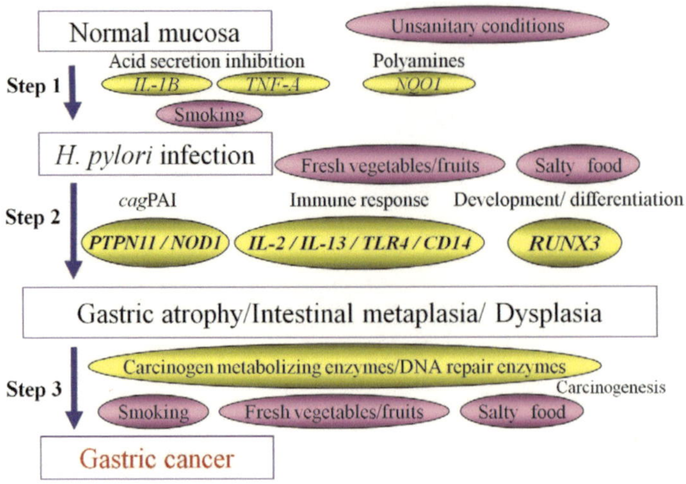

Fig. 1. Steps in *Helicobacter pylori*-induced gastric cancer.

secretion (Beales et al., 1998), and *H. pylori* infected patients showed a marked increase in IL-1β mRNA in mucosa (Wang et al., 1999). A recent study demonstrated that IL-1β decreased gastrin level (Chakravorty et al., 2009), elucidating the mechanism of the acid secretion reduction due to *H. pylori* infection. IL-1β induces TNF-α, and vice versa. Although IL-1β and TNF-α have several roles, polymorphisms connected to both molecules are classified as one group in this chapter (Table 1).

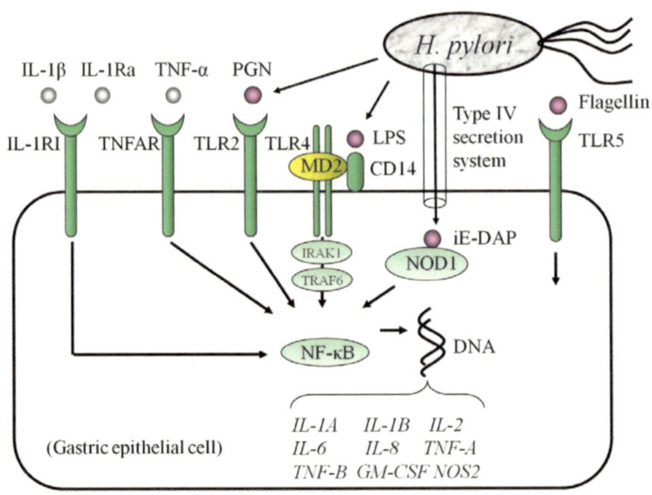

Fig. 2. Signal pathways from *Helicobacter pylori* infection to pro-inflammatory gene expression.

IL-1A

IL-1A making a cluster in chromosome 2q14 with *IL-1B* and *IL-1RN* has two single nucleotide polymorphisms (SNPs) of C-889T and G4845T, as well as a 46-bp variable number of tandem repeats (VNTR) polymorphism (Bailly et al., 1993). It was reported that the combination *IL-1A* -889TT and *IL-1B* -511T (-511TT or -511TC) was related to high plasma levels of IL-1β (Hullkonen et al., 2000). The association with *H. pylori* infection was examined only for a Japanese population (Hamajima et al., 2001), providing no association of *IL-1A* C-889T (Table 1). In the study, the association with 46-bp VNTR polymorphism was not examined, because the polymorphism was not found among Japanese (Hamajima et al., 2002a). Polymorphism G4845T was reported to be linked with C-889T (Armitage et al., 2000).

IL-1B

Three polymorphisms of *IL-1B* T-511C, C-31T, and C3954T located in chromosome 2q14, have been studied for many diseases. It is known that -511*T* and -511*C* are tightly linked with -31*C* and -31*T*, respectively (Hamajima et al., 2001a). An electrophoretic mobility-shift assay demonstrated that C-31T was a functional polymorphism (El-Omar et al., 2000), while C3954T is unlikely to be functional.

We conducted four studies for Japanese and Japanese Brazilians, all of which showed a similar result, that those with -31*TT* had a higher risk of *H. pylori* seropositivity (Hamajima et al., 2001a; Hamajima et al., 2002b; Uno et al., 2002). The risk elevation was marked for smokers except one study (Hamajima et al., 2002b). Since cigarette smoke includes about 4,000 chemicals, many genes may be upregulated or downregulated. A study on C-31T in Brazil showed a higher seropositive rate for those with -31*TT* genotype, though not significant (Queiroz et al., 2009). Concerning T-511C polymorphism, no associations were found among Japanese (Kato et al., 2001) and Koreans (Kim et al., 2006), while a Chinese study reported a significant association with -511*T* allele (-511*TT* + -511*TC*) (Liou, 2007), which was linked to -31*C* allele.

IL-1RI

There are two receptors for IL-1β; IL-1RI and IL-1RII. The former transduces the signal, but the latter does not. IL-1RI in 2q12 has reportedly four polymorphisms; C-116T (RFLP-A), C-90T, T49C, and RFLP-B at an unknown site (Bergholdt et al., 1995). There were no reports on the association between these polymorphisms and *H. pylori* seropositivity, except our study for C-116T indicating no association (Hamajima et al., 2003a).

IL-1RN

IL-1RN has an 86-bp VNTR polymorphism. Among 241 Japanese, the allele frequency was 4.1% for 2 repeat allele, 0.2% for 3 repeat allele, 94.6% for 4 repeat allele, and 1.0% for 5 repeat allele (Hamajima et al., 2001a). No significant differences in *H. pylori* soropositivity among different genotypes of *IL-1RN* 86-bp VNTR were observed for Japanese, Koreans, and Chinese (Hamajima et al., 2001a; Kim et al., 2006; Liou et al., 2007). Since the minor alleles are rare for the three ethnic groups, statistical power of these studies was not enough.

TNF-A

TNF-A and *TNF-B* genes are located between HLA-B and HLA-DR on 6p21.3. In the promoter area of *TNF-A*, G-238A, G-244A, G-308A, C-857T, C-863A, and T-1031C were reported (Kamizono et al., 2000; Yamaguchi et al., 2001). Among East Asians, -238*A*, -244*A* and -308*A* alleles were rare (2.0%, 0.0% and 1.7%, respectively in Japanese (Kamizono et al., 2000; Yamaguchi et al., 2001)), and C-863A was tightly linked with T-1031C (Higuchi et al., 1998). The functions of these alleles were controversial, but -308*A* was regarded as a high expression allele (D'Alfonso et al., 1994).

Subjects (Reference)	aOR or *HP%*					
IL-1A C-889T	*CC*		*CT/TT*			
241 Japanese (Hamajima, 2001a)	62%	(n=201)	68%	(n=39) / (n=1)		
IL-1B C-31T	*CC*		*CT*		*TT*	
241 Japanese (Hamajima, 2001a)	1	(n=42)	2.32*	(n=133)	2.46*	(n=66)
55 smokers	1	(n=16)	6.18*	(n=27)	22.9*	(n=12)
465 Japanese (Uno, 2002)	1	(n=116)	0.97	(n=183)	1.73*	(n=163)
80 ever smokers	1	(n=23)	1.68	(n=34)	5.29*	(n=22)
547 Japanese (Hamajima, 2002a)	1	(n=116)	1.32	(n=237)	1.35	(n=178)
127 smokers	1	(n=23)	1.12	(n=60)	1.01	(n=41)
963 Jpn. Brazil. (Uno, 2002)	1	(n=226)	1.30	(n=432)	1.45*	(n=289)
124 smokers	1	(n=ND)	2.45	(n=ND)	3.49*	(n=ND)
541 Brazil. (Queiroz, 2009)	64%	(n=112)	71%	(n=265)	67%	(n=164)
IL-1B T-511C	*TT*		*TC*		*CC*	
499 Japanese (Kato, 2001)	52%	(n=113)	54%	(n=243)	53%	(n=143)
474 Koreans (Kim, 2006)	86%	(n=131)	86%	(n=259)	88%	(n=84)
663 Chinese (Liou, 2007)	67%	(n=148)	64%	(n=343)	55%*	(n=172)
IL-1RI C-116T	*CC*		*CT*		*TT*	
241 Japanese (Hamajima, 2003a)	65%	(n=93)	58%	(n=114)	72%	(n=32)
IL-1RN VNTR	*4rpt/4rpt*		*2rpt*		*Others*	
241 Japanese (Hamajima, 2001a)	62%	(n=217)	-		67%	(n=24)
474 Koreans (Kim, 2006)	-		80%	(n=60)	87%	(n=414)
663 Chinese (Liou, 2007)	-		66%	(n=53)	61%	(n=540)
540 Brazil. (Queiroz, 2009)	67%	(n=378)	70%	(n=162)	-	
TNF-A T-1031C	*TT*		*TC*		*CC*	
1,374 Japanese (Hamajima, 2003a)	1	(n=952)	0.92	(n=385)	0.43*	(n=34)
963 Jpn. Brazil. (Atsuta, 2006)	1.18	(n=648)	0.96	(n=269)	1	(n=31)
TNF-A C-857T	*CC*	*CT*	*TT*			
1,374 Japanese (Hamajima, 2003a)	1	(n=931)	1.06	(n=373)	1.69	(n=42)
963 Jpn. Brazil. (Atsuta, 2006)	1	(n=613)	1.17	(n=301)	1.21	(n=36)
TNF-A -1031 & -857	*CC&CC*	*TT&CC*	*TC&CT*	*TT&TT*		
1,374 Japanese (Hamajima, 2003a)	1(n=34)	2.37*(n=595)	2.84*(n=76)	3.63*(n=42)		
963 Jpn. Brazil. (Atsuta, 2006)	1(n=30)	1.08 (n=377)	1.03 (n=67)	1.27 (n=35)		
253 ever smokers	1(n=11)	2.01 (n=102)	1.76 (17)	2.30 (n=5)		
TNF-A G-308A	*GG*		*GA*		*AA*	
393 Germans (Kunstmann, 1999)	52%	(n=277)	56%	(n=89)	56%	(n=18)
792 Italians (Zambon, 2005)	54%	(n=ND)	61%*	(n=ND)	-	(n=ND)
474 Koreans (Kim, 2006)	86%	(n=400)	89% for *GA*(n=59)/*AA*(n=2)			
539 Brazil. (Queiroz, 2009)	70%	(n=403)	66%	(n=123)	46%	(n=13)
TNF-B A252G	*AA*	*AG*	*GG*			
1,374 Japanese (Hamajima, 2003a)	1	(n=501)	1.05	(n=656)	1.05	(n=204)

*: statistically significant (p<0.05), Jpn. Brazil.: Japanese Brazilians, and ND: not described.

Table 1. Genetic polymorphis of molekuls potentially related with gastric acid secretion, reported on the associations with Helicobacter pyloriinfections: sex-age-ajusted odd ratio (aOR) or seropositive percentage (HP%)

Among the studies reported on the *TNF-A* polymorphisms (Queiroz et al., 2009; Kim et al., 2006; Hamajima et al., 2003b; Atsuta et al., 2006; Kunsmann et al, 1999; Zambon et al., 2005), significant associations were found for T-1031C and for the combination of T-1031C and A-857T among 1,374 Japanese (Hamajima et al., 2003), as well as for G-308A among 792 Italians (Zambon et al., 2005). If -1031*T* and -857*T* are the high expression alleles, the findings of the studies on TNF-A seemed rather consistent to indicate that high TNF-α expression favors persistent *H. pylori* infection.

TNF-B

TNF-B A252G, whose *G* allele is strongly linked with *TNF-A* -857*C* allele in Japanese (Hamajima et al., 2003b), was not associated with seropositivity, as shown in Table 1. Another polymorphism, *TNF-B* Thr26Asn, was found to link completely with A252G.

2.1.2 Genetic polymorphisms of molecules associated with innate immune responses

Innate immune responses have not completely been understood. The polymorphisms of the molecules possibly involved in the innate immune responses are selected in this section (Table 2).

CD14

CD14, located in chromosome 5q31.1, has a polymorphism C-159T. Serum soluble CD14 was reported to be significantly higher in those with -159*TT* (n=42, median=4.5μg/ml) than in those with -159*CC* (n=67, median=4.1μg/ml) (Baldini et al., 1999). Although the polymorphism seemed functional, no association was found with *H. pylori* seropositivity (Hamajima et al., 2003a).

CXCR2

CXCR2 in 2q35 was reported to have three polymophisms; C785T causing a silent codon change in leucine, and T1208C and G1440A in the 3′ untranslated region of exon 3 (Renzoni et al., 2000). These polymorphisms are tightly linked, forming a haplotype with 785C, 1208T, and 1440G. Accordingly, any polymorphism of the three may be used for a pilot association study on disease risk. No significant difference was observed in the seropositive rate among the three genotypes of C785T in Japan (Hamajima et al., 2003a).

IL-2

T-330G of *IL-2* gene on chromosome 4q26-27 was reported to be a functional polymorphism; the production was higher in -330*GG* genotype than in *TT* genotype (Williams et al., 1988; Hoffmann et al., 2001). The -330*TT* was at a higher risk of gastric atrophy (Togawa et al., 2005) and less frequent among Asians (38% out of 29 individuals) than among Caucasians (51% out of 199 individuals) (Hoffmann et al., 2002). While the polymorphism was not associated with *H. pylori* seropositivity among Japanese (Togawa et al., 2005), -330*TT* genotype was significantly associated with the seropositivity relative to -330*C* allele (*CC*+*CT*) among Brazilians (Queiroz et al., 2009).

IL-4

IL-4 C-33*T* on chromosome 5q31.1 was reported to be functional; IL-4 protein production was higher in -33*TT* genotype than in -33*CC* genotype (Nakashima et al., 2002). Our dataset showed no association with *H. pylori* seropositivity in Japanese (Togawa et al., 2005).

IL-8

IL-8 located in chromosome 4q12-q21 was reported to have nine polymorphisms (four in 5′ upstream regions, four at introns, and one in 3′ downstream region). Among Europeans, two haplotypes, one with -1722del*T*, -251*A*, 396*G*, 781*T*, 1633*T*, and 2767*T* termed del*TAGTTT* in the order of those polymorphisms, and the other with del*TTTCCA*, are dominant with frequencies of 0.41 and 0.52, respectively. The haplotypes are more diverse among Africans; delTAGCCA (frequency 0.36), del*TATCCA* (0.19), ins*TATCCA* (0.18), and del*TTTCCA* (0.10), respectively (Hull et al., 2001), but the genotyping of T-251*A* and T396G is sufficient for classifying the haplotypes even among Africans. Among Japanese, there was a strong linkage between the two polymorphisms; 396*TT* was found in 90.0% of 110 individuals with -251*TT*, 396*TG* in 90.5% of 95 individuals with -251*TA*, and 396*GG* in 100% of 22 individuals with -251*AA* (Hamajima et al., 2003c), indicating that T-251A is a good marker for Japanese.

Although a study on IL-8 expression found that the *A* allele had a higher expression than the *T* allele (Hull et al., 2001). Plasma IL-8 levels was found to be higher in A allele carriers among those with *H. pylori* seronegative, but lower among the seropositives without gastric atrophy (Naito et al., 2010). Although no significant association was found with the seropositivity, the point estimate of the adjusted odds ratio was less than unity for the *A* allele carriers (Hamajima et al., 2003c).

IL-10

IL-10 G-1082A and T-819C polymorphisms were reported to influence the expression of *IL-10* mapped on 1q31-32; -1082A and -819T are high expression alleles (Turner et al., 1997; Helminen et al., 2001). There is a large difference in -1082*G* allele frequency among different regions; 0.51 in Belfast, 0.52 in Glasgow, and 0.47 in Strasbourg (Donger et al., 2001), but 0.04 among Japanese(Ito et al., 2000). We found that there was no significant association between T-819C and *H. pylori* seropositivity.

As mentioned, a high level of IL-10 and a lower level of IL-8 create favorable conditions for prolonging the *H. pylori* infection in human gastric mucosa. Accordingly, the combination of *IL-8* -251*TT* (the low expression genotype) and *IL-10* -819*TT* (the high expression genotype) was expected to be favorable for persistent *H. pylori* infection. Among three studies, one study demonstrated that the other combinations were at a significantly lower risk of the persistent infection (Hamajima et al., 2003c), but another study was opposite (Hamajima et al., 2003a). When smokers were selected, the genotype combinations other than *IL-8* -251*TT* and IL-10 -819*TT* were at a lower risk in the three studies, though not significant for two studies (Table 2).

IL-13

IL-13 is a Th2 cytokine, whose gene is located in 5q31. Closely linked polymorphisms, A-1512C, C-1111T, and Arg130Gln, have been examined for disease risk (Beghe et al., 2009). Although the association between gastric atrophy development and C-1111T was observed (Togawa et al., 2005), there was no association with the seropositivity.

MPO

Myeloperoxidase (MPO) is a lysosomal enzyme in polymorphonuclear leukocytes and monocytes. It produces hypochlorous acid to kill a wide range of organisms. While mutations, Arg569Trp, Val173Cys, or Met251Thr of *MPO* located in 17q23.1 cause fatal diseases such as chronic granulomatous disease due to severe enzyme activity deficiency (Nauseef et al., 1994), *MPO* G-463A exhibits less influential, but the transcription level of *A* allele was reported to be one twenty-fifth of G allele (Piedrafita et al., 1996). Two studies showed the *A* allele carriers were at a lower risk of the seropositivity, though not significant (Hamajima et al, 2001b; Katsuda et al, 2003). Intuitively, low enzyme activity seemed to provide a favorable situation, but the results were opposite.

NF-KB2

NF-KB2 encoding NF-κB2 (p100) has a Ins/Del polymorphism at -10*G* (or 1867GG/G), as well as two polymorphisms with a rare minor allele (Shinohara et al., 2001). Although the function of Ins/Del -10*G* has not been demonstrated, no association was found with *H. pylori* seropositivity (Hamajima et al., 2003a).

NOS2

Nitric oxide synthase (NOS) was three isozymes; neuronal constitutive NOS (nNOS) encoded by *NOS1*, inducible NOS (iNOS) encoded by *NOS2*, and endothelial constitutive NOS (enNOS) encoded by *NOS3*. There were several polymorphisms reported for *NOS2* in chromosome 17cen-q11.2, such as C-1173T, G-954C, (TAAA)n, and (CCTTT)n. A C150T (Ser608Leu) polymorphism at exon 16 was reported to have an association with type 1 diabetes (Johannsen et al., 2001), but the association with *H. pylori* was not observed among Japanese (Goto et al., 2006a). There were no studies with the other polymorphisms of NOS2.

NQO1

NQO1 is an obligate two-electron reductase, whose gene is located in chromosome 16q22 (Ross et al., 2000). The gene has a functional polymorphism C609T (Pro187Ser); the *T* allele has no enzyme activity (Siegel et al., 1999). The *CC* genotype was found that to favor persistent *H. pylori* infection among Japanese (Goto et al., 2005).

ODC

ODC in chromosome 2p25, encoding ornitine decarboxylase, has a functional polymorphism G317A in intron 1; the expression was higher in the *A* allele than in the *G* allele (Guo et al., 2000). Aspirin chemoprevention of colorectal adenoma recurrence was reported to be more effective among those with 317*AA* than those with the other genotypes. The 317*AA* genotype was 5-7% in Europe and the United States (Hubner et al., 2008), while it was 36% in Japan (Goto et al., 2007). The association with *H. pylori* seropositivity was not observed among Japanese (Goto et al., 2007).

TLR2

Arg677Trp, Arg753Gln, and Ins/Del at -196 to -174 were reported as polymorphisms of *TLR2* on chromosome 4q32 (Queiroz et al., 2009; Tahara et al., 2007). Although the minor allele was rare, the association with Arg753Gln was examined among Brazilians. They found no association with the polymorphism (Queiroz et al., 2009).

TLR4

In *TLR4* on chromosome 9q32-33, two polymorphisms, Asp299Gly and Thr399Ile, have been reported. The 299Gly/399Ile allele is less sensitive to LSP than 299Asp/399Thr allele, resulting in lower NF-κB activity (Arbour et al., 2000). The LPS-hyposensitive allele was found to be 5.9% among 879 blood donors in England (Read et al., 2001), but not found

Subjects [Reference]	aOR or *HP%*					
CD14 T-159C	*TT*		*TC*		*CC*	
1,374 Japanese (Hamajima, 2003a)	1	(n=413)	0.94	(n=678)	1.16	(n=413)
CXCR2 C785T	*CC*		*CT*		*TT*	
241 Japanese (Hamajima, 2003a)	65%	(n=110)	63%	(n=100)	56%	(n=25)
IL-2 T-330G	*GG*		*GT*		*TT*	
454 Japanese (Togawa, 2005)	1	(n=45)	1.10	(n=196)	1.15	(n=202)
541 Brazil. (Queiroz, 2009)	70%	(n=27)	63%	(n=221)	72%*	(n=293)
IL-4 C-33T	*CC*		*CT*		*TT*	
454 Japanese (Togawa, 2005)	1	(n=42)	1.43	(n=183)	1.25	(n=227)
IL-8 T-251A	*TT*		*TA*		*AA*	
454 Japanese (Hamajima, 2003c)	1	(n=234)	0.86	(n=177)	0.70	(n=37)
IL-10 T-819C	*TT*		*TC*		*CC*	
454 Japanese (Hamajima, 2003c)	1	(n=220)	0.67	(n=177)	0.82	(n=37)
IL-8 & *IL-10*	*TT&TT*	*Others*				
454 Japanese (Hamajima, 2003c)	1	(n=115)	0.62*	(n=327)		
65 smokers	1	(n=ND)	0.13*	(n=ND)		
241 Japanese (Hamajima, 2003a)	1	(n=57)	1.04	(n=178)		
55 smokers	1	(n=ND)	0.45	(n=ND)		
679 Japanese (Hamajima, 2003a)	1	(n=164)	1.49*	(n=507)		
158 smokers	1	(n=ND)	0.89	(n=ND)		
IL-13 C-1111T	*CC*		*CT*		*TT*	
454 Japanese (Togawa, 2005)	1	(n=310)	0.73	(n=127)	1.09	(n=11)
MPO G-463A	*GG*		*GA/AA*			
241 Japanese (Hamajima, 2001b)	1	(n=192)	0.69	(n=47)/(n=2)		
454 Japanese (Katsuda, 2003)	1	(n=354)	0.84	(n=77)/(n=6)		
NF-KB2 -10G	*InsIns*	*InsDel*	*DelDel*			
1,374 Japanese (Hamajima, 2003a)	1	(n=513)	1.03	(n=648)	1.15	(n=199)
NOS2 C150T (Ser608Leu) *CC*		*CT*		*TT*		
454 Japanese (Goto, 2006a)	No association					
NQO1 C609T (Pro187Ser) *TT*		*TC*		*CC*		
241 Japanese (Goto, 2005a)	1	(n=48)	1.13	(n=107)	2.42*	(n=86)
454 Japanese (Goto, 2005a)	1	(n=83)	1.57	(n=210)	1.70	(n=153)
ODC A317G	*AA*		*AG*		*GG*	
465 Japanese (Goto, 2007)	1	(n=167)	1.09	(n=229)	1.02	(n=69)
TLR2 Arg753Gln	*ArgArg*	*ArgGln*	*GlnGln*			
541 Brazil. (Queiroz, 2009)	68%	(n=531)	70%	(n=10)	-	(n=0)
TLR4 Asp299Gly	*AspAsp*	*AspGly*	*GlyGly*			
541 Brazil. (Queiroz, 2009)	68%	(n=490)	71%	(n=51)	-	(n=0)
TLR4 G3725C	*GG*		*GC*		*CC*	
1,592 Japanese (Hishida, 2009a)	1	(n=827)	0.95	(n=474)	0.72	(n=90)
TLR5 Arg392Ter	*ArgArg*	*ArgTer*	*TerTer*			
541 Brazil. (Queiroz, 2009)	68%	(n=504)	71%	(n=34)	67%	(n=3)

* Statistically significant (p<0.05), Jpn. Brazil.: Japanese Brazilians, Brazil.: Brazilians

Table 2. Genetic polymorphisms of molecules potentially involved in innate responses, reported on the associations with Helicobacter pylori infection: sex-age-adjusted odds ratio (aOR) or seropositive percentage (HP%)

among 275 Japanese (Tahara et al., 2007). For Japanese, G3725C in 3'UTR was reported to have an association with periodontitis. We found that the polymorphism had an association with severe gastric atrophy, but did not with persistent *H. pylori* infection (Hishida et al., 2009a).

TLR5

A polymorphism *TLR5* Arg392Ter on chromosome 1q41-42 was examined for the association among Brazilans (Queiroz et al., 2009). There was no significant association in the study.

2.1.3 Genetic polymorphisms of molecules associated with adhesion to epithelial cells

BabA of *H. pylori* binds of H type I and Lewis b antigen carbohydrate structure on human epithelial cells. H type I is synthesized from Type I precursor with secretor enzyme encoded by *FUT2*, and further metabolized to Lewis b with Lewis enzyme encoded by *FUT3*. Both enzymes are fucosyltransferase.

FUT2 (secretor gene)

Although many polymorphisms were reported, main alleles of *FUT2* located in 19q13.3 are *Se1* (357*C*, 385*A*, 571*C*, 628*C*), *Se2* (357*T*, 385*A*, 571*C*, 628*C*), *sej* (357*T*, 385*T*, 571*C*, 628*C*), *se3* (357*C*, 385*A*, 571*T*, 628*C*), *se4* (357*C*, 385*A*, 571*C*, 628*T*), and *se5* (combined with a pseudogene). Se1 and Se2 exhibit full enzyme activity, while sej shows very low activity, and se3, se4, and se5 reveal no activity. Accordingly, *Se1* and *Se2* are denoted by *Se*, and the others by *se*. Among Caucasians, *se3* and *se4* are common *se* alleles, whereas in East Asians *se5* and *sej* are main se alleles (Narimatsu et al., 1998). Since those with *sese* genotype cannot synthesize H type I nor Lewis b, they were expected to have the lower seropositive rate. Our first study fitted the expectation (Ikehara et al., 2001), but it was not confirmed in the second and third datasets (Hamajima et al., 2002b). Those with *sese* genotype was reported to be resistance for Norwalk virus infection (Lindesmith L et al., 2003).

Subjects [Reference]	aOR					
FUT2	*SeSe*		*Sese*		*sese*	
241 Japanese (Ikehara, 2001)	1	(n=61)	0.79	(n=127)	0.35*	(n=51)
679 Japanese (Hamajima, 2002c)	1	(n=170)	1.51*	(n=328)	1.50	(n=181)
464 Japanese (Hamajima, 2002c)	1	(n=139)	1.57	(n=218)	1.29	(n=107)
FUT3	*LeLe*		*Lele*		*lele*	
241 Japanese (Hamajima, 2002c)	1	(n=124)	1.95*	(n=98)	2.80	(n=17)
679 Japanese (Hamajima, 2002c)	1	(n=353)	0.98	(n=251)	1.31	(n=59)
424 Japanese (Hamajima, 2002c)	1	(n=235)	1.06	(n=155)	1.40	(n=33)

* Statistically significant ($p<0.05$)

Table 3. Genetic polymorphisms of other miscellaneous molecules, reported on the associations with Helicobacter pylori infection: sex-age-adjusted odds ratio (aOR) or seropositive percentage (HP%)

FUT3 (Lewis gene)

FUT3 has three polymorphisms; T59G, G508A, and T1067A. An *Le* allele is defined as one with 59*T*, 508*G*, and 1067*T*, an *le1* allele with 59*G*, 508*A*, and 1067*T*, an *le2* allele with 59*G*, 508*G*, and 1067*A*, and an *le3* allele with 59*G*, 508*G*, and 1067*T*. The *le1* and *le2*, denoted by *le*, lack enzyme activity. Since *le3* shows almost full enzyme activity, it is grouped into *Le* (Narimatsu et al., 1998). The *LeLe* genotype, which may disturb the synthesis of H type I by FUT2 through sharing the same substrate (type I precursor), showed the lower seropositivity in the first dataset, while the finding was not reproduced by the second and third datasets (Hamajima et al., 2002b) (Table 3).

2.2 Genetic predisposition to *Helicobacter pylori*-induced gastric precancerous lesions

The presence of gastric lesions outside the tumor was recognized as gastric precancerous lesions in gastrectomy specimens or biopsies taken by flexible gastroscopes, which lead to the development of a model of gastric carcinogenesis generally accepted. Long-term follow-up of cohorts in high-risk populations has documented the dynamics of gastric precancerous process. Severe gastric atrophy, corpus-predominant gastritis, intestinal metaplasia and dysplasia are well-recognized predominant predispositions to gastric cancer (Correa P, 1988; Uemura et al., 2001).

There seems to be a considerable variation in the extent of these gastric damages due to *H. pylori* infection from one subject to another, suggesting that genetic factors are playing important roles in the long-term outcome of *H. pylori* infection.

Although biological mechanisms underlying the genesis of gastric precancerous conditions remain largely unknown, both direct effects by the virulence factors of *H. pylori*, such as cytotoxin-associated gene A (CagA), and indirect effects derived from pro-inflammatory immune response by the host seem to be involved (Takahashi et al., 2007) (Table 4).

2.2.1 Cag pathogenicity island-related genes and their polymorphisms

The main effects of *H. pylori* virulence factors on the development of gastric precancerous lesions may be represented by the CagA. CagA is a 120 to 145-kDa *H. pylori* protein encoded by the *cagA* gene, which is localized at one end of the *cag* pathogenicity island (*cag*PAI), a 40-kb DNA segment considered to be horizontally transfected to the *H. pylori* genome (Censini et al., 1996; Akopyants et al., 1998). CagA is delivered from *H. pylori* bacterium into host cell cytoplasms through the type IV secretion system and undergoes tyrosine phosphorylation. In the injected gastric epithelial cells, CagA induces cellular spreading and elongation called the 'hummingbird phenotype', which is thought to play important roles in *H. pylori*-induced gastric carcinogenesis. In this CagA-dependent morphologic transformation of gastric epithelial cells, a key molecule SHP-2 (src homology 2 domain-containing protein tyrosine phosphatase-2) is required. Binding of tyrosine phosphorylated CagA to the SH2 domains of SHP-2 causes a conformational change in SHP-2 itself which leads to the aberrant activation of SHP-2 phosphatase. SHP-2 plays a major role in intracellular signaling provoked by various growth factors, hormones or cytokines, and is widely expressed in both embryonic and adult tissues (Higashi et al., 2002). SHP-2 is required for full activation of the Ras-MAP kinase cascade in response to growth factor-receptor interaction and plays an important role in cell morphogenesis as well as cell mortility (Higashi et al., 2002), which might partly explain the mechanism for the formation of hummingbird phenotype.

Meanwhile, CagA is shown to disrupt the tight junctions and causes loss of epithelial apical-basolateral polarity through the specific interaction of CagA with partitioning-defective-1 (PAR1)/ microtubule affinity-regulating kinase-2 (MARK2) (Sadaat et al., 2007) (Figure 3). PAR1b is localized to the basolateral membrane in normal polarized epithelial cells, while atypical protein kinase C (aPKC) complex is localized specifically to the apical membrane. When CagA is delivered and injected into normal polarized gastric epithelial cells, CagA inhibits the kinase activity of PAR1b by binding directly to its kinase domain, which subsequently leads to junctional and polarity defects followed by the disorganization of the epithelial monolayer (Sadaat et al., 2007). PAR1b exists as a homodimer in the cells, and two CagA protein bind to a PAR1b dimer, which is also essential for stable CagA-SHP2 interaction.

Recently, a cytosilic pattern recognition receptor, nucleotide-binding oligomerization domain protein 1 (NOD1), was found to respond to peptidoglycan delivered by *H. pylori* cagPAI (Viala et al., 2004). NOD1 is known to sense the essential gamma-D-glutamyl-meso-diaminopimelic acid (i.E.-DAP) dipeptide, which is uniquely contained in peptidoglycan of all gram negative and certain gram-positive bacteria (Neel et al., 2003).

As the precise relationship of gastric precancerous lesions like gastric atrophy (GA) and intestinal metaplasia (IM) with these cagPAI-associated molecules is largely left unknown, further investigations are required to clarify the roles of these cagPAI-related molecules in the genesis of gastric precancerous lesions.

PTPN11 (Protein tyrosine phosphatase, non-receptor type, 11)

The *PTPN11* G/A polymorphism at intron 3 (rs2301756), is a G-to-A single nucleotide substitution at 223 bp upstream of exon 4 in the *PTPN11* gene encoding SHP-2 at chromosome 12q24.1. The biological function of this polymorphism has not yet been reported. The first dataset showed that one (11.1%) out of 9 infected individuals with the *AA* genotype had gastric atrophy, while 134 (56.1%) among 239 infected with the G allele had atrophy (Goto et al., 2006a). Our recent report of 1,636 non-cancer Japanese subjects demonstrated that the risk of severe gastric atrophy was significantly reduced for those with at least one A allele of this *PTPN11* G/A polymorphism at intron 3 (OR = 0.62, 95% CI = 0.42-0.90), confirming the association of this *PTPN11* gene polymorphism with the risk of gastric precancerous lesions in *H. pylori*-infected subjects (Hishida et al., 2009a). If the polymorphism is functional or linked to a functional one, the association can be biologically explained by the difference in the strength of signal transduction through the CagA-SHP2 complex. According to the NCBI dbSNP, the frequencies of the *G* allele of rs2301756, high risk allele for gastric atrophy, is 0.802 among 1,484 Japanese and 0.917 among 48 Chinese, while the corresponding was 0.348 among 46 African American and 0.064 among 46 Caucasians, indicating that Japanese and Chinese become high risk ethnic groups through CagA-positive *H. pylori* infection, if the hypothesis that the *G* allele confers stronger signals via the CagA-SHP2 interaction is true.

NOD1

Recent report revealed that the carriage of the *NOD1* G796A (E266K) mutation increases the susceptibility for gastric atrophy strikingly: OR = 34.2 in NOD1 796*AA* and OR = 13.35 in *NOD1* 796*GA* compared to subjects with *NOD1* 796*GG* (Kara et al., 2010).

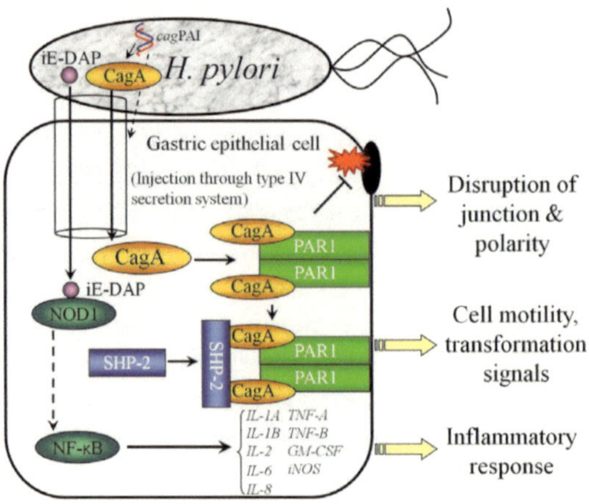

Fig. 3. Signal pathways induced by the *Helicobacter pylori cag* pathogenicity island related molecules.

2.2.2 Immune related genes and their polymorphisms

For the effects of pro-inflammatory immune response by the hosts, TLR4 is known to recognize lipopolysaccharide (LPS) of gram-negative bacteria and is proved to play important roles in *H. pylori* infection through the interaction of macrophage/monocyte TLR4 with *H. pylori* LPS. The initial recognition of LPS and subsequent signaling by TLR4 is supported by several accessory proteins: LPS first binds to lipopolysaccharide-binding protein (LBP) which works as an opsonin for CD14 which then acts as a catalyst for the binding of LPS to MD-2. The signal induced by LPS/MD-2/TLR4 complex is transmitted through myeloid differentiation factor 88 (MyD88), interleukin (IL)-1 receptor associated kinase (IRAK), tumor necrosis factor (TNF) receptor-associated factor 6 (TRAF6) and inhibitory κB kinase (IKK) to nuclear factor (NF)- κB, leading to the production of pro-inflammatory cytokines such as IL-1A, IL-1B, IL-6 or TNF-A. The human immune system is also balanced by the anti-inflammatory cytokines like IL-10, IL-4 or IL-13 which are controlled by regulatory T-cells. In these inflammatory processes, augmented expression of inducible nitric oxide synthase (iNOS) is shown to play important roles in the generation of oxygen radicals, while overexpressed cyclooxygenase-2 (COX-2) is demonstrated to contribute to the proliferation of the gastric epithelium through the up-regulation of cell-cycles as well as to the propagation of gastric inflammation *via* the prostaglandin pathways. The induction of iNOS is also supposed to be modulated by the activity of protein kinase C-eta (PRKCH) via the phosphorylation of nuclear factor-kappa B (NF-kB) or activator protein-1 (AP-1) (Pham et al., 2003a; Pham et al., 2003b).

Oxidative DNA damage is also supposed to play important roles in the pathogenesis of *H. pylori*-induced gastric mucosal damage, where 8-OHdG is a potential sensitive marker of DNA oxidation (Farinati et al., 2008). The damaged bases in DNA are mainly repaired by the base excision repair (BER) system; the accumulation of 8-Hydroxy-2'-deoxyguanosine (8-OHdG) or 2-hydroxyadenine (2-OH-A) in DNA is prevented by the co-operation of mutT human homolog-1 (MTH1), 8-hydroxyguanine DNA glycosylase (OGG1) and mutY human homolog (MUTYH) (Nakabeppu et al., 2004). The number of studies that investigated the contribution of these molecules involved in inflammatory response, such as innate immune response, oxygen radical production, oxidative DNA damage repair processes, together with cell-cycle regulation and/or cell proliferation in the genesis of *H. pylori*-induced gastric precancerous lesions is also limited, requiring further biological investigations in the near future.

TLR4

One study in Caucasians showed that the *TLR4* +896 A/G polymorphism (rs4986790) was associated with the risk of gastric atrophy, where the *TLR4* +896 *G* carriers had an 11-fold increased risk of gastric atrophy with hypochlorhydria (Hold et al., 2007). Subsequent Japanese study also clarified the possible association between another genetic variation in *TLR4* gene, the *TLR4* +3725G/C polymorphism (rs11536889), and the risk of severe gastric atrophy in Japanese (Hishida et al., 2009a), suggesting the significance of genetic variations in host innate immunity due to *TLR4* polymorphisms also in East Asian populations.

CD14

There is one single nucleotide polymorphism in the promoter region of the *CD14* gene, *CD14* C-159T polymorphism, which is critical for *CD14* expression (Zhang et al., 1994). Recent study by one Japanese group demonstrated that *CD14* promoter -159TT and *T* carrier were associated with lower risk of gastric atrophy in *H. pylori*-infected subjects who were 61 years or older (Tahara et al., 2007).

IL-2 and IL-13

IL-2 T-330G polymorphism was demonstrated to be a functional polymorphism (Williams et al., 1988), with higher IL-2 production in *GG* genotype than in *TT* genotype (Hoffmann et al., 2001). Those with *TT* genotype were shown to be at a higher risk of gastric atrophy (Togawa et al., 2005), who were less frequent in Asians (38% out of 29 individuals) than in Caucasians (51% out of 199 individuals) (Hoffmann et al., 2002).
IL-13 gene in chromosome 5q31 has several polymorphisms; at least 3 polymorphisms at the promoter region, 2 polymorphisms at intron 1, Arg130Gln, and 4 polymorphisms at 3′ UTR of exon 4 have been reported (Howard et al., 2001). The -1111*TT* genotype was shown to harbor increased binding ability of nuclear proteins, and was also reported to be associated with asthma (Howard et al., 2001; Van der Pouw Kraan et al, 1999). As for the risk of gastric atrophy, -1111*TT* was found to be a low risk genotype (Togawa et al., 2005). The biological mechanism involved was not yet clarified.

IL-4R

One study of Venezuelan subjects revealed that those with homozygotes with the low activity allele (*GG*) of the A398G polymorphism in the *IL-4R* gene (rs1805010) had a modestly increased risk of gastric atrophy (OR = 1.52, 95% CI = 1.05-2.21) (Kato et al., 2006), suggesting the role of genetic variability in the anti-inflammatory mediators in the genesis of *H. pylori*-induced gastric precancerous lesions.
iNOS C150T (rs2297518) and *PRKCH* rs3783799 G/A polymorphisms: *PRKCH* is shown to be involved in oxidative stress, by activating iNOS and nitric oxide production (Pham et al., 2003). The associations of the polymorphisms in these two genes (*iNOS* C150T [rs2297518] and *PRKCH* rs3783799 G/A polymorphisms) with the risk of gastric atrophy were investigated in Japanese population, which revealed that those with *PRKCH* rs3783799 AA genotype were at significantly higher risk of severe gastric atrophy (OR = 2.37, 95% CI = 1.11-5.05) (Goto et al., 2010), while there were no significant association between the *iNOS* C150T polymorphism and risk of gastric atrophy (Goto et al., 2006b).

2.2.3 Other miscellaneous genes and their polymorphisms

Recently, it was reported that the loss expression of sonic hedgehog (Shh), a regulatory gene essential for developmental patterning, and aberrant expressions of *caudal-type homeobox transcription factor 2* (*CDX2*), a master regulatory gene of intestinal development and differentiation, in *H. pylori*-induced atrophic gastritis are the early events correlated with the occurrence of intestinal metaplasia, which can be reversible by the eradication of *H. pylori*. In accordance with these findings, CDX2 expression has been demonstrated to be associated with intestinal phenotypes in gastric cancers (Shiotani et al., 2008).

Another important tumor suppressor gene in intestinal-type gastric cancer is *runt-related gene 3* (*RUNX3*) encoding a subunit of polyomavirus enhancer binding protein 2 (Li et al., 2002), since expression of *RUNX3* is greatly reduced in intestinal metaplasias in human stomachs (Oshio et al., 2004) and *RUNX3-/-* mouse gastric epithelial cells have a potential to differentiate into CDX-2 positive intestinal type cells (Oshio et al., 2004). Li and colleagues (Li et al., 2002; Levanon et al., 2003) reported that the gastric mucosa of *RUNX3* null mice showed hyperplasia, indicating that loss of *RUNX3* leads to gastric carcinogenesis in humans. Consistent with this, an analysis of RUNX3 in human stomach cancer cell lines and primary human tumours revealed hemizygosity in 40% of the tumours examined, and silencing by promoter hypermethylation in 60% of the tumours, and this figure increased up to 90% in the advanced stage tumours. It is shown that the *RUNX3-/-* mouse gastric mucosa exhibits hyperplasias due to the stimulated proliferation and suppressed apoptosis in the cells, suggesting that RUNX3 is an attractive candidate as a tumor suppressor of gastric cancer. The CpG island of *RUNX3* P2 promoter is hypermethylated in human and mouse gastric cancer cell lines and in primary human tumors (Li et al, 2002; Waki et al., 2003), also suggesting the tumor suppressor function of RUNX3 in the etiology of stomach cancer.

Heat-shock protein (HSP) 70 plays essential roles in cellular response to a variety of environmental stresses by acting as molecular chaperons in the folding of newly synthesized proteins in cells and assist in the folding of damaged proteins (Becker et al., 1994). HSP expression in the gastric mucosa is shown to be attenuated by *H. pylori* infection and aspirin intake, and one HSP inducer geranylgeranylacetone (GGA) reportedly protects gastric mucosa from iNOS induced by *H. pylori* infection (Yeo et al., 2004), suggesting that HSP has important roles in protecting gastric mucosa against *H. pylori* or aspirin induced injuries.

Gastric carcinogenesis can also be regarded as a multistep process that initiates with the disregulation of normal controls of apoptoisis and cell proliferation, in which FAS receptor-ligand system is shown to be a key regulator of apoptosis (Hsu et al., 2008).

Pepsinogen C (PGC), alternatively called pepsinogen II or gastricsin, an inactive precursor of pepsin C, is an aspartic protease specifically produced by the gastric chief cells, cardiac cells, pylori cells and Brunner's glands from late infant stages to adulthood period. PGC is considered to be a differentiation marker of gastric epithelium, whose changes in expression may reflect the severity of gastric mucosal damage (Samloff et al., 1982).

RUNX3

Among *H. pylori* seropositive subjects, we found a significant association between *RUNX3* rs760805 T/A polymorphism and the risk of gastric atrophy with the age- and sex-adjusted OR of 1.51 (95% CI 1.11-2.05, P=0.008) in *TA*, 1.59 (95% CI 1.08-2.33, P=0.019) in *AA*, and 1.53 (95% CI 1.14-2.05, P=0.004) in *TA+AA*, compared with *TT* genotype (Hishida et al., 2009b). This finding was in accordance with the recent biological report that RUNX3 expression correlated with chief cell differentiation in human gastric cancers (Ogasawara et al., 2009).

Polymorphism	Function	Rs number	Subjects (Reference)	OR and/or GA%
IL-1B C-31T	5'UTR	rs1143627	253 Japanese (Atsuta, 2006)	*CC* (54%),*CT* (52%),*TT* (56%)
"			455 Jpn.Brazil. (Uno, 2004)	*CC*,*CT*:0.61,*TT*:0.58 *CC* (36%), *CT* (31%), *TT* (21%)
"			1,328Venezuelan (Kato, 2007)	*TT*,*CT*:1.01,*CC*:0.91
IL-2 T-330G	5'UTR	rs2069762	244 Japanese (Togawa, 2005)	*GG*,*TG*:1.64,*TT*:2.78 *GG (38%),*TG* (50%),*TT* (62%)
IL-4 C-33T	5'UTR	rs2070874	249 Japanese (Togawa, 2005)	*CC*,*CT*:2.47,*TT*:1.80 *CC* (38%),*CT* (60%),*TT* (53%)
IL-4 T-590C	5'UTR	rs2243250	1,301 Venezuelan (Kato, 2006)	*TT*,*CT*:0.82,*CC*:0.81
IL-4R C-3223T	5'UTR	rs2057768	1,301 Venezuelan (Kato, 2006)	*CC*,*CT*:0.97,*TT*:1.01
IL-4R A398G	Non-synonimous (Ile50Val)	rs1805010	1,301 Venezuelan (Kato, 2006)	*AA*,*AG*:1.14,*GG*:1.52*
IL-6 G-174C	5'UTR	rs1800795	1,315 Venezuelan (Kato, 2007)	*GG*,*CG*:0.98,*CC*: 0.57
IL-8 T-251A	5'UTR	rs4073	1,347 Venezuelan (Kato, 2007)	*TT*,*AT*:0.98,*AA*:1.07
IL-10 G-1082A	5'UTR	rs1800896	1,301Venezuelan (Kato, 2006)	*GG*,*AG*:1.05,*AA*:1.14
IL-13 C-1111T	5'UTR	rs1800925	248 Japanese (Togawa, 2005)	*CC*,*CT*+*TT*:0.41 *CC (59%),*CT*+*TT* (45%)
TNF-A T-1031C	5'UTR	rs4647198	455 Jpn.Brazil. (Atsuta, 2006)	*CC* (29%),*TC* (33%),*TT* (34%)
C-857T	5'UTR	rs1799724	456 Jpn.Brazil. (Atsuta, 2006)	*CC* (32%),*CT* (36%),*TT* (39%)
-1031&-857			455 Jpn.Brazil. (Atsuta, 2006)	*CC&CC* (29%),*TT&CC* (33%),*TC&CT* (43%),*TT&TT* (39%)
G-308A	5'UTR	rs1800629	1,327 Venezuelan (Kato, 2006)	*GG*,*AG*+*AA*:1.27
MCP1 G-2518A	5'UTR	rs1024611	1,311 Venezuelan (Kato, 2007)	*AA*,*AG*:1.02, *GG*:1.18
PTPN11 G/A at intron3	intron	rs2301756	248 Japanese (Goto, 2006a)	*GG*,*GA*:0.70,*AA*:0.09 *GG (59%),*GA* (49%),*AA* (11%)
"			979 Japanese (Hishida, 2009a)	*GG*,*GA*+*AA*:0.62[‡] *GG (22%),*GA*+*AA* (15%)[‡]
NOD1 G796A	Non-synonimous (Glu266Lys)	rs2075820	150 Turks (Kara, 2010)	*GG*,*GA*: 13.35*,*AA*:34.2*
TLR4 A+896G	Non-synonimous (Asp299Gly)	rs4986790	103 Caucasians (Hold, 2007)	*AA*,*AG*:11.0* *AA* (36%),*AG* (87%)[§]
"			717 Venezuelan (Kato, 2007)	*GlyGly*/ *AspGly*,*AspAsp*: 1.53
TLR4 G+3725C	3'UTR	rs11536889	980 Japanese (Hishida, 2009b)	GG,GC+CC:1.33 GG(18%),GC+CC(22%)‡
CD14 C-159T(C-260T)	5'UTR	rs2569190	717 Venezuelan (Kato, 2007)	*CC*,*CT*+*TT*:1.06
PRKCH rs3783799 G/A	intron	rs3783799	1,638 Japanese (Goto, 2010)	*GG*,*GA*:0.99,*AA*:2.37*
iNOS C150T	Non-synonimous (Ser608Leu)	rs2297518	250 Japanese (Goto, 2006a)	*CC*,*CT*+*TT*:0.75
RUNX3 T/A at intron3	intron	rs760805	938 Japanese (Hishida, 2009)	*TT*,*TA*:1.51*,*AA*:1.59*TT* (46%),*TA* (56%),*AA* (56%)
HSP70-2 A/B (A1267G)	Synonimous (Gln351Gln)	rs1061581	137 Japanese (Tahara, 2009)	*BB* (45%),*AA*+*AB* (67%)[‡]
FAS G-1377A	5'UTR	rs2234767	109 Taiwanese (Hsu, 2008)	No association
FAS A-670G	5'UTR	rs1800682	109 Taiwanese (Hsu, 2008)	No association
FASL T-844C	5'UTR	rs763110	109 Taiwanese (Hsu, 2008)	*TT*,*TC*+*CC*:9.4*
PGC Ins/Del	Ins/Del	(unknown)	86 Chinese (Pham, 2003)	*DD* (90%),others(50%)*
NQO1 C609T	Non-synonimous (Pro187Ser)	rs1800682	396 Japanese (Goto, 2005a)	*TT*,*CT*:1.25,*CC*:1.23
GSTM1	Ins/Del	(unknown)	396 Japanese (Goto, 2005a)	*Null*,*Present*:1.35
GSTT1	Ins/Del	rs71748309	396 Japanese (Goto, 2005a)	*Null*,*Present*:0.87
ACE Ins/Del	Ins/Del	rs1799752	271 Japanese (Goto, 2005c)	*II*,*ID*:1.12,*DD*:0.99
RANTES C-471T	5'UTR	rs2107538	344 Germans (Hellmig, 2005)	No association
SDHC JST173800 C/G	3'UTR	rs3813632	249 Japanese (Goto, 2006c)	*CC*,*GC*:1.26,*GG*:0.51 *CC* (53%), *GC* (59%), *GG* (38%)
IFNGR1 G-611A	5'UTR	rs1327474	805 Portugese (Canedo, 2008)	*GG*,*GA*:1.2,*AA*:1.2
IFNGR1 C-56T	5'UTR	rs2234711	814 Portugese (Canedo, 2008)	*CC*,*CT*:1.4,*TT*:1.3

Table 4. Polymorphisms associated with gastric atrophy *Helicobacter pylori* seropositives.

Polymorphisms of other miscellaneous genes

HSP 70-2

It is shown that the *AA* genotype of *HSP 70-2* A/B polymorphism (PsiI polymorphism, corresponding to A1267G polymorphism) had the highest level of mRNA expression compared with the other genotypes (*AB* or *BB*). Recently one Japanese group reported that the BB genotype of *HSP 70-2* gene is significantly associated with the reduced risk of severe gastric atrophy in *H. pylori* infected older subjects (Tahara et al., 2009), indicating the importance of this HSP polymorphism in the genesis of *H. pylori*-induced gastric precancerous lesions.

FASL

Lately one study group in Taiwan investigated the relations between precancerous gastric lesions and polymorphisms in the promoter regions of the death pathway genes FAS and FASL (FAS G-1377A, FAS A-670G and FASL T-844C) in 109 *H. pylori*-infected Taiwanese individuals, and found that FASL -844 *C* allele significantly increased the risk of atrophy in the gastric corpus, with an adjusted OR of 5.0 (95% CI = 1.5-6.8) (Hsu et al., 2008).

PGC

Recent study among Chinese demonstrated that subjects with *PGC Del/Del* genotype of the *PGC ins/del* polymorphism were at significantly higher risk of atrophic gastritis (OR=3.11; 95%CI 1.44-6.71), and *H. pylori*-seropositive subjects with *PGC Del/Del* genotype had significantly elevated risk of atrophic gastritis (OR=11.16; 95%CI 1.37-90.84) with the interaction of 6.48 (Sun et al., 2009), suggesting the positive link between *PGC* gene polymorphism and *H. pylori*-induced gastric atrophy.

2.3 Genetic factors for *Helicobacter pylori*-induced gastric carcinogenesis

To date, many genetic polymorphisms have been examined on the associations with gastric cancer in case-control studies with the mixed cases (*H. pylori*-related and *H. pylori*-unrelated) and controls at different stages (unexposed to *H. pylori*, exposed but uninfected, infected but without gastric atrophy, and with gastric atrophy), as shown in Fig. 5. Since those case-control studies compared genotype frequencies between the mixed cases and heterogeneous controls, the estimated odds ratios did not reflect any distinct step to gastric cancer. Controls unexposed to *H. pylori* have the same genotype frequency as the average among the exposed, which reduces the difference in the genotype frequency between the uninfected and infected. In order to measure the associations between genotypes and *H. pylori* infection, the studies are to be conducted at a region where the exposure to the bacterium was highly prevalent. Usual case-control studies could provide the estimates for the final step (ie, literal carcinogenesis), when genotype frequency is different between gastric atrophy and gastric cancer, and the same among the uninfected, infected, and those with gastric atrophy.

Table 5 lists the polymorphisms reported on gastric cancer risk, adopted from Gonzalez et al.(Gonzalez et al., 2002) and recent studies(Ebert et al., 2005; Geddert et al., 2005; Li et al., 2005; Tsukino et al., 2002; Sugimoto et al., 2005; Gao et al., 2002; Wu et al., 2002; Goto et al., 2005; Lai et al., 2005a; Lee et al., 2004; Savage et al., 2004; Lai et al., 2005b; Lacasana-Navarro et al., 2006; Kim et al., 2005; Hamajima et al., 2002a; Duarte et al., 2005). The ORs are listed in case of being significant. Accordingly, it should be noted that there were many insignificant studies behind Table 5.

There are several studies to demonstrate the risks of both gastric atrophy and gastric cancer in comparison with the same controls without gastric atrophy. Individuals with IL-8 -251A allele had OR=1.50 with 95% confidence interval (95%CI)=0.98-2.23 for gastric atrophy and OR=1.50 with 95%CI=1.00-2.25, indicating that the risk elevation was due to the risk for gastric atrophy, not for the step from gastric atrophy to gastric cancer.(Taguchi et al., 2005) The direct comparisons between controls with gastric atrophy and cases with gastric cancer were reported; no associations for *p53* Arg72Pro (Hiyama et al., 2002; Chung et al., 2006), and for *PTPN11* G/A at intron 3 (Goto et al., 2006a).

Lifestyle factors may interact with the genotypes in the final step. Biologically, the interactions of smoking, fresh vegetables/fruits and salty food with polymorphisms of carcinogen-metabolic enzyme and DNA repair enzymes are very plausible.

Polymorphism	Country(Reference)	OR (95%CI)
ACE I/D	Germany (Ebert, 2005)	*DD, DI*:0.55 (0.31-0.96),
		II:0.20 (0.08-0.54)
cyclinD1 G870A	Germany(Geddert, 2005)	significant association (p=0.003)
CYP1A1 Ile/Val	China(Li, 2005)	*IleIle, ValVal*:4.84 (1.24-22.07)
CYP2C6 *1/*4	Japan(Tsukino, 2002)	*1*1/*1*4, *4*4:3.14 (1.05-9.41)
CYP2C19 *1/*2/*3	Japan(Sugimoto, 2005)	* 1*1, no*1:1.98 (1.07-3.65)
CYP2E1 RsaI	Japan*	
	Brazil*	
	China(Gao, 2002)	
E-cadherin C-160A	Taiwan(Wu, 2002)	*CC, AA*:0.20 (0.06-0.56)
EGF A61G	Japan(Goto, 2005)	
GSTM1 present/null	UK*	*present, null*:2.9 (1.25-6.73)
	Japan*	*present, null*:1.70 (1.05-2.8)
	Iran*	*present, null*:2.3 (1.15-4.95)
	Poland*	
	China(Li, 2005)	*present, null*:2.81 (1.39-5.71)
	Taiwan(Lai, 2005)	*present, null*:1.75 (1.04-2.96)
GSTM3 IVS6del3	Poland*	
GSTP1 I105V	Japan*	
	Poland*	
GSTT1 present/null	China*	*present, null*:2.5 (1.01-6.2)
	Poland*	*present, null*:3.1 (1.5-6.5)
		among current smokers
	Japan*	
IL-1B C-1473G	Korea (Lai, 2005)	
C-511T	Poland(El-Omar, 2000)	*CC, CT*:1.8 (1.3-2.4),
		TT:2.6 (1.7-3.9)
	Portugal*	*CC, CT/TT*:1.7 (1.1-2.7)
	Taiwan(Wu, 2003)	
C3954T	Poland(El-Omar, 2000)	
IL-1RN 86-bp VNTR	Poland(El-Omar, 2000)	*4rpt4rpt, 2rp2rp*:3.7 (2.4-5.7)
	Taiwan(Wu, 2003)	
IL-1B C-511T+	Portugal*	*CC+LL/L2rpt*,
IL-1RN 86-bp VNTR		*CT/TT+2rpt2rp*:9.0 (3.5-23.0)
IL-2 G-384T, G114T	China(Savage, 2004)	
IL-4 C-590T	Taiwan(Wu, 2003; Lai, 2005)	
RP1/RP2	Taiwan(Lai, 2005)	
IL-4R Ile50Val	Taiwan(Wu, 2003)	
Gln576Arg	Taiwan(Wu, 2003)	
IL-10 G-1082A	Taiwan(Wu, 2003)	*AA, AG*:2.14 (1.07-4.30)
	China(Savage, 2004)	

T-819C	Taiwan[Wu, 2003]	*TT, TC*:1.83 (1.23-2.71), *CC*:1.95 (1.03-3.69)
	China[Savage, 2004]	
MK G-2669A	Taiwan[Lai, 2005]	
MTHFR C677T	China*	*CC, TT*:1.87 (1.00-3.48)
	Mexico[Lacasana-Navarro, 2006]	*CC, TT*:1.62 (1.00-2.59)
C677T, A1298C	Korea[Kim, 2005]	
MUC1 VNTR	Portugal*	*Large, Small*: 4.3 (1.8-10.5)
MUC6 VNTR	Portugal*	*Large, Small*: p<0.05
*MYCL1 Eco*RI	Japan*	*LL, LS*:1.55 (1.03-2.34)
	Japan*	*LL, LS/SS*:3.09 (1.33-7.21)
NAT1	UK*	*slow, rapid*:2.6 (1.3-5.3)
	Japan*	
NAT2	UK*	
	Japan*	
NQO1 C609T	Japan[Hamajima, 2002d]	
OGG1 Ser327Cys	Japan*	
	Brazil*	
p16^{INK4A} C540G	Germany[Geddert, 2005]	
C570G	Taiwan[Lai, 2005]	
p21 codon31	Taiwan[Lai, 2005]	
p53 codon72	Taiwan[Lai, 2005]	significant association (p=0.02)
PPARγ Pro12Ala(C/G)	China[Liao, 2006]	*CC, CG/GG*:2.5 (1.1-5.8)
TFF2 VNTR	Portugal*	
TNF-A G-308A	Korea*	
	Taiwan[Wu, 2003]	
G-238A	Korea*	
	Taiwan[Wu, 2003]	
XRCC1 Arg194Trp	Brazil[Duarte, 2005]	
Arg399Gln	Brazil[Duarte, 2005]	
Arg194Trp+ Arg399Gln	China*	*TrpTrp+ArgArg, ArgArg+ ArgGln/GlnGln*:1.73 (1.12-2.69)
XRCC3 Thr241Met	Brazil[Duarte, 2005]	

* Studies cited in the review by Gonzalez et al. (2002).

L: alleles longer than *2rpt*

Table 5. Polymorphisms reported on the associations with gastric risk> only singnificant are with odds ratio (OR) and 95% confidence interval (95%CI).

3. Conclusion

It is clear that *H. pylori*-related gastric cancer develops through several steps including the infection, gastric atrophy, (histologically intestinal metaplasia, dysplasia) and cancer. Lifestyle factors such as smoking and diet could influence one or more steps. On the other hand, genotypes may be step-specific because the biological process is distinct in the different steps. Accumulated findings on the associations between gastric cancer risk and polymorphism genotypes demonstrated that the strength of associations varied among the studies. Since usual case-control studies examined the mixed effects on these steps, the inconsistent findings may be natural. In addition, the diversity of lifestyle interacting with the genotypes among the different study subjects may enlarge the inconsistency. In order to elucidate the genetic traits of *H. pylori*-related gastric cancer, the studies on each step taking into account of the lifestyle factors will be requested. Such studies will produce useful information for gastric cancer prevention.

4. Acknowledgement

The author wishes to thank Drs. Nobuyuki Hamajima, Kazuo Tajima, Keitaro Matsuo and all the staffs involved in the studies for the gastric cancer molecular epidemiology & prevention in Japan.

5. References

Akopyants NS, Clifton SW, Kersulyte D, et al. (1998). Analyses of the *cag* pathogenicity island of *Helicobacter pylori*. Mol Microbiol, Vol. 28, pp. 37-53.

Armitage GC, Wu Y, Wang H-Y, et al. (2000). Low prevalence of a periodontitis-associated interleukin-1 composite genotype in individuals of Chinese heritage. *J Periodontol*, Vol. 71, pp. 164-171.

Arbour NC, Lorenz E, Schutter BC et al. (2000). *TLR4* mutations are associated with endotoxin hyporesponsiveness in humans. *Nat Genet*, Vol. 25, pp. 187-191.

Atsuta Y, Ito LS, Oba-Shinjo SM et al. (2006). Associations of *TNF-A*-1031*TT* and -857*TT* genotypes with *Helicobacter pylori* seropositivity and gastric atrophy among Japanese Brazilians. *Int J Clin Oncol*, Vol. 11, pp. 140-145.

Bailly S, di Giovine FS, Blakemore AIF, et al. (1993). Genetic polymorphism of human interleukin-1α. *Eur J Immunol*, Vol. 23, pp. 1240-1245.

Baldini M, Lohman IC, Halonen M, et al. (1999). A polymorphism in the 5′ flanking region of the *CD14* gene is associated with circulating souble CD14 levels and with total serum immunoglobulin E. *Am J Respir Cell Mol Biol*, Vol. 20, pp. 976-983.

Beales IL & Calam J. (1998). Interleukin 1 beta and tumour necrosis factor alpha inhibit acid secretion in cultured rabbit parietal cells by multiple pathways. *Gut*, Vol. 42, pp. 227-234.

Becker J & Craig JE. (1994). Heat-shock proteins as molecular chaperones. Eur J Biochem, Vol. 219, pp. 11-23.

Beghe B, Hall IP, Garker SG et al. (2010). Polymorphisms in IL13 pathway genes in asthma and chronic obstructive pulmonary disease. *Allegy*, Vol. 65, pp. 474-81.

Bergholdt R, Karlsen AE, Johannesen J et al. (1995). Characterization of polymorphisms of an interleukin 1 receptor type 1 gene (IL1RI) promoter region (P2) and their relation to insulin-dependent diabetes mellitus (IDDM). *Cytokine*, Vol. 7, pp. 727-733.

Censini S, Lange C, Xiang Z, et al. (1996). *cag*, a pathogenicity island of *Helicobacter pylori*, encodes type I-specific and disease-associated virulence factors. *Proc Natl Acad Sci USA*, Vol. 93, pp. 14648-14653.

Chakravorty M, De DD, Choudhury A, et al. (2009). *IL1B* promoter polymorphism regulates the expression of gastric acid stimulating hormone gastrin. *Int J Biochem Cell Biol*, Vol. 41, pp. 1502-1510.

Chamaillard M, Hashimoto M, Horie Y, et al. (2003). An essential role for Nod1 in host recognition of bacterial peptidoglycan containing diaminopimelic acid. *Nat Immunol*, Vol. 4, pp. 702-707.

Chung WC, Lee KM, Lee BI, et al. (2006). *P53* genetic polymorphism of gastric cancer in Korea. *Korean J Intern Med*, Vol. 21: pp. 28-32.

Correa P. (1988). A Human Model of Gastric Carcinogenesis. *Cancer Res*, Vol. 48, pp. 3554-3560.

D'Alfonso S & Richiardi PM (1994). A polymorphic variation in a putative regulation box of the *TNFa* promoter region. *Immunogenet*, Vol. 39, pp. 150-155.

Danesh J.(1999). *Helicobacter pylori* infection and gastric cancer: systematic review of the epidemiological studies. *Aliment Pharmacol Ther*, Vol. 13, pp. 851-856.

Donger C, Georges J-L, Nicaud V et al. (2001). New polymorphisms in the *interleukin-10* gene - relationships to myocardinal infarction. *Eur J Clin Invest*, Vol. 31, pp. 9-14.

Duarte MC, Colombo J, Rossit ARB, et al. (2005). Polymorphisms of DNA repair genes *XRCC1* and *XRCC2*, interaction with environmental exposure and risk of chronic gastritis and gastric cancer. World J Gastroenterol, Vol. 11, pp. 6593-600.

Ebert MP, Lendeckel U, Westphal S, et al. (2005). The *angiotensin I-converting enzyme* gene insertion/deletion polymorphism in linked to early gastric cancer. *Cancer Epidemiol Biomarkers Prev*, Vol. 14, pp. 2987-2989.

El-Omar EM, Carrington M, Chow,W-H, et al. (2000). Interleukin-1 polymorphisms associated with increased risk of gastric cancer. *Nature*, Vol. 404, pp. 398-402.

El-Omar EM, Ng MT & Hold GL. (2008). Polymorphisms in Toll-like receptor genes and risk of cancer. Oncogene, Vol. 27, pp. 244-252.

Eslick GD, Lim LL, Byles JE, et al. (1999). Association of *Helicobacter pylori* infection with gastric carcinoma: a meta-analysis. *Am J Gastroenterol*, Vol. 94, pp. 2373-2379.

Farinati F, Cardin R, Bortolami M, et al. (2008). Oxidative DNA damage in gastric cancer: cagA status and *OGG1* gene polymorphism. *Int J Cancer*, 123: 51-55.

Ferwerda B, McCall MB, Verheijen K, et al. (2008). Functional consequences of *Toll-like receptor 4* polymorphisms. Mol Med, Vol. 14, pp. 346-352.

Fukamachi H, Ito K & Ito Y. (2004). Runx3-/- gastric epithelial cells differentiate into intestinal type cells. Biochem Biophys Res Commun, Vol. 321, pp. 58-64.

Fukase K, Kato M, Kikuchi S, et al. (2008). Effect of eradication of *Helicobacter pylori* on incidence of metachronous gastric carcinoma after endoscopic resection of early gastric cancer: an open-label, randomised controlled trial. *Lancet*, Vol. 372, pp. 392-397.

Gao C, Takezaki T, Wu J, et al. (2002). Interaction between *cytochrome-450 2E1* polymorphisms and environmental factors with risk of esophageal and stomach cancers in Chinese. *Cancer Epidemiol Biomarkers Prev*, Vol. 11, pp. 29-34.

Geddert H, Kiel S, Zotz RB, et al. (2005). Polymorphism of *p16INK4A* and *cyclic D1* in adenocarcinomas of the upper gastrointestinal tract. *J Cancer Res Clin Oncol*, Vol. 131, pp. 803-808.

Gonzalez CA, Sala N & Capella G. (2002). Genetic susceptibility and gastric cancer risk. *Int J Cancer*, Vol. 100, pp. 249-260.

Goto Y, Hamajima N, Honda H et al. (2005a). Association between *Helicobacter pylori* seropositivity and *NAD(P)H:quinone oxidoreductase 1* (*NQO1*) C609T polymorphism observed for outpatients and health checkup examinees. Gastric Cancer, Vol. 8, pp. 12-17.

Goto Y, Ando T, Goto H, et al. (2005b). No association between *EGF* gene polymorphism and gastric cancer. *Cancer Epidemiol Biomarkers Prev*, Vol. 14, pp. 2454-2456.

Goto Y, Ando T, Naito M, et al. (2006a). *Inducible nitric oxide synthase* polymorphism is associated with the increased risk of differentiated gastric cancer in a Japanese population. *World J. Gastroenterol*, Vol.12, pp. 6361-6365.

Goto Y, Ando T, Yamamoto K et al. (2006b). Association between serum pepsinogens and polymorphism of *PTPN11* encoding SHP-2 among Helicobacter pylori seropositive Japanese. *Int J Cancer*, Vol. 118, pp. 203-208.

Goto Y, Nishio K, Ishida Y et al. (2007). No association between *Helicobacter pylori* seropositivity and ornithine decarboxylase (ODC) A317G polymorphism, and no modification by *NAD(P)H:quinone oxidoreductase 1* (*NQO1*) C609T. Nagoya J Med Sci, Vol. 69, pp. 17-22.

Goto Y, Hishida A, Matsuo K, et al. (2010). *PRKCH* gene polymorphism is associated with the risk for severe gastric atrophy. Gastric Cancer, Vol. 13, pp.90-94.

Guo Y, Harris RB, Rosson D, et al. (2000). Functional analysis of human ornithine decarboxylase alleles. *Cancer Res*, Vol. 60, pp. 6314-6317.

Hamajima N, Naito M, Kondo T, et al. (2006). Genetic factors involved in the development of Helicobacter pylori-related gastric cancer. *Cancer Sci*, Vol 97, pp. 1129-1138.

Hamajima N, Matsuo K, Saito T et al. (2001a). *Interleukin 1* polymorphisms, lifestyle factors, and *Helicobacter pylori* infection. *Jpn J Cancer Res*, Vol. 92, pp. 383-389.

Hamajima N, Matsuo K, Suzuki T et al. (2001b). Low expression myeloperoxidase negatively associated with *Helicobacter pylori* infection. *Jpn J Cancer Res*, Vol. 92, pp. 488-493.

Hamajima N, Saito T, Matsuo K et al. (2002a). Genotype frequencies for 50 polymorphisms for 241 Japanese non-cancer patients. *J Epidemiol*, Vol. 12, pp. 229-236.

Hamajima N, Ito H, Matsuo K, et al. (2002b) *Helicobacter pylori* seropositivity, the interleukin 1B polymorphism, and smoking among first-visit outpatients. *Asian Pac J Cancer Prev*, Vol. 3, pp. 23-28.

Hamajima N, Shibata A, Ikehara Y et al. (2002c). Lack of consistency in the association of *Helicobacter pylori* seropositivity with Se and Le polymorphisms among Japanese. *Gastric Cancer*, Vol. 5, 194-200.

Hamajima N, Matsuo K, Iwata H, et al.(2002d). *NAD(P)H: quinone oxidoreductase 1* (*NQO1*) C609T polymorphism and the risk of eight cancers in Japan. *Int J Clin Oncol*, Vol. 7, pp. 103-8.

Hamajima N. (2003a). Persistent *Helicobacter pylori* infection and genetic polymorphisms of the host. *Nagoya J Med Sci*, Vol. 66, pp. 103-117.

Hamajima N, Shibata A, Katsuda N, et al. (2003b). The highest *Helicobacter pylori* seropositive rate among those with *TNF-A-857TT* and -1031*TT* genotypes. Gastric Cancer, Vol. 6, pp. 230-236.Hamilton SR, Aaltonen LA. (2000). *Pathology and Genetics. Tumours of the Digestive System. WHO Classification of Tumours.* IARC Press, Lyon.

Hamajima N, Katsuda N, Matsuo K et al. (2003c). High anti-*Helicobacter pylori* antibody seropositivity associated with the combination of *IL-8* -251*TT* and *IL-10* -819*TT* genotype. *Helicobacter*, Vol. 8, 105-110.

Helminen ME, Kilpinen S, Virta M,et al. (2001). Susceptibility to primary Epstein-Barr virus infection is associated with interleukin-10 gene promoter polymorphism. *J Infect Dis*, Vol. 184, pp. 777-780.

Higuchi T, Seki N, Kamizono S, et al. (1998). Polymorphism of the 5'-flanking region of the human *tumor necrosis factor (TNF)-alpha* gene in Japanese. *Tissue Antigens,* Vol. 51, pp. 605-612.

Hishida A, Matsuo K, Goto Y et al. (2009a). *Toll-like receptor 4* +3725 G/C polymorphism, *Helicobacter pylori* seropositivity, and the risk of gastric atrophy and gastric cancer in Japanese. *Helicobacter,* Vol. 14, 47-53.

Hishida A, Matsuo K, Goto Y, et al. (2009b). Associations of a *PTPN11* G/A polymorphism at intron 3 with *Helicobacter pylori* seropositivity, gastric atrophy and gastric cancer in Japanese. BMC Gastroenterol; Vol. 51.

Hishida A, Matsuo K, Goto Y, et al. (2009c). Significant association of *RUNX3* T/A polymorphism at intron 3 (rs760805) with the risk of gastric atrophy in *Helicobacter pylori* seropositive Japanese. J Gastroenterol, Vol. 44, pp. 1165-1171.

Hiyama T, Tanaka S, Kitadai Y, et al. (2002). *p53* codon 73 polymorphism in gastric cancer susceptibility in patients with Helicobacter pylori-assoicated chronic gastritis. *Int J Cancer,* Vol. 100, pp. 304-8.Hoffmann SC, Stanley EM, Darrin Cox E, et al. (2001). Association of cytokine polymorphic inheritance and in vitro cytokine production in anti-CD3/CD28-stimulated peripheral blood lymphocytes. *Transplantation,* Vol. 72, pp. 1444-1450.

Hoffmann SC, Stanley EM, Darrin Cox E, et al. (2002). Ethnicity greatly influences cytokine gene polymorphism distribution. *Am J Transplant*, Vol. 2, pp. 560-567.

Hold GL, Rabkin CS, Chow WH, et al. (2007). A Functional Polymorphism of *Toll-like Receptor 4* Gene Increases Risk of Gastric Carcinoma and Its Precursors. Gastroenterology, Vol. 132, pp. 905-912.

Hsu P, Lu P, Wang E, et al. (2008). Polymorphisms of death pathway genes *FAS* and *FASL* and risk of premalignant gastric lesions. Anticancer Res, Vol. 28, pp. 97-104.

Hubner RA, Muir KR, Liu F-F, et al. (2008). Ornithine decarboxylase G316A genotype is prognostic for colorectal adenoma recurrence and predicts efficacy of aspirin chemoprevention. Clin Cancer Res, Vol. 14, pp. 2303-2309.

Hull J, Ackerman H, Isles K et al. (2001). Unusual haplotypic structure of IL8, a susceptibility locus for a common respiratory virus. *Am J Hum Genet*, Vol. 69, pp. 413-419.

Hullkonen J, Laippata P, Hurme M, et al. (2000). A rare allele combination of the interleukin-1 gene complex is associated with high interleukin-1β plasma levels in healthy individuals. *Eur Cytokine Netw*, Vol. 11, pp. 251-255.

Ikehara Y, Nishihara S, Yasutomi H et al.(2001). Polymorphisms of two *fucosyltransferase* genes (Lewis and Secretor genes) involving type I Lewis antigens are associated with the presence of anti-*Helicobacter pylori* IgG antibody. Cancer Epidemiol Biomarkers Prev, Vol. 10, pp. 971-977.

Ito M, Takahashi H, Fuse K et al. (2000). Polymorphisms of *tumor necrosis factor-a* and *interleukin-10* genes in Japanese patients with idiopathic dilated cardiomyopathy. Jpn Heart J, Vol. 41, pp. 183-191.

Johannesen J, Pie A, PociotF et al. (2001). Linkage of the human inducible nitric oxide synthase gene to type 1 diabetes. *J Clin Endocrinol Metab,* Vol. 86, pp. 2792-2796.

Kamizono S, Hiromatsu Y, Seki N et al. (2000). A polymorphism of the 5′ flanking region of *tumour necrosis factor a* gene is associated with thyroid-associated ophthalmopathy in Japanese. *Clin Endocrinol,* Vol. 52, pp. 759-764.

Kara B, Akkiz H, Doran F, et al. (2010). The significance of E266K polymorphism in the *NOD1* gene on *Helicobacter Pylori* infection: an effective force on pathogenesis? Clin Exp Med, Vol. 10, pp. 107-12.

Kato I, Canzian F, Franceshi S, et al. (2006). Genetic polymorphism in anti-inflammatory cytokine signaling and the prevalence of gastric precancerous lesions in Venezuela. *Cancer Causes Control,* Vol. 17, pp. 1183-1191.

Kato S, Onda M, Yamada S, et al. (2001). Association of the *interleukin-1β* genetic polymorphism and gastric cancer risk in Japanese. *J Gastroenterol,* Vol. 36, pp. 696-699.

Katsuda N, Hamajima N, Tamakoshi A et al. (2003). Helicobacter pylori seropositivity and the Myeloperoxidase G-463A polymorphism in combination with interleukin-1B in Japanese health checkup examinees. *Jpn J Clin Oncol,* Vol. 33, pp. 192-197.

Kim JK, Kim S, Han HJ, et al. (2005). Polymorphisms of *5,10-methylenetetrahydrofolate reductase* and risk of stomach cancer in a Korean population. Anticancer Res, Vol. 25, pp. 2249-52.

Kim N, Cho S-I, Yim J-Y et al. (2006). The effects of genetic polymorphisms of *IL-1* and *TNF-A* on *Helicobacter pylori*-induced gastroduodenal diseases in Korea. *Helicobacter,* Vol. 11, pp. 105-112.

Knuefermann P, Nemoto S, Baumgarten G, et al. (2002). Cardiac inflammation and innate immunity in septic shock. Is there a role for Toll-like receptors? *Chest,* Vol. 121, pp. 1329-1336

Kunstmann E, Epplen C, Elitok E et al. (1999). *Helicobacter pylori* infection and polymorphisms in the *tumor necrosis factor* region. *Electrophoresis,* Vol. 20, pp. 1756-1761.

Lacasana-Navarro M, Galvan-Portillo M, Chen J, et al. (2006). *Methylenetetrahydrofolate reductase* 677C>T polymorphism and gastric cancer susceptibility in Mexico. *Eur J Cancer,* Vol. 42, pp. 528-33.

Lai K-C, Chen W-C, Jeng L-B, et al. (2005a). Association of genetic polymorphisms of *MK, IL-4, p16, p21, p53* genes and human gastric cancer in Taiwan. Eur J Surg Oncol, Vol. 31, pp. 1135-40.

Lai KC, Chen WC, Tsai FJ, et al. (2005b). *Glutathione S-trasferase M1* gene null genotype and gastric cancer risk in Taiwan. Hepatogastroenterology, Vol. 52, pp. 1916-1919.

Lee Y-A, Ki C-S, Kim H-J, et al. (2004). Novel *interleukin 1β* polymorphism increased the risk of gastric cancer in Korean population. J Gastroenterol, Vol. 39, pp. 429-433.

Levanon D, Brenner O, Otto F, et al. (2003). Runx3 knockouts and stomach cancer. *EMBO Rep,* Vol. 4, pp. 560–564.

Li H, Chen X-L & Li H-Q. (2005). Polymorphism of *CYPIA1* and *GSTM1* genes associated with susceptibility of gastric cancer in Shandong province of China. *World J Gastroenterol,* Vol. 11; 5757-5762.

Liou J-M, Lin J-T, Wang H-P, et al. (2007). *IL-1B* -511 polymorphism is associated with increased host susceptibility to *Helicobacter pylori* infection in Chinese. *Helicobacter,* Vol. 12, pp. 142-149.

Maeda S, Akanuma M, Mitsuno Y, et al. (2001). Distinct Mechanism of *Helicobacter pylori*-mediated NF-kB Activation between Gastric Cancer Cells and Monocytic Cells. *J Biol Chem,* Vol. 48, pp. 44856-44864.

Naito M, Eguchi H, Goto Y et al. (2010). Association between circulating IL-8 levels, *IL-8* T-251A genotypes and *Helicobacter pylori* infection. Epidemiol Infect, Vol. 138, pp 512-518.

Nakabeppu Y, Tsuchimoto D, Ichinoe A, et al. (2004). Biological significance of the defense mechanisms against oxidative damage in nucleic acids caused by reactive oxygen species: from mitochondria to nuclei. *Ann NY Acad Sci,* Vol. 1011, pp. 101-111.

Nakashima H, Miyake K, Inoue Y et al. (2002). Association between *IL-4* genotype and *IL-4* production in the Japanese population. *Genes Immun,* Vol. 3, pp. 107-109.

Narimatsu H, Iwasaki H, Nakayama F et al. (1998). Lewis and secretor gene dosages affect CA19-9 and DU-PAN-2 serum levels in normal individuals and colorectal cancer patients. *Cancer Res,* Vol. 58, pp. 512-518.

Nauseef WM, Brigham S & Cogley M. (1994). Hereditary myeloperoxidase deficiency due to a missense mutation of arginine 569 to tryptophan. *J Biol Chem,* Vol. 269, pp. 1212-1216.

Neel BG, Gu H & Pao L. (2003). The 'Shp'ing news: SH2 domain-containing tyrosine phosphatases in cell signaling. *Trends Biochem Sci,* Vol. 28, pp. 284-293.

Opal SM & DePalo VA. (2000). Anti-inflammatory cytokines. *Chest,* 117: 1162-1172.

Oshimo Y, Oue N, Mitani Y, et al. (2004). Frequent loss of RUNX3 expression by promoter hypermethylation in gastric carcinoma. *Pathobiology,* Vol. 71, pp. 137-143.

Parkin DM, Whelan SL, Ferlay J, Raymond L, Young J. (1997). *Cancer Incidence in Five Continents* (Volume VII), IARC Press, Lyon.

Parkin DM, Pisani P, Ferlay J. (1999). Estimates of the worldwide incidence of 25 major cancers in 1990. *Int J Cancer,* Vol. 80: pp.827–841.

Pham TN, Rahman P, Tobin YM, et al. (2003a). Elevated serum nitric oxide levels in patients with inflammatory arthritis associated with co-expression of inducible nitric oxide synthase and protein kinase C-eta in peripheral blood monocyte-derived macrophages. J Rheumatol, Vol. 30, pp. 2529-2534.

Pham TN, Brown BL, Dobson PR, et al. (2003b). Protein kinase C-eta (PKC-eta) is required for the development of inducible nitric oxide synthase (iNOS) positive phenotype in human monocytic cells. *Nitric Oxide,* Vol. 9, pp. 123-134.

Piedrafita FJ, Molander RB, Vansant G, et al. (1996).An Alu element in the myeloperoxidase promoter contains a composite SP1-thyroid hormone-retinoic acid response element. *J Biol Chem,* Vol. 271, pp. 14412-14420.

Queiroz DMM, Saraiva IEB, Rocha GA, et al. (2009). *IL-2* -330G polymorphism allele is associated with decreased risk of *Helicobacter pylori* infection in adulthood. *Microbes Infect,* Vol.11, pp. 980-987.

Read RC, Pullin J, Gregory S et al. (2001). A functional polymorphism of *toll-like receptor 4* is not associated with likelihood of severity of meningococcal disease. J Infect Dis, Vol. 184, pp. 640-642.

Renzoni E, Lympany P, Sestini P et al. (2000). Distribution of novel polymorphisms of the interleukin-8 and CXC receptor 1 and 2 genes in systemic sclerosis and cryptogenic fibrosing alveolitis. *Arthritis Rheum,* Vol. 43, pp. 1633-1640.

Ross D, Kepa JK, Winski SL, et al. (2000). NAD(P)H:quinone oxidoreductase 1 (NQO1): chemoprotection, bioactivation, gene regulation and genetic polymorphisms. Chem Biol Interact, Vol. 129, pp. 77-97.

Sadaat I, Higashi H, Obuse C, et al. (2007). *Helicobacter pylori* CagA targets PAR1/MARK kinase to disrupt epithelial cell polarity. Nature, Vol. 447, pp. 330-333.

Samloff IM. (1982). Pepsinogen I and II: purification from gastric mucosa and radioimmunoassay in serum. Gastroenterology, Vol. 82, pp. 26-33.

Savage SA, Abnet CC, Haque K, et al. (2004). Polymorphisms in *interleukin -2, -6,* and *-10* are not associated with gastric cardia or esophageal cancer in a high-risk Chinese population. *Cancer Epidemiol Biomarkers Prev,* Vol. 13, pp. 1547-1549.

Siegel D, McGuinness SM, Winski SL, et al (1999). Genotype-phenotype relationships in studies of a polymorphism in *NAD(P)H:quinone oxidoreductase 1.* Pharmacogenetics, Vol. 9, pp. 113-121.

Shinohara Y, Iwasaki H, Ota N, et al. (2001). Novel single nucleotide polymorphisms of the human nuclear factor kappa-B 2 gene identified by sequencing the entire gene. *J Hum Genet,* 46, 50-51.

Shiotani A, Kamada T, Yamanaka Y, et al. (2008). Sonic hedgehog and CDX2 expression in the stomach. J *Gastroenterol Hepatol,* Vol. 23 (Suppl 2), pp. S161-166.

Sugimoto M, Furuta T, Shirai N, et al. (2005). Poor metabolizer genotype status of *CYP2C19* is a risk factor for developing gastric cancer in Japanese patients with *Helicobacter pylori* infection. *Aliment Pharmacol Ther,* Vol. 22, pp. 1033-1040.

Sun LP, Guo XL, Zhang Y, et al. (2009). Impact of *pepsinogen C* polymorphism on individual susceptibility to gastric cancer and its precancerous conditions in a Northeast Chinese population. *J Cancer Res Clin Oncol,* Vol. 135, pp. 1033-1039.

Taguchi A, Ohmiya N, Shirai K, et al.(2005). Interleukin-8 promoter polymorphism increases the risk of atrophic gastritis and gastric cancer in Japan. *Cancer Epidemiol Biomarkers Prev,* Vol.14, pp. 2487-93.

Tahara T, Arisawa T, Wang F et al. (2007a). *Toll-like receptor 2* -196 to 174del polymorphism influences the susceptibility of Japanese people to gastric cancer. Cancer Sci, Vol. 98, pp. 1790-1794.

Tahara T, Arisawa T, Shibata T, et al. (2007b). Absence of common polymorphisms of *Toll like receptor 4* (*TLR4*):Asp299Gly, Thr399Ile in patientas with gastrointestinal diseases in Japan. J Clin Biochem Nutr, Vol. 40, pp. 62-65.

Tahara T, Arisawa T, Shibata T, et al. (2007c). Association of polymorphism of *TLR4* and *CD14* genes with gastroduodenal diseases in Japan. Inflammopharmacology 2007; 15: 124-128.

Tahara T, Shibata T, Arisawa T, et al. (2009). The *BB* genotype of heat-shock protein (HSP) 70-2 gene is associated with gastric pre-malignant condition in *H. pylori*-infected older patients. Anticancer Res, Vol. 29, pp. 3453-3458.

Takaishi S & Wang TC. (2007). Providing AID to p53 mutagenesis. *Nat Med,* Vol. 13, pp. 404-406.

Tartaglia M, Niemeyer CM, Shannon KM, et al. (2004). SHP-2 and myeloid malignancies. *Curr Opin Hematol,* 11: 44-50.

Togawa S, Joh T, Itoh M et al. (2005). Interleukin-2 gene polymorphisms associated with increased risk of gastric atrophy from *Helicobacter pylori* infection. *Helicobacter,* Vol. 10, pp. 172-178.

Tsuji S, Tsujii M, Murata H, et al. (2006). *Helicobacter pylori* eradication to prevent gastric cancer: Underlying molecular and cellular mechanisms. *World J Gastroenterol,* Vol. 12, pp.1671-1680.

Tsukino H, Kuroda Y, Qio D, et al. (2002). Effects of *cytochrome p450* (*CYP*) *2A6* gene deletion and *CYP2E1* genotypes on gastric adenocarcinoma. *Int J Cancer,* Vol. 100, pp. 425-428.

Turner DM, Williams DM, Sankaran D, et al. (1997). An investigation of polymorphism in the *interleukin-10* gene promoter. Eur J Immunogenet, Vol. 24, pp. 1-8.

Uemura N, Okamoto S, Yamamoto S, et al. (2001). *Helicobacter pylori* infection and the development of gastric cancer. N Engl J Med 2001; 345: 784-789.

Uno M, Hamajima N, Ito LS, et al. (2002). *Helicobacter pylori* seropositivity and IL-1B C-31T polymorphism among Japanese Brazilians. *Int J Mol Med,* Vol. 10, pp. 321-326.

Viala J, Chaput C, Boneca IG, et al. (2004). Nod1 responds to peptidoglycan delivered by the *Helicobacter pylori cag* pathogenicity island. *Nat Immunol,* Vol. 5, pp. 1166-1174.

Wambura C, Aoyama N, Shirasaka D, et al. (2002). Effect of *Helicobacter pylori*-induced cyclooxygenase-2 on gastric epithelial cell kinetics: implication for gastric carcinogenesis. Helicobacter, Vol. 7, pp. 129-138.

Wang M, Furuta T, Takashima M et al. (1999). Relation between interleukin-1 beta messanger RNA in gastric fundic mucosa and gastric juice pH in patients with infected with *Helicobacter pylori*. *J Gastroenterol,* Vol. 34, Suppl 11, pp. 10-17.

Williams TM, Eisenberg L, Burlein JE, et al. (1988). Two regions within the human *IL-2* gene promoter are important for inducible IL-2 expression. *J Immunol,* Vol. 141, pp. 662-666.

Wong BC, Lam SK, Wong WM, et al. (2004). *Helicobacter pylori* eradication to prevent gastric cancer in a high-risk region of China: a randomized controlled trial. *JAMA,* Vol. 291, pp. 187-194.

Wu M-S, Huang S-P, Chang Y-T, et al. (2002). Associaition of the -160 C > A promoter polymorphism of *E-cadherin* gene with gastric carcinoma risk. Cancer, Vol. 94, pp. 1443-1448.

Yamaguchi E, Itoh A, Hizawa N (2001). The gene polymorphism of *tumor necrosis factor-β*, but not that of tumor necrosis factor-α, is associated with the prognosis of sarcoidosis. *Chest,* Vol. 119, pp. 753-761.

Yeo M, Park HK, Kim DK, et al. (2004). Restoration of heat-shock protein70 suppresses gastric mucosal inducible nitric oxide synthase expression induced by *Helicobacter pylori*. *Proteomics,* Vol. 4, pp. 3335-3342.

Zambon C-F, Basso D, Navaglia F et al. (2005). Pro- and anti-inflammatory cytokines gene polymorphisms and *Helicobacter pylori* infection: interactions influence outcome. *Cytokine,* Vol. 29, pp. 141-152.

13

A Double-Edged Sword: Roles of Helicobacter Pylori in Gastric Carcinoma

Li-Jun Xue [1], Quan-Sheng Su[1], Xiao-Bei Mao[1], Qing Lin[1], Xiao-Bei Liu[1], Chang Liu[2], Yong Lin[1], Ji-Hong Yang[1], Hong-Ju Yu[1] and Xiao-Yuan Chu[1]
[1]Departments of Oncology and
[2]Gastroenterology, Jinling Hospital, Nanjing University School of Medicine, 305 East Zhong-shan Road, Nanjing, Jiangsu Province, China

1. Introduction

Gastric carcinoma (GC) remains one of the most malignant tumors either in morbidity or mortality rates around the world (IARC, 2002). Development of GC is influenced by multiple factors including genetic, biological, social, and psychological ones, etc.., however, the function mechanisms of which are too sophisticated and still under explorations (Matysiak-Budnik & Mégraud, 2006). Similar to other malignant tumors, GC leads to death mainly due to system or organ failure because of cancer advancement and metastasis. Chemotherapy-based regimens combined with radiological and immunomodulating therapies are fundamental but unsatisfactory because most GC patients are in advanced stage when diagnosed, although radical operation throws those at early stage a light of prolonged survival and even clinical cure (Quiros & Bui, 2009). As for prophylaxis, many reports have mentioned the protective role of eradication of *Helicobacter pylori*, which has been identified as a definite carcinogen for GC, but few evidences proved a successful *H. pylori* vaccine showing effects on GC prevention, just as Hepatitis B virus vaccine on prevention of primary hepatocellular carcinoma (IARC, 1994; Murakami et al., 2005; Cai et al., 2005; Di Bisceglie 2009).

H. pylori, a stomach colonizing spiral gram-negative bacterium, interacts with the host in a multiplicity of ways during its adhesion, colonization, invasion, and induction of inflammatory and immune responses (Peek 2005). The great majority of researchers link *H. pylori* infection with development or even recurrence of GC according to some clinical trials, meta-analyses, and *in vitro* experiments (Wong et al., 2004; Fukase et al., 2008). However, a few recent studies have disclosed the other side of the coin, in which positive *H. pylori* status appears to be associated with better outlook in GC patients (Meimarakis et al., 2006; Marrelli et al., 2009). Therefore, *H. pylori* probably factually play a bi-directional role in GC just like a double-edged sword. To learn about both edges of *H. pylori* infection will provides us with new sights in vaccine design, prevention, and even therapy of GC.

Herein, we try to re-elucidate the relationship between *H. pylori* and GC from novel angles, in which GC consists of *H. pylori*-related (Hp-GC) and non-*H. pylori*-related (nHp-GC) ones, and in which roles of the infection are divided into two parts including harmful and beneficial ones.

2. H. pylori virulence factors

H. pylori infection usually initiates from bacterial invasion, colonization, and expression and translocation of virulence factors, and persists through induction and maintenance of complex responses at certain levels in the host (Peek 2005). Herein, virulence factors extensively mean pathogenic components and contain those contributing to bacterial survival within the host, which are ever called as maintenance factors sometimes. According to the complete genome published and continuously updated since 1997, *H. pylori* (26695 strain) is of about 1.67 Mb in length with 1576 protein-coding genes, many of which encode virulent products associated with *H. pylori* pathogenesis (Tomb et al., 1997).

The cytotoxin-associated gene (cag) pathogenicity island (PAI), one of most well known virulence components, is of about 35 Kb with 26 open reading frames and is present in about 60% *H. pylori* strains in Europe and United States (Tomb et al., 1997; Peek 2005). Among all Cag PAI products, the CagA (Cag26) has been identified with relatively clear functions in development of GC (Huang et al., 2003). The involved carcinogenic mechanisms of CagA mainly include activation of certain signalling pathways such as Ras, SHP2, ERK, MAPK and JAK/STAT3, activation of C-terminal Src kinase and inhibition of Src activity, enhancement of epithelial gene transcription, disruption of cellular polarity, and morphological changes and final transformation of gastric epithelial cells (GECs) (Mimuro et al., 2002; Higashi et al., 2002; Selbach et al., 2002; Bagnoli et al., 2005; Lee et al., 2010).

Vacuolating toxin (vacA) of about 3.9 Kb is an independent key virulence determinant for *H. pylori* pathogenesis (Tomb et al., 1997). Around 60% of *H. pylori* strains produce detectable amounts of VacA *in vitro*, although this gene is present in all strains (Konturek et al., 2009). Cytotoxic activity of VacA varys considerably in different strains due to various gene subtypes based on sequence diversities in the N-terminal (allele types s1a, s1b, s1c, or s2) and middle regions (allele types m1 or m2) (Atherton et al., 1995; Peek 2005). It has been demonstrated that infection with vacA s1 and m1 strains are associated with an increased risk of GC (Gerhard et al., 1999). VacA plays a role in carcinogenesis probably through inducing vacuolation and cellular detachment, permeabilizing epithelial cells, promoting apoptosis, and suppressing T-cell proliferation and activation (Peek 2005).

Outer membrane proteins (OMP) represent a large family of adhesins and participate in *H. pylori* infection mainly by mediating bacterial adherence and colonization in gastric mucosa (Odenbreit 2005). As one of OMP members, blood-group antigen-binding adhesin (BabA) can bind the blood-group antigen Lewis b on host epithelial cell membranes, and those strains possessing the encoding gene babA2 are associated with high risk of GC (Oliveira et al., 2003; Konturek et al., 2009). Lipopolysaccharide (LPS), another cell wall component, can disrupt stomach mucosa and involve in the organism survival and persistence of *H. pylori* infection (Grebowska et al., 2008). Moreover, the LPS O-antigen mimics human Lewisx and Lewisy blood-group antigens, which also mediate bacterial adhesion and colonization and alternatively cause immune cross-reactivity (Moran 1996; Appelmelk et al., 2001).

There are still many other important virulence factors related with *H. pylori* infection and even carcinogenesis. Urease, an approximately 560-kDa hexameric enzyme consisting of 30-kDa UreA and 64-kDa UreB subunits, is produced abundantly by all *H. pylori* isolates (Turbett et al., 1992). Urease is independently essential for colonization and persistent survival of the germ because it crucially contributes to local pH homeostasis within the stomach lumen (Stingl et al., 2002; Mollenhauer-Rektorschek et al., 2002). The induced by contact with epithelium factor Antigen (IceA), with two major allelic sequence variants of IceA1 and IceA2, is an independent strain-specific *H. pylori* locus significantly associated with distal GC (Kidd et al., 2001). IceA1 leads to relatively severer gastric inflammation and tissue damage following production induced by bacterial contact with GECs, which exists in 72% of the *H. pylori* isolates in a Chinese population (Sheu et al., 2002). Flagella are bacterial motile structures with two types of filaments, that are encoded by flaA and flaB genes and functionaly regulated by flgE and flbA genes (Dunn et al., 1997). Normal expression and interaction of these virulence factors are required for bacterial motility or colonization during *H. pylori* infection.

Notably, *H. pylori* plays pathogenic or carcinogenic roles as an integrity, although its multiple virulence components have their own special contributions at various infection stages. The co-interactions among the virulence factors are likewise important for pathogenesis but may be so complex or always ignored and need further explorations. In addition, cross-interactions between *H. pylori* and the host are very vital for infection or carcinogenesis, which mainly contain inflammatory and immune responses, and genetic or phenotypic alterations (McNamara & El-Omar, 2008).

3. Inflammatory responses

H. pylori infection is firstly characterized by acute or chronic activation of inflammatory cells and release of multiple cytokines including pro-inflammatory and inflammatory ones (Peek 2005). The spectrum and relative levels of cytokines, to a certain extent, reflect the intensity of the host response to infection, which may result in different outcomes including gastric mucosal inflammation, injury, ulcer, and even cancer.

Cytokines such as tumor necrosis factor α (TNF-α), interleukin-1β (IL-1β) / IL-1 receptor antagonist (IL-1RN), IL-6, IL-8 and IL-10 are always significantly up-regulated in stomach mucosa, gastric fluids and the sera of *H. pylori*-infected patients and play vital functions in gastritis, metaplasia, dysplasia and carcinogenesis (McNamara & El-Omar, 2008). TNF-α and IL-1 are the most relevant factors consistently confirmed in animal models and various populations. TNF-α can markedly potentiate apoptosis, activate signalling pathways, influence mucosal inflammation and stimulate gastric acid secretion (Ierardi et al., 2003). Moreover, *H. pylori* causes sensitization of GECs for TNF-related apoptosis-inducing ligand (TRAIL)-mediated apoptosis, besides direct induction of apoptosis and inhibition of DNA synthesis (Tsai & Hsu, 2010). The *H. pylori* infection strengthens IL-1 functions in the carcinogenic process through complex pathways. IL-1β and IL-1RN as key pro-inflammatory genotypes of IL-1, which is a powerful gastric acid suppressor, can increase the risk of atrophic gastritis (AG) and both intestinal and diffuse types of non-cardia GC (Starzyńska et al., 2006; Rad et al., 2004). IL-1β with significantly higher level in neoplasm than in normal mucosa, involves in the carcinogenesis by stimulating hyper-proliferation in GECs via tyrosine kinase signalling (Beales 2002). *H. pylori*-induced gastritis is possibly driven in an IL-6-dependent fashion (Jackson et al., 2006). IL-6 participates in activation of the STAT3 signalling pathway by the translocated CagA in host cells, which may play a role in gastric carcinogenesis (Bronte-Tinkew et al., 2009). IL-6 level in the serum is related with GC status and its level in the tumor correlates significantly with lymphatic invasion and the depth of invasion (Kai et al., 2005). As for IL-8, its level in cancer tissues is more than double fold in advanced GC than that in early GC irrespective of *H. pylori* status (Yamaoka et al., 2001). IL-8 modulates gastric acid secretion, promotes the proliferation, enhances the FasL-induced apoptosis, and mutually and dependently activates NF-κB (Konturek et al., 2002; Varro et al., 2004; Guo et al., 2006). Moreover, IL-8 as a potent leukocyte chemoattractant, contributes to mucosal tissue injury and induces the upregulation and phosphorylation of EGFR and subsequent signalling events, which plays an fundamental role in carcinogenic mechanisms (Kassai et al., 1999; Beswick & Reyes, 2008). IL-10 inhibits the FasL-induced apoptosis in GECs though without significant effect on the transcription of Fas (Guo et al., 2006). IL-11 activates the STAT3 like IL-6 and concomitantly increases proliferation of GECs (Jackson et al., 2007).

Some other molecules including cyclooxygenase-2 (COX-2), prostaglandin E2 (PGE2), nitric oxide (NO), inducible NO synthase (iNOS), monocyte chemoattractant protein 1 (MCP1), and hepatocyte growth factor (HGF) and c-MET also relate to GC-associated inflammatory responses (Zhuang X et al., 2001; Futagami et al., 2008; Snider & Cardelli, 2009; Cho et al., 2010). COX-2 as a key mediator in inflammation and cancer formation, together with PGE2, one of its major products, are remarkably up-regulated in *H. pylori*-related gastritis, GC, and precancerous lesions including atrophy, intestinal metaplasia (IM) and dysplasia of the stomach (Dong et al., 2009; Walduck et al., 2009; Zhang et al., 2009). COX-2 can be induced by gastrin, growth factors, inflammatory cytokines and reactive oxygen species in GECs (Seo et al., 2007). The overexpression of COX-2 may continue to exist in metaplastic or dysplastic mucosa even after successful *H. pylori* eradication, which increases the risk for carcinogenesis and indicates that COX-2 has a crucial role in not only Hp-GC but also nHp-GC (Tsuji et al., 2006). COX-2 overexpression is even thought as a biomarker of intestinal type and earlier stage of GC and an independent prognostic factor for worse survival (Park et al., 2009). COX-2 induces carcinogenesis mainly by inhibiting apoptosis, increasing proliferation and enhancing angiogenesis through multiple pathways including Wnt signalling, p38MAPK / ATF-2 pathway, TLR2 / TLR9 and c-Src-dependent NF-κB activation, MMP-9 and VEGF activation, proteinase-activated receptor-2 signalling, PPARγ inhibition, and so on (Leung et al., 2003; Chang et al., 2004 & 2005; Huang et al., 2006; Li et al., 2009; Zhang et al., 2009;). PGE2, a downstream mediator with central roles in the mentioned COX-2 pathways, plays important functions in both inflammation and carcinogenesis. PGE2 participates in IL-8 production in GECs, facilitates *H. pylori* colonization and persistent infection, and suppresses the immune functions of CD4 (+) T-helper 1 cells by silencing IL-2 gene transcription, which may help accelerate the tumor formation (Takehara et al., 2006; Toller et al., 2010).

During chronic *H. pylori* infection, there are still excessive amounts of reactive oxygen and nitrogen species containing NO and iNOS, which play crucial roles in the stepwise process of GC (Son et al., 2001; Tiwari et al., 2010). NO as an important endogenous carcinogenic factor, correlates with gastric hypoacidity, inhibits p53 expression, increases genetic and epigenetic changes by mediating mutation or DNA methylation, and perturbs the balance between apoptosis and proliferation in GECs (McGee & Mobley, 2000; Lamarque et al., 2003; Shiotani et al., 2004; Chen et al., 2006; Katayama et al., 2009;). Being one of independent prognostic factors, the iNOS overexpression is induced by *H. pylori* infection with involvements of TNF-α, Ras, AP-1, c-Fos and c-Jun, and related to apoptosis, angiogenesis, tumor progression, and poor survival in GC especially of the intestinal type (Tatemichi et al., 1998; Rieder et al., 2003; Chen et al., 2006; Cho et al., 2010). MCP-1 is significantly higher at mRNA level in poorly differentiated GC, which has effect on COX-2 expression and subsequent PGE2 and VEGF production (Futagami et al., 2008). HGF is more frequently detected in GC tissue than in normal mucosa and shows a concentration-dependent increase under the stimulation of gastrin (Konturek et al., 2001 & 2003). Being the receptor of HGF, c-Met is activated by *H. pylori*, involved in malignant transformation of gastric mucosa and invasive growth of tumor cells, and strongly implicated in late-stage cancer progression and worse prognosis (Zhuang X et al., 2001; Churin et al., 2003; Snider & Cardelli, 2009). In addition, *H. pylori*-mediated GEC invasion depends on c-Met activation, besides on increased activities of MMP-2 and MMP-9 (Oliveira et al., 2006). The c-Met interacts with CagA and suppresses the phosphatidylinositol 3-kinase/Akt pathway, which then leads to β-catenin activation and NF-κB signalling (Suzuki et al., 2009).

4. Immune responses

Another critical aspect of interactions between *H. pylori* and the host are immune responses, which consist of special and unspecialized ones. In fact, immune and inflammatory responses overlap each other especially in roles of many cytokines mentioned above during the infection and carcinogenesis. Herein we mainly focus on important alterations in antibody responses, status of immune cells, balance of cytokines, autoimmune reactions and immune tolerance.

4.1 Antibody responses

A significantly higher seroprevalence has been found in *H. pylori*-infected patients with gastritis, duodenal ulcer, or GC (Przyklenk et al., 1990). Some scientists have concluded that higher *H. pylori* seroprevalence is present in GC patients at early stages of tumor development compared those at advanced stages, whereas others have not (Lin et al., 1993; Klaamas et al., 1996; Komoto et al., 1998). Seropositivity of anti-*H. pylori* IgG is highly prevalent with 76% at 0-4 years and 99% by > or = 18 years of age in a rural population of Africa, where the immunological response is Th2-dominant, which may partly explain the lower risk of Hp-GC (Mbulaiteye et al., 2006). The immune serum-treated *H. pylori* cannot be eliminated *in vitro* by primary human macrophages, although serum enhances the bacteria uptake (Keep et al., 2010). Antibodies are not only dispensable for protection, but they impair both the elimination of bacteria and the development of gastritis. This effect appears to be IgA-dependent and is not a function of specific IgM or IgG antibodies (Akhiani 2005).
The major antibodies responsive to *H. pylori* include IgA and IgG. GC patients elicit different anti-*H. pylori* IgG and IgA responses than the patients with atrophic and superficial gastritis (Manojlovic et al., 2008). IgA>IgG ratio and lower IgG is significantly more frequent in patients with GC and gastric lymphoma than those with gastritis and duodenal ulcer. Correspondingly, higher IgG and IgA levels are often observed in patients with duodenal ulcer or non-atrophic gastritis (Manojlovic et al., 2004 & 2008). As for subclass of IgG response, the IgG1 is lower in GC and AG patients than in gastritis ones; IgG2 is lower for patients with GC localized in the corpus. The IgG1 response in GC patients is correlated with *H. pylori* CagA status (Vorobjova et al., 2006). CagA-positive *H. pylori* strains also seem to markedly frequently induce an IgA response than CagA-negative strains. The presence of serum IgA antibodies likely indicates more severe late outcome of *H. pylori* infection (Rautelin et al., 2000). Anti-CagA antibodies are always higher in GC and AG compared with non-atrophic gastritis. As reported, Hp-GC patients are of 2-3 folds higher in CagA

seropositivity than age-matched *H. pylori*-positive non-GC controls. In addition, anti-CagA antibodies are significantly more prevalent among individuals with elevated titres of *H. pylori*-related IgA than in those only with IgG, with the exception of a small subgroup who later develop GC (Rautelin et al., 2000).

Heat shock protein (HSP) 60 may be associated with *H. pylori*-related gastritis and gastric carcinogenesis. The positivity rate for anti-HSP60 antibody is markedly higher not only in *H. pylori*-positive patients than in *H. pylori*-negative ones, but also in GC patients, especially of the diffuse type, than in *H. pylori*-positive non-GC patients (Tanaka et al., 2009). The isocitrate dehydrogenase (ICD) of *H. pylori*, as an antigen interacting with the host immune system subsequent to a possible autolytic release, significantly elicits humoral immune response and reveals high serum antibody titers in patients with gastritis and ulcer (Hussain et al., 2008). In addition, the *H. pylori*-induced inflammation leads to aberrant glycosylation and demasking of core peptide epitope of mucin 1 (MUC1), which could enhance the host immune responses (Klaamas et al., 2007). IgG immune response to tumor-associated MUC1 is up-regulated among *H. pylori*-infected individuals and related with a higher degree of inflammation in gastric mucosa. The level of anti-MUC1 IgG is positively correlated with that of anti-*H. pylori* IgG in both blood donors and patients with benign diseases, whereas the anti-MUC1 IgM level is not (Klaamas et al., 2007). Moreover, the anti-MUC1 IgG level is notablely higher in GC patients than in blood donors, irrespective of *H. pylori* status or cancer stage. In some individuals, the *H. pylori* infection may stimulate specific response to tumor-associated MUC1 peptide thus modulating tumor immunity (Klaamas et al., 2007).

4.2 Status of immune cells

The infiltration of T, B and macrophage cells always increases at the gastric site of infection with *H. pylori*. The status of T cells and macrophage are closely associated with local and system protective immune responses including native and acquired ones, whereas B cells mainly play more roles in antibody responses and deregulated and exhaustive *H. pylori*-induced T cell-dependent B-cell activation even supports the onset of stomach B-cell lymphoma (D'Elios et al., 2005).

The tumor-infiltrating lymphocytes (TIL) from primary tumors have been isolated and analyzed to characterize the anti-tumor immune responses in GC patients (van den Engel et al., 2006). The CD3 (+) T cell population contains 50% CD4 (+) and 39% CD8 (+) cells. The number of CD19 (+) B cells significantly increases but that of CD3 (+) T cells significantly decreases in intestinal compared to diffuse type of GC. Most of T cell cultures derived from isolated TILs in Hp-GC patients secrete both IFN-γ and IL-5 when stimulated with autologous tumor cells (van den Engel et al., 2006).

There is a significant tendency of Th1/Th2 polarization in patients with *H. pylori* infection, especially of those with CagA positive strains (Wang et al., 2007). Protection against *H. pylori* infection including inhibition of *bacterial* colonization, is mainly mediated by CD4 (+) Th1 cell -mediated immunity (Inoue et al., 2009). Th1-mediated cellular immunity is associated with earlier stages of GC, while Th2-mediated humoral immunity dominates the advanced stages and is negatively associated with an abundance of regulatory T-cells (Treg) (Wang et al., 2007).

Treg cells of positive CD4, CD25 and Foxp3, suppress the host immune response to *H. pylori* infection and have been identified as the major regulatory factor of adaptive immune responses (Kandulski et al., 2010). Vaccine-induced protection against *H. pylori* correlates with an augmented local recall response in the gastric mucosa, reduced amount of Treg, and increased proportions of neutrophils and CD4 (+) T cells (Becher et al., 2010). The CD4 (+) T cells isolated from stomachs of vaccinated mice can proliferate *in vitro* in response to *H. pylori* antigen, and secrete Th1 cytokines, particularly IFN-γ. The efficiency of these vaccines relates to the alteration of gastric immune responses, from a homogeneous Th1 response to a mixed Th1 and Th2 response (Ernst et al., 2001). The functions of Treg cells are either mediated by direct cell-cell contact or by secretions of the immune-modulating TGF-β1 and IL-10 cytokines (Kandulski et al., 2010). Treg is involved in bacterial persistence, increased in *H. pylori*-associated gastritis, and even positively related with the grade of chronic inflammation and the number of lymphoid follicles (Jang 2010). Treg is also markedly elevated in patients with GC compared to those with chronic gastritis and gastric dysplasia. Additionally, *H. pylori* may direct immunosuppression of T cells and regulate the host immune responses through activation of Treg and dendritic cells (Blanchard et al., 2004).

Macrophages are essential components of innate immunity, and their apoptosis will impair the host mucosal defense to microbes (Asim et al., 2010). *H. pylori* infection leads to a rapid infiltration of macrophages into the mouse stomach. *H. pylori* also activates TLR-2 and TLR-4 in macrophages, and subsequently induces the secretion of distinct cytokines including IL-2, IL-6 and IFN-α (Obonyo et al., 2007). However, the bacteria remain viable when internalized by GECs or even macrophages, which indicates the killing defects in the host due to inhibition of the phagosome maturation (Keep et al., 2010). In addition, *H. pylori* induces the formation of a specific phospho-c-Fos c-Jun activator protein-1 (AP-1) complex in gastric macrophages by an ERK-dependent way, that causes apoptosis and contributes to immune escape of the germ (Asim et al., 2010).

Several *H. pylori* proteins can impair macrophage and T cell functions *in vitro* through unclear mechanisms (Zabaleta et al., 2004). VacA, known as a toxic protein with vacuolating activity, can induce apoptosis in GECs, affect antigen presentation by B lymphocytes, inhibit T cell activation and proliferation, and modulate the T cell-mediated cytokine responses, which mainly target the adapted immune system (Gebert et al., 2004). CagA is also capable of preventing hydroxyurea-induced B-cell apoptosis by reducing p53 accumulation (Umehara et al., 2003). The arginase may impair T cell functions through inhibiting proliferation and the TCR zeta-chain (CD3zeta) expression, besides its role in urea production (Zabaleta et al., 2004).

4.3 Network of cytokines

H. pylori-stimulated host inflammatory and immune responses lead to release of a large amount of cytokines, which contribute to the loss of balance between cell proliferation and apoptosis prior to many gastric lesions including AG and GC. There is a shift from Th1 (IFN-γ, TNF-α and IL-12) towards Th2 (IL-4, IL-10 and IL-6)-type immune response in patients with GC and dysplasia (Marotti et al., 2008). IL-13 is recently described as a central mediator of Th2-dominant immune response and may be implicated in different outcomes of *H. pylori* infection (Marotti et al., 2008). TGF-β and IL-10 are two vital anti-inflammatory cytokines that regulate mucosal immunity in various infectious diseases (Wu et al., 2007). The local and systemic T-cell response in Hp-GC patients is mainly characterized by production of IL-10 (Lundin et al., 2007). When stimulated with *H. pylori* antigens, T cells from both peripheral blood and gastric mucosa produce significantly higher amounts of IL-10 in Hp-GC patients than in *H. pylori*-infected asymptomatic subjects. In addition, the frequency of activated CD8 (+) T cells is markedly reduced in stomach mucosa of GC patients compared to asymptomatic individuals (Lundin et al., 2007). Therefore, the increased production of the suppressive cytokine IL-10 in Hp-GC patients may lead to a diminished local cytotoxic anti-tumor T-cell response and even contributes to cancer progression.

A predominant *H. pylori*-specific Th1 response associates with peptic ulcer, whereas combined secretion of both Th1 and Th2 cytokines are present in simple gastritis (D'Elios et al., 2005). In *H. pylori*-infected mice, the local Th1-type response might alter the systemic Th1/Th2-type cytokine balance under particular physiopathological conditions of active tissue and/or vascular formation, such as pregnancy (Rossi et al., 2004). *H. pylori* neutrophil-activating protein is able to recruit leukocytes and stimulate neutrophils or monocytes to release IL-12, a key cytokine for the differentiation of naive Th cells into the Th1 phenotype (D'Elios et al., 2007). During *H. pylori* infection, activated macrophages produce IL-18, which stimulates the IFN-γ secretion by NK and T cells (Kawabata et al., 2001). Nevertheless, Th1 immune response in the stomach may destroy the proliferation / apoptosis balance and promote the severity of *H. pylori*-induced gastric lesions (Xia et al., 2001; Vivas et al., 2008).

In the host, the innate immune response usually represents by TLRs and Nod-like receptors that recognize their specific ligands, activate transcription factors including NF-kB, AP-1 and CREB-1, and induce inflammatory cytokines such as IL-8, IL-12, IL-6, IL-1β, IL-18, TNF-α and IL-10 (Sánchez-Zauco et al., 2010). Amounts of the tumor suppressor p53 and the major innate immune hub protein TRAF-6 reduce in *H. pylori*-infected gastric cells, and coincide with a partially cagPAI-dependent decrease in the expression and activity of deubiqutinating enzyme USP7, which indicates that *H. pylori* may also influence some immunity-associated cytokines through interfering in the host ubiquitin pathways (Coombs et al., 2010).

During *H. pylori* infection, significant overexpression of MHC II antigen-presenting genes, IL-7R ubiquitin-D, CXCR4, lactoferrin immune response-related genes, CXCL-2 and -13, CCL18 chemokine ligand, and VCAM-1 genes have been established (Galamb et al., 2008). In addition, IL-23p19 up-regulation is confirmed in gastric biopsies from both *H. pylori* infected-mice and patients with chronic gastritis (Vivas et al., 2008). CCR6 is markedly upregulated in CD3 (+) T cells infiltrating the gastric mucosa and has been reported to mediate lymphocyte homeostasis and immune responses in mucosal tissue (Wu et al., 2007; Tsai & Hsu, 2010). CCL20, the ligand to CCR6, selectively expresses in inflamed stomach tissues and is upregulated in response to *H. pylori* in GECs stimulated by IL-1β and TNF-α. Furthermore, recombinant CCL20 induces lymphocyte chemotaxis migration in fresh gastric T cells *in vitro* (Wu et al., 2007). The interaction between CCR6 and CCL20 plays a potential role in recruiting T cells to inflamed gastric epithelium during *H. pylori* infection (Tsai & Hsu, 2010).

4.4 Autoimmune and immune tolerance

H. pylori has evolved means to structurally alter its surface characteristics to evade innate and adaptive immune responses (Nilsson et al., 2006). *H. pylori* expresses mimicry of some ABO blood group antigens (Moran et al., 2010). Additionally, CagA, VacA and BabA can mimic and bind to specific receptors or surface molecules on GECs and platelets (Höcker & Hohenberġer 2003; Takahashi et al., 2004; Hennig et al., 2004; Baldari et al., 2005). It has been shown that anti-CagA, anti-VacA and anti-BabA antibodies targeting both *H. pylori* components and host mimic molecules can be detected in the majority of GC patients with increased levels (Rudi et al., 1997; Vaucher et al., 2000; Sokic-Milutinovic et al., 2004). *H. pylori* LPS is of underacylation and underphosphorylation and has significantly lower endotoxic and immuno-activities, which may lead to the infection chronicity (Moran et al., 2010). *H. pylori* produces LPS O-antigen units that can be posttranslationally fucosylated to generate Lewis antigens, which are also found on human GECs, and this molecular mimicry induces autoreactive antibodies (Nilsson et al., 2006). Circulating anti-Lewis antibody is detected in the sera of GC patients but not in *H. pylori*-negative control subjects (Hynes et al., 2005). Absorption of the sera with outer membrane vesicles decreases anti-Lewis autoantibody level. The ability of these vesicles to absorb anti-Lewis autoantibody indicates that they partly play a role in putative autoimmune aspects of *H. pylori* pathogenesis (Hynes et al., 2005).

As reported, C57BL/6 mice infected with CagA (+) *H. pylori* during the neonatal period tend to be protected from preneoplastic lesions, compared to those infected with the same strain at 5-6 weeks of age (Arnold et al., 2011). This protection results from the development of *H. pylori*-specific peripheral immunologic tolerance, which is mediated by long-lived inducible Treg and controls the local CD4 (+) T-cell responses that trigger premalignant transformation. Moreover, both the biased ratio of Treg to T-effector cells in the neonatal period and prolonged low-dose exposure to antigens contribute to the development of immune tolerance to *H. pylori* (Arnold et al., 2011). In addition, exposure of cells to most microbial pathogens can up-regulate HSPs, whereas *H. pylori* decreases expression of HSPs including HSP8, HSP70, HSP60, and heat shock factor 1 (HSF-1). The down-regulation of HSPs may be a mechanism of immune evasion that promotes chronic *H. pylori* infection (Axsen et al., 2009). NO / iNOS as one part of the host innate defense system, determines the killing efficiency of *H. pylori* by macrophages. *H. pylori* up-regulates arginase II (Arg2) expression, resulting in reduction of NO / iNOS production and decreased killing of the germ by macrophages, which implicates another potential mechanism of the immune evasion of *H. pylori* (Lewis et al., 2010).

5. Genetic and phenotypic alterations

Some polymorphisms of certain genes including IL-1, IL-4, IL-6, IL-8, IL-10, TNF, iNOS and COX-2, which likely differ in various host species, play important roles in the inflammation, immune responses, and gastric carcinogenesis, besides in susceptibility to *H. pylori* infection. The GC risk-associated alleles are more prevalent in certain subjects of special human races, geographic regions, and *H. pylori* infection status. Thus, genetic and phenotypic backgrounds of *H. pylori* may interact with mentioned host factors and influence the related biological or pathological processes.

5.1 IL-1

IL-1β and IL-1RN polymorphisms relate to the development of GC and *H. pylori* infection markedly increases the risk, which supports the association of these polymorphisms with risk of Hp-GC (Al-Moundhri et al., 2006). Either infection with vacA s1 (+), vacA m1 (+) and cagA (+) strains or the host genotype of IL-1β -511T homozygous for IL-1RN2/2 allele is associated with an increased GC risk (Figueiredo et al., 2002). Individuals with polymorphisms in IL-1 and TNF-α genes have the highest risk of GC, when they are simultaneously infected by virulent *H. pylori* strains of cagA (+), vacA s1 (+), vacA m1 (+) and babA2 (+). As for IL-1 gene, the odds of developing GC are greatest in those with combination of high-risk bacterial / host genotypes such as vacA s1 / IL-1β -511T, vacA m1 / IL-1β -511T, cagA (+) / IL-1β -511T, vacA s1 / IL-1RN2/2, vacA m1 / IL-1RN2/2, and cagA (+) / IL-1RN2/2 (Figueiredo et al., 2002).

IL-1β -511T/-31C (+) and IL-1RN2 (+) polymorphisms are associated with severe degrees of inflammation, prevalence of IM and AG, and increased expression of IL-1β, which plays a central role in GC development (Rad et al., 2004). The combined prevalence of *H. pylori* infection and IL-1β -511T genotype has a strong association with GC risk in both Latino and Chinese populations (Morgan et al., 2006; Feng et al., 2008). The IL-1β -511T/T carrier status enhances hypermethylation of multiple CpG island loci and increases the risk for Hp-GC of non-cardiac type as an independent risk factor in a Chinese population (Li et al., 2007; Yoo et al., 2010). IL-1β -511C allele is related with increased risk of AG and GC in Peru (Gehmert et al., 2009). IL-1β -511C/C polymorphism enhances IL-1β production in the antrum, and involves in the development of nHp-GC in North Indian (Kumar et al., 2009). In a Korean population, combined effects of *H. pylori* infection and IL-1β -511C/-31T polymorphisms with enhanced mucosal IL-1β production contribute to the development of intestinal-type GC (Chang et al., 2005). IL-1β -511CC/-31TT variants also increase GC risk in a Chinese population, especially of those with *H. pylori* infection (Yang et al., 2004). Nevertheless, IL-1β -511/-31 alleles are not associated with GC risk in Japan and IL-1β -511T-to-C genotype is not associated with GC in a multistep carcinogenesis model (Kato et al., 2001; Sugimoto et al., 2007). In addition, none of the variants of IL-1β -511C>T, -31T>C, -1464G>C and -3737C>T, is individually or in its haplotype configuration linked to GC in a Caucasian population (Wex et al., 2010).

IL-1β -31C/+3954T haplotypes are more likely detected with IM or dysplasia of the stomach and relate to GC risk in African Americans, but not in Caucasians, Swedes and Italians (Palli et al., 2005; Camargo et al., 2006; Persson et al., 2009; Zabaleta et al., 2011). In Mexico, IL-1β -31C allele increases high-grade dysplasia and is an independent risk factor for GC (Garza-González et al., 2003). The IL-1β -31CC carriers have an increased risk of intestinal-type GC among CagA-positive subjects, compared to those with IL-1β -31TT. Among CagA-negative subjects, however, there is no mentioned association (Sicinschi et al., 2006). IL-1β 1473C>G is significantly associated with GC among Koreans (Lee et al., 2004). In Japan, IL-1β +3953 polymorphism can influence the cancer risk of gastric corpus (Sakuma et al., 2005). Carriers of IL-1β +3954T or IL-1RN2 heterozygote allele cause increased GC risk in a Costa Rican population, although IL-1β -31, IL-1β -511 and IL-10 polymorphisms do not (Alpízar-Alpízar et al., 2005).

IL-1RN1/2 genotype is significantly and independently associated with GC (Erzin et al., 2008). IL-1RN2 allele relates to GC especially in *H. pylori*-positive patients of an Omani Arab population (Al-Moundhri et al., 2006). In Italy, multivariate analyses have shown a notable increase in GC risk for the IL-1RN2 / IL-1β -31T haplotype carriers (Palli et al., 2005). *H. pylori*-infected individuals with carriers of IL-1RN2 show high risks for both intestinal and diffuse types of GC in Asia (Chen et al., 2004). IL-1RN2 and IL-1β -511T may contribute to intestinal GC in the absence of concomitant *H. pylori* infection (Ruzzo et al., 2005). IL-1RN2/2 and IL-1β -31C genotypes relate to higher GC risk in Caucasians (Garza-González et al., 2003). The IL-1RN2/2 genotype is strongly associated with early-stage GC, and involves in the development of nHp-GC in North Indian (Glas et al., 2004; Kumar et al., 2009). IL-1RN 2R/2R and Ex5-35C genotypes are related to an increased risk of Hp-GC of non-cardia type (Crusius et al., 2008). However, IL-1β -511, IL-1RN and IL-2 polymorphisms do not significantly contribute to GC in Korean patients (Shin et al., 2008). In Mexico, IL-1RN2/2 is also not associated with either high-grade dysplasia or risk of GC (Garza-González et al., 2003).

5.2 IL-10

As for subtypes of GC in Taiwanese Chinese, the high IL-10 producer genotype is significantly linked with the risk of cardia type or advanced stage (Wu et al., 2003). The ATA/GCC haplotype of IL-10 -1082/-819/-592 significantly increases GC risk compared with ATA/ATA haplotype (Sugimoto et al., 2007). The -1082G/-819C/-592C alleles (GCC haplotype) usually lead to higher mucosal IL-10 mRNA level than ATA haplotype and are associated with colonization by more virulent *H. pylori* strains of cagA (+), vacA s1 (+), and babA2 (+) (Rad et al., 2004). IL-10 -1082 AG+GG but not -819 or -592 polymorphisms, markedly increase GC risk in China, especially in patients with *H. pylori* infection (Xiao et al., 2009). In a low prevalence province of China, the -1082G* allele is related with significantly increased risk of Hp-GC, whereas the higher susceptibility to GC in -1082 AG+GG genotype does not show a synergism with *H. pylori* status in another population of northern China (Bai et al., 2008). In Korean, the frequency of -1082G carriers is higher in diffuse-type GC or benign gastric ulcer (BGU), regardless of *H. pylori* infection (Kang et al., 2009). Moreover, IL-10 -819CC and IL-1RN 9589TT genotypes are of inverse association with *H. pylori* seropositivity among cases with chronic AG, an established precursor of GC (Gao et al., 2009). The IL-10 819C allele is related with IM in *H. pylori*-positive subjects of a Singapore-Chinese population (Zhu et al., 2009).

In *H. pylori*-infected Japanese, the frequency of -592AA homozygote showing concomitant carriage of HLA DRB1*0405-DQB1*0401 is notably higher in intestinal-type GC. In addition, the HLA class II and -592A/C polymorphism synergistically affect the susceptibility to GC (Ando et al., 2009). IL-10 -592C/A, IL-1β +3954T/C and IL-1RN*2/L are individually associated with GC in Costa Rican regions, and a combination of these cytokine polymorphisms with *H. pylori* vacA s1b / m1 genotypes further increased the risk (Con et al., 2009). IL-10 -592/-1082 alleles are not linked with high-grade dysplasia or GC risk in a Mexican population, though relate to high GC risk in Caucasians; whereas carriers with two or more risk-associated alleles of IL-10 -592C, IL-1β -31C and IL-1RN2 are at increased risk for intestinal-type GC in Mexico, compared to those with 0 or 1 mentioned allele (Garza-González et al., 2003). In Korean, the presence of IL10 -592C/A as opposed to A/A is one of risk factors for IM. The -592CC is associated with more than doubling of the risk for intestinal-type GC. Furthermore, a synergistic effect has been observed between IL-10 -592A/A and IL-8 -251A/A with respect to the development of GC or BGU (Kang et al., 2009). IL-10 -819C and -592C alleles are associated with increased GC risk in Japan, but -1082 polymorphism not (Sugimoto et al., 2007). The -819TT genotype relates to IM and non-cardia GC in an Italian population (Zambon et al., 2005).

Data from Korea have even suggested that the association between IL-10 genetic polymorphisms and GC risk is modified by soybean product intake (Ko et al., 2009). The combined effect between low intake of soybean products and -1082AG/GG, -819TC/CC or -592GG/GA variants will increase the risk for GC. As for subgroups, the CCG haplotype has an increased risk of GC relative to ATA haplotype among subjects with low intake of soybean products (Ko et al., 2009).

5.3 IL-4, IL-6 and IL-8

There is a moderately increased risk for Hp-GC of non-cardia type in IL-4R -29429T variant (Crusius JB et al., 2008). In Taiwanese Chinese, a higher risk of developing cardia or diffuse-type GC is observed for the carrier of IL-4 -590CT/CC genotype (Wu et al., 2003). IL-4 -168C and -590T alleles and IL-6 -174G/G haplotype significantly relate to the risk of non-cardia

GC (Sugimoto et al., 2010). The IL-6 -174G allele is markedly higher in patients with GC than those with chronic gastritis (Gatti et al., 2007).

IL-8 -251A allele significantly increases the risk of gastric dysplasia in Venezuelan subjects, especially of those infected with CagA (+) *H. pylori*, which suggests a role of interactions between host and bacterial genetic factors in the development of precancerous lesions (Kato et al., 2006). Similarly in a Mexican population, the -251A genotype has a significant effect on the prevalence of dysplasia and may be related to distal GC, especially when *H. pylori* CagA is present (Garza-Gonzalez et al., 2007). IL-8 -251A/T allele and polymorphisms in vacA gene are involved in limiting the infection outcome to gastritis and peptic ulcer or in favoring cancer onset in Iranian patients (Kamali-Sarvestani et al., 2006). The -251T>A polymorphism is usually associated with higher IL-8 expression, severe neutrophil infiltration and increased risk of AG and GC in Japan, but not with GC risk in a Portuguese population (Taguchi et al., 2005; Canedo et al., 2008). The IL-8 -251A polymorphism may be associated with progression of AG in *H. pylori*-infected patients, and increase the risks for GC and gastric ulcer in Japanese people (Ohyauchi et al., 2005). The -251A/A genotype, which is more common in *H. pylori*-positive patients with GC or BGU than in *H. pylori*-positive controls, increases the risk for upper-third location, diffuse, poorly differentiated, lymph node and liver metastasis, and p53-mutated subtypes of GC (Taguchi et al., 2005; Kang et al., 2009). The high-risk IL-8 -251T allele is related with >2-fold increased risk for GC of diffused and mixed types (Lee et al., 2005). In addition, the -251T/T genotype significantly relates to increased risk of GC with high frequency of microsatellite instability (Shirai et al., 2006).

5.4 TNF

Polymorphisms of TNF-α -857TT and -1031TT, besides CD14, CXC chemokine receptor 2 (CXCR2), IL-1 RI, NF-κB2, and TLR-4, have the potential to influence persistent *H. pylori* infection (Hamajima et al., 2003). TNF-α -857T/-863A/-1031C alleles are associated with increased risks for gastric ulcer and GC in Japan (Sugimoto et al., 2007). In a Korean population, the -857C/T variant is independently and significantly related to an increased risk of GC regardless of smoking status. However, all haplotype-pairs including TCT or CCC of -863C/A and -1031T/C are linked with a higher GC risk only among smokers (Yang et al., 2009). TNF-α -308 genotypes correlate to higher risk of GC in Caucasians, but not to high-grade dysplasia or increased risk of GC in Mexican population (Garza-González et al., 2003). The -308A allele increases the risk for GC development but is only weakly associated with the early-stage diffuse-type GC (Glas et al., 2004). The -308G/A haplotype relates to an increased IL-8 expression and the susceptibility to GC in several studies. In Poland, GC risk is dramatically relevant to the TNF-α -308G>A and IFN-γ R2 Ex7-128C>T polymorphisms, but not to IL-1α -889C>T and IL-12α IVS2-798T>A, IVS2-701C>A and Ex7+277G>A variants (Hou et al., 2007). Risk of GC is also markedly elevated in Chinese subjects carrying the TNF-α -308 AG genotype (Lu et al., 2005). In addition, polymorphisms in TNF-β (*A and +252G/G) and HSP70-1 (*C and +190C/G) show a significant gene-dose effect as risk markers from preneoplastic lesions to GC in Mexican (Partida-Rodríguez et al., 2010).

5.5 Other cytokine genes

NOS2 -954G/C (especially -954GC+CC) polymorphism but not Ser608Leu is associated with higher risk of GC in a Brazilian population (Jorge et al., 2010). The iNOS C150T is related with the risk of Hp-GC, but not with gastric atrophy or *H. pylori* seropositivity in a Japanese population. Considering the location of GC, there are significant differences between the controls and non-cardia group for iNOS -150C/T and C/T + T/T (Goto et al., 2006). The iNOS promoter polymorphism of long CCTTT repeat notably upregulates its mRNA level and leads to increased risk of intestinal-type GC in Japanese women, especially of those with IL-1β -31 polymorphism and without smoking history (Tatemichi et al., 2005).

In the high incidence Hexi area of Gansu Province in China, COX-2 -899G>C polymorphism may be a risk factor for GC, and the -899C carrier genotype and *H. pylori* infection possibly have a synergistic effect on GC. However, COX-2 587G>A is not related with GC risk (Zhu et al., 2011). COX-2 -1195AA polymorphism also plays an important role in developing GC in another high-risk Chinese population (Zhang et al., 2006). COX-2 -765G>C polymorphism might be a marker for genetic susceptibility to GC in northern India, regardless of *H. pylori* infection (Saxena et al., 2008). Moreover, the lymphotoxin-α NcoI A/G heterozygous genotype correlates to *H. pylori* infection in noncardia GC patients of Chinese Han population (Li et al., 2005). And in Cauca population, the glutathione S-transferase M1 homozygous deletion polymorphism is related to increased GC risk (Torres et al., 2004).

6. Beneficial edge of the sword

In recent years, increasing data have indicated that patients with Hp-GC prospectively have a better outlook than those with nHp-GC (Meimarakis et al., 2006; Marrelli et al., 2009). *H. pylori* infection must play certain roles as the other edge of the sword, which is beneficial for the host and counteracts its harmfulness in pathological lesions including gastritis, GC, and lymphoma. However, up to date, the corresponding studies and results are still limited because of multiple influencing factors including traditional unilateral opinions.

The positive interaction between *H. pylori* and the host should be the radical factor in leading to changes of local and system immune responses. There is a high *H. pylori* prevalence but a low GC risk in *H. pylori*-infected than in uninfected Mexican children, which may be attributed to significantly higher infiltration of macrophages and T and B cells, a balanced increase of CD4, CD8, and CD20 lymphocytes, but decreased levels of activated mast cells, neutrophil and mononuclear cells (Muñoz et al., 2007). During *H. pylori* infection, both the number of local CD4 (+) T cells and MHC II expression by the GECs increase, and GECs can process and present antigens to CD4 (+) T cells as a new kind of local antigen presenting cells (APC) (Barrera et al., 2002). Therefore, *H. pylori* infection in the host may alter natural immune mechanisms against cancer.

The humeral immune response induced by *H. pylori* is predominately IgG1 subclass (suggestive of a Th2 response) and likely protects against the development of GC, although it is not essential for bacterial eradication (Segal et al., 2001). As reported, the antibody level of anti- Thomsen-Friedenreich antigen (TAg) in GC patients is significantly lower than that in normal blood donors (Klaamas et al., 2002). However, TAg-specific IgG immune response is up-regulated exclusively in *H. pylori*-infected individuals, which may contribute to the significantly better survival of Hp-GC patients at early stage than that of nHp-GC ones at the same stage. Better survival is also noted in *H. pylori* seropositive IgM strong responders at approximately 40-60 months of observation, though the anti-T IgM level is not significantly related to the survival (Kurtenkov et al., 2003). In addition, the stimulation of *H. pylori*-related autoantibodies in antigen processing and presentation and subsequent T-cell activation and proliferation improves host immune status. On the other hand, in an autoimmune response, autoantibodies can induce the cross-reaction against those localized or circulating GC cells, which are characterized by mimic or absorbed *H. pylori* antigens, and lead to the killing and even suppressing of metastasis of cancer cells (Xue et al., 2008). Thus, it is hypothesized that autoimmune responses induced by *H. pylori* components may help improve the prognosis of GC patients.

Several models, including delayed type hypersensitivity in immune mice, and spontaneous clearance of *H. pylori* from IL-10 and phagocyte oxidase mice, provide evidence that severe inflammation may be sufficient to eradicate the germ (Blanchard et al., 2004). *H. pylori* LPS can dramatically initiate inflammatory responses and cause severe pathological changes not only *in vitro* but also *in vivo*. However, increased levels of TNF-α and IL-10, as well as a strong antigen specific Th1 response including, IFN-γ, IL-2 and high IgG2a serum titers are simultaneously observed in mice inoculated with *H. pylori* LPS+ sonicate. Mice that received LPS- sonicate are strongly Th2 biased in their immune response, with significantly more IL-4 than IFN-γ and serum IgG1 titers higher than IgG2a (Taylor et al., 2006). Accordingly, *H. pylori*-induced inflammatory responses potentially have positive functions in resisting certain cancer-advancement-related biological processes post the development of GC and showing better outlook in those patients, although they have played fundamental roles during the phase of cancer formation.

Interestingly, the COX-2 expression induced by *H. pylori* still seems to be able to attenuate the degree of AG, the initial event of GC, though it plays a role in gastric carcinogenesis (Hahm et al., 2002). COX-2-dependent PGE2 also shows a protective effect during the oncogenic process of Hp-GC in that it can prevent *H. pylori*-induced gastric preneoplasia and reverse preexisting lesions by suppressing IFN-γ expression (Toller et al., 2010). As confirmed, the protective effect is always accompanied by increased bacterial colonization in models, which is attributed to the IL-2-dependent immunosuppressive effects of PGE2 on CD4 (+) Th1 cells in migration, proliferation and cytokine secretion. Therefore, PGE2 has an important immunomodulatory role during *H. pylori* infection, preventing excessive local immune responses and the associated immunopathology by inhibiting the effector functions of pathogenic Th1 cells (Toller et al., 2010).

Certain genetic and phenotypic polymorphisms also show beneficial effects in improving the prognosis of GC patients, which might differ in various populations and need further confirmation. IL-6 -572G carrier is found to have a protective effect against IM development as compared with C/C (Kim et al., 2008). IL-8 -251AA genotype confers a decreased risk for Hp-GC of non-cardia type, mainly of the intestinal type (Crusius et al., 2008). IL-10 -592C/C is an independent factor associated with a decreased risk of intestinal-type GC by multivariate analysis (Kang et al., 2009). When analyzed together with host genetic factors, the presence of the IL-1β -31TT genotype emerges as a protective factor against gastric malignant disorders (Erzin et al., 2008). Based on a review of 25 case-control studies in Caucasian, Asian and African populations, IL-1β and NAT1 variants are most consistently associated with increased GC risk, which may account for up to 48% of attributable risk of GC, but HLA-DQ, TNF and CYP2E polymorphisms may confer certain protection against GC (González et al., 2002). However, a comprehensive analysis of 207 SNPs of 11 Cytokine genes including IL-1α, IL-1β, IL-1RN, IL-4, IL-4R, IL-8, IL-10, IL-12, TNF-α, TNF-β, and IFN-γ, has revealed that just variations in IL-4 (984 and 2983 AA/GA) and IL-1RN (-1102 and 6110 CG/GA) diplotypes are negatively associated with the risk of Hp-GC (Seno et al., 2007).

7. Conclusion

The majority of GC relates to chronic inflammation induced by *H. pylori* infection, in which many bacterial virulence factors including Cag PAI, VacA, OMP, LPS, urease, IceA, and flagella components participate with fundamental roles through a complex network of inflammatory cytokines, multiple signalling pathways, and even some genetic or phenotypic polymorphisms of the host. Gastric carcinogenesis, especially of the intestinal-type tumor, is a multistep process of mucosal alterations leading from gastritis via glandular atrophy, IM and dysplasia to invasive carcinoma (Bornschein et al., 2010). There is a potential 'point of no return' during this process, which means a situation when certain alterations are no longer reversible by *H. pylori* eradication and progression to GC have to continue (Vieth et al., 2006; Bornschein et al., 2010). Thus, the gastric carcinogenesis is actually divided into two phases; one is of reversible pre-the-'point of no return', and the other is of irreversible post-the-'point of no return'. During the first phase, *H. pylori* works with more roles as a confirmed carcinogen according to traditional opinion; whereas in the second phase, the inflammation has been switched to *H. pylori*-independent carcinogenesis with GC as the destination.

Considering the host-bacterium cross-talk background and described double functions of both inflammatory / immune responses and genetic / phenotypic polymorphisms, a novel angle should be adopted to analyze the roles of *H. pylori* as a double-edged sword in GC. *H. pylori* is more harmful in promoting carcinogenesis prior to the 'point of no return', however, may be more beneficial for improving the host outlook post the development of GC. Based on this theory, *H. pylori* eradication may be performed at proper stage to protect against GC, and more efficient vaccines of prophylaxis and therapeutic ones might be designed and used to prevent the advancement of GC and improve the prognosis, which needs further confirmation by large from-bench-to-bed studies.

8. Acknowledgement

This work is supported by a grant from the National Natural Science Foundation of China (No.30901733).

9. References

Akhiani AA. The role of type-specific antibodies in colonization and infection by *Helicobacter pylori*. Curr Opin Infect Dis. 2005;18(3):223-7.

Al-Moundhri MS, Al-Nabhani M, Al-Bahrani B, Burney IA, Al-Madhani A, Ganguly SS, Al-Yahyaee SA, Grant CS. Interleukin-1beta gene (IL-1B) and interleukin 1 receptor antagonist gene (IL-1RN) polymorphisms and gastric cancer risk in an Omani Arab population. Gastric Cancer. 2006;9(4):284-90.

Alpízar-Alpízar W, Pérez-Pérez GI, Une C, Cuenca P, Sierra R. Association of interleukin-1B and interleukin-1RN polymorphisms with gastric cancer in a high-risk population of Costa Rica. Clin Exp Med. 2005;5(4):169-76.

Ando T, Ishikawa T, Kato H, Yoshida N, Naito Y, Kokura S, Yagi N, Takagi T, Handa O, Kitawaki J, Nakamura N, Hasegawa G, Fukui M, Imamoto E, Nakamura C, Oyamada H, Isozaki Y, Matsumoto N, Nagao Y, Okita M, Nakajima Y, Kurokawa M, Nukina M, Ohta M, Mizuno S, Ogata M, Obayashi H, Park H, Kitagawa Y,

Nakano K, Yoshikawa T. Synergistic effect of HLA class II loci and cytokine gene polymorphisms on the risk of gastric cancer in Japanese patients with *Helicobacter pylori* infection. Int J Cancer. 2009;125(11):2595-602.

Appelmelk BJ, Vandenbroucke-Grauls CMJE. Lipopolysaccharide Lewis Antigens. In: Mobley HLT, Mendz GL, Hazell SL, editors. *Helicobacter pylori*: Physiology and Genetics. Washington (DC): ASM Press; 2001. Chapter 35.

Arnold IC, Lee JY, Amieva MR, Roers A, Flavell RA, Sparwasser T, Müller A. Tolerance rather than immunity protects from *Helicobacter pylori*-induced gastric preneoplasia. Gastroenterology. 2011;140(1):199-209.

Asim M, Chaturvedi R, Hoge S, Lewis ND, Singh K, Barry DP, Algood HS, de Sablet T, Gobert AP, Wilson KT. *Helicobacter pylori* induces ERK-dependent formation of a phospho-c-Fos c-Jun activator protein-1 complex that causes apoptosis in macrophages. J Biol Chem. 2010;285(26):20343-57.

Atherton JC, Cao P, Peek RM Jr, Tummuru MK, Blaser MJ, Cover TL. Mosaicism in vacuolating cytotoxin alleles of *Helicobacter pylori*. Association of specific vacA types with cytotoxin production and peptic ulceration. J Biol Chem. 1995;270(30):17771-7.

Axsen WS, Styer CM, Solnick JV. Inhibition of heat shock protein expression by *Helicobacter pylori*. Microb Pathog. 2009;47(4):231-6.

Bagnoli F, Buti L, Tompkins L, Covacci A, Amieva MR. *Helicobacter pylori* CagA induces a transition from polarized to invasive phenotypes in MDCK cells. Proc Natl Acad Sci USA 2005; 102(45): 16339-44.

Bai XL, Sun LP, Liu J, Chen W, Zhang Y, Yuan Y. [Correlation of interleukin-10-1082G/a single nucleotide polymorphism to the risk of gastric cancer in north China: a case-control study]. Ai Zheng. 2008;27(1):35-40.

Baldari CT, Lanzavecchia A, Telford JL. Immune subversion by *Helicobacter pylori*. Trends Immunol 2005; 26(4): 199-207.

Barrera C, Espejo R, Reyes VE. Differential glycosylation of MHC class II molecules on gastric epithelial cells: implications in local immune responses. Hum Immunol. 2002;63(5):384-93.

Beales IL. Effect of interlukin-1beta on proliferation of gastric epithelial cells in culture. BMC Gastroenterol. 2002;2:7.

Becher D, Deutscher ME, Simpfendorfer KR, Wijburg OL, Pederson JS, Lew AM, Strugnell RA, Walduck AK. Local recall responses in the stomach involving reduced regulation and expanded help mediate vaccine-induced protection against *Helicobacter pylori* in mice. Eur J Immunol. 2010;40(10):2778-90.

Beswick EJ, Reyes VE. Macrophage migration inhibitory factor and interleukin-8 produced by gastric epithelial cells during *Helicobacter pylori* exposure induce expression and activation of the epidermal growth factor receptor. Infect Immun. 2008;76(7):3233-40.

Blanchard TG, Drakes ML, Czinn SJ. Helicobacter infection: pathogenesis. Curr Opin Gastroenterol. 2004;20(1):10-5.

Bornschein J, Kandulski A, Selgrad M, Malfertheiner P. From gastric inflammation to gastric cancer. Dig Dis. 2010;28(4-5):609-14.

Bronte-Tinkew DM, Terebiznik M, Franco A, Ang M, Ahn D, Mimuro H, Sasakawa C, Ropeleski MJ, Peek RM Jr, Jones NL. *Helicobacter pylori* cytotoxin-associated gene A activates the signal transducer and activator of transcription 3 pathway *in vitro* and *in vivo*. Cancer Res. 2009;69(2):632-9.

Cai X, Carlson J, Stoicov C, Li H, Wang TC, Houghton J. Helicobacter felis eradication restores normal architecture and inhibits gastric cancer progression in C57BL/6 mice. Gastroenterology. 2005;128(7):1937-52.

Camargo MC, Mera R, Correa P, Peek RM Jr, Fontham ET, Goodman KJ, Piazuelo MB, Sicinschi L, Zabaleta J, Schneider BG. Interleukin-1beta and interleukin-1 receptor antagonist gene polymorphisms and gastric cancer: a meta-analysis. Cancer Epidemiol Biomarkers Prev. 2006;15(9):1674-87.

Canedo P, Castanheira-Vale AJ, Lunet N, Pereira F, Figueiredo C, Gioia-Patricola L, Canzian F, Moreira H, Suriano G, Barros H, Carneiro F, Seruca R, Machado JC. The interleukin-8-251*T/*A polymorphism is not associated with risk for gastric carcinoma development in a Portuguese population. Eur J Cancer Prev. 2008;17(1):28-32.

Chang YJ, Wu MS, Lin JT, Chen CC. *Helicobacter pylori*-Induced invasion and angiogenesis of gastric cells is mediated by cyclooxygenase-2 induction through TLR2/TLR9 and promoter regulation. J Immunol. 2005;175(12):8242-52.

Chang YJ, Wu MS, Lin JT, Sheu BS, Muta T, Inoue H, Chen CC. Induction of cyclooxygenase-2 overexpression in human gastric epithelial cells by *Helicobacter pylori* involves TLR2/TLR9 and c-Src-dependent nuclear factor-kappaB activation. Mol Pharmacol. 2004;66(6):1465-77.

Chang YW, Jang JY, Kim NH, Lee JW, Lee HJ, Jung WW, Dong SH, Kim HJ, Kim BH, Lee JI, Chang R. Interleukin-1B (IL-1B) polymorphisms and gastric mucosal levels of IL-1beta cytokine in Korean patients with gastric cancer. Int J Cancer. 2005;114(3):465-71.

Chen A, Li CN, Hsu PI, Lai KH, Tseng HH, Hsu PN, Lo GH, Lo CC, Lin CK, Hwang IR, Yamaoka Y, Chen HC. Risks of interleukin-1 genetic polymorphisms and *Helicobacter pylori* infection in the development of gastric cancer. Aliment Pharmacol Ther. 2004;20(2):203-11.

Chen CN, Hsieh FJ, Cheng YM, Chang KJ, Lee PH. Expression of inducible nitric oxide synthase and cyclooxygenase-2 in angiogenesis and clinical outcome of human gastric cancer. J Surg Oncol. 2006;94(3):226-33.

Cho SO, Lim JW, Kim KH, Kim H. Involvement of Ras and AP-1 in *Helicobacter pylori*-induced expression of COX-2 and iNOS in gastric epithelial AGS cells. Dig Dis Sci. 2010;55(4):988-96.

Churin Y, Al-Ghoul L, Kepp O, Meyer TF, Birchmeier W, Naumann M. *Helicobacter pylori* CagA protein targets the c-Met receptor and enhances the motogenic response. J Cell Biol. 2003;161(2):249-55.

Con SA, Takeuchi H, Con-Chin GR, Con-Chin VG, Yasuda N, Con-Wong R. Role of bacterial and genetic factors in gastric cancer in Costa Rica. World J Gastroenterol. 2009;15(2):211-8.

Coombs N, Sompallae R, Olbermann P, Gastaldello S, Göppel D, Masucci MG, Josenhans C. *Helicobacter pylori* affects the cellular deubiquitinase USP7 and ubiquitin-regulated components TRAF6 and the tumour suppressor p53. Int J Med Microbiol. 2011;301(3):213-24.

Crusius JB, Canzian F, Capellá G, Peña AS, Pera G, Sala N, Agudo A, Rico F, Del Giudice G, Palli D, Plebani M, Boeing H, Bueno-de-Mesquita HB, Carneiro F, Pala V, Save VE, Vineis P, Tumino R, Panico S, Berglund G, Manjer J, Stenling R, Hallmans G, Martínez C, Dorronsoro M, Barricarte A, Navarro C, Quirós JR, Allen N, Key TJ, Binghan S, Caldas C, Linseisen J, Kaaks R, Overvad K, Tjønneland A, Büchner FC, Peeters PH, Numans ME, Clavel-Chapelon F, Trichopoulou A, Lund E, Jenab M, Rinaldi S, Ferrari P, Riboli E, González CA. Cytokine gene polymorphisms and the risk of adenocarcinoma of the stomach in the European prospective investigation into cancer and nutrition (EPIC-EURGAST). Ann Oncol. 2008;19(11):1894-902.

D'Elios MM, Amedei A, Benagiano M, Azzurri A, Del Prete G. *Helicobacter pylori,* T cells and cytokines: the "dangerous liaisons". FEMS Immunol Med Microbiol. 2005;44(2):113-9.

D'Elios MM, Montecucco C, de Bernard M. VacA and HP-NAP, Ying and Yang of *Helicobacter pylori*-associated gastric inflammation. Clin Chim Acta. 2007;381(1):32-8.

Di Bisceglie AM. Hepatitis B and hepatocellular carcinoma. Hepatology. 2009;49(5 Suppl):S56-60.

Dong LM, Shu XO, Gao YT, Milne G, Ji BT, Yang G, Li HL, Rothman N, Zheng W, Chow WH, Abnet CC. Urinary prostaglandin E2 metabolite and gastric cancer risk in the Shanghai women's health study. Cancer Epidemiol Biomarkers Prev. 2009;18(11):3075-8.

Dunn BE, Cohen H, Blaser MJ. *Helicobacter pylori*. Clin Microbiol Rev. 1997;10(4):720-41.

Ernst PB, Pappo J. T-cell-mediated mucosal immunity in the absence of antibody: lessons from *Helicobacter pylori* infection. Acta Odontol Scand. 2001;59(4):216-21.

Erzin Y, Koksal V, Altun S, Dobrucali A, Aslan M, Erdamar S, Goksel S, Dirican A, Kocazeybek B. Role of host interleukin 1beta gene (IL-1B) and interleukin 1 receptor antagonist gene (IL-1RN) polymorphisms in clinical outcomes in *Helicobacter pylori*-positive Turkish patients with dyspepsia. J Gastroenterol. 2008;43(9):705-10.

Feng Y, Zhang J, Dai L, Zhang J, Wang P, Zang J, Li Y, Wang K. Inflammatory cytokine gene polymorphisms in gastric cancer cases' and controls' family members from Chinese areas at high cancer prevalence. Cancer Lett. 2008;270(2):250-9.

Figueiredo C, Machado JC, Pharoah P, Seruca R, Sousa S, Carvalho R, Capelinha AF, Quint W, Caldas C, van Doorn LJ, Carneiro F, Sobrinho-Simões M. *Helicobacter pylori* and interleukin 1 genotyping: an opportunity to identify high-risk individuals for gastric carcinoma. J Natl Cancer Inst. 2002;94(22):1680-7.

Fukase K, Kato M, Kikuchi S, Inoue K, Uemura N, Okamoto S, Terao S, Amagai K, Hayashi S, Asaka M; Japan Gast Study Group. Effect of eradication of *Helicobacter pylori* on incidence of metachronous gastric carcinoma after endoscopic resection of early gastric cancer: an open-label, randomized controlled trial. Lancet 2008; 372(9636):392-7.

Futagami S, Tatsuguchi A, Hiratsuka T, Shindo T, Horie A, Hamamoto T, Ueki N, Kusunoki M, Miyake K, Gudis K, Tsukui T, Sakamoto C. Monocyte chemoattractant protein 1 and CD40 ligation have a synergistic effect on vascular endothelial growth factor production through cyclooxygenase 2 upregulation in gastric cancer. J Gastroenterol. 2008;43(3):216-24.

Galamb O, Gyõrffy B, Sipos F, Dinya E, Krenács T, Berczi L, Szõke D, Spisák S, Solymosi N, Németh AM, Juhász M, Molnár B, Tulassay Z. *Helicobacter pylori* and antrum erosion-specific gene expression patterns: the discriminative role of CXCL13 and VCAM1 transcripts. Helicobacter. 2008;13(2):112-26.

Gao L, Weck MN, Nieters A, Brenner H. Inverse association between a pro-inflammatory genetic profile and *Helicobacter pylori* seropositivity among patients with chronic atrophic gastritis: enhanced elimination of the infection during disease progression? Eur J Cancer. 2009;45(16):2860-6.

Garza-Gonzalez E, Bosques-Padilla FJ, Mendoza-Ibarra SI, Flores-Gutierrez JP, Maldonado-Garza HJ, Perez-Perez GI. Assessment of the toll-like receptor 4 Asp299Gly, Thr399Ile and interleukin-8 -251 polymorphisms in the risk for the development of distal gastric cancer. BMC Cancer. 2007;7:70.

Garza-González E, Hold G, Pérez-Pérez GI, Bosques-Padilla FJ, Tijerina-Menchaca R, Maldonado-Garza HJ, el-Omar E. [Role of polymorphism of certain cytokines in gastric cancer in Mexico. Preliminary results] Rev Gastroenterol Mex. 2003;68(2):107-12.

Gatti LL, Burbano RR, Zambaldi-Tunes M, de-Lábio RW, de Assumpção PP, de Arruda Cardoso-Smith M, Marques-Payão SL. Interleukin-6 polymorphisms, *Helicobacter pylori* infection in adult Brazilian patients with chronic gastritis and gastric adenocarcinoma. Arch Med Res. 2007;38(5):551-5.

Gebert B, Fischer W, Haas R. The *Helicobacter pylori* vacuolating cytotoxin: from cellular vacuolation to immunosuppressive activities. Rev Physiol Biochem Pharmacol. 2004;152:205-20.

Gehmert S, Velapatiño B, Herrera P, Balqui J, Santivañez L, Cok J, Vargas G, Combe J, Passaro DJ, Wen S, Meyer F, Berg DE, Gilman RH. Interleukin-1 beta single-nucleotide polymorphism's C allele is associated with elevated risk of gastric cancer in *Helicobacter pylori*-infected Peruvians. Am J Trop Med Hyg. 2009;81(5):804-10.

Gerhard M, Lehn N, Neumayer N, Borén T, Rad R, Schepp W, Miehlke S, Classen M, Prinz C. Clinical relevance of the *Helicobacter pylori* gene for blood-group antigen-binding adhesin. Proc Natl Acad Sci USA. 1999; 96(22):12778-83.

Glas J, Török HP, Schneider A, Brünnler G, Kopp R, Albert ED, Stolte M, Folwaczny C. Allele 2 of the interleukin-1 receptor antagonist gene is associated with early gastric cancer. J Clin Oncol. 2004;22(23):4746-52.

González CA, Sala N, Capellá G. Genetic susceptibility and gastric cancer risk. Int J Cancer. 2002;100(3):249-60.

Goto Y, Ando T, Naito M, Goto H, Hamajima N. Inducible nitric oxide synthase polymorphism is associated with the increased risk of differentiated gastric cancer in a Japanese population. World J Gastroenterol. 2006;12(39):6361-5.

Grebowska A, Moran AP, Matusiak A, Bak-Romaniszyn L, Czkwianianc E, Rechciński T, Walencka M, Płaneta-Małecka I, Rudnicka W, Chmiela M. Anti-phagocytic activity of *Helicobacter pylori* lipopolysaccharide (LPS)--possible modulation of the innate immune response to these bacteria. Pol J Microbiol. 2008;57(3):185-92.

Guo T, Qian JM, Zhang JZ, Li XB, Zhao YQ. [Effects of *Helicobacter pylori* and *Helicobacter pylori*-related cytokines on apoptosis of gastric epithelial cells and mechanisms thereof] Zhonghua Yi Xue Za Zhi. 2006;86(38):2670-3.

Hahm KB, Lim HY, Sohn S, Kwon HJ, Lee KM, Lee JS, Surh YJ, Kim YB, Joo HJ, Kim WS, Cho SW. *In vitro* evidence of the role of COX-2 in attenuating gastric inflammation and promoting gastric carcinogenesis. J Environ Pathol Toxicol Oncol. 2002;21(2):165-76.

Hamajima N. Persistent *Helicobacter pylori* infection and genetic polymorphisms of the host. Nagoya J Med Sci. 2003;66(3-4):103-17.

Hennig EE, Mernaugh R, Edl J, Cao P, Cover TL. Heterogeneity among *Helicobacter pylori* strains in expression of the outer membrane protein BabA. Infect Immun 2004; 72(6): 3429-35.

Higashi H, Tsutsumi R, Muto S, Sugiyama T, Azuma T, Asaka M, Hatakeyama M. SHP-2 tyrosine phosphatase as an intracellular target of *Helicobacter pylori* CagA protein. Science 2002;295(5555):683-6.

Höcker M, Hohenberġer P. *Helicobacter pylori* virulence factors--one part of a big picture. Lancet 2003; 362 (9391):1231-3.

Hou L, El-Omar EM, Chen J, Grillo P, Rabkin CS, Baccarelli A, Yeager M, Chanock SJ, Zatonski W, Sobin LH, Lissowska J, Fraumeni JF Jr, Chow WH. Polymorphisms in Th1-type cell-mediated response genes and risk of gastric cancer. Carcinogenesis. 2007;28(1):118-23.

Huang JQ, Zheng GF, Sumanac K, Irvine EJ, Hunt RH. Meta-analysis of the relationship between cagA seropositivity and gastric cancer. Gastroenterology 2003;125(6):1636–44.

Huang L, Zhang KL, Li H, Chen XY, Kong QY, Sun Y, Gao X, Guan HW, Liu J. Infrequent COX-2 expression due to promoter hypermethylation in gastric cancers in Dalian, China. Hum Pathol. 2006;37(12):1557-67.

Hussain MA, Naveed SA, Sechi LA, Ranjan S, Alvi A, Ahmed I, Ranjan A, Mukhopadhyay S, Ahmed N. Isocitrate dehydrogenase of *Helicobacter pylori* potentially induces humoral immune response in subjects with peptic ulcer disease and gastritis. PLoS One. 2008;3(1):e1481.

Hynes SO, Keenan JI, Ferris JA, Annuk H, Moran AP. Lewis epitopes on outer membrane vesicles of relevance to *Helicobacter pylori* pathogenesis. Helicobacter. 2005;10(2):146-56.

Ierardi E, Di Leo A, Barone M, Marangi S, Burattini O, Panarese A, Margiotta M, Francavilla R, Panella C, Francavilla A, Cuomo R. Tumor necrosis factor alpha and apoptosis in *Helicobacter pylori* related progressive gastric damage: a possible mechanism of immune system involvement in epithelial turnover regulation. Immunopharmacol Immunotoxicol. 2003;25(2):203-11.

Inoue K, Shiota S, Yamada K, Gotoh K, Suganuma M, Fujioka T, Ahmed K, Iha H, Nishizono A. Evaluation of a new tumor necrosis factor-alpha-inducing membrane protein of *Helicobacter pylori* as a prophylactic vaccine antigen. Helicobacter. 2009;14(5):135-43.

International Agency for Research on Cancer. Cancer incidence in five continents. IARC Sci Publ 2002;VIII:1-781.

International Agency for Research on Cancer. Infection with *Helicobacter pylori*. In: IARC monographs on the evaluation of carcinogenic risks to humans. Schistosomes, liver flukes and *Helicobacter pylori*. Lyon: IARC,1994; 61:177-244.

Jackson CB, Judd LM, Menheniott TR, Kronborg I, Dow C, Yeomans ND, Boussioutas A, Robb L, Giraud AS. Augmented gp130-mediated cytokine signalling accompanies human gastric cancer progression. J Pathol. 2007;213(2):140-51.

Jang TJ. The number of Foxp3-positive regulatory T cells is increased in *Helicobacter pylori* gastritis and gastric cancer. Pathol Res Pract. 2010;206(1):34-8.

Jorge YC, Duarte MC, Silva AE. Gastric cancer is associated with NOS2 -954G/C polymorphism and environmental factors in a Brazilian population. BMC Gastroenterol. 2010;10:64.

Kai H, Kitadai Y, Kodama M, Cho S, Kuroda T, Ito M, Tanaka S, Ohmoto Y, Chayama K. Involvement of proinflammatory cytokines IL-1beta and IL-6 in progression of human gastric carcinoma. Anticancer Res. 2005;25(2A):709-13.

Kamali-Sarvestani E, Bazargani A, Masoudian M, Lankarani K, Taghavi AR, Saberifiroozi M. Association of H pylori cagA and vacA genotypes and IL-8 gene polymorphisms with clinical outcome of infection in Iranian patients with gastrointestinal diseases. World J Gastroenterol. 2006;12(32):5205-10.

Kandulski A, Malfertheiner P, Wex T. Role of regulatory T-cells in *H. pylori*-induced gastritis and gastric cancer. Anticancer Res. 2010;30(4):1093-103.

Kang JM, Kim N, Lee DH, Park JH, Lee MK, Kim JS, Jung HC, Song IS. The effects of genetic polymorphisms of IL-6, IL-8, and IL-10 on *Helicobacter pylori*-induced gastroduodenal diseases in Korea. J Clin Gastroenterol. 2009;43(5):420-8.

Kassai K, Yoshikawa T, Yoshida N, Hashiramoto A, Kondo M, Murase H. *Helicobacter pylori* water extract induces interleukin-8 production by gastric epithelial cells. Dig Dis Sci. 1999;44(2):237-42.

Katayama Y, Takahashi M, Kuwayama H. *Helicobacter pylori* causes runx3 gene methylation and its loss of expression in gastric epithelial cells, which is mediated by nitric oxide produced by macrophages. Biochem Biophys Res Commun. 2009;388(3):496-500.

Kato I, van Doorn LJ, Canzian F, Plummer M, Franceschi S, Vivas J, Lopez G, Lu Y, Gioia-Patricola L, Severson RK, Schwartz AG, Muñoz N. Host-bacterial interaction in the development of gastric precancerous lesions in a high risk population for gastric cancer in Venezuela. Int J Cancer. 2006;119(7):1666-71.

Kato S, Onda M, Yamada S, Matsuda N, Tokunaga A, Matsukura N. Association of the interleukin-1 beta genetic polymorphism and gastric cancer risk in Japanese. J Gastroenterol. 2001;36(10):696-9.

Kawabata T, Ichikura T, Majima T, Seki S, Chochi K, Takayama E, Hiraide H, Mochizuki H. Preoperative serum interleukin-18 level as a postoperative prognostic marker in patients with gastric carcinoma. Cancer. 2001;92(8):2050-5.

Keep S, Borlace G, Butler R, Brooks D. Role of immune serum in the killing of *Helicobacter pylori* by macrophages. Helicobacter. 2010;15(3):177-83.

Kidd M, Peek RM, Lastovica AJ, Israel DA, Kummer AF, Louw JA. Analysis of iceA genotypes in South African *Helicobacter pylori* strains and relationship to clinically significant disease. Gut. 2001;49(5):629-35.

Kim N, Park YS, Cho SI, Lee HS, Choe G, Kim IW, Won YD, Park JH, Kim JS, Jung HC, Song IS. Prevalence and risk factors of atrophic gastritis and intestinal metaplasia in a Korean population without significant gastroduodenal disease. Helicobacter. 2008;13(4):245-55.

Klaamas K, Held M, Wadström T, Lipping A, Kurtenkov O. IgG immune response to *Helicobacter pylori* antigens in patients with gastric cancer as defined by ELISA and immunoblotting. Int J Cancer. 1996;67(1):1-5.

Klaamas K, Kurtenkov O, Rittenhouse-Olson K, Brjalin V, Miljukhina L, Shljapnikova L, Engstrand L. Expression of tumor-associated Thomsen-Friedenreich antigen (T Ag) in *Helicobacter pylori* and modulation of T Ag specific immune response in infected individuals. Immunol Invest. 2002;31(3-4):191-204.

Klaamas K, Kurtenkov O, von Mensdorff-Pouilly S, Shljapnikova L, Miljukhina L, Brjalin V, Lipping A. Impact of *Helicobacter pylori* infection on the humoral immune response to MUC1 peptide in patients with chronic gastric diseases and gastric cancer. Immunol Invest. 2007;36(4):371-86.

Ko KP, Park SK, Cho LY, Gwack J, Yang JJ, Shin A, Kim CS, Kim Y, Kang D, Chang SH, Shin HR, Yoo KY. Soybean product intake modifies the association between interleukin-10 genetic polymorphisms and gastric cancer risk. J Nutr. 2009;139(5):1008-12.

Komoto K, Haruma K, Kamada T, Tanaka S, Yoshihara M, Sumii K, Kajiyama G, Talley NJ. *Helicobacter pylori* infection and gastric neoplasia: correlations with histological gastritis and tumor histology. Am J Gastroenterol. 1998;93(8):1271-6.

Konturek PC, Kania J, Kukharsky V, Ocker S, Hahn EG, Konturek SJ. Influence of gastrin on the expression of cyclooxygenase-2, hepatocyte growth factor and apoptosis-related proteins in gastric epithelial cells. J Physiol Pharmacol. 2003;54(1):17-32.

Konturek PC, Konturek SJ, Brzozowski T. *Helicobacter pylori* infection in gastric cancerogenesis. J Physiol Pharmacol. 2009;60(3):3-21.

Konturek PC, Konturek SJ, Sulekova Z, Meixner H, Bielanski W, Starzynska T, Karczewska E, Marlicz K, Stachura J, Hahn EG. Expression of hepatocyte growth factor, transforming growth factor alpha, apoptosis related proteins Bax and Bcl-2, and gastrin in human gastric cancer. Aliment Pharmacol Ther. 2001;15(7):989-99.

Konturek SJ, Starzynska T, Konturek PC, Karczewska E, Marlicz K, Lawniczak M, Jaroszewicz-Heigelman H, Bielanski W, Hartwich A, Ziemniak A, Hahn EG. *Helicobacter pylori* and CagA status, serum gastrin, interleukin-8 and gastric acid secretion in gastric cancer. Scand J Gastroenterol. 2002;37(8):891-8.

Kumar S, Kumar A, Dixit VK. Evidences showing association of interleukin-1B polymorphisms with increased risk of gastric cancer in an Indian population. Biochem Biophys Res Commun. 2009;387(3):456-60.

Kurtenkov O, Klaamas K, Sergeyev B, Chuzmarov V, Miljukhina L, Shljapnikova L. Better survival of *Helicobacter pylori* infected patients with early gastric cancer is related to a higher level of Thomsen-Friedenreich antigen-specific antibodies. Immunol Invest. 2003;32(1-2):83-93.

Lamarque D, Tran Van Nhieu J, Breban M. [What are the gastric modifications induced by acute and chronic *Helicobacter pylori* infection?] Gastroenterol Clin Biol. 2003;27(3 Pt 2):391-400.

Lee IO, Kim JH, Choi YJ, Pillinger MH, Kim SY, Blaser MJ, Lee YC. *Helicobacter pylori* CagA phosphorylation status determines the gp130-activated SHP2/ERK and JAK/STAT signal transduction pathways in gastric epithelial cells. J Biol Chem. 2010;285(21):16042-50.

Lee KA, Ki CS, Kim HJ, Sohn KM, Kim JW, Kang WK, Rhee JC, Song SY, Sohn TS. Novel interleukin 1beta polymorphism increased the risk of gastric cancer in a Korean population. J Gastroenterol. 2004;39(5):429-33.

Lee WP, Tai DI, Lan KH, Li AF, Hsu HC, Lin EJ, Lin YP, Sheu ML, Li CP, Chang FY, Chao Y, Yen SH, Lee SD. The -251T allele of the interleukin-8 promoter is associated with increased risk of gastric carcinoma featuring diffuse-type histopathology in Chinese population. Clin Cancer Res. 2005;11(18):6431-41.

Leung WK, To KF, Go MY, Chan KK, Chan FK, Ng EK, Chung SC, Sung JJ. Cyclooxygenase-2 upregulates vascular endothelial growth factor expression and angiogenesis in human gastric carcinoma. Int J Oncol. 2003;23(5):1317-22.

Lewis ND, Asim M, Barry DP, Singh K, de Sablet T, Boucher JL, Gobert AP, Chaturvedi R, Wilson KT. Arginase II restricts host defense to *Helicobacter pylori* by attenuating inducible nitric oxide synthase translation in macrophages. J Immunol. 2010;184(5):2572-82.

Li C, Xia B, Yang Y, Li J, Xia HH. TNF gene polymorphisms and *Helicobacter pylori* infection in gastric carcinogenesis in Chinese population. Am J Gastroenterol. 2005;100(2):290-4.

Li C, Xia HH, Xie W, Hu Z, Ye M, Li J, Cheng H, Zhang X, Xia B. Association between interleukin-1 gene polymorphisms and *Helicobacter pylori* infection in gastric carcinogenesis in a Chinese population. J Gastroenterol Hepatol. 2007;22(2):234-9.

Li Q, Liu N, Shen B, Zhou L, Wang Y, Wang Y, Sun J, Fan Z, Liu RH. *Helicobacter pylori* enhances cyclooxygenase 2 expression via p38MAPK/ATF-2 signalling pathway in MKN45 cells. Cancer Lett. 2009;278(1):97-103.

Lin JT, Wang JT, Wang TH, Wu MS, Chen CJ. *Helicobacter pylori* infection in early and advanced gastric adenocarcinoma: a seroprevalence study in 143 Taiwanese patients. Hepatogastroenterology. 1993;40(6):596-9.

Lu W, Pan K, Zhang L, Lin D, Miao X, You W. Genetic polymorphisms of interleukin (IL)-1B, IL-1RN, IL-8, IL-10 and tumor necrosis factor {alpha} and risk of gastric cancer in a Chinese population. Carcinogenesis. 2005;26(3):631-6.

Lundin BS, Enarsson K, Kindlund B, Lundgren A, Johnsson E, Quiding-Järbrink M, Svennerholm AM. The local and systemic T-cell response to *Helicobacter pylori* in gastric cancer patients is characterised by production of interleukin-10. Clin Immunol. 2007;125(2):205-13.

Manojlovic N, Babic D, Filipovic-Ljeshovic I, Pilcevic D. Anti *Helicobacter pylori* IgG and IgA response in patients with gastric cancer and chronic gastritis. Hepatogastroenterology. 2008;55(82-83):807-13.

Manojlovic N, Nikolic L, Pilcevic D, Josifovski J, Babic D. Systemic humoral anti-*Helicobacter pylori* immune response in patients with gastric malignancies and benign gastroduodenal disease. Hepatogastroenterology. 2004;51(55):282-4.

Marotti B, Rocco A, De Colibus P, Compare D, de Nucci G, Staibano S, Tatangelo F, Romano M, Nardone G. Interleukin-13 mucosal production in *Helicobacter pylori*-related gastric diseases. Dig Liver Dis. 2008;40(4):240-7.

Marrelli D, Pedrazzani C, Berardi A, Corso G, Neri A, Garosi L, Vindigni C, Santucci A, Figura N, Roviello F. Negative *Helicobacter pylori* status is associated with poor prognosis in patients with gastric cancer. Cancer 2009;115(10):2071-80.

Matysiak-Budnik T & Mégraud F. *Helicobacter pylori* infection and gastric cancer. Eur J Cancer 2006; 42: 708-16.

Mbulaiteye SM, Gold BD, Pfeiffer RM, Brubaker GR, Shao J, Biggar RJ, Hisada M. *H. pylori*-infection and antibody immune response in a rural Tanzanian population. Infect Agent Cancer. 2006; 1:3.

McGee DJ, Mobley HL. Pathogenesis of *Helicobacter pylori* infection. Curr Opin Gastroenterol. 2000;16(1):24-31.

McNamara D, El-Omar E. *Helicobacter pylori* infection and the pathogenesis of gastric cancer: a paradigm for host-bacterial interactions. Dig Liver Dis. 2008;40(7):504-9.

Meimarakis G, Winter H, Assmann I, Kopp R, Lehn N, Kist M, Stolte M, Jauch KW, Hatz RA. *Helicobacter pylori* as a prognostic indicator after curative resection of gastric carcinoma: a prospective study. Lancet Oncol 2006; 7(3): 211-22.

Mimuro H, Suzuki T, Tanaka J, Asahi M, Haas R, Sasakawa C. Grb2 is a key mediator of *Helicobacter pylori* CagA protein activities. Mol Cell. 2002; 10(4):745-55.

Mollenhauer-Rektorschek M, Hanauer G, Sachs G, Melchers K. Expression of UreI is required for intragastric transit and colonization of gerbil gastric mucosa by *Helicobacter pylori*. Res Microbiol. 2002;153(10):659-66.

Moran AP. The role of endotoxin in infection: *Helicobacter pylori* and Campylobacter jejuni. Subcell Biochem. 2010;53:209-40.

Moran, AP. The role of lipopolysaccharide in *Helicobacter pylori* pathogenesis. Aliment. Pharmacol. Ther. 1996;10 (suppl. 1), 39-50.

Morgan DR, Dominguez RL, Keku TO, Heidt PE, Martin CF, Galanko JA, Omofoye OA, Sandler RS. Gastric cancer and the high combination prevalence of host cytokine genotypes and *Helicobacter pylori* in Honduras. Clin Gastroenterol Hepatol. 2006;4(9):1103-11.

Muñoz L, Camorlinga M, Hernández R, Giono S, Ramón G, Muñoz O, Torres J. Immune and proliferative cellular responses to *Helicobacter pylori* infection in the gastric mucosa of Mexican children. Helicobacter. 2007;12(3):224-30.

Murakami K, Kodama M, Sato R, Okimoto T, Watanabe K, Fujioka T. *Helicobacter pylori* eradication and associated changes in the gastric mucosa. Expert Rev Anti Infect Ther 2005; 3(5): 757-64.

Nilsson C, Skoglund A, Moran AP, Annuk H, Engstrand L, Normark S. An enzymatic ruler modulates Lewis antigen glycosylation of *Helicobacter pylori* LPS during persistent infection. Proc Natl Acad Sci USA. 2006;103(8):2863-8.

Obonyo M, Sabet M, Cole SP, Ebmeyer J, Uematsu S, Akira S, Guiney DG. Deficiencies of myeloid differentiation factor 88, Toll-like receptor 2 (TLR2), or TLR4 produce specific defects in macrophage cytokine secretion induced by *Helicobacter pylori*. Infect Immun. 2007;75(5):2408-14.

Odenbreit S. Adherence properties of *Helicobacter pylori*: impact on pathogenesis and adaptation to the host. Int J Med Microbiol. 2005;295(5):317-24

Ohyauchi M, Imatani A, Yonechi M, Asano N, Miura A, Iijima K, Koike T, Sekine H, Ohara S, Shimosegawa T. The polymorphism interleukin 8 -251 A/T influences the susceptibility of *Helicobacter pylori* related gastric diseases in the Japanese population. Gut. 2005;54(3):330-5.

Oliveira AG, Santos A, Guerra JB, Rocha GA, Rocha AM, Oliveira CA, Cabral MM, Nogueira AM, Queiroz DM. babA2- and cagA-positive *Helicobacter pylori* strains are associated with duodenal ulcer and gastric carcinoma in Brazil. J Clin Microbiol. 2003;41(8):3964-6.

Oliveira MJ, Costa AC, Costa AM, Henriques L, Suriano G, Atherton JC, Machado JC, Carneiro F, Seruca R, Mareel M, Leroy A, Figueiredo C. *Helicobacter pylori* induces gastric epithelial cell invasion in a c-Met and type IV secretion system-dependent manner. J Biol Chem. 2006;281(46):34888-96.

Palli D, Saieva C, Luzzi I, Masala G, Topa S, Sera F, Gemma S, Zanna I, D'Errico M, Zini E, Guidotti S, Valeri A, Fabbrucci P, Moretti R, Testai E, del Giudice G, Ottini L, Matullo G, Dogliotti E, Gomez-Miguel MJ. Interleukin-1 gene polymorphisms and gastric cancer risk in a high-risk Italian population. Am J Gastroenterol. 2005;100(9):1941-8.

Park ES, Do IG, Park CK, Kang WK, Noh JH, Sohn TS, Kim S, Kim MJ, Kim KM. Cyclooxygenase-2 is an independent prognostic factor in gastric carcinoma patients receiving adjuvant chemotherapy and is not associated with EBV infection. Clin Cancer Res. 2009;15(1):291-8.

Partida-Rodríguez O, Torres J, Flores-Luna L, Camorlinga M, Nieves-Ramírez M, Lazcano E, Perez-Rodríguez M. Polymorphisms in TNF and HSP-70 show a significant association with gastric cancer and duodenal ulcer. Int J Cancer. 2010;126(8):1861-8.

Peek RM Jr. Pathogenesis of *Helicobacter pylori* infection. Springer Semin Immun. 2005; 27:197-215.

Persson C, Engstrand L, Nyrén O, Hansson LE, Enroth H, Ekström AM, Ye W. Interleukin 1-beta gene polymorphisms and risk of gastric cancer in Sweden. Scand J Gastroenterol. 2009;44(3):339-45.

Przyklenk B, Bauernfeind A, Bornschein W, Emminger G, Heilmann K, Schweighart S. The role of Campylobacter (Helicobacter) pylori in disorders of the gastrointestinal tract. Infection. 1990;18(1):3-7.

Quiros RM, Bui CL. Multidisciplinary approach to esophageal and gastric cancer, Surg. Clin. North Am. 2009;89(1): 79-96 , viii.

Rad R, Dossumbekova A, Neu B, Lang R, Bauer S, Saur D, Gerhard M, Prinz C. Cytokine gene polymorphisms influence mucosal cytokine expression, gastric inflammation, and host specific colonisation during *Helicobacter pylori* infection. Gut. 2004;53(8):1082-9

Rautelin HI, Oksanen AM, Karttunen RA, Seppälä KM, Virtamo JR, Aromaa AJ, Kosunen TU. Association of CagA-positive infection with *Helicobacter pylori* antibodies of IgA class. Ann Med. 2000;32(9):652-6.

Rieder G, Hofmann JA, Hatz RA, Stolte M, Enders GA. Up-regulation of inducible nitric oxide synthase in *Helicobacter pylori*-associated gastritis may represent an increased risk factor to develop gastric carcinoma of the intestinal type. Int J Med Microbiol. 2003;293(6):403-12.

Rossi G, Romagnoli S, Lauretti L, Pancotto L, Taccini E, Rappuoli R, Del Giudice G, Ruggiero P. *Helicobacter pylori* infection negatively influences pregnancy outcome in a mouse model. Helicobacter. 2004;9(2):152-7.

Rudi J, Kolb C, Maiwald M, Zuna I, von Herbay A, Galle PR, Stremmel W. Serum antibodies against *Helicobacter pylori* proteins VacA and CagA are associated with increased risk for gastric adenocarcinoma. Dig Dis Sci 1997; 42(8):1652-9.

Ruzzo A, Graziano F, Pizzagalli F, Santini D, Battistelli V, Panunzi S, Canestrari E, Catalano V, Humar B, Ficarelli R, Bearzi I, Cascinu S, Naldi N, Testa E, Magnani M. Interleukin 1B gene (IL-1B) and interleukin 1 receptor antagonist gene (IL-1RN) polymorphisms in *Helicobacter pylori*-negative gastric cancer of intestinal and diffuse histotype. Ann Oncol. 2005;16(6):887-92.

Sakuma K, Uozaki H, Chong JM, Hironaka M, Sudo M, Ushiku T, Nagai H, Fukayama M. Cancer risk to the gastric corpus in Japanese, its correlation with interleukin-1beta gene polymorphism (+3953*T) and Epstein-Barr virus infection. Int J Cancer. 2005;115(1):93-7.

Sánchez-Zauco NA, Giono-Cerezo S, Maldonado-Bernal C. [Toll-like receptors, pathogenesis and immune response to *Helicobacter pylori*]. Salud Publica Mex. 2010;52(5):447-54.

Saxena A, Prasad KN, Ghoshal UC, Bhagat MR, Krishnani N, Husain N. Polymorphism of -765G > C COX-2 is a risk factor for gastric adenocarcinoma and peptic ulcer disease in addition to H pylori infection: a study from northern India. World J Gastroenterol. 2008;14(10):1498-503.

Segal I, Ally R, Mitchell H. *Helicobacter pylori*--an African perspective. QJM. 2001;94(10):561-5.

Selbach M, Moese S, Hauck CR, Meyer TF, Backert S. Src is the kinase of *Helicobacter pylori* CagA protein *in vitro* and *in vivo*. J Biol Chem 2002; 277(9): 6775-8.

Seno H, Satoh K, Tsuji S, Shiratsuchi T, Harada Y, Hamajima N, Sugano K, Kawano S, Chiba T. Novel interleukin-4 and interleukin-1 receptor antagonist gene variations associated with non-cardia gastric cancer in Japan: comprehensive analysis of 207 polymorphisms of 11 cytokine genes. J Gastroenterol Hepatol. 2007;22(5):729-37.

Seo JH, Kim KH, Kim H. Role of proteinase-activated receptor-2 on cyclooxygenase-2 expression in *H. pylori*-infected gastric epithelial cells. Ann N Y Acad Sci. 2007;1096:29-36.

Sheu SM, Sheu BS, Yang HB, Li C, Chu TC, Wu JJ. Presence of iceA1 but not cagA, cagC, cagE, cagF, cagN, cagT, or orf13 genes of *Helicobacter pylori* is associated with more severe gastric inflammation in Taiwanese. J Formos Med Assoc. 2002;101(1):18-23.

Shin WG, Jang JS, Kim HS, Kim SJ, Kim KH, Jang MK, Lee JH, Kim HJ, Kim HY. Polymorphisms of interleukin-1 and interleukin-2 genes in patients with gastric cancer in Korea. J Gastroenterol Hepatol. 2008;23(10):1567-73.

Shiotani A, Iishi H, Kumamoto M, Nakae Y. *Helicobacter pylori* infection and increased nitrite synthesis in the stomach. Inflammation and atrophy connections. Dig Liver Dis. 2004;36(5):327-32.

Shirai K, Ohmiya N, Taguchi A, Mabuchi N, Yatsuya H, Itoh A, Hirooka Y, Niwa Y, Mori N, Goto H. Interleukin-8 gene polymorphism associated with susceptibility to non-cardia gastric carcinoma with microsatellite instability. J Gastroenterol Hepatol. 2006;21(7):1129-35.

Sicinschi LA, Lopez-Carrillo L, Camargo MC, Correa P, Sierra RA, Henry RR, Chen J, Zabaleta J, Piazuelo MB, Schneider BG. Gastric cancer risk in a Mexican population: role of *Helicobacter pylori* CagA positive infection and polymorphisms in interleukin-1 and -10 genes. Int J Cancer. 2006;118(3):649-57.

Snider JL, Cardelli JA. *Helicobacter pylori* induces cancer cell motility independent of the c-Met receptor. J Carcinog. 2009;8:7

Sokic-Milutinovic A, Wex T, Todorovic V, Milosavljevic T, Malfertheiner P. Anti-CagA and anti-VacA antibodies in *Helicobacter pylori*-infected patients with and without peptic ulcer disease in Serbia and Montenegro. Scand J Gastroenterol 2004; 39(3): 222-6.

Son HJ, Rhee JC, Park DI, Kim YH, Rhee PL, Koh KC, Paik SW, Choi KW, Kim JJ. Inducible nitric oxide synthase expression in gastroduodenal diseases infected with *Helicobacter pylori*. Helicobacter. 2001;6(1):37-43.

Starzyńska T, Ferenc K, Wex T, Kähne T, Lubiński J, Lawniczak M, Marlicz K, Malfertheiner P. The association between the interleukin-1 polymorphisms and gastric cancer risk depends on the family history of gastric carcinoma in the study population. Am J Gastroenterol. 2006;101(2):248-54.

Stingl K, Uhlemann EM, Schmid R, Altendorf K, Bakker EP. Energetics of *Helicobacter pylori* and its implications for the mechanism of urease-dependent acid tolerance at pH 1. J Bacteriol. 2002;184(11):3053-60.

Sugimoto M, Furuta T, Shirai N, Nakamura A, Xiao F, Kajimura M, Sugimura H, Hishida A. Different effects of polymorphisms of tumor necrosis factor-alpha and interleukin-1 beta on development of peptic ulcer and gastric cancer. J Gastroenterol Hepatol. 2007;22(1):51-9.

Sugimoto M, Furuta T, Shirai N, Nakamura A, Kajimura M, Sugimura H, Hishida A. Effects of interleukin-10 gene polymorphism on the development of gastric cancer and peptic ulcer in Japanese subjects. J Gastroenterol Hepatol. 2007;22(9):1443-9.

Sugimoto M, Yamaoka Y, Furuta T. Influence of interleukin polymorphisms on development of gastric cancer and peptic ulcer. World J Gastroenterol. 2010;16(10):1188-200.

Suzuki M, Mimuro H, Kiga K, Fukumatsu M, Ishijima N, Morikawa H, Nagai S, Koyasu S, Gilman RH, Kersulyte D, Berg DE, Sasakawa C. *Helicobacter pylori* CagA phosphorylation-independent function in epithelial proliferation and inflammation. Cell Host Microbe. 2009;5(1):23-34.

Taguchi A, Ohmiya N, Shirai K, Mabuchi N, Itoh A, Hirooka Y, Niwa Y, Goto H. Interleukin-8 promoter polymorphism increases the risk of atrophic gastritis and gastric cancer in Japan. Cancer Epidemiol Biomarkers Prev. 2005;14(11 Pt 1):2487-93.

Takahashi T, Yujiri T, Shinohara K, Inoue Y, Sato Y, Fujii Y, Okubo M, Zaitsu Y, Ariyoshi K, Nakamura Y, Nawata R, Oka Y, Shirai M, Tanizawa Y. Molecular mimicry by *Helicobacter pylori* CagA protein may be involved in the pathogenesis of *H. pylori*-associated chronic idiopathic thrombocytopenic purpura. Br J Haematol 2004; 124(1): 91-6.

Takehara H, Iwamoto J, Mizokami Y, Takahashi K, Ootubo T, Miura S, Narasaka T, Takeyama H, Omata T, Shimokobe K, Ito M, Matsuoka T. Involvement of cyclooxygenase-2--prostaglandin E2 pathway in interleukin-8 production in gastric cancer cells. Dig Dis Sci. 2006;51(12):2188-97.

Tanaka A, Kamada T, Yokota K, Shiotani A, Hata J, Oguma K, Haruma K. *Helicobacter pylori* heat shock protein 60 antibodies are associated with gastric cancer. Pathol Res Pract. 2009;205(10):690-4.

Tatemichi M, Ogura T, Nagata H, Esumi H. Enhanced expression of inducible nitric oxide synthase in chronic gastritis with intestinal metaplasia. J Clin Gastroenterol. 1998;27(3):240-5.

Tatemichi M, Sawa T, Gilibert I, Tazawa H, Katoh T, Ohshima H. Increased risk of intestinal type of gastric adenocarcinoma in Japanese women associated with long forms of CCTTT pentanucleotide repeat in the inducible nitric oxide synthase promoter. Cancer Lett. 2005;217(2):197-202.

Taylor JM, Ziman ME, Huff JL, Moroski NM, Vajdy M, Solnick JV. *Helicobacter pylori* lipopolysaccharide promotes a Th1 type immune response in immunized mice. Vaccine. 2006;24(23):4987-94.

Tiwari SK, Manoj G, Sharma V, Sivaram G, Saikant R, Bardia A, Sharma VK, Abid Z, Khan AA, Habeeb MA, Habibullah CM, Kumar BS, Nandan A. Relevance of *Helicobacter pylori* genotypes in gastric pathology and its association with plasma malondialdehyde and nitric oxide levels. Inflammopharmacology. 2010;18(2):59-64.

Toller IM, Hitzler I, Sayi A, Mueller A. Prostaglandin E2 prevents Helicobacter-induced gastric preneoplasia and facilitates persistent infection in a mouse model. Gastroenterology. 2010;138(4):1455-67, 1467.e1-4.

Tomb JF, White O, Kerlavage AR, Clayton RA, Sutton GG, Fleischmann RD, Ketchum KA, Klenk HP, Gill S, Dougherty BA, Nelson K, Quackenbush J, Zhou L, Kirkness EF, Peterson S, Loftus B, Richardson D, Dodson R, Khalak HG, Glodek A, McKenney K, Fitzegerald LM, Lee N, Adams MD, Hickey EK, Berg DE, Gocayne JD, Utterback TR, Peterson JD, Kelley JM, Cotton MD, Weidman JM, Fujii C, Bowman C, Watthey L, Wallin E, Hayes WS, Borodovsky M, Karp PD, Smith HO, Fraser CM, Venter JC. The complete genome sequence of the gastric pathogen *Helicobacter pylori*. Nature.1997;388(6642):539-47.

Torres MM, Acosta CP, Sicard DM, et al. [Genetic susceptibility and risk of gastric cancer in a human population of Cauca, Colombia] Biomedica. 2004;24(2):153-62.

Tsai HF & Hsu PN. Interplay between *Helicobacter pylori* and immune cells in immune pathogenesis of gastric inflammation and mucosal pathology. Cell Mol Immunol. 2010;7(4):255-9.

Tsuji S, Tsujii M, Murata H, Nishida T, Komori M, Yasumaru M, Ishii S, Sasayama Y, Kawano S, Hayashi N. *Helicobacter pylori* eradication to prevent gastric cancer: underlying molecular and cellular mechanisms. World J Gastroenterol. 2006;12(11):1671-80.

Turbett GR, Høj PB, Horne R, Mee BJ. Purification and characterization of the urease enzymes of Helicobacter species from humans and animals. Infect Immun. 1992;60(12):5259-66.

Umehara S, Higashi H, Ohnishi N, Asaka M, Hatakeyama M. Effects of *Helicobacter pylori* CagA protein on the growth and survival of B lymphocytes, the origin of MALT lymphoma. Oncogene. 2003;22(51):8337-42.

van den Engel NK, Winter H, Rüttinger D, Shau I, Schiller M, Mayer B, Moudgil T, Meimarakis G, Stolte M, Jauch KW, Fox BA, Hatz RA. Characterization of immune responses in gastric cancer patients: a possible impact of *H. pylori* to polarize a tumor-specific type 1 response? Clin Immunol. 2006;120(3):285-96.

Varro A, Noble PJ, Pritchard DM, Kennedy S, Hart CA, Dimaline R, Dockray GJ. *Helicobacter pylori* induces plasminogen activator inhibitor 2 in gastric epithelial cells through nuclear factor-kappaB and RhoA: implications for invasion and apoptosis. Cancer Res. 2004;64(5):1695-702.

Vaucher C, Janvier B, Nousbaum JB, Grignon B, Pezennec L, Robaszkiewicz M, Gouerou H, Picard B, Fauchere JL. Antibody response of patients with *Helicobacter pylori*-related gastric adenocarcinoma: significance of anti-cagA antibodies. Clin Diagn Lab Immunol 2000; 7(3): 463-7.

Vieth M, Stolte M. Elevated risk for gastric adenocarcinoma can be predicted from histomorphology. World J Gastroenterol. 2006;12(38):6109-14.

Vivas JR, Regnault B, Michel V, Bussière FI, Avé P, Huerre M, Labigne A, D' Elios MM, Touati E. Interferon gamma-signature transcript profiling and IL-23 upregulation in response to *Helicobacter pylori* infection. Int J Immunopathol Pharmacol. 2008;21(3):515-26.

Vorobjova T, Ren Z, Dunkley M, Clancy R, Maaroos HI, Labotkin R, Kull K, Uibo R. Response of IgG1 and IgG2 subclasses to *Helicobacter pylori* in subjects with chronic inflammation of the gastric mucosa, atrophy and gastric cancer in a country with high *Helicobacter pylori* infection prevalence. APMIS. 2006;114(5):372-80.

Walduck AK, Weber M, Wunder C, Juettner S, Stolte M, Vieth M, Wiedenmann B, Meyer TF, Naumann M, Hoecker M. Identification of novel cyclooxygenase-2-dependent genes in *Helicobacter pylori* infection *in vivo*. Mol Cancer. 2009;8:22.

Wang SK, Zhu HF, He BS, Zhang ZY, Chen ZT, Wang ZZ, Wu GL. CagA+ H pylori infection is associated with polarization of T helper cell immune responses in gastric carcinogenesis. World J Gastroenterol. 2007;13(21):2923-31.

Wex T, Leodolter A, Bornschein J, Kuester D, Kähne T, Kropf S, Albrecht C, Naumann M, Roessner A, Malfertheiner P. Interleukin 1 beta (IL1B) gene polymorphisms are not associated with gastric carcinogenesis in Germany. Anticancer Res. 2010;30(2):505-11.

Wong BC, Lam SK, Wong WM, Chen JS, Zheng TT, Feng RE, Lai KC, Hu WH, Yuen ST, Leung SY, Fong DY, Ho J, Ching CK, Chen JS; China Gastric Cancer Study Group. *Helicobacter pylori* Eradication to Prevent Gastric Cancer in a High-Risk Region of China: A Randomized Controlled Trial. JAMA. 2004;291(2):187-194

Wu MS, Lin JT, Hsu PN, Lin CY, Hsieh YT, Chiu YH, Hsueh PR, Liao KW. Preferential induction of transforming growth factor-beta production in gastric epithelial cells and monocytes by *Helicobacter pylori* soluble proteins. J Infect Dis. 2007;196(9):1386-93.

Wu MS, Wu CY, Chen CJ, Lin MT, Shun CT, Lin JT. Interleukin-10 genotypes associate with the risk of gastric carcinoma in Taiwanese Chinese. Int J Cancer. 2003;104(5):617-23.

Wu YY, Tsai HF, Lin WC, Hsu PI, Shun CT, Wu MS, Hsu PN. Upregulation of CCL20 and recruitment of CCR6+ gastric infiltrating lymphocytes in *Helicobacter pylori* gastritis. Infect Immun. 2007;75(9):4357-63.

Xia HH, Talley NJ. Apoptosis in gastric epithelium induced by *Helicobacter pylori* infection: implications in gastric carcinogenesis. Am J Gastroenterol. 2001;96(1):16-26.

Xiao H, Jiang Y, Li R, Xia B. [Association of IL-10 gene polymorphisms with gastroduodenal diseases in Hubei Han population]. Zhonghua Yi Xue Yi Chuan Xue Za Zhi. 2009;26(4):423-6.

Xue LJ, Su QS, Yang JH, Lin Y. Autoimmune responses induced by *Helicobacter pylori* improve the prognosis of gastric carcinoma. Med Hypotheses. 2008;70(2):273-6.

Yamaoka Y, Kodama T, Kita M, Imanishi J, Kashima K, Graham DY. Relation between cytokines and *Helicobacter pylori* in gastric cancer. Helicobacter. 2001;6(2):116-24.

Yang J, Hu Z, Xu Y, Shen J, Niu J, Hu X, Guo J, Wei Q, Wang X, Shen H. Interleukin-1B gene promoter variants are associated with an increased risk of gastric cancer in a Chinese population. Cancer Lett. 2004;215(2):191-8.

Yang JJ, Ko KP, Cho LY, Shin A, Gwack J, Chang SH, Shin HR, Yoo KY, Kang D, Park SK. The role of TNF genetic variants and the interaction with cigarette smoking for gastric cancer risk: a nested case-control study. BMC Cancer. 2009;9:238.

Yoo EJ, Park SY, Cho NY, Kim N, Lee HS, Kim D, Kang GH. Influence of IL1B polymorphism on CpG island hypermethylation in *Helicobacter pylori*-infected gastric cancer. Virchows Arch. 2010;456(6):647-52.

Zabaleta J, Camargo MC, Ritchie MD, Piazuelo MB, Sierra RA, Turner SD, Delgado A, Fontham ET, Schneider BG, Correa P, Ochoa AC. Association of haplotypes of inflammation-related genes with gastric preneoplastic lesions in African Americans and Caucasians. Int J Cancer. 2011;128(3):668-75.

Zabaleta J, McGee DJ, Zea AH, Hernández CP, Rodriguez PC, Sierra RA, Correa P, Ochoa AC. *Helicobacter pylori* arginase inhibits T cell proliferation and reduces the expression of the TCR zeta-chain (CD3zeta). J Immunol. 2004;173(1):586-93.

Zambon CF, Basso D, Navaglia F, Belluco C, Falda A, Fogar P, Greco E, Gallo N, Rugge M, Di Mario F, Plebani M. Pro- and anti-inflammatory cytokines gene polymorphisms and *Helicobacter pylori* infection: interactions influence outcome. Cytokine. 2005;29(4):141-52.

Zhang LJ, Wang SY, Huo XH, Zhu ZL, Chu JK, Ma JC, Cui DS, Gu P, Zhao ZR, Wang MW, Yu J. Anti-*Helicobacter pylori* therapy followed by celecoxib on progression of gastric precancerous lesions. World J Gastroenterol. 2009;15(22):2731-8.

Zhang XM, Miao XP, Tan W, Sun T, Guo YL, Zhao D, Lin DX. [Genetic polymorphisms in the promoter region of cyclooxygenase-2 and their association with risk of gastric cancer]. Zhongguo Yi Xue Ke Xue Yuan Xue Bao. 2006;28(2):119-23.

Zhu F, Loh M, Hill J, Lee S, Koh KX, Lai KW, Salto-Tellez M, Iacopetta B, Yeoh KG, Soong R; Singapore Gastric Cancer Consortium. Genetic factors associated with intestinal metaplasia in a high risk Singapore-Chinese population: a cohort study. BMC Gastroenterol. 2009;9:76.

Zhu KX, Li YM, Li X, Zhou WC, Shan Y, Liu T. Study on the association of COX-2 genetic polymorphisms with risk of gastric cancer in high incidence Hexi area of Gansu province in China. Mol Biol Rep. 2011;38(1):649-55.

Zhuang X, Lin S, Zheng J, Wang L, Sun G, Li Y. The prognostic research of expression and relationship between *Helicobacter pylori* of c-met oncogene correlation with gastric mucosal proliferation. Zhonghua Nei Ke Za Zhi. 2001;40(6):381-4.

Part 4

Current and Future Treatment

14

Gastric Carcinoma Neoadjuvant and Adjuvant Therapy

Yüksel Ürün[1], Ali Ayberk Beşen[2] and Hüseyin Abalı[2]
[1]*Ankara University School of Medicine, Department of Internal Medicine, Division of Medical Oncology,*
[2]*Baskent University School of Medicine,Department of Internal Medicine, Division of Medical Oncology, Turkey*

1. Introduction

1.1 Epidemiology

In the last 80 years, the incidence of gastric cancer and gastric cancer-related mortality has decreased significantly. However, gastric cancer is the 4th most common cancer and the 2nd common cause of cancer associated mortality in the world (Crew, K.D. Neugut, A.I., 2006, Ferlay, J., et al., 2010, Ferlay, J., et al., 2010, Jemal, A., et al., 2010, Krejs, G.J., 2010, Malvezzi, M., et al., 2010, Sasako, M., et al., 2010, Shin, H.R., et al., 2010). Gastric cancer according to anatomic location in the stomach, proximal (cardia) and distal (noncardia) is divided into 2 groups. Although decreasing, distal located tumors are still the most common type in developing countries. While there is an increase in proximal located tumors, the distal located gastric cancers have been decreasing in western societies (Ferlay, J., et al., 2010, Krejs, G.J., 2010, Malvezzi, M., et al., 2010). More than 90% of gastric cancers are adenocarcinomas and can be either intestinal, or diffuse type (Crew, K.D. Neugut, A.I., 2006, Krejs, G.J., 2010).

The incidence vary significantly throughout the world. More than half of all gastric cancers in the world are seen in eastern Asia (Sasako, M., et al., 2010). Korea and Japan had the highest incidence countries. While its incidence is 60/100.000 for men and 25/100.000 for women in Korea and Japan (Long, N., et al., 2010), it is around 5/100.000 for Australia and New Zealand (Crew, K.D. Neugut, A.I., 2006, Ferlay, J., et al., 2010, Krejs, G.J., 2010, Malvezzi, M., et al., 2010, Sasako, M., et al., 2010, Shin, H.R., et al., 2010). Often seen in whites aged 60-80, the male to female ratio is 2:1, which rises up to 5:1 for proximal tumors (Krejs, G.J., 2010). The main risk factors related to the development of gastric cancer are Helicobacter pylori infection, dietary factors, tobacco use and obesity (Crew, K.D. Neugut, A.I., 2006, Krejs, G.J., 2010, Sasako, M., et al., 2010). Having been the most important cancer-related mortality in the United States in the 1930s for both sexes, its incidence and mortality rates have dramatically decreased over the years. For the year 2010, 21.000 new cases and 11.000 deaths from stomach cancer are estimated in the United States (Jemal, A., et al., 2010). As the 4th most common cause of cancer-related deaths, gastric cancer incidence and mortality rates among the European countries also show significant variations (Ferlay, J., et al., 2010, Krejs, G.J., 2010, Malvezzi, M., et al., 2010). The incidence of stomach cancer in men is 8/100.000 and in women 3-4/100.000 in European Union (EU) countries. For Russia, these rates are 25 and 10 and for United Kingdom (UK) 5-6, and 2-3, respectively. Although decreased in major European countries, mortality rates still high in eastern and southern Europe with an estimated new cases of 150.000 and gastric cancer-related mortality 116.000 for the year 2008 (Ferlay, J., et al., 2010).

1.2 Surgical therapy

There is no doubt that the only curative treatment option for gastric cancer is gastrectomy and regional lymph node dissection (Swan, R. Miner, T.J., 2006, Tanizawa, Y. Terashima, M., 2010), although the most appropriate surgery and lymph node dissection are still controversial. The debate about surgical approach and extent of lymph node dissection continuing. In early gastric cancer, which is confined to the mucosa or submucosa, in Japan and Korea in particular, endoscopic mucosal dissection and endoscopic submucuosal resection is the usual management (Deprez, P.H., et al., 2010, Kim, J.J., et al., 2007).

Although there are some discussions, subtotal gastrectomy and total gastrectomy is considered to be similar in terms of survival. The complex lymph nodes of stomach are classified by Japanese Gastric Cancer Association. According to this classification regional lymph nodes are divided to 3 groups according to the location of the primary tumor and lymph node dissection is separated into the D0, D1, D2 and D3. Perigastric lymph nodes have been recognized as D1 and the ones around the main branches of the celiac axis as D2 (Japanese Gastric Cancer, A., 1998). The extent of lymph node dissection in gastric cancer surgery is one of the most controversial issues. D2 dissection was performed as a standard approach in Japan, Korea, and some Western countries. D1 dissection is done in many western countries. One of the most well-known studies on this subject is the work of Dutch Gastric Cancer Group. In this study comparing D1 and D2 dissections, a 5-year overall survival and risk of relapse were similar, but perioperative mortality and complication rates were statistically significantly higher in D2 arm (Bonenkamp, J.J., et al., 1999). In a meta-analysis, the benefit of the addition of paraaortic lymphadenectomy (PALD) to D2 dissection was discussed and concluded that additional PALD didn't show survival benefit and was evaluated as less secure (Chen, X.Z., et al., 2010).

D2 dissection and D2 with PALD were compared. While surgery related complication rate were similar between D2 and PALD groups, 5-year overall survival rates were 69.2% in D2 arm and 70.3% in PALD arm [HR (hazard ratio) 1.03, CI (confidence interval) 0.77-1.37, p = 0.85] (Sasako, M., et al., 2008).

The 15 year results of Dutch study was recently published. The median follow-up was 15.2 years. D1 arm had higher locoregional relapse rate and higher gastric cancer related death rate (182, 48%) than D2 arm (123, 37%) (p =0.01). However, the overall survival rate of the D1 arm at 15 years (21%, 85 of 380) and D2 arm (29%, 98 of 331) were similar (p = 0.34) (Songun, I., et al., 2010). You can see key elements of related trials in Table 1.

In the meta-analysis of Yang and colleagues, it was shown that splenectomy didn't have benefit and is not recommended as a routine practice (Yang, K., et al., 2009). However, current National Comprehensive Cancer Network (NCCN) guideline recommends D1 (perigastric lymph nodes) and D2 (along in with named vessels of celiac axis) dissection, with a goal of at least 15 lymph nodes removed at moderate to high volume centers (Ajani, J.A., 2011). Although D2 procedure has a higher postoperative mortality and morbidity, it is being applied as a standard approach with confidence at many large centers.

Study	Intervention	Patients (n)	Postoperative Morbidity	Postoperative Mortality	5-Year Survival
Dutch trial (1989-1993)	D1 vs. D2	380/331	25.0%/43.0% (p<0,001)	4.0%/10.0% (p<0,004)	45.0%/47.0%, HR 1.00 (95% CI, 0.82-1.22)
MRC trial (1987-1994)	D1 vs. D2	200/200	28.0%/46.0% (p<0,001)	6.5%/13.0% (p=0,04)	35.0%/33.0%, HR 1.10 (95% CI, 0.87-1.39)
Taiwanese trial	D1 vs. D3	110/111	7.3%/17.1% (p<0,012)	0%/0%	53.6%/59.5%, HR 0.49 (95% CI, 0.32-0.77)
IGCSG trial (1999-2002)	D1 vs. D2	76/86	10.5%/16.3% (p<0,29)	0%/1.3% N.S	Under analysis

Table 1. Major randomized controlled trials comparing D1 with D2/D3 (Tanizawa, Y. Terashima, M., 2010)

1.3 Prognostic factors and relapse pattern

Based on 10 year results of the "German Gastric Cancer Study," (Siewert, J.R., et al., 1998) they evaluated prognostic factors and they showed that lymph node ratio (ratio between positive and removed nodes; p<0.0001), residual tumor category (R0, Rl, R2; p <0.0001), pT-category (pTl, pT2, pT3 and pT4; p<0.0001, postoperative complications (p<0.0001), distant metastases (MO, Ml; p=0.003) affected prognosis. In a prospective multicenter study; it was shown that nodal status, depth of invasion, limited or extended lymphadenectomy (D1 vs. D2-D3), tumor location (lower vs. upper) and age were independent predictors of recurrence (Marrelli, D., et al., 2005). It was also shown that T (T2 vs. T3, risk ratio 3.55, 95% CI 1.98-6.44 and p: 0.001) and histological type (intestinal vs. diffuse/mixed, risk ratio 2.11, 95% CI 1.25-2.95 and p: 0.021) were independent prognostics indicator in node negative gastric cancer patients (Baiocchi, G.L., et al., 2010). Depth of tumor invasion and nodal involvement are considered the most important prognostic factors (Marrelli, D., et al., 2005). Although in many cases surgical treatment is the primary treatment, usually locoregional, hematogenous, and peritoneal recurrences are seen and in patients with developing relapse an effective treatment option isn't available (Marrelli, D., et al., 2005). Studies have demonstrated that at least half of all patients who undergo curative resection will have locoregional, peritoneal or distant recurrence (Table 2) (Baiocchi, G.L., et al., 2010, Bonenkamp, J.J., et al., 1999, Buzzoni, R., et al., 2006, D'Angelica, M., et al., 2004, de Manzoni, G., et al., 2003, Kattan, M.W., et al., 2003, Marrelli, D., et al., 2005, Otsuji, E., et al., 2004, Wang, S.Y., et al., 2009), meaning that surgery alone was unable to eradicate all locoregional disease in the majority of patients.
Therefore in addition to surgical resection, the need for systemic and local therapies are apparent. Various preoperative, perioperative and postoperative regimens, chemotherapy (CT), radiotherapy (RT) or combining therapy, have been designed to eradicate microscopic disease.

Reference	Types of relapse (%)			
	Locoregional	Peritoneal	Distant	Multiple-sites
(Marrelli, D., et al., 2005)	23.7	16.2	17.2	7.8
(Buzzoni, R., et al., 2006)	15.8	N.S	34.5	N.S
(Otsuji, E., et al., 2004)	16.0	54.0	31.0	N.S
(Wang, S.Y., et al., 2009)	9.5	23.3	20.6	46.6
(de Manzoni, G., et al., 2003)	32.7	18.1	40	9
(D'Angelica, M., et al., 2004)	25.9	13.6	28.1	32.5
(Sakuramoto, S., et al., 2007)*	11.5	15.8	11.3	N.S.
(Macdonald, J.S., et al., 2001)*	29.0	72.0	18.0	N.S.

N.S.: not specified *Site of first relapse,

Table 2. Type of relapse after curative resection

The majority of patients with gastric cancer are diagnosed at advanced stages. Even in patients are diagnosed at an early stage, 5-year survival rate of patients undergoing surgery alone is low. While the 5 year survival rates are about 70.0% in patients with stage IA, it is 20.0% in patients with stage III (Edge, S. Byrd, D., 2010). Therefore, it is clear that treatments in addition to surgery for gastric cancer are needed. For this reason, a lot of studies in terms of neoadjuvant, perioperative, or adjuvant RT, CT or combined approaches have been tried.

1.4 Possible therapeutic strategies to improve outcome of surgical therapy

CT, RT or combinations of the 2 can therotically be applied before (neoadjuvant) or after (adjuvant) the curative surgery. Being applied earlier in time, neoadjuvant therapy is expected to down stage the disease and increase the rate of curative resection and eradicate possible micrometastases, which are undetectable at the beginning of the treatment. In addition, pre-surgical patients usually have better performance status and can be expected to tolerate treatments better. However on the other hand, patients with initially resectable disease could loose their chance of curative surgery and postsurgical mortality may be increased. One other pitfall of neoadjuvant therapy is imperfectness of clinical staging. There is a possibility to give unnecessay oncological treatments to patients with very early stages of cancer who would not have otherwise receive based on pathological staging . Prior to surgery, yet the normal anatomy and blood flow, target volumes of RT could be more easily detected. However, more patients have metastatic disease at surgery than patients undergoing preoperative reviews. Two randomized important studies on this subject were the Magic and Holland trials (Cunningham, D., et al., 2006, Hartgrink, H.H., et al., 2004).

In the adjuvant setting, pathological staging is known. There is no danger of giving unnecessary treatment. However, patients can tolerate adjuvant therapies less and CT or RT could not be applied at effective doses. In addition, blood flow to the gastric bed may be decreased after surgery which leads to tissue hypoxia. Hypoxic tumor cells do not proliferate to the extend at which non-hypoxic tumors do. Since many chemotherapeutics and RT are more effective on hypoxic cells, adjuvant therapeutic strategies may be less effective than expected.

2. Neoadjuvant trials

2.1 Neoadjuvant radiotherapy

Neoadjuvant randomized clinical trial evaluating the efficacy of RT alone is limited. Zhang et al. randomized 370 patients with *gastric adenocarcinoma of cardia* to surgery alone or RT and surgery group. In the RT arm patients, underwent surgery 2-4 weeks after 40 Gy. The rate of tumor resectability and ratio of T2 tumor were more in RT arm with 11.0% decrease of T4 tumors. Five- and 10-year survival rates for RT plus surgery and surgery alone groups were 30.1%, 19.7% and 20.2%, 13.3%; respectively and these differences were statistically significant. No significant difference was observed between 2 group in term of surgical complication rates (Zhang, Z.X., et al., 1998).

In another study preoperative RT in resectable gastric cancer, there were 51 patients in both RT plus surgery and surgery alone arms and the total doses of RT was 20 Gy and was given in 5 fractions. Although, statistically insignificant, 5- and 10-year survival rates were 39.0%, 32.0% and 30.0%, 18.0% for the preoperative RT and surgery alone groups, respectively. Although concentrated preoperative RT was safe, wasn't enough to provide survival advantage (Skoropad, V., et al., 2002).

Fiorica et al. were evaluated 9 randomized trials (with these two above study, 4 neoadjuvant and 5 adjuvant trials). In this meta-analysis; 3-year (HR 0.57, CI 95% 0.43 - 0.76; p= 0.0001) and 5-year (HR 0.62 CI 95% 0.46 - 0.84; p= 0.002) survival advantage were observed with preoperative RT. Although there was increasing trend in postoperative mortality for preoperative RT group, these difference wasn't statistically significant (HR 0.61 CI 95% 0.24 - 1.57; p= 0.31) (Fiorica, F., et al., 2007).

2.2 Neoadjuvant chemo(-radio)therapy

The CT regimens have been used in patients with metastatic disease has led the way for regimens which could be used as neoadjuvant CT. The first randomized controlled neoadjuvant CT trial was Dutch randomized FAMTX (5-Fluorouracil, doxorubicin and Methotrexate) trial. There were 56 patients and FAMTX regimen was used. The ratio of resectability was similar and at median follow-up of 83 months the median survival is 18 months for FAMTX group vs. 30 months in surgery alone group (p=0.17). This trial could not show a beneficial effect of pre-operative FAMTX, even preoperative CT tends to have negative effect (Hartgrink, H.H., et al., 2004). However, it is clear that FAMTX regimen isn't an effective treatment option for today. In addition, fewer patients have been taken than planned in this study, 25.0% of patients did not receive the planned treatment because of toxicity associated with CT.

The MAGIC trial is one of the most important neoadjuvant CT studies. In this study ECF (epirubicin, cisplatin, and infusional 5-fluorouracil) regimen, which is more effective than FAMTX regimen in patients with metastatic disease, was used. ECF CT regimen was compared surgery alone. Patients with resectable adenocarcinoma of the stomach, esophagogastric junction, or lower esophagus were ranomized to either perioperative CT and surgery (250 patients) or surgery alone (253 patients). CT consisted of 3 preoperative and 3 postoperative cycles of intravenous epirubicin (50 mg per square meter of body-surface area) and cisplatin (60 mg per square meter) on day 1, and a continuous intravenous infusion of fluorouracil (200 mg per square meter per day) for 21 days (Cunningham, D., et al., 2006). Of patients, 90.7% completed preoperative CT, but only 103 of 208 (49.5%) who completed preoperative CT and surgery also completed postoperative treatment. The curative resection rates were similar; 69.3% in the perioperative CT group and 66.4% in the surgery group. There was a greater proportion of stage T1 and T2 tumors and less advanced nodal disease in the perioperative-CT group. The perioperative-CT group had a higher likelihood of overall survival (hazard ratio for death, 0.75; 95% CI, 0.60 to 0.93; p= 0.009; 5-year survival rate, 36% vs. 23%) and of progression-free survival (hazard ratio for progression, 0.66; 95% CI, 0.53 to 0.81; p<0.001).

3.1 Adjuvant chemotherapy

Numerous clinical trials concerning adjuvant CT for gastric cancer have been conducted with different CT regimens. The results of adjuvant CT trials are conflicting as well, majority being negative with disparities between asian and western ones. Geographic

Author	Patient (n)	Neoadjuvant approach	PR %	pCR %	R0 resection %	OS (months)	OS for R0 resection patients (months)
(Menges, M., et al., 2003)	25	3 or 4 cycles of C, 5-FU, FA	73.0	0	65.0	15.5	23.0
(Schuhmacher, C.P., et al., 2001)	42	3 or 4 cycles of Et-D-C	N.S.	0	73.8	19.1	28.4*
(Ajani, J.A., et al., 2006)	43	2 cycles of induction C, 5-FU, FA followed concurrent RT and weekly infusional 5-FU	N.S.	26.0	77.0	23.2	N.R.
(Hartgrink, H.H., et al., 2004)	59 (29 vs.30)	4 cycles of *FAMTX* vs. surgery alone	32.0#		62.0 vs. 63.0	18.2 vs.30.3	30.0 vs. 66.0
(Biffi, R., et al., 2010)	69 (34 vs. 35)	4 cycles of T-C-5FU Arm A (preoperative) Arm B (postoperative)	55.0	11.7	85.0 vs. 91.0	N.S.	N.S.
(Schuhmacher, C., et al., 2010)	144 (72 vs.72)	2 cycles of C, 5-FU, FA vs. surgery alone	5.8	30.4	81.9* vs.66.7	64.6 vs. 52.5	N.S.
(Cunningham, D., et al., 2006)	503 (250 vs. 253)	3 preoperative and 3 postoperative cycles of E, C, 5-FU vs. surgery alone	N.S.	N.S.	69.3 vs. 66.4	36.0 vs. 23.0* (5 year survival rate)	N.S.

*Statistically significant, C:cisplatin, FU:fluorouracil, FA: folinic asid, RT: radiotherapy, D: doxorubicin, Et:etoposide, N.S.: not specified, N.R.:not reached, MTX: methoterxate, #PR or pCR, PR: partial response, pCR: pathologic complete response, E:epirubicin, T:docetaxel, *FAMTX:* fluorouracil, doxorubicin, methoterxate

Table 3. Major randomized controlled Neoadjuvant trials

variation, small sample sized studies, differences in the surgical techniques account for these conflicting results. However, this does not mean that adjuvant chemotherapies are useless. Compared to current counterparts, CT regimens used in those old studies are relatively-weaker regimes. Many studies are undepowered. Many meta-analyses investigating the role of adjuvant CT for gastric cancer have been performed to overcome such inconsistencies.

Author	Year	No. of studies	Patients	OR/HR (95%CI)
(Hermans, J., et al., 1993)	1993	11	2096	0.88 (0.78-1.08)
(Earle, C.C. Maroun, J.A., 1999)	1999	13	1990	0.80 (0,66-0,97)*
(Mari, E., et al., 2000)	2000	21	3658	0,82 (0,75-0,89)*
(Liu, T.S., et al., 2008)	2008	23	4919	0,85 (0,80-0,90)*
(Paoletti, X., et al., 2010)	2010	17	3838	0,82 (0,76-0,90)*

OR: Odds ratio, * statistically significant values for survival

Table 4. Meta-analyses of adjuvant chemotherapy in gastric cancer

A meta-analysis was conducted on 13 randomized trials of adjuvant CT in gastric cancer concluded that adjuvant CT might produce a small survival benefit with a borderline statistical significance (Earle, C.C. Maroun, J.A., 1999). The trials in this meta-analysis were all performed in Western countries. Marie et al reviewed 20 clinical trials of adjuvant CT compared with surgery alone published between 1983 and 1999. Reviewers suggested that CT reduced the risk of death by 18% (HR 0.82, 95% CI: 0.75-0.89) and addition of anthracyclines to 5-FU did not show a statistically significant improvement when compared with other regimens (Mari, E., et al., 2000). The meta-analysis published in 2008 by Liu et al. based on 23 randomized clinical trial included 4919 patients (2441 in the adjuvant CT arm, 2478 in the observation arm). The study showed relative risk on death of 0.85 (95%CI: 0.80-0.90) which favored the survival role of adjuvant CT. The authors of this meta-analysis concluded that NNT (number needed to treat) was 14, indicating that 14 patients would need to receive adjuvant therapy to prevent one death (Liu, T.S., et al., 2008). However, meta-analyses mentioned above were restricted since they were based on the review of the literature rather than original individual patient data. Recently, an individual patient level meta-analysis of randomized control trials was published by GASTRIC (Global Advanced/Adjuvant Stomach Tumor Research International Collaboration) Group. The meta-analysis based on 17 trials (including 3838 patients) comparing adjuvant CT with surgery alone for resectable gastric carcinoma. In the study four groups of CT regimens were defined: 1) monochemotherapy agents 2) fluorouracil, mitomycin C and other therapies without anthracyclines 3) fluorouracil, mitomycin C, and anthracyclines 4) other polychemotherapy regimens. The study revealed statistically significant benefit associated with adjuvant CT both for overall survival (OS) (HR, 0.82; 95% CI, 0.76-0.90) and disease-free survival (DFS) (HR, 0.82; 95% CI, 0.75-0.90, P<.001, for both). There was no significant difference between 4 CT regimens in terms of OS and DFS. The reviewers suggested that, adjuvant fluorouracil -based CT, even as monotherapy, had improved overall survival after curative resection of gastric cancer (Paoletti, X., et al., 2010). Also in the meta-analyses of Sun et al. the pooled HR for overall survival was 0.78 (95 per cent confidence interval 0.71 to 0.85) in favor of CT (Sun, P., et al., 2009).

S-1 is an orally active combination of tegafur, gimercil and oteracil that has an appropriate bio-availability for using after gastrectomy. The Japanese randomized phase 3 trial assessed the efficacy of S-1 monotherapy as adjuvant CT in resected gastric cancer. In the study conducted by Sakuramoto et al. 1059 patients with stage 2-3 gastric cancer randomized to surgery only or adjuvant therapy with S-1 after extended (D2) gastrectomy. In the interim analysis after median follow-up of 2 years both overall survival and relapse-free survival differed between two groups favoring adjuvant CT arm, so the data and safety monitoring committee recommended early discontinuation of the trial. The study disclosed that the hazard ratio for death in the S1 group, as compared to surgery only group was 0.68 (95% CI, 0.52-0.87, P=0.003) and 3-year overall survival of 80.1% vs. 70.1% respectively. The authors suggested that S-1 was potent adjuvant CT for East Asian patients who underwent D2 dissection for locally advanced gastric cancer (Sakuramoto, S., et al., 2007). After this trial adjuvant CT without radiation therapy has been the standard in Japan.

In conclusion, adjuvant CT may be considered in patients with locally advanced gastric cancer after curative surgery who had not received neoadjuvant treatment and not candidate for chemoradition therapy.

3.2 Adjuvant radiotherapy

One randomized clinical trial evaluated the role of adjuvant RT after curative resection in gastric cancer (without concurrent CT). According to the trial performed by British Stomach Cancer Group 436 patients with resected gastric cancer were stratified to no adjuvant treatment or adjuvant RT or adjuvant CT with adriamycin, 5-FU and mitomycin C. The five year survival rates were as follows: for surgery alone 20%, for surgery plus RT 12.0%, for surgery plus CT 19.0%. No advantage in terms of survival in either adjuvant arm was observed, but RT offered an advantage in reducing local recurrence as compared to surgery only group (local recurrence rates were 27.0% versus 10.0% favoring surgery plus RT (Hallissey, M.T., et al., 1994).

3.3 Adjuvant chemoradiotherapy

Gastric cancer can recur loco-regionally, or systemically. The review from Memorial Sloan-Kettering Cancer (MSKCC) demonstrated patterns of relapse of 1172 patients who underwent potentially curative surgery from July 1985 through June 2000 (D'Angelica, M., et al., 2004). Among 496 patients who had a recurrence, whole data on recurrence was obtained in 367 patients. Loco-regional sites were a component of relapse in 54.0% of patients including the anastomosis, lymph nodes and the gastric bed. Distant sites and peritoneal relapse were documented in 51.0% and 29.0% of patients, respectively. Since adjuvant RT alone did not appear to confer advantage in terms of survival, RT combined with CT was evaluated in randomized clinical trials. The rationale to use CRT in the adjuvant setting in gastric cancer is not only to control loco-regional recurrence but also distant metastases. First, when used concurrently with RT chemotherapeutic agents may act as a radio-sensitizer. Second, CT may improve systemic control by eliminating microscopic distant metastasis. Various mechanisms are responsible for the interaction between CT and RT. Ionizing radiation induces DNA base damage, alkali-labile sites, single-strand breaks, and double strand breaks. Double strand breaks are the most important damage among them and causes tumor-kill whether remains unrepaired. Chemotherapeutic agents that inhibit DNA repair, including fluorouracil, cisplatin, irinotecan, can improve radiation cytotoxicity synergistically. CT can also act by restraining post-radiation damage repair. The phase of the cell cycle is another determinant of radio-sensitivity. While cells in G2-M phase are most radiosensitive, cells in the S phase of the cell cycle are the most radio-resistant (Terasima, T. Tolmach, L.J., 1961). CT and RT also produce synergistic effect by targeting different phases of the cell cycle when used concurrently. Moreover, drugs such as taxanes has the ability to block the cell cycle at the G2-M phase so that enhances the radiation effect (Tishler, R.B., et al., 1992).

Several randomized trials assessed the effectiveness of chemo-radiation after curative surgery. Dent et al. performed randomized trial including 142 patients with all stages of gastric carcinoma. The patients in Division I (T1-3, N1-2, and M0) were assigned to control and RT plus 5-FU group. Division II (T4, M1) was randomized into three groups; a control group, RT plus 5-FU, thiotepa for six months. After 4.5 year's follow-up the control and treatment groups did not differ with respect to survival rate in neither Division I nor Division II (Dent, D.M., et al., 1979). In the randomized trial conducted by Bleiberg and colleagues, 115 patients who underwent curative and palliative surgery were stratified into four treatment groups. Patients received RT alone or in combination with short-term and/or long term 5-FU infusion. Statistically differences were determined in terms of overall survival but the difference in survival disappeared when comparisons adjusted for prognostic factors (Bleiberg, H., et al., 1989). In the study by Moertel and co-workers 62 patients with resectable but poor prognosis gastric carcinoma were randomized to surgery versus surgery plus adjuvant treatment with 5-FU plus radiation. Although both five-year survival rates and local-regional recurrence favored treatment arm results did not reach statistical significance (Moertel, C.G., et al., 1984).

The largest trial evaluating the use of postoperative chemoradiation was U.S. Intergroup 0116 trial (Macdonald, J.S., et al., 2001). In this study 556 patients with curatively resected gastric or gastroesophageal junction adenocarcinoma (stage Ib through IV M0) were randomized to surgery alone or adjuvant combined chemoradiotherapy (CRT). The adjuvant treatment consisted of one course of 5-FU 425 mg/m2/d and leucovorin 20 mg/m2/d, daily for five days, followed one month later by 45 Gy of radiation during 5 weeks with 5-FU 425 mg/m2/d and leucovorin 20 mg/m2/d on days 1 through 4 and last 3 days of radiation. One month after completion of RT 2 more 5-day cycles of CT (5-FU 425 mg/m2/d plus leucovorin 20 mg/m2/d) were administered. After a median follow-up of 5 years, the median duration of survival was 36 and 27 months in the CRT and surgery-only groups, respectively. The 3-year survival rates were 50% versus 41% favoring adjuvant treatment. The 3-year rates of relapse free survival increased from 31.0% to 48.0% in the CRT group. Improvements both in overall and relapse free survival were statistically significant. Grades 3 and 4 toxic effects (mostly, hematologic and gastrointestinal) occurred in 41.0% and 32.0% of chemo-RT groups, respectively. Three patients (%1) died as a result of toxic effect of the treatment. The extent of the surgical resection was an important issue in the study protocol. Although, D2 dissection was recommended, only 10.0% of patients underwent a D2 dissection, 54.0% of the patients underwent D0 dissection (in which all of the N1 nodes were not resected). When patients relapse patterns were examined, local-regional recurrence was higher in the surgery only group, despite the higher distant metastasis rates detected in the CRT group (statistical assessment of the relapse sites were not included in the study). The study demonstrated that the benefit of CRT in the adjuvant setting was mainly apparent by reducing loco-regional recurrence. At the end of the study Macdonald et al. suggested that, postoperative CRT should be considered for all patients at high risk for recurrence of adenocarcinoma of the stomach or gastro-esophageal junction who undergone curative resection.

4. Intra-peritoneal chemotherapy

Peritoneal spread of tumor cells is frequently seen in the course of gastric carcinoma. The expected median survival time is approximately 3 to 6 months when peritoneal carcinomatosis and ascites become evident (Sakata, Y., et al., 1998). The rationale to use peritoneal route to prevent and/or treat the peritoneal spread is to deliver higher concentrations of CT within peritoneal cavity without marked systemic toxicity. Several randomized trials assessed the role of intra-peritoneal CT with different aspects regarding the timing of drug administration, the type of chemotherapeutic agents and the impact of hyperthermia. At least two meta-analyses of randomized clinical trials on adjuvant intra-peritoneal CT for curatively resected gastric cancer showed clinical benefit of this treatment. The meta-analysis by Xu and colleagues included eleven trials involving 1161 cases (Xu, D.Z., et al., 2004). All included trials were randomized, controlled trials that compared surgery plus intra-peritoneal CT with or without activated carbon particles with surgery alone. No other adjuvant treatment including oral or parenteral CT, RT or chemo-immunotherapy was used in the adjuvant group. In the study 609 patients were assigned to the treatment group and 552 to the control group. Most of the studies used mitomycin C with or without carbon particles as a chemotherapeutic agent. The pooled odds ratio was 0.51 with a 95% confidence interval (0.40-0.65). Moreover, in the subgroup analysis trials that used intra-peritoneal hyperthermic chemoperfusion or CT with activated carbon particles was more effective than the trials without hyperthermia and carbon particles. The other meta-analysis performed by Yan and coworkers also involved 13 randomized control trials that compared surgery plus intra-peritoneal CT to surgery alone (Yan, T.D., et al., 2007). The trials included patients with locally advanced gastric cancer without distant metastasis. In the study intra-peritoneal chemotherapies grouped in five categories according to the timing of the procedure and whether hyperthermia was used. The 1st group was composed of trials assessing the role of hyperthermic intra-operative intra-peritoneal CT (HIIC). The 2nd group involved trials investigating normothermic intra-operative intra-peritoneal CT (NIIC). The 3rd group was composed of trials exploring the efficiency of early postoperative intra-peritoneal CT (EPIC). The 4th group included combined forms and the 5th group included the trials of delayed postoperative intra-peritoneal CT (DPIC). The study showed significant survival benefit in favor of HIIC (Hamazoe, R., et al., 1994) (HR:0.60; 95% CI;0.43-0.83) and HIIC combined with EPIC (Gao Z, J.Z., Zhou F, 2002, Wei, G., et al., 2005) (HR:0.45;95%CI:0.29-0.68). The improved survival provided by NIIC did not reach statistical significance (Rosen, H.R., et al., 1998, Takahashi, T., et al., 1995, Yonemura, Y., et al., 2001) (HR:0.67;95% CI:044-1.01; p=0.06), no benefit was found either with EPIC (HR:0.64;95% CI:037-1.10) or DPIC (HR:0.89;95% CI:0.51-1.55). The meta-analysis did not show significant difference in perioperative mortality between the 2 arms. The incidence of intra-abdominal abscess was significantly higher among patients in the intra-peritoneal CT arm. Though none of the individual trial showed increased incidence in terms of neutropenia the meta-analysis found intra-peritoneal chemotherapy associated with increased risk of neutropenia. The authors of the meta-analysis concluded that HIIC with or without EPIC after resection of advanced gastric cancer was associated with improved overall survival at the expense of increased risk of intra-abdominal abscess and neutropenia.

5. Current standard of care in the world

Surgical resection with lymph node dissection is the primary treatment of early gastric cancer. Total gastrectomy is preferred for tumors arising from proximal stomach or tumors infiltrating stomach diffusely. For distal gastric cancers subtotal gastrectomy is procedure of choice due to fewer complications, lower morbidity and similar survival compared with total gastrectomy (Bozzetti, F., et al., 1999). Endoscopic mucosal resection is the standard treatment in Japan for early gastric cancer limited to mucosa without lymph node involvement (Soetikno, R., et al., 2005).

The extent of lymph node dissection still remains to be a matter of debate. Although gastrectomy with D2 lymphadenectomy is the standard treatment in Japan, in Western studies extensive lymphadenectomy have not provided survival benefit when compared with D1 lymph node dissection (Bonenkamp, J.J., et al., 1999). D2 dissection is more and more adopted in western societies.

In United Kingdom and most of the parts of Europe perioperative CT with ECF regimen became the standard of care, based on the results of the MAGIC trial. This approach is also recommended with level 1 evidence in United States (U.S.) for patients with T2 or higher tumors.

The results of INT-0116 trial changed standard of care in United States from observation to chemo-radiation after curative resection of gastric cancer without evidence of metastasis. Patients with T3, T4 or node positive tumors are recommended to be treated with RT (45-50 Gy) concurrent with 5-FU plus 5-FU (with leucovorin) after curative resection in U.S., although this approach has not been accepted in most of Europe and Japan.

In Japanese population adjuvant CT with S-1 was detected to improve survival after gastric resection with D2 lymph-node dissection in stage II-III gastric cancer. Though it seems to be feasible adjuvant treatment option in East Asian patients, there is not enough data to recommend this approach in Western population.

6. Future directions

Despite advances both in adjuvant and metastatic setting, overall survival in gastric cancer remains to be poor. New agents and new schedules which have been proved to be effective are being integrated into trials of neoadjuvant or adjuvant trials. Emerging data from clinical trials evaluating combination chemotherapies and new molecular targeted therapies has shown clinical benefit especially in metastatic disease. The efficacy of these novel therapies should be confirmed in well designed prospective randomized clinical trials.

Newer chemotherapeutic agents, namely taxanes, oral fluoropyrimidines (UFT, S1, capecitabine) and irinotecan have widely searched in advanced stages of gastric cancer. Naturally, it is expected that the most effective and tolerable chemotherapeutic strategies in the metastatic setting should be evaluated in earlier stages. In the V325 trial by Van Cutsem et al. the combination of docetaxel, cisplatin and 5-FU (DCF), was significantly superior than cisplatin plus 5-FU (CF) in terms of OS, time to tumor progression and response rate (Van Cutsem, E., et al., 2006). In the phase II randomized trial (NEOTAX) DCF combination CT will be evaluated as a neoadjuvant therapy in locally advanced gastric adenocarcinoma (Clinicaltrials.gov number is NCT00343239). The objective of this study is to determine the impact of DCF combination CT on R0 resection rate in gastric cancer. Patient recruitment is over and the first results are expected in January 2012.

In the large CRITICS trial, the question of whether adjuvant CRT with weekly cisplatin and capecitabine after 3 cycles of neoadjuvant ECC (epirubicin, cisplatin and capecitabine) and surgery in comparison with 3 more cycles of the neoadjuvant schedule (clinicaltrials.gov no: NCT00407186). Nearly 800 patients are expected to be recruited and the first results are awaited in 2013.

The rationale to combine targeted therapies with CT is to improve the efficacy with acceptable toxicity. Epidermal growth factor receptor 2 (also known as HER-2) has become important target in gastric cancer. Trastuzumab, a fully humanized monoclonal antibody against HER-2, was recently evaluated in metastatic gastric cancer. In randomized phase 3 ToGA trial patients were randomly assigned to receive trastuzumab plus CT (capecitabine plus cisplatin or fluorouracil plus cisplatin) or CT alone. The study revealed that median overall survival was 13.8 months in those assigned to trastuzumab plus CT as compared with 11.1 months in those received CT alone (HR: 0.74; 95% CI:0.60-0.91; P=0.046). The authors suggested that trastuzumab plus CT substantially improved OS in patients with high expression of HER-2 protein (immunohistochemistry 2+ and FISH + or immunohistochemistry 3+) compared with patients with low expression of HER-2 (immunohistochemistry 0 or 1+ and FISH+). It was also reported that combining trastuzumab with CT did not cause additional toxic effect (Bang, Y.J., et al., 2010). It is currently not known whether the benefit achieved in metastatic gastric cancer will be translated to adjuvant setting. It was also shown that replacing cisplatin with oxaliplatin and fluorouracil with capecitabine is not inferior than the classical ECF (epirubicin, cisplatin, fluorouracil)(Okines, A.F., et al., 2009). A study of capecitabine in combination with trastuzumab and oxaliplatin in patients with resectable gastric cancer, namely TOXAG (Trastuzumab, Oxaliplatin, and Xeloda for Adjuvant Gastric Cancer) was recently designed to evaluate the impact of trastuzumab in adjuvant and adjuvant strategy.

Bevacizumab, recombinant humanized monoclonal antibody that targets vascular endothelial growth factor, was recently studied in combination with irinotecan and cisplatin in patients with metastatic gastric adenocarcinoma in a phase II multicenter study (Shah, M.A., et al., 2006). The study revealed that, time to disease progression improved by 75% in compared to historical controls. Rates of rare but important complications of bevacizumab, namely gastrointestinal perforation and hemorrhage, was also found similar to rates of several recent large advanced phase studies. The authors of this study concluded that bevacizumab could be added to CT safely and was active in the treatment of advanced gastric adenocarcinoma. A randomized phase III trial will assess the safety and efficacy of neoadjuvant and adjuvant CT including epirubicin, cisplatin and capecitabine with or without bevacizumab in patients with untreated resectable gastric or gastroesophageal junction cancer (MAGIC-B Study) (clinicaltrials.gov no: NCT00407186). Planning to have

1100 patients, the results of this study may clarify the role of bevacizumab in adjuvant/neoadjuvant setting.
There are also adjuvant studies exploring the role of S-1, a newer oral fluoropyrimidine analog.

7. References

Ajani, J. A. Gastric Cancer. 2011.

Ajani, J. A., et al. Phase II trial of preoperative chemoradiation in patients with localized gastric adenocarcinoma (RTOG 9904): quality of combined modality therapy and pathologic response. J Clin Oncol. 2006;24(24):3953-3958.

Baiocchi, G. L., et al. A multicentric Western analysis of prognostic factors in advanced, node-negative gastric cancer patients. Ann Surg. 2010;252(1):70-73.

Bang, Y. J., et al. Trastuzumab in combination with chemotherapy versus chemotherapy alone for treatment of HER2-positive advanced gastric or gastro-oesophageal junction cancer (ToGA): a phase 3, open-label, randomised controlled trial. Lancet. 2010;376(9742):687-697.

Biffi, R., et al. Surgical outcome after docetaxel-based neoadjuvant chemotherapy in locally-advanced gastric cancer. World J Gastroenterol. 2010;16(7):868-874.

Bleiberg, H., et al. Adjuvant radiotherapy and chemotherapy in resectable gastric cancer. A randomized trial of the gastro-intestinal tract cancer cooperative group of the EORTC. Eur J Surg Oncol. 1989;15(6):535-543.

Bonenkamp, J. J., et al. Extended lymph-node dissection for gastric cancer. N Engl J Med. 1999;340(12):908-914.

Bozzetti, F., et al. Subtotal versus total gastrectomy for gastric cancer: five-year survival rates in a multicenter randomized Italian trial. Italian Gastrointestinal Tumor Study Group. Ann Surg. 1999;230(2):170-178.

Buzzoni, R., et al. Pathological features as predictors of recurrence after radical resection of gastric cancer. Br J Surg. 2006;93(2):205-209.

Chen, X. Z., et al. Meta-analysis of effectiveness and safety of D2 plus para-aortic lymphadenectomy for resectable gastric cancer. J Am Coll Surg. 2010;210(1):100-105.

Crew, K. D.&Neugut, A. I. Epidemiology of gastric cancer. World J Gastroenterol. 2006;12(3):354-362.

Cunningham, D., et al. Perioperative chemotherapy versus surgery alone for resectable gastroesophageal cancer. N Engl J Med. 2006;355(1):11-20.

D'Angelica, M., et al. Patterns of initial recurrence in completely resected gastric adenocarcinoma. Ann Surg. 2004;240(5):808-816.

de Manzoni, G., et al. Pattern of recurrence after surgery in adenocarcinoma of the gastro-oesophageal junction. Eur J Surg Oncol. 2003;29(6):506-510.

Dent, D. M., et al. Prospective randomized trial of combined oncological therapy for gastric carcinoma. Cancer. 1979;44(2):385-391.

Deprez, P. H., et al. Current practice with endoscopic submucosal dissection in Europe: position statement from a panel of experts. Endoscopy. 2010.

Earle, C. C.&Maroun, J. A. Adjuvant chemotherapy after curative resection for gastric cancer in non-Asian patients: revisiting a meta-analysis of randomised trials. Eur J Cancer. 1999;35(7):1059-1064.

Edge SB, Byrd DR , Compton CC, eds. AJCC Cancer Staging Manual. 7th ed. New York, NY: Springer (118)Ferlay, J., Parkin, D. M.&Steliarova-Foucher, E. Estimates of cancer incidence and mortality in Europe in 2008. Eur J Cancer. 2010;46(4):765-781.

Ferlay, J., et al. Estimates of worldwide burden of cancer in 2008: GLOBOCAN 2008. Int J Cancer. 2010.

Fiorica, F., et al. The impact of radiotherapy on survival in resectable gastric carcinoma: a meta-analysis of literature data. Cancer Treat Rev. 2007;33(8):729-740.

Gao Z, J. Z., Zhou F. Clinical surgery of early intraperitoneal hyperthermic chemoperfusion for gastric cancer patients after operation. Zhonggou Zhongliu Linchuang. 2002;29:294–295.

Hallissey, M. T., Dunn, J. A., Ward, L. C.&Allum, W. H. The second British Stomach Cancer Group trial of adjuvant radiotherapy or chemotherapy in resectable gastric cancer: five-year follow-up. Lancet. 1994;343(8909):1309-1312.

Hamazoe, R., Maeta, M.&Kaibara, N. Intraperitoneal thermochemotherapy for prevention of peritoneal recurrence of gastric cancer. Final results of a randomized controlled study. Cancer. 1994;73(8):2048-2052.

Hartgrink, H. H., et al. Neo-adjuvant chemotherapy for operable gastric cancer: long term results of the Dutch randomised FAMTX trial. Eur J Surg Oncol. 2004;30(6):643-649.

Hermans, J., et al. Adjuvant therapy after curative resection for gastric cancer: meta-analysis of randomized trials. J Clin Oncol. 1993;11(8):1441-1447.

Japanese Gastric Cancer, A. Japanese Classification of Gastric Carcinoma - 2nd English Edition. Gastric Cancer. 1998;1(1):10-24.

Jemal, A., Siegel, R., Xu, J.&Ward, E. Cancer statistics, 2010. CA Cancer J Clin. 2010;60(5):277-300.

Kattan, M. W., Karpeh, M. S., Mazumdar, M.&Brennan, M. F. Postoperative nomogram for disease-specific survival after an R0 resection for gastric carcinoma. Journal of Clinical Oncology. 2003;21(19):3647-3650.

Kim, J. J., et al. EMR for early gastric cancer in Korea: a multicenter retrospective study. Gastrointest Endosc. 2007;66(4):693-700.

Krejs, G. J. Gastric cancer: epidemiology and risk factors. Dig Dis. 2010;28(4-5): 600-603.

Liu, T. S., Wang, Y., Chen, S. Y.&Sun, Y. H. An updated meta-analysis of adjuvant chemotherapy after curative resection for gastric cancer. Eur J Surg Oncol. 2008;34(11):1208-1216.

Long, N., et al. Cancer epidemiology and control in north-East Asia - past, present and future. Asian Pac J Cancer Prev. 2010;11 Suppl 2:107-148.

Macdonald, J. S., et al. Chemoradiotherapy after surgery compared with surgery alone for adenocarcinoma of the stomach or gastroesophageal junction. N Engl J Med. 2001;345(10):725-730.

Malvezzi, M., et al. An age-period-cohort analysis of gastric cancer mortality from 1950 to 2007 in Europe. Ann Epidemiol. 2010;20(12):898-905.

Mari, E., et al. Efficacy of adjuvant chemotherapy after curative resection for gastric cancer: a meta-analysis of published randomised trials. A study of the GISCAD (Gruppo Italiano per lo Studio dei Carcinomi dell'Apparato Digerente). Ann Oncol. 2000;11(7):837-843.

Marrelli, D., et al. Prediction of recurrence after radical surgery for gastric cancer: a scoring system obtained from a prospective multicenter study. Ann Surg. 2005;241(2):247-255.

Menges, M., et al. Low toxic neoadjuvant cisplatin, 5-fluorouracil and folinic acid in locally advanced gastric cancer yields high R-0 resection rate. J Cancer Res Clin Oncol. 2003;129(7):423-429.

Moertel, C. G., et al. Combined 5-fluorouracil and radiation therapy as a surgical adjuvant for poor prognosis gastric carcinoma. J Clin Oncol. 1984;2(11):1249-1254.

Okines, A. F., et al. Meta-analysis of the REAL-2 and ML17032 trials: evaluating capecitabine-based combination chemotherapy and infused 5-fluorouracil-based combination chemotherapy for the treatment of advanced oesophago-gastric cancer. Ann Oncol. 2009;20(9):1529-1534.

Otsuji, E., et al. Time to death and pattern of death in recurrence following curative resection of gastric carcinoma: analysis based on depth of invasion. World J Surg. 2004;28(9):866-869.

Paoletti, X., et al. Benefit of adjuvant chemotherapy for resectable gastric cancer: a meta-analysis. JAMA. 2010;303(17):1729-1737.

Rosen, H. R., et al. Adjuvant intraperitoneal chemotherapy with carbon-adsorbed mitomycin in patients with gastric cancer: results of a randomized multicenter trial of the Austrian Working Group for Surgical Oncology. J Clin Oncol. 1998;16(8):2733-2738.

Sakata, Y., et al. Late phase II study of novel oral fluoropyrimidine anticancer drug S-1 (1 M tegafur-0.4 M gimestat-1 M otastat potassium) in advanced gastric cancer patients. Eur J Cancer. 1998;34(11):1715-1720.

Sakuramoto, S., et al. Adjuvant chemotherapy for gastric cancer with S-1, an oral fluoropyrimidine. N Engl J Med. 2007;357(18):1810-1820.

Sasako, M., et al. Gastric Cancer Working Group report. Jpn J Clin Oncol. 2010;40 Suppl 1:i28-37.

Sasako, M., et al. D2 lymphadenectomy alone or with para-aortic nodal dissection for gastric cancer. N Engl J Med. 2008;359(5):453-462.

Schuhmacher, C., et al. Neoadjuvant chemotherapy compared with surgery alone for locally advanced cancer of the stomach and cardia: European Organisation for Research and Treatment of Cancer randomized trial 40954. J Clin Oncol. 2010;28(35):5210-5218.

Schuhmacher, C. P., et al. Neoadjuvant therapy for patients with locally advanced gastric carcinoma with etoposide, doxorubicin, and cisplatinum. Closing results after 5 years of follow-up. Cancer. 2001;91(5):918-927.

Shah, M. A., et al. Multicenter phase II study of irinotecan, cisplatin, and bevacizumab in patients with metastatic gastric or gastroesophageal junction adenocarcinoma. J Clin Oncol. 2006;24(33):5201-5206.

Shin, H. R., Masuyer, E., Ferlay, J.&Curado, M. P. Cancer in Asia - Incidence rates based on data in cancer incidence in five continents IX (1998-2002). Asian Pac J Cancer Prev. 2010;11 Suppl 2:11-16.

Siewert, J. R., Bottcher, K., Stein, H. J.&Roder, J. D. Relevant prognostic factors in gastric cancer: ten-year results of the German Gastric Cancer Study. Ann Surg. 1998;228(4):449-461.

Skoropad, V., Berdov, B.&Zagrebin, V. Concentrated preoperative radiotherapy for resectable gastric cancer: 20-years follow-up of a randomized trial. J Surg Oncol. 2002;80(2):72-78.

Soetikno, R., Kaltenbach, T., Yeh, R.&Gotoda, T. Endoscopic mucosal resection for early cancers of the upper gastrointestinal tract. J Clin Oncol. 2005;23(20):4490-4498.

Songun, I., et al. Surgical treatment of gastric cancer: 15-year follow-up results of the randomised nationwide Dutch D1D2 trial. Lancet Oncol. 2010;11(5):439-449.

Sun, P., Xiang, J. B.&Chen, Z. Y. Meta-analysis of adjuvant chemotherapy after radical surgery for advanced gastric cancer. Br J Surg. 2009;96(1):26-33.

Swan, R.&Miner, T. J. Current role of surgical therapy in gastric cancer. World J Gastroenterol. 2006;12(3):372-379.

Takahashi, T., et al. Prophylaxis and treatment of peritoneal carcinomatosis: intraperitoneal chemotherapy with mitomycin C bound to activated carbon particles. World J Surg. 1995;19(4):565-569.

Tanizawa, Y.&Terashima, M. Lymph node dissection in the resection of gastric cancer: review of existing evidence. Gastric Cancer. 2010;13(3):137-148.

Terasima, T.&Tolmach, L. J. Changes in x-ray sensitivity of HeLa cells during the division cycle. Nature. 1961;190:1210-1211.

Tishler, R. B., Geard, C. R., Hall, E. J.&Schiff, P. B. Taxol sensitizes human astrocytoma cells to radiation. Cancer Res. 1992;52(12):3495-3497.

Van Cutsem, E., et al. Phase III study of docetaxel and cisplatin plus fluorouracil compared with cisplatin and fluorouracil as first-line therapy for advanced gastric cancer: a report of the V325 Study Group. J Clin Oncol. 2006;24(31):4991-4997.

Wang, S. Y., et al. Clinical impact of positive surgical margin status on gastric cancer patients undergoing gastrectomy. Ann Surg Oncol. 2009;16(10):2738-2743.

Wei, G., et al. [Efficacy of intraoperative hypotonic peritoneal chemo-hyperthermia combined with early postoperative intraperitoneal chemotherapy on gastric cancer]. Ai Zheng. 2005;24(4):478-482.

Xu, D. Z., et al. Meta-analysis of intraperitoneal chemotherapy for gastric cancer. World J Gastroenterol. 2004;10(18):2727-2730.

Yan, T. D., et al. A systematic review and meta-analysis of the randomized controlled trials on adjuvant intraperitoneal chemotherapy for resectable gastric cancer. Ann Surg Oncol. 2007;14(10):2702-2713.

Yang, K., et al. Effectiveness and safety of splenectomy for gastric carcinoma: a meta-analysis. World J Gastroenterol. 2009;15(42):5352-5359.

Yonemura, Y., et al. Intraoperative chemohyperthermic peritoneal perfusion as an adjuvant to gastric cancer: final results of a randomized controlled study. Hepatogastroenterology. 2001;48(42):1776-1782.

Zhang, Z. X., et al. Randomized clinical trial on the combination of preoperative irradiation and surgery in the treatment of adenocarcinoma of gastric cardia (AGC)--report on 370 patients. Int J Radiat Oncol Biol Phys. 1998;42(5):929-934.

15

Establishment of the Standard Prophylactic Strategy for Peritoneal Recurrence and Proposal of the Optimal Therapeutic Protocol for Gastric Cancer

Shimada S[1], Kuramoto M[1], Ikeshima S[1], Matsuo A[1], Ikuta Y[1], Kuhara H[1] and Baba H[2]
[1]*Department of Surgery, Yatsushiro Social Insurance General Hospital*
[2]*Department of Gastroenterological Surgery, Graduate School of Medical Sciences, Kumamoto University, Kumamoto*
Japan

1. Introduction

Advances in diagnosis and surgical techniques have improved the conditions of patients with gastric cancer. Peritoneal dissemination, however, is still the most frequent cause of death, and the prognosis of patients with peritoneal metastasis of gastric cancer is extremely poor (Balfour, 1973; Hioki et al.,2010; Maruyama, 1987; Makino et al., 2010; M. Yamamoto et al., 2009). In patients with serosal invasion, about half develop peritoneal recurrence and die from the disease within the first 2 years of follow-up, even if curative resection is performed (Abe et al., 1995; Ikeguchi et al., 1994; Kaibara et al., 1987; Moriguchi et al., 1992; Ribero et al., 1998). Furthermore, it has been reported that the survival span of the patients with cytology-positive peritoneal lavage fluid and without the macroscopic peritoneal dissemination (CY+/P-) of gastric cancer was almost the same as that of patients with P+ (Boku, et al., 1990; Shimada et al., 2003), and the 5-year survival rate of patients with CY+/P- is only 2% (Bando et al., 1999). Accordingly, the treatment recommendations for gastric cancer in the event of positive cytology range from palliative chemotherapy to attempts at neo-adjuvant therapies followed by surgical resection. However, the results of published randomized clinical trials of adjuvant perioperative intra-peritoneal chemotherapy have not fully demonstrated any significant improvement in survival as compared with surgery alone, especially in the cases with P+ (Cunliffe & Sugarbaker, 1989; Cheong et al., 2007; Hagiwara et al., 1992; Ikeguchi et al., 2005; Kunisaki et al., 2002; Sauter et al., 1994). Therefore, a reliable and appropriate standard prophylactic regimen for peritoneal recurrence in patients with gastric cancer needs be established.

Clinical and pathologic factors that have been found to correlate with the presence of positive cytology are usually at an advanced stage of the disease (Burke et al., 1998; Iitsuka et al., 1979; Koga et al., 1984; Ribeiro et al.,2006; Yawata et al.,1998). The most likely cause is the presence of intra-peritoneal free cancer cells from the serosal surface of the primary cancer and their implantation on the peritoneum. Furthermore, our previous study proved that lymph node dissection opened the lymphatic channel and spread viable cancer cells into the peritoneal cavity (Marutsuka et al., 2003). This could explain the main reason for the peritoneal recurrence after curative surgery for patients with non serosa-invasive gastric cancer.

Peritoneal dissemination is probably completed by the implantation of peritoneal free cancer cells exfoliated from serosa-invasive tumors. Consequently, it is very important to prevent peritoneal metastasis prior to the fixation and progression of free cancer cells to the peritoneum in patients with advanced gastric cancer. This is because the presence of intra-peritoneal free cancer cells without macroscopic dissemination could possibly indicate a condition wherein the implantation of cancer cells on the intra-peritoneal wall has not yet occurred.

Based on this assumption, we have been advocating the adoption of 'extensive intra-operative peritoneal lavage' (EIPL) (Shimada et al., 2002; K. Yamamoto et al., 2005) as a reliable and practical intra-operative technique as an adjuvant therapy for preventing the implantation of cancer cells on the intra-peritoneal wall after a potentially curative resection combined with intra-peritoneal chemotherapy (EIPL-IPC). EIPL is very simple and can be performed anywhere and at anytime. It is a rather efficient method for reducing the number of intra-peritoneal free cancer cells to zero potentially, when the cancer cells are analyzed by a detection system using real-time reverse transcriptase-polymerase chain reaction (RT-PCR), and intra-peritoneal chemotherapy subsequent to EIPL could be effective for eradicating the remaining cancer cells. We have confirmed the clinical effectiveness of EIPL by ultra-rapid quantitative RT-PCR protocol (Marutsuka et al., 2003). Very few intra-peritoneal free cancer cells could be detected in the washing fluid after 6 to 8 washes. Finally, our recent prospective randomized controlled clinical trial clearly revealed that EIPL therapy significantly improved the 5-year survival rate of advanced gastric patients with intra-peritoneal free cancer cells (Kuramoto et al., 2009).

In this manuscript, the risk factors on peritoneal recurrence from clinicopathological features of gastric carcinoma and the contribution of EIPL method to the remarkable improvement in the 5-year survival for patients with CY+/P- on clinical trials is reviewed, and the optimal treatment protocol for patients with gastric cancer is proposed.

2. Clinicopathological features and risk factors on peritoneal recurrence for gastric carcinoma

Results of specific preoperative studies, intraoperative findings, postoperative pathologic staging, clinical management, and follow-up data from 2117 patients underwent gastric resection with D2 lymph nodes dissection for primary gastric carcinoma were registered prospectively (Shimada S, et al.). Preoperative diagnosis was made on the basis of endoscopic, radiologic, and endoscopic ultrasonographic (EUS) (Kida et al., 1998) findings. Pathologic diagnosis and classifications were based on the Japanese Classification of Gastric Carcinoma by the Japanese Research Society for Gastric Cancer (Japanese Research Society for Gastric Cancer, 1999).

The incidences of lymph node metastasis from tumors with mucosal (M), submucosal (SM), and advanced gastric cancer were 2.5%, 20.2%, and 71.2%, respectively. The detailed pathological analysis revealed that all M tumors with lymph node metastasis (n=14) had ulceration or ulceration scar (UL+) in the lesions even if the lesion was smaller than 1.5 cm in diameter. On the other hand, no M tumor without ulceration or ulceration scar (UL-)

(n=328) had any lymph node metastasis. In advanced gastric cancer, approximately 57% of the metastatic tumors had distant lymph nodes metastasis. Serosal invasion was also popular in advanced gastric cancer; approximately 50% of the advanced tumors had serosal invasion.

Fig 1 showed cancer-specific 5-year survival rates of gastric cancer according to the tumor depth. Gastric resection with D2 lymph nodes dissection for primary gastric carcinoma yielded good prognosis in M and SM tumors; 98% and 95% of the cancer-specific 5-year survival rates, respectively. There were no apparent prognostic factors in patients with M tumors. In patients with SM tumors, the cancer-specific 5-year survival of those with lymph node metastasis was significantly lower than that of those without such metastasis (77.6% vs 98.2%; $P < 0.001$). An sharp decrease in survival was seen between patients with two positive nodes and those with three positive nodes, and the cancer-specific 5-year survival rate of patients with three or more metastatic lymph nodes was significantly lower than that of those with one or two nodes ($P = 0.041$). Multivariate analyses revealed that the involvement of three or more lymph nodes was the sole independent prognostic determinant ($P = 0.016$); the level of nodal metastasis was not an independent prognostic factor ($P = 0.384$). In advanced gastric cancer, serosal invasion was the strong prognostic factor as well as the factor of more than three lymph nodes metastasis. These results suggest that gastric cancer patients with lymph nodes metastasis and serosal invasion should be given special weight of additional therapy after surgery (Fig. 1).

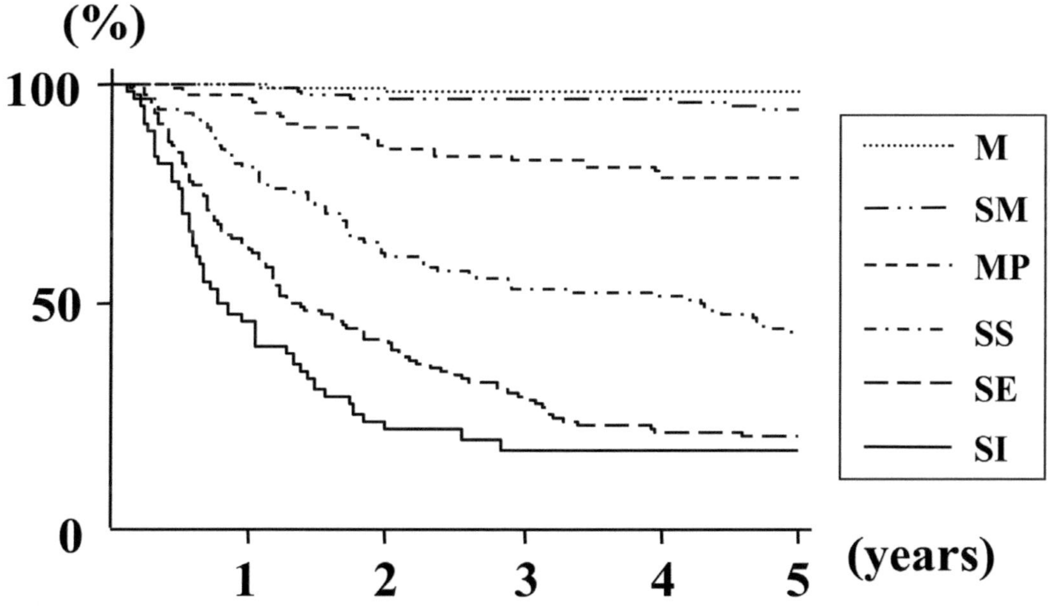

Fig. 1. Cancer-specific 5-year survival rates of gastric cancer according to the tumor depth. M: mucosal tumor, SM: submucosal tumor, MP: tumor with muscularis proprial invasion, SS: tumor with subserosal invasion, SE: tumor with serosal invasion, SI: tumor invasion of adjacent structures (Shimada et al., 2003)

3. Real-time detection system for Intra-peritoneal free cancer cells

An ultra-rapid quantitative RT-PCR protocol, which is a combined system of an ultra-rapid RT-PCR, using a fully automated mRNA extractor and a real-time one-step RT-PCR system with a hybridization probe format, has been established to diagnose intra-peritoneal cancer cells spread during a surgical operation (Marutsuka et al., 2003). This new method enabled us to obtain the results of RT-PCR within approximately 70 minutes after sampling. Furthermore, we carried out multiple-marker RT-PCR assays in a combination of carcinoembryonic antigen (CEA) and cytokeratin 20 (CK20) to eliminate false positive results and to improve specificity. This assay system was able to detect at least 10 cancer cells in 1×10^7 of leukocytes, indicating comparable sensitivity to conventional nested-RT-PCR. Accordingly, the accurate diagnosis of the spread of intra-peritoneal cancer cells was done during the actual operation (Fig. 2).

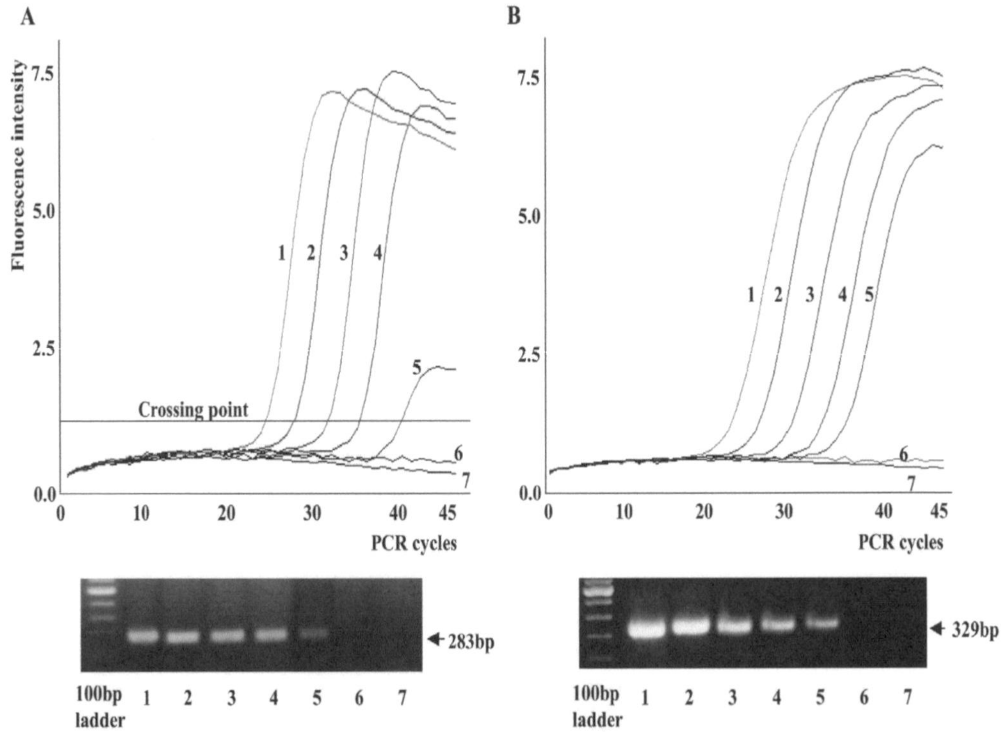

Fig. 2. Sensitivity of ultra-rapid quantitative RT-PCR assay by LightCycler™ using CEA (A) and CK20 (B) mRNA marker. Curves and lanes 1-5 were serially diluted 10^5 cells to 10^1 cells of WiDr colon carcinoma cell in 10^7 leukocytes from healthy volunteer, respectively; curve and lane 6: 10^7 leukocytes from healthy volunteer; curve and lane 7: no template. This assay system could detect at least 10 WiDr colon carcinoma cells in 10^7 leukocytes. The PCR products were analyzed by 2% agarose gel electrophresis, and they were matched to the expected sizes of CEA and CK20. 'Crossing points' were used to establish an external standard curve for quantification. Forty-five rounds of amplification were completed within 30min. (Marutsuka et al., 2003)

4. Mechanisms of peritoneal recurrence after operation for non-serosa-invasive gastric cancer

Even though curative surgery has been performed for patients with non- serosa-invasive gastric cancer, some patients die of peritoneal recurrence (Abe et al., 1995; Bozzetti et al., 1986; Fink & Longmire, 1991; Shimada et al., 2001a; Yoo et al., 2000). As shown in Table 1, even in patients with early gastric cancer, three out of 420 died of peritoneal recurrence.

	Mucosal tumor	Submucosal tumor
No. of patients	621	430
Lymph node metastasis (%)	14 (2.3)	84 (19.5)
Cancer death (5-year survival rate: %)	6 (99.0)	26 (94.0)
Recurrence		
Hematogenous	6	19
Lymphatic	0	4
Peritoneal	0	3

Table 1. Lymph node metastasis and cancer death in early gastric carcinoma treated by D2 gastrectomy

Our investigations based on the intraoperative ultra-rapid RT-PCR system elucidated the cause (Marutsuka et al., 2003). Peritoneal lavage samples from 63 patients with non-serosa-invasive gastric carcinoma were obtained at laparotomy and immediately after lymph node dissection. To identify the free cancer cells in the samples, CEA and CK20 specific RT-PCR were performed using LightCycler™ method in combination with an automated mRNA extractor. In the peritoneal lavage samples from non-serosa-invasive cases after lymph node dissection, a CEA mRNA product was detected in 15 of 63 patients (23.8%) (Fig. 3). This was not evident in the mucosal (M) tumors, but was identified in three (14.3%), five (33.3%), and seven (53.8%) patients with submucosal (SM), muscularis propria (MP), and subserosal (SS) tumor, respectively. As regards CK20 mRNA, the product was identified in 14 of 63 patients (22.2%). Just like CEA mRNA, CK20 mRNA was not detected in the mucosal tumors, but was identified in three (14.3%), five (33.3%), and six patients (46.2%) with SM, MP, and SS tumor, respectively. Both CEA mRNA and CK20 mRNA were detected in three (14.3%), four (26.7%), and six (46.2%) with SM, MP, and SS tumor, respectively. In consequence, the number of free cancer cells, calculated by the standard curve for cancerous cells, were 3.5 ± 3.7 (mean ± SD), 12.1 ± 9.6, and 124.8 ± 224.0 cells/100ml in the lavage after lymph node dissection from SM, MP, and SS tumor, respectively.

This study using the intraoperative ultra-rapid RT-PCR system revealed that free cancer cells were found in 14.3% and 26.7% of the lavage fluid after lymph node dissection from patients with SM and MP tumors, respectively. Statistical analysis demonstrated that lymph node metastasis was the independent predictor for the existence of intra-peritoneal free cancer cells after lymph node dissection.

From our previous study on 1272 cases of gastric carcinoma, 1/257 cases (0.4%) of SM and 6/136 cases (4.4%) of MP cases developed peritoneal metastasis after potentially curative operation (Shimada et al., 2001a, 2003). Among them, 86% of the patients had lymph node metastasis and/or lymphatic invasion. Our results determined that lymph node dissection is the main factor for spreading viable free cancer cells into the peritoneal cavity. Thus, it was proved that lymph node dissection opens the lymphatic channel and spreads viable cancer cells into the peritoneal cavity.

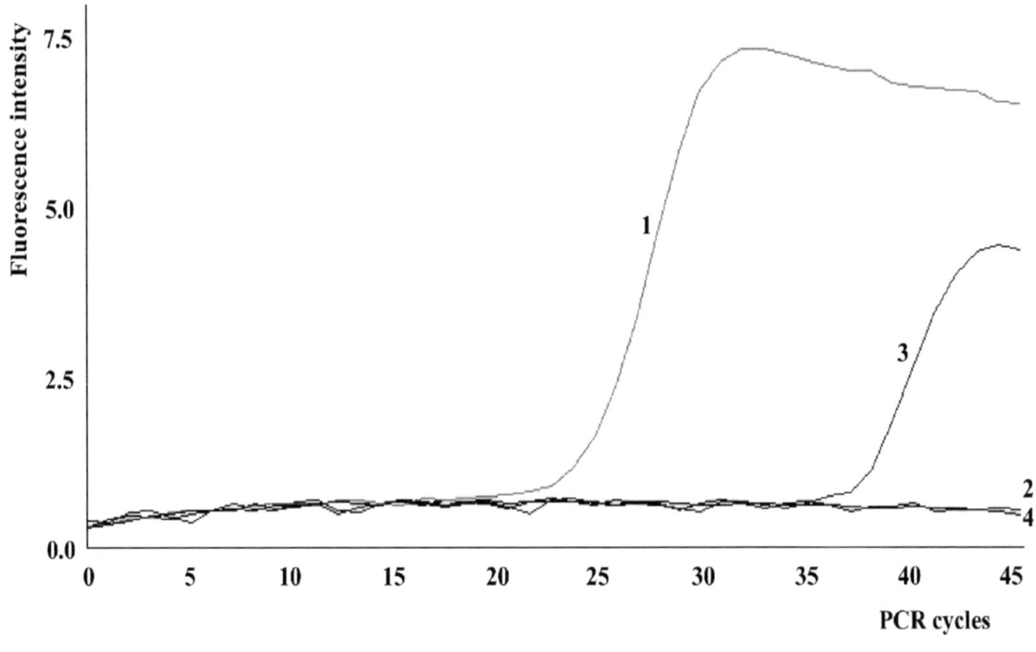

Fig. 3. Representative results of ultra-rapid RT-PCR by LightCycler™ in a patient with SM tumor of well-differentiated adenocarcinoma with lymph node metastasis and lymphatic invasion. Curve 1: WiDr colon cancer cells as positive control; curve 2: intraperitoneal lavage sample at laparotomy; curve 3: intraperitoneal lavage sample immediately after lymph nodes dissection; curve 4: no template as negative control. (Marutsuka et al., 2003)

5. EIPL therapy

To date, there are no definitive effective therapies for peritoneal carcinomatosis. Therefore, attention has been paid to detecting peritoneal free cancer cells in patients with advanced gastric carcinoma without overt peritoneal metastasis, and attempts to prevent peritoneal metastasis (S. Fujimoto et al.,1999; T. Fujimoto et al., 2002; Hamazoe et al., 1994; Hayes et al., 1999; Rosen et al, 1998; C.C. Wu et al., 1997, Yonemura et al., 1995; Yu et al., 1998).

The status of CY+/P- includes the condition where peritoneal implantation has not occurred yet. We have proposed that EIPL is a quite formidable method for reducing the number of cells to potentially zero, just like the so-called 'limiting dilution' approach. EIPL was performed in five cases of serosa-invasive (SE) gastric carcinoma with CY+/P-, and its efficacy was evaluated by the ultra-rapid quantitative RT-PCR protocol (Shimada et al., 2002). Sequential washing of intra-peritoneal free cancer cells of $3.8 \times 10^5 \pm 1.4 \times 10^5$/100ml of lavage decreased the number to 2.8 ± 1.5 cells by 6 to 8 washes. Free cancer cells were not detected in the washing fluid after that (Fig. 4).

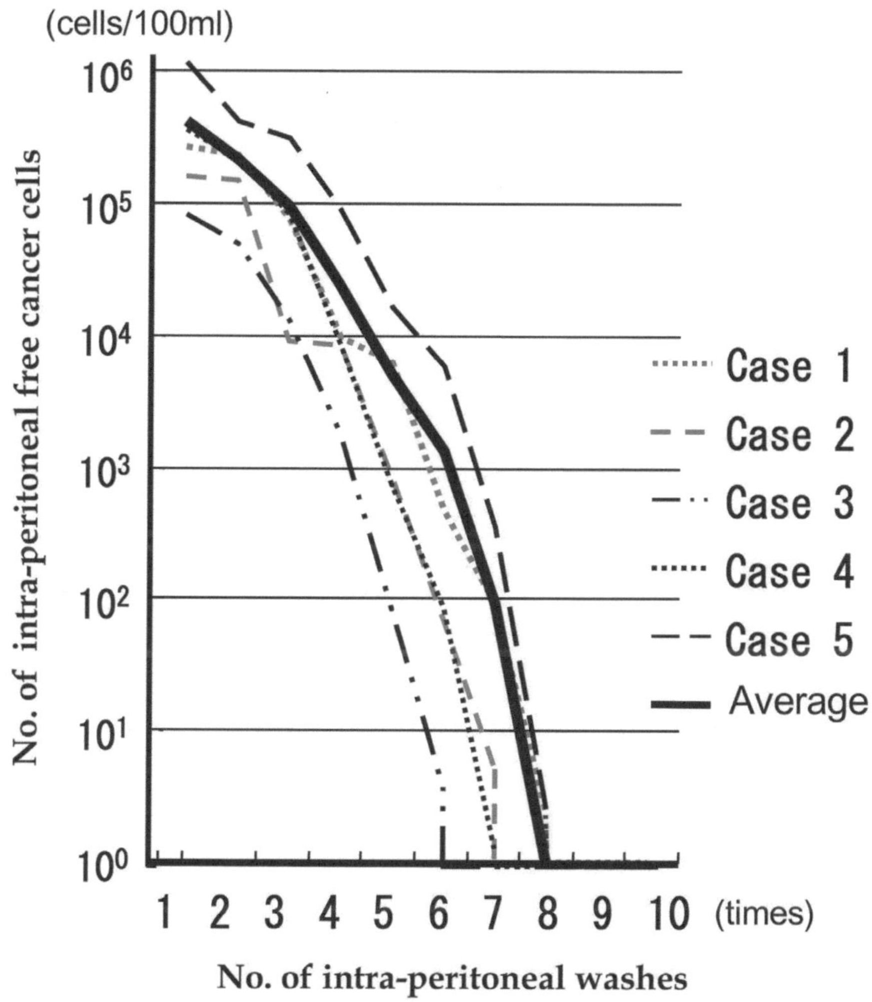

Fig. 4. Changes in numbers of intra-peritoneal free cancer cells in five gastric cancer patients with CY+ treated by EIPL therapy. The numbers of free cancer cells in 100 ml of samples from the first to the 10th wash using each 1 litter of saline were quantitated by ultra-rapid RT-PCR. The free cancer cells in the lavage fluids were serially diluted by 8 litters of saline and disappeared in washing fluids after the 8th wash.

On the other hand, $2.8 \times 10^4 \pm 4.5 \times 10^4$ of intra-peritoneal free cancer cells still remained in 100ml of the lavage when not treated with EIPL. Our preliminary subset analysis based on 24 consecutive patients with CY+/P- who underwent curative surgical treatment for advanced gastric cancer, and were followed up for 2 years or until death, has shown a statistically significant ($P = 0.017$) improvement of a two-year survival rate when treated with EIPL as compared with when not treated with EIPL (Shimada et al., 2002).

6. Five-year survival rates of patients who had EIPL therapy through a prospective randomized clinical trial

Following a pioneering study (Shimada et al., 2002; K. Yamamoto et al., 2005), we performed the EIPL therapy for advanced gastric cancer patients with CY+/P- in order to clearly clarify the distinct 5-year survival effects through a prospective randomized multicenter trial (Kuramoto et al., 2009). A total of 88 gastric cancer cases with CY+/P- from 1522 patients with advanced gastric cancer at multicenter were enrolled in this study, and were randomly allocated to three groups: surgery alone group, surgery plus intra-peritoneal chemotherapy (IPC) group, and surgery plus EIPL and IPC (EIPL-IPC) group. In EIPL-IPC group, 100mg of cisplatin (CDDP) was administered into the peritoneal cavity, after the EIPL treatment. Peritoneal lavage for the surgery alone group and the IPC group was done with 3 liters (1 liter, three times) before the closure of the abdominal wall or intra-peritoneal chemotherapy, respectively.

The overall five-year survival rate of the patients with EIPL-IPC was 43.8%, and this data was significantly higher than that of the IPC group (4.6%, $P < 0.0001$) and the surgery alone group (0 %, $P < 0.0001$) (Fig. 5). Among various recurrent patterns, the EIPL-IPC group had a significantly lower incidence of peritoneal recurrence than either of the other groups ($P < 0.0001$). Univariate and multivariate analyses clearly revealed that EIPL was the most significant impact factor.

The results of the present prospective randomized multicenter study far exceeded our expectations and showed a remarkably much better prognosis than previous studies on gastric cancer patients with CY+/P-. For example, a study on the median survival time (MST) of 91 patients with CY+/P- who had potentially curative resection stated survival to be only 386 days (Kodera et al., 1999), and the 5-year overall survival rate has been 13% (Rosenberg et al., 2006). In this study, the surgery alone group as well as the IPC group also showed similar results to the reports just cited. Surprisingly, however, in the CY+/P- group the overall five-year survival rate and MST were 42.1% and 35 months, respectively, and showed remarkably significant ($P < 0.0001$) improvement of both survival and MST. The results appeared so convincing and promising to us as to serve as a solid basis for employing the EIPL-IPC therapy with a great degree of confidence and high expectations.

7. Proposal of the optimal and practical therapeutic strategy for gastric cancer

Based on the data presented in this review, the authors propose the following treatment protocol for gastric cancer (Fig. 6). Accurate diagnosis of mucosal or submucosal cancer is made macroscopically including an EUS examination. Mucosal and submucosal invasion is correctly diagnosed in 75 to 85% of patients using EUS. All mucosal lesions with UL- should be treated by endoscopic submucosal dissection (ESD). If histologic examination of the ESD specimen reveals complete resection, the treatment is considered to be perfect and the patient only needs follow-up. If histologic examination reveals an incomplete resection, laparoscopic local resection is required. For a mucosal tumor with UL+, laparoscopic gastrectomy with D1 is indicated. All macroscopic SM and advanced cancer cancer (MP, SS, SE and SI) should be treated by gastrectomy with D2 (Shimada et al., 2001a).

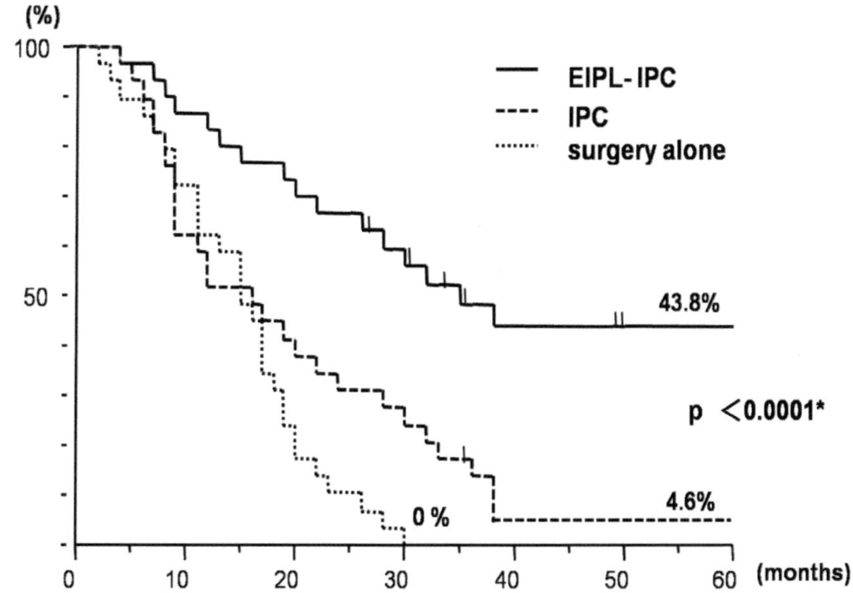

Number at risk

EIPL- IPC	30	27	22	16	11	9	8
IPC	29	22	12	8	1	1	1
surgery alone	29	23	7	1	0	0	0

Fig. 5. The survival curves for 88 patients stratified according to the treatment. *By log-rank test. (Kuramoto et al., 2009)

Although a Dutch report has described the high post-operative morbidity and hospital mortality after gastrectomy with D2 lymph node dissection (Bonenkamp et al., 1995), D2 resections appear to be feasible and safe in Japanese (Japanese Research Society for Gastric Cancer, 1999; Kuramoto et al., 2009; Maruyama, 1987; Nakamura et al., 1992; Ohgaki et al., 1999; Sano et al., 2004; Shimada et al., 2001b; C.W. Wu et al., 2008) and certain Western patients (Harrison et al., 1998; Lim et al., 2007). In our study, operative morbidity and hospital mortality was 1.5% (16 of 1051) and 0.5% (5 of 1051) respectively. Certain factors in the Dutch patients such as a more advanced tumor stage or larger physical build to the Japanese patients in this study might have influenced the high morbidity and mortality. The present study on patients with gastric cancer suggested that the potential benefits of D2 operation outweigh the risk of increased postoperative morbidity and mortality. Therefore, advanced gastric cancer should be treated by gastrectomy with D2, and D2+α may be necessary for patients with apparent N2 and/or N3 lymph nodes metastasis. Complete extirpation of gastric cancer with a sufficient resection margin from the tumor and the removal of metastatic lymph nodes is the only treatment that offers hope of cure for patients with gastric cancer (Balfour, 1973; Harrison et al., 1998; Japanese Research Society for Gastric Cancer, 1999; Maruyama, 1987; Shimada et al., 2003; Zhang et al., 2010). However, as a matter of course, excessive gastrectomy and lymph node dissection have to be avoided for the adverse effects they have on a patient's subsequent quality of life.

From the viewpoint of prophylactic strategy against peritoneal recurrence, the findings presented in this paper should greatly transform the surgical treatment for gastric cancer, including non-serosa-involved tumors. The authors strongly advocate for the adoption of the new treatment protocol for gastric cancer as shown in Fig. 6.

After the appropriate tumor resection and lymph node dissection, our novel EIPL regimen serves an extremely important role for gastric patients with high peritoneal recurrent risks such as serosal invasion and lymph node metastasis. The innovative EIPL method is very practical and the theoretical basis creates high expectation as to the effects of cyto-reduction, potentially to nil. Furthermore, the EIPL therapy is simple, very little time-consuming, inexpensive, it is not curtailed by place or time, and does not need any special techniques or devices in order to be applied. In addition, even if a few cancer cells were to remain after EIPL therapy, these cells might find it difficult to survive and/or to disseminate due to the effects of IPC or postoperative systemic chemotherapy with S1 (Ishizoe et al., 2006; Shirasaka et al., 2000; Sugimachi et al., 1999) .

Conventional cytological examination with Papanicolou staining (Papanicolaou, 1963) has been reported to lack sensitivity, and it is suggested that occult free cancer cells are present at the time of the operation in such cases. Therefore, improvements have been made by many investigators using immunological methods with selected monoclonal antibodies or real-time RT-PCR for the detection of free cancer cells in the peritoneal washes (Benevolo et al., 1998; Broll et al., 2001; Dicken et al., 2006; Kodera et al., 2002; Saito et al., 2007; P. Vogel et al., 1999; I. Vogel & Kalthoff, 2001). These methods have allowed the identification of cytology false-negative cases in gastric cancer. However, because these means are not generally available at the actual time of the operation, a cytological examination is commonly performed to detect the existence of free cancer cells in the peritoneal cavity. From these cautionary points of view, it is only prudent that the EIPL-IPC therapy would be employed for all patients with serosa-involved gastric cancer and regardless of CY+/P-.

On the other hand, although curative surgery has been used for patients with non-serosa-involved gastric cancer, some die of peritoneal recurrence. One of the reasons postulated for peritoneal dissemination in non-serosa-involved gastric cancer is that the lymph node dissection might open lymphatic channels and spread viable cancer cells to the peritoneal cavity (Fink & Longmire, 1991). We have demonstrated that free cancer cells were found in the lavage fluid after the lymph node dissection in 26.7% of patients with muscle-involved tumors, suggesting that the surgical operation itself causes the peritoneal dissemination of the these cancer cells (Marutsuka et al., 2003). Therefore, EIPL therapy is also strongly recommended for non-serosa-involved gastric carcinomas suspected of lymphatic invasion through surgery, or positive real-time RT-PCR for detection of free cancer cells in the peritoneal washes after D2 operation for non-serosa-involved tumor, including early gastric carcinoma (Fig. 6).

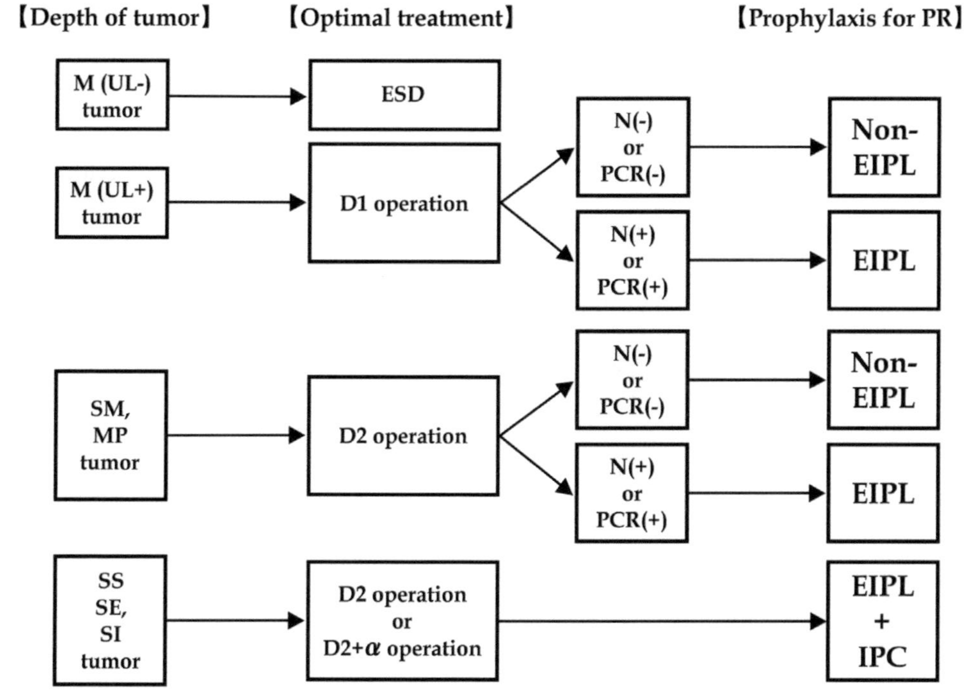

Fig. 6. A practical and optimal treatment protocol for gastric cancer. PR: peritoneal recurrence, M: mucosal tumor, SM: submucosal tumor, MP: tumor with muscularis proprial invasion, SS: tumor with subserosal invasion, SE: tumor with serosal invasion, SI: tumor invasion of adjacent structures, UL+: tumor with ulceration or ulceration scar, UL-: tumor without ulceration or ulceration scar, ESD: endoscopic submucosal dissection, D1 operation: gastrectomy with dissection of group 1 lymph node, D2 operation: gastrectomy with dissection of group 1 and 2 lymph node, N(+): positive lymph node metastasis through surgery, N(-): no evidence of lymph node metastasis, PCR: real-time reverse transcriptase-polymerase chain reaction, EIPL: extensive intraoperative peritoneal lavage, IPC: intra-peritoneal chemotherapy

8. Conclusion

EIPL therapy was developed as a prophylactic strategy for peritoneal recurrence, with the goal of improving the prognosis for patients with gastric cancer. In the present article, the risk factors on peritoneal recurrence from clinicopathological features of gastric carcinoma and the therapy's contribution to a remarkable improvement in the 5-year survival for gastric cancer patients with positive lavage cytology on prospective randomized controlled clinical trials was reviewed. From the viewpoint of prophylactic strategy against peritoneal recurrence, we propose the optimal and practical treatment protocol for gastric cancer.

9. References

Abe, S., Yoshimura, H., Tabara, H., Tachibana, M., Monden, N., Nakamura, T., & Nagaoka, S. (1995). Curative resection of gastric cancer: limitation of peritoneal lavage cytology in predicting the outcome. *Journal of Surgical Oncology,* Vol.59, No.4, pp. 226-9

Balfour, D.C. (1973). Factors of significance in the prognosis of cancer of the stomach. *Annals of Surgery,* Vol.105, pp. 733-40

Bozzetti, F., Bonfanti, G., Morabito, A., Bufalino, R., Menotti, V., Andreola, S., Doci, R., & Gennari, L. (1986). A multifactorial approach for the prognosis of patients with carcinoma of the stomach after curative resection. *Surgery, Gynecology & Obstetrics ,* Vol.162, No.3, pp. 229-34

Boku, T., Nakane, Y., Minoura, T., Takada, H., Yamamura, M., Hioki, K., & Yamamoto, M. (1990). Prognostic significance of serosal invasion and free intraperitoneal cancer cells in gastric cancer. *The British Journal of Surgery,* Vol.77, No.4, pp. 436-9

Bonenkamp, J.J., Songun, I., Hermans, J., Sasako, M., Welvaart, K., Plukker, J.T., van Elk, P., Obertop, H., Gouma, D.J., & Taat, C.W. (1995). Randomised comparison of morbidity after D1 and D2 dissection for gastric cancer in 996 Dutch patients. *Lancet,* Vol.345, No. 8952, pp. 745-8

Benevolo, M., Mottolese, M., Cosimelli, M., Tedesco, M., Giannarelli, D., Vasselli, S., Carlini, M., Garofalo, A., & Natali, P.G. (1998). Diagnostic and prognostic value of peritoneal immunocytology in gastric cancer. *Journal of clinical oncology,* Vol.16, No.10, pp. 3406-11

Burke, E.C., Karpeh, M.S. Jr., Conlon, K.C., & Brennan, M.F. (1998). Peritoneal lavage cytology in gastric cancer: an independent predictor of outcome. *Annals of Surgical Oncology,* Vol.5, No.5, pp. 411-5

Bando, E., Yonemura, Y., Takeshita, Y., Taniguchi, K., Yasui, T., Yoshimitsu, Y., Fushida, S., Fujimura, T., Nishimura, G., & Miwa, K. (1999). Intraoperative lavage for cytological examination in 1297 patients with gastric carcinoma. *American Journal of Surgery,* Vol.178, No.3, pp. 256-62

Broll, R., Weschta, M., Windhoevel, U., Berndt, S., Schwandner, O., Roblick, U., Schiedeck, T.H., Schimmelpenning, H., Bruch, H.P., & Duchrow, M. (2001). Prognostic significance of free gastrointestinal tumor cells in peritoneal lavage detected by immunocytochemistry and polymerase chain reaction. *Langenbeck's Archives of Surgery,* Vol.386, No.4, pp. 285-92

Cunliffe, W.J., & Sugarbaker, P.H. (1989). Gastrointestinal malignancy: rationale for adjuvant therapy using early postoperative intraperitoneal chemotherapy. *British Journal of Surgery,* Vol.76, No.10, pp. 1082-90

Cheong, J.H., Shen, J.Y., Song, C.S., Hyung, W.J., Shen, J.G., Choi, S.H., & Noh, S.H. (2007). Early postoperative intraperitoneal chemotherapy following cytoreductive surgery in patients with very advanced gastric cancer. *Annals of Surgical Oncology,* Vol.14, No.1, pp. 61-8

Dicken, B.J., Graham, K., Hamilton, S.M., Andrews, S., Lai, R., Listgarten, J., Jhangri, G.S., Saunders, L.D., Damaraju, S., & Cass, C. (2006). Lymphovascular invasion is associated with poor survival in gastric cancer: an application of gene-expression and tissue array techniques. *Annals of Surgery,* Vol.243, No.1, pp. 64-73

Fink, A., & Longmire, W. (1991). Carcinoma of stomach. In: *Textbook of Surgery,* Subiston, D.C., (Ed.), 814-27, W.B. Saunders, Philadelphia, USA

Fujimoto, S., Takahashi, M., Mutou, T., Kobayashi, K., & Toyosawa, T. (1999). Successful intraperiotneal hyperthermic chemoperfusion for the prevention of postoperative peritoneal recurrence in patients with advanced gastric carcinoma. *Cancer,* Vol.85, No.3, pp. 529-34

Fujimoto, T., Zhang, B., Minami, S., Wang, X., Takahashi, Y., & Mai, M. (2002). Evaluation of intraoperative intraperitoneal cytology for advanced gastric carcinoma. *Oncology,* Vol.62, No.3, pp. 201-8

Hagiwara, A., Takahashi, T., Kojima, O., Sawai, K., Yamaguchi, T., Yamane, T., Taniguchi, H., Kitamura, K., Noguchi, A., & Seiki, K. (1992). Prophylaxis with carbon-absorbed mitomycin against peritoneal recurrence of gastric cancer. *Lancet,* Vol.339, No. 8794, pp. 629-31

Hamazoe, R., Maeta, M., & Kaibara, N. (1994). Intraperitoneal thermochemotherapy for prevention of peritoneal recurrence of gastric cancer. Final results of a randomized controlled study. *Cancer,* Vol.73, No.8, pp. 2048-52

Harrison, L.E., Karpeh, M.S., & Brennan, M.F. (1998). Extended lymphadenectomy is associated with a survival benefit for node-negative gastric cancer. *Journal of Gastrointestinal Surgery,* Vol.2, No.2, pp. 126-31

Hayes, N., Wayman, J., Wadehra, V., Scott, D.J., Raimes, S.A., & Griffin, S.M. (1999). Peritoneal cytology in the surgical evaluation of gastric carcinoma. *British Journal of cancer,* Vol.79, No. 3-4, pp. 520-4

Hioki, M., Gotohda, N., Konishi, M., Nakagohri, T., Takahashi, S., & Kinoshita, T. (2010). Predictive factors improving survival after gastrectomy in gastric cancer patients with peritoneal carcinomatosis. *World Journal of Surgery,* Vol.34, No.3, pp. 555-62

Iitsuka, Y., Kaneshima, S., Tanida, O., Takeuchi, T., & Koga, S. (1979). Intraperitoneal free cancer cells and their viability in gastric cancer. *Cancer,* Vol.44, No.4, pp. 1476-80

Ikeguchi, M., Oka, A., Tsujitani, S., Maeta, M., & Kaibara, N. (1994). Relationship between area of serosal invasion and intraperitoneal free cancer cells in patients with gastric cancer. *Anticancer Research,* Vol.14, No. 5B, pp. 2131-4

Ikeguchi, M., Matsumoto, S., Yoshioka, S., Murakami, D., Kanaji, S., Ohro, S., Yamaguchi, K., Saito, H., Tatebe, S., Kondo, A., Tsujitani, S., & Kaibara, N. (2005). Laparoscopic-assisted intraperiotneal chemotherapy for the patients with scirrhous gastric cancer. *Chemotherapy,* Vol.51, No.1, pp. 15-20

Ishizone, S., Maruta, F., Saito, H., Koide, N., Sugiyama, A., Nakayama, J., & Miyagawa, S. (2006). Efficacy of S-1 for patients with peritoneal metastasis of gastric cancer. *Chemotherapy,* Vol.52, No. 6, pp. 301-7

Japanese Research Society for Gastric Cancer. (1999). *Japanese Classification of Gastric Carcinoma,* First English Edition, Kanehara, Tokyo, Japan

Koga, S., Kaibara, N., Iitsuka, Y., Kudo, H., Kimura, A., & Hiraoka, H. (1984). Prognostic significance of intraperitoneal free cancer cells in gastric cancer patients. *Journal of Cancer Research and Clinical Oncology,* Vol.108, No.2, pp. 236-8

Kaibara, N., Iitsuka, Y., Kimura, A., Kobayashi, Y., Hirooka, Y., Nishidoi, H., & Koga, S. (1987). Relationship between area of serosal invasion and prognosis in patients with gastric carcinoma. *Cancer,* Vol.60, No.1, pp. 136-9

Kida, M., Tanabe, S., Watanabe, M., Kokutou, M., Kondou, I., Yamada, Y., Sakaguchi, T., & Saigenji, K. (1998). Staging of gastric cancer with endoscopic ultrasonography and endoscopic mucosal resection. *Endoscopy,* Vol.30, No.1, pp. 64-8

Kodera, Y., Yamamura, Y., Shimizu, Y., Torii, A., Hirai, T., Yasui, K., Morimoto, T., & Kato, T. (1999). Peritoneal washing cytology: prognostic value of positive findings in patients with gastric carcinoma undergoing a potentially curative resection. *Journal of Surgical Oncology,* Vol.72, No.2, pp. 60-5

Kodera, Y., Nakanishi, H., Ito, S., Yamamura, Y., Kanemitsu, Y., Shimizu, Y., Hirai, T., Yasui, K., Kato, T., & Tatematsu, M. (2002). Quantitative detection of disseminated free cancer cells in peritoneal washes with real-time reverse transcriptase-polymerase chain reaction. *Annals of Surgery,* Vol.235, No.4, pp. 499-506

Kunisaki, C., Shimada, H., Nomura, M., Akiyama, H., Takahashi, M., & Matsuda, G. (2002). Lack of efficacy of prophylactic peritoneal perfusion on subsequent peritoneal recurrence and survival in patients with advanced gastric cancer. *Surgery,* Vol.131, No.5, pp. 521-8

Kuramoto, M., Shimada, S., Ikeshima, S., Matsuo, A., Yagi, Y., Matsuda, M., Yonemura, Y., & Baba, H. (2009). Extensive intraoperative peritoneal lavage as a standard prophylactic strategy for peritoneal recurrence in patients with gastric carcinoma. *Annals of Surgery,* Vol.250, No.2, pp. 242-6

Lim, S., Muhs, B.E., Marcus, S.G., Newman, E., Berman, R.S., & Hiotis, S.P. (2007). Results following resection for stage IV gastric cancer; are better outcomes observed in selected patients subgroups? *Journal of Surgical Oncology,* Vol.95, No.2, pp. 118-22

Maruyama, K. (1987). The most important prognostic factors for gastric cancer patients. A study using univariate and multivariate analyses. *Scandinavian Journal of Gastroenterology,* Vol.22, pp. 63-8

Moriguchi, S., Maehara, Y., Korenaga, D., Sugiuchi, K., & Nose, Y. (1992). Risk factors which predict pattern of recurrence after curative surgery for patients with advanced gastric cancer. *Surgical Oncology,* Vol.1, No.5, pp. 341-6

Marutsuka, T., Shimada, S., Shiomori, K., Hayashi, N., Yagi, Y., Yamane, T., & Ogawa, M. (2003). Mechanisms of peritoneal metastasis after operation for non-serosa-invasive gastric carcinoma: an ultrarapid detection system for intraperitoneal free cancer cells and a prophylactic strategy for peritoneal metastasis. *Clinical Cancer Research,* Vol.9, No.2, pp. 678-85

Makino, T., Fujiwara, Y., Takiguchi, S., Miyata, H., Yamasaki, M., Nakajima, K., Nishida, T., Mori, M., & Doki, Y. (2010). The utility of pre-operative peritoneal lavage examination in serosa-invading gastric cancer patients. *Surgery,* Vol.148, No.1, pp. 96-102

Nakamura, K., Ueyama, T., Yao, T., Xuan, Z.X., Ambe, K., Adachi, Y., Yakeishi, Y., Matsukuma, A., & Enjoji, M. (1992). Pathology and prognosis of gastric carcinoma. Findings in 10,000 patients who underwent primary gastrectomy. *Cancer,* Vol.70, No.5, pp. 1030-7

Ohgaki, M., Takahashi, T., Hagiwara, A., Yamasaki, J., & Togawa, T. (1999). Effect of Extensive lymphnode dissection on the survival of early gastric cancer. *Hepato-Gastroenterol,* Vol.46, No.27, pp. 2096-9

Papanicolaou, G.N. (1963). Atlas of Exfoliative Cytology, *Harvard University Press,* Cambridge, USA

Ribeiro, U. Jr., Gama-Rodrigues, J.J., Safatle-Ribeiro, A.V., Bitelman, B., Ibrahim, R.E., Ferreira, M.B., Laudanna, A.A., & Pinotti, H.W. (1998). Prognostic significance of intraperitoneal free cancer cells obtained by laparoscopic peritoneal lavage in patients with gastric cancer. *Journal of Gastrointestinal Surgery,* Vol.2, No.3, pp. 244-9

Rosen, H.R., Jatzko, G., Repse, S., Potrc, S., Neudorfer, H., Sandbichler, P., Zacherl, J., Rabl, H., Holzberger, P., Lisborg, P., & Czeijka, M. (1998). Adjuvant intraperitoneal chemotherapy with carbon-adsorbed mitomycin in patients with gastric cancer: results of a randomized multicenter trial of the Austrian Working Group for Surgical Oncology. *Journal of Clinical Oncology,* Vol.16, No.8, pp. 2733-8

Ribeiro, U. Jr., Safatle-Ribeiro, A.V., Zilberstein, B., Mucerino, D., Yagi, O.K., Bresciani, C.C., Jacob, C.E., Iryia, K., & Gama-Rodrigues, J. (2006). Does the intraoperative peritoneal lavage cytology add prognostic information in patients with potentially curative gastric resection? *Journal of Gastrointestinal Surgery,* Vol.10, No.2, pp. 170-7

Rosenberg, R., Nekarda, H., Bauer, P., Schenck, U., Hoefler, H., & Siewert, J.R. (2006). Free peritoneal tumor cells are an independent prognostic factor in curatively resected stage 1B gastric carcinoma. *The British Journal of Surgery,* Vol.93, No.3, pp. 325-31

Sauter, T., Hofbauer, F., & Depisch, D. (1994). Adjuvant intraperitoneal cisplatin chemotherapy does not improve long-term survival after surgery for advanced gastric cancer. *Journal of Clinical Oncology,* Vol.12, No.5, pp. 970-4

Sugimachi, K., Maehara, Y., Horikoshi, N., Shimada, Y., Sakata, Y., Mitachi, Y., & Taguchi, T. (1999). An early phase II study of oral S-1, a newly developed 5-fluorouracil derivative for advanced and recurrent gastrointestinal cancers. The S-1 Gastrointestinal Cancer Study Group. *Oncology,* Vol.57, No.3, pp. 202-10

Shirasaka, T., Yamamitsu, S., Tsuji, A., & Taguchi, T. (2000). Conceptual changes in cancer chemotherapy: from an oral fluoropyrimidine prodrug, UFT, to a novel oral fluoropyrimidine prodrug, S-1, and low-dose FP therapy in Japan. *Investigational New Drugs,* Vol.18, No.4, pp. 315-29

Shimada, S., Yagi, Y., Shiomori, K., Honmyo, U., Hayashi, N., Matsuo, A., Marutsuka, T., & Ogawa, M. (2001a). Characterization and proposal of the optimal therapeutic strategy for early gastric cancer. *Surgery,* Vol.129, No.6, pp. 714-9

Shimada, S., Yagi, Y., Honmyo, U., Shiomori, K., Yoshida, N., & Ogawa, M. (2001b). Involvement of more than three lymph nodes predicts poor prognosis of early gastric carcinoma. *Gastric Cancer,* Vol.4, No.2, pp. 54-9

Shimada, S., Tanaka, E., Marutsuka, T., Honmyo, U., Tokunaga, H., Yagi, Y., Aoki, N., & Ogawa, M. (2002). Extensive intraoperative peritoneal lavage and chemotherapy for gastric cancer patients with peritoneal free cancer cells. *Gastric Cancer,* Vol.5, No.3, pp. 168-72

Shimada, S., Yagi, Y., Shiomori, K., Shiomori, K., Marutsuka, T., Hirota, M., Honmyo, U., & Ogawa, M. (2003). Proposal of the optimal and practical therapeutic strategy for gastric cancer. In *Biological Response to Planned and Unplanned injuries: Cellular, molecular and genetic aspects,* Ogawa, M., (Ed.), 389-7, International Congress Series, Elsevier, Amsterdam, Netherlands

Sano, T., Sasako, M., Yamamoto, S., Nashimoto, A., Kurita, A., Hiratsuka, M., Tsujinaka, T., Kinoshita, T., Arai, K., Yamamura, Y., & Okajima, K. (2004). Gastric cancer surgery: morbidity and mortality results from a prospective randomized controlled trial comparing D2 and extended para-aortic lymphadenectomy--Japan Clinical Oncology Group study 9501. Journal of Clinical Oncology, Vol.22, No.14, pp. 2767-73

Saito, H., Osaki, T., Murakami, D., Sakamoto, T., Kanaji, S., Ohro, S., Tatebe, S., Tsujitani, S., & Ikeguchi, M. (2007). Prediction of sites of recurrence in gastric carcinoma using immunohistochemical parameters. *Journal of Surgical Oncology,* Vol.95, No.2, pp. 123-8

Vogel, P., Rüschoff, J., Kümmel, S., Zirngibl, H., Hofstädter, F., Hohenberger, W., & Jauch, K.W. (1999). Immunocytology improves prognostic impact of peritoneal tumour cell detection compared to conventional cytology in gastric cancer. *European Journal of Surgical Oncology,* Vol.25, No.5, pp. 515-9

Vogel, I., & Kalthoff, H. (2001). Disseminated tumor cells. Their detection and significance for prognosis of gastrointestinal and pancreatic carcinomas. *Virchows Archiv,* Vol.439, No.2, pp. 109-17

Wu, C.C., Chen, J.T., Chang, M.C., Ho, W.L., Chen, C.Y., Yeh, D.C., Liu, T.J., & P'eng, F.K. (1997). Optimal surgical strategy for potentially curable serosa-involved gastric carcinoma with intraperitoneal free cancer cells. *Journal of the American College of Surgeons,* Vol.184, No.6, pp. 611-7

Wu, C.W., Chiou, J.M., Ko, F.S., Lo, S.S., Chen, J.H., Lui, W.Y., & Whang-Peng, J. (2008). Quality of life after curative gastrectomy for gastric cancer in a randomised controlled trial. British Journal of Cancer, Vol.98, No.1, pp. 54-9

Yonemura, Y., Ninomiya, I., Kaji, M., Sugiyama, K., Fujimura, K., Sawa, T., Katayama, K., Tanaka, S., Hirono, Y., & Miwa, K. (1995). Prophylaxis with intraoperative chemohyperthermia against peritoneal recurrence of serosal invasion-positive gastric cancer. *World Journal of Surgery,* Vol.19, No.3, pp. 1-6

Yawata, A., Adachi, M., Okuda, H., Naishiro, Y., Takamura, T., Hareyama, M., Takayama, S., Reed, J.C., & Imai, K. (1998). Prolonged cell survival enhances peritoneal dissemination of gastric cancer cells. *Oncogene,* Vol.16, No.20, pp. 2681-6

Yu, W., Whang, I., Suh, I., Averbach, A., Chang, D., & Sugarbaker, P.H. (1998). Prospective randomized trial of early postoperative intraperitoneal chemotherapy as an adjuvant to resectable gastric cancer. *Annals of Surgery,* Vol.228, No.3, pp. 347-54

Yoo, C.H., Noh, S.H., Shin, D.W., Choi, S.H., & Min, J.S. (2000). Recurrence following curative resection for gastric carcinoma. *The British Journal of Surgery,* Vol.87, No.2, pp. 236-42

Yamamoto, K., Shimada, S., Hirota, M., Yagi, Y., Matsuda, M., & Baba, H. (2005). EIPL(extensive intraoperative peritoneal lavage) therapy significantly reduces peritoneal recurrence after pancreatectomy in patients with pancreatic cancer. *International Journal of Oncology,* Vol.27, No.5, pp. 1321-8

Yamamoto, M., Matsuyama, A., Kameyama, T., Okamoto, M., Okazaki, J., Utsunomiya, T., Tsutsui, S., Fujiwara, M., & Ishida, T. (2009). Prognostic re-evaluation of peritoneal lavage cytology in Japanese patients with gastric carcinoma. *Hepato-gastroenterology,* Vol.56, No.89, pp. 261-5

Zhang, H., Liu, C., Wu, D., Meng, Y., Song, R., Lu, P., & Wang, S. (2010). Does D3 surgery offer a better survival outcome compared to D1 surgery for gastric cancer? A result based on a hospital population of two decades as taking D2 surgery for reference. *BMC Cancer,* Vol.10, pp. No.6, 308

16

Hepatic Metastases from Gastric Carcinoma

Guido Alberto Massimo Tiberio, Nazario Portolani
and Stefano Maria Giulini
University of Brescia
Italy

1. Introduction

"Aprioristic passive attitude": this is the mode that correctly defines the standard approach to gastric cancer patients presenting with hepatic metastases.

This behaviour is deeply motivated by the aggressive biology of the disease that so often frustrates any therapeutic approach. In fact, at diagnosis liver metastases are often multiple and associated to other extra-hepatic metastatic sites [D'Angelica et al., 2004; Dicken et al., 2005]. Furthermore, in the rare cases submitted to ablative treatments, hepatic and systemic recurrence has been experienced in the majority of cases.

However, considering survival performances extrapolated from a cohort of 1452 patients submitted to hepatic resection for noncolorectal nonendocrine liver metastases [Adam et al.,2006], it was observed that metastases from gastric adenocarcinoma performed in an intermediate way, ranking 10th in a list of 18 primaries. In fact, in selected cases an aggressive treatment can achieve unexpected results: 5-year survival rates from 10% to 40% have consistently been reported in surgical series considering patients with liver metastases as sole metastatic site.

An aggressive attitude, however, doesn't really penetrate into clinical practice and passivity still prevails, as depicted by an Italian survey reporting over 60% of patients not receiving specific treatments, including 30% of cases affected by 1 or 2 small metastases, and by therapeutic indication being influenced by patients' determination [Tiberio et al., 2008]. This attitude is rather diffused if a recent review reported 436 surgically treated cases [Kerkar, 2010] and a French survey recruited 101 patients from 41 centres [Chiche, 2005], numbers to be faced, for example, to more than 14700 resections for metastases from colo-rectal cancer enrolled in *LiverMetSurvey* as to December 2010.

With this contribution we will attempt to promote a pragmatic approach to these patients, knowing that only a μετάνοια (change of mind) may lead to the recognition of cases that can benefit from a tailored treatment and thus to better results. This attitude seems particularly important in these days in which promising therapeutic improvements are announced by state-of-art multimodal treatments favouring local and systemic control of the disease.

2. Clinical considerations

The dimension of the phenomenon is difficult to assess. It is influenced by a number of factors such as the incidence of gastric cancer in different geographical areas, the characteristics and quality of different health-care systems, the deployment of effective mass-screening programs capable to detect -and cure- gastric malignancies in an early phase. It seems reasonable to assume that the incidence of hepatic metastases from gastric cancer during the course of the disease figures around 10%-20% in eastern countries like Japan and South Korea, rises to 30%-40% in Western Europe and Anglo-Saxon world were an increase of advanced stages at diagnosis is recorded despite a steady and significant reduction of the incidence of gastric carcinoma in the last 20 years [Fayçal et al., 2005] and lies unmeasured -but probably over 50%- in other less monitored countries.

According to the presentation, hepatic metastases can be synchronous or metachronous. Synchronous metastases are detected during routine work-up of gastric primaries or -unexpectedly- at surgical exploration, but in some cases their detection leads to diagnosis of gastric cancer. They must be differentiated from the direct infiltration of liver parenchyma originating from gastric cancer itself (T4). They can originate from unresectable gastric cancers but also from resectable primaries.

Metachronous metastases are detected in up to 25-30% of patients submitted to curative gastrectomy. Eighty percent of them appear within the first 2 postoperative years, but it must be known that a wide consensus exists in considering synchronous those lesions diagnosed during the very first postoperative period (~ 6 months).

At diagnosis metastases-related symptoms and signs are generally observed when hepatic metastases are discovered first and lead to the diagnosis of gastric cancer; in the other cases patients are asymptomatic or may display the signs and symptoms of gastric tumor.

Clinical examination searches for epigastric or hypochondriac masses and hepatomegaly; at rectal or vaginal examination signs of peritoneal carcinosis are looked-for.

When Tumor markers CA 19-9, CEA and CA 72-4 are simultaneously positive they are strongly suggestive of liver involvement [Marrelli et al., 2004].

At US and CT imaging metastases from gastric cancer display aspecific hypo-dense and hypo-vascularised patterns and can't be distinguished from hepatic metastases originating from other gastro-enteric primaries.

An adequate radiological report must enumerate their number, measures and location, the latter in reference to Couinaud' segmentation. A good report allows the stadiation of hepatic disease according to the Japanese Gastric Cancer Association [10], a simple and practical classification, with direct therapeutic impact (table 1). In fact, H-3 hepatic involvement generally excludes ablative treatments, which are considered only for H-1 or H-2 cases.

H-0	No liver metastases
H-1	Liver metastases limited to one lobe of the liver
H-2	Isolated diverse metastases in both lobes of the liver
H-3	Multiple distributed metastases in both lobes of the liver

Table 1. Classification of hepatic metastases from gastric cancer as proposed by the Japanese Gastric Cancer Association, 1998.

3. Therapeutic approach

3.1 Systemic chemotherapy

At diagnosis liver metastases are often multiple and associated to other extra-hepatic metastatic sites such as peritoneal dissemination, extensive lymph-node and/or systemic metastases. In these conditions nothing more than palliative or supportive treatments can be proposed, without appreciable long term results. Chemotherapy achieves median survival ranging from 7 to 15 months but long term survival remains anecdotal [Cocconi et al., 2003; Lee et al., 2007; Cao et al., 2009]. In particular, considering the few trials evaluating systemic chemotherapy in the subset of patients with liver-only metastatic involvement, 5-years survival rates do not reach 2% [Yoshida et al., 2004].

3.2 Surgical treatment

Resection of liver metastases from gastric cancer is indicated in absence of extra-hepatic disease, if a complete ablation of the metastases can be achieved while preserving postoperative liver function [Ambiru et al, 2001; Okano et al., 2002]; it must also be associated to curative gastrectomy in case of synchronous lesions. In these conditions hepatectomy is a low-risk procedure, with negligible mortality and morbidity rates.
The surgical literature shows that several clinical and pathological parameters correlate with survival; among these, staging factors of the primary tumor, metastases-related and surgery-related variables have been reported more often than others (table 2).

Author	No.	T	N	G	H	Ø metastasis	Timing*	Margin§	MST (months)	No. survivors > 5 Years
Ochiai '94	21	√	√	-	-	n.a.	n.a.	n.a.	18	2 (19 %)
Miyazaki '97	21	-	-	-	√	n.a.	-	√	n.a.	2 (9.5 %)
Fujii '01	10	-	-	-	-	√	√	n.a.	16	1 (10 %)
Ambiru '01	40	-	-	-	-	-	√	-	12	6 (15 %)
Imamura '01	17	-	√	√	-	n.a	√	√	12	0
Okano '02	19	-	-	√	√	-	√	n.a.	21	4 (21 %)
Zacherl '02	15	-	-	-	√	-	√	-	8.8	2 (13 %)^
Saiura '02	10	-	-	-	-	-	-	n.a.	25	2 (20 %)
Shirabe '03	36	-	ly	-	√	-	-	-	n.a.	4 (11 %)
Roh '05	11	n.a.	-	-	n.a.	-	-	-	19	2 (18 %)
Chiche '05	101	-	-	-	√	√	-	√	14,5	11 (10 %)
Sakamoto '07	37	√	-	-	√	√	-	-	31	2 (5,4 %)
Koga '07	42	√	-	-	√	-	-	-	34	8 (19%)
Tsujimoto '10	17	√	ly	n.a.	-	-	-	n.a.	34	5 (29%)

MST: mean survival time Timing: synchronous vs.metachronous; § resection margin: + vs -; √ = prognostic factor; n.a.= not available; ly = lymphatic invasion; ^ = alive after 3 years.

Table 2. Prognostic factors and survival from series of patients submitted to surgical treatment of hepatic metastases.

However, data concerning long-term survivors demonstrate that, if we exclude bi-lobar spread of metastases (H 3), none of the reported predictive factors -alone or in combination- can deprive a patient of the possibility of long-term survival after hepatic resection, raising concern about the clinical value of prognostic factors emerging from small and super-selected populations submitted to liver resection.

3.2.1 Results from unselected populations

The correct approach to these particular patients can be extrapolated from a handful of key papers that addressed the topic analyzing unselected populations of gastric cancer patients presenting hepatic metastases as sole site of metastatic disease (table 3). From a cohort of 58 patients, the Korean group of Cheon and coll. did not extrapolate any primary-related or metastasis-related factor showing prognostic significance. On the very same line is the group of Makino and coll. from Japan, who studied 63 patients.
Ueda and colleagues, again from Japan, studied a cohort of 73 patients presenting synchronous metastases. Their data show that factors influencing survival where the extent of hepatic involvement (H1-2 vs H3) and macroscopic peritoneal dissemination (P0 vs P1) detected at surgical exploration. When focusing on the subgroup of H1-2 and P0 patients, they showed that number (1 vs >1) and size of hepatic metastases and N status of gastric cancer (N0-1 vs N2-3) influenced survival. An Italian survey performed under the auspices of the Italian Research Group on Gastric Cancer [Tiberio et al., 2008] studied an unselected cohort of 73 patients presenting metachronous metastases after curative D ≥ 2 gastrectomy. It was found that the factors T, N and G of the gastric primary, when rated T3b-T4, N+ and G3, independently display a clear negative prognostic value with cumulative effect.
These parameters may be helpful in order to appropriately select the therapeutic approach or, at least, to submit the cases to multidisciplinary evaluation, being aware that the prognosis of these patients is directly influenced by therapeutic choices. In fact, all the 4 above mentioned studies strongly highlight that the main factor influencing long-term survival (p ranging from 0.01 to 0.001) is the therapeutic approach to the liver metastases, in particular when hepatectomy is performed.

Author	No	Timing	Prognostic factors
Cheon 2008	58	Synchronous + metachronous	R0 resection of hepatic metastases
Ueda 2009	72	Synchronous	H; P; R0 Resection of hepatic metastases
Tiberio 2008	73	Metachronous	T; N; G of gastric primary; Resection of hepatic metastases
Hwang 2009	73	Metachronous	Stage of gastric primary Extrahepatic metastases; H Treatment of hepatic metastases

Table 3. Prognostic factors from series considering unselected populations.

In the Italian study hepatectomy was associated to a five-fold increase in survival of the less favourable patients (>1 negative prognostic factor) and achieved a 5-year survival rate of

20%. Furthermore, Cheon and coll. and Ueda and coll. evidenced that the possibility to perform a radical operation (R0 vs R1) affects long-term survival and report overall 5-year survival rates of 20% and 60%, respectively. It is worth of note that in synchronous cases radical surgery was intended not only in regard to hepatic lesions, to be resected as prescribed by good surgical practice, but also in regard to gastric tumors, to be treated by standard curative D ≥ 2 gastrectomy (table 4).
Data reported in table 2 and 4 show that surgical therapy offers interesting and sound results. On a more realistic level, we must however recognize that these patients, despite all efforts, generally die of cancer progression. Hepatic recurrence is observed in about 70% of cases and in about half of them is associated to extra-hepatic relapse (table 5); if the literature and our experience do not permit an insight into the role of repeated hepatectomies in case of exclusive hepatic recurrence, this observation raises concern about the timing of treatment, in order to avoid superfluous operations. A simple time-test can achieve an acceptable selection once a potential candidate to curative surgery is encountered. It can be easily suggested in case of metachronous lesions with favourable location but it can be contraindicated in case of critically located metastases and, in general, in case of synchronous metastases, especially if associated to symptomatic or resectable gastric primaries. The French school [Adam et al., 2006] strongly suggests a multidisciplinary approach to these patients and, in particular, favours a systemic chemotherapy, to be started at diagnosis whenever possible, in order to offer its advantages to the greatest number of patients and to effectively select cases for surgery.

Author	No	Timing	MST (months)	1-; 3-; 5- year survival rates
Cheon (2008)	58	Synchr. + Metachr.	Overall: 16	No hepatic resection: 29.4%; 0%; 0%
				Hepatic resection ± RFA: 75,3%; 31.7%; 20.8%
Makino (2010)	63	Synchr. + Metachr.	Overall: 16	No hepatic resection: 53.2%; 4.2%; 0%
			Hepatic resection: 31.2	Hepatic resection: 82,3%; 46,4%; 37.1%
Ueda (2008)	72	Synchr.	n.a.	No hepatic resection: 36.4%; 0%; 0%
				Hepatic resection ± HAIC: 80%; 60%; 60%
Tiberio (2008)	73	Metachr.	Overall: 7	
			BST: 5	BST: 22%; 2%; 0%
			Chemotherapy: 12	Chemotherapy: 45%; 6%; 0%
			Hepatic resection: 23	Hepatic resection: 81%; 20%; 20%

n.a. = not available; RFA = radio-frequency-ablation; HAIC = hepatic artery infusion chemotherapy; BST = best supportive treatment;

Table 4. Survival from series considering unselected populations

Author	No.	Hepatic recurrence (%)	Overall recurrence (%)
Miyazaki 1997	21	76.2	81
Fujii 2001	10	50	80
Ambiru 2001	40	72.5	77.5
Ambiru 2001	40	72.5	77.5
Okano 2002	19	63.2	73.7
Okano 2002	19	63.2	73.7
Saiura 2002	10	-	80
Shirabe 2003	36	61.1	83.3
Roh 2005	11	72.7	91
Sakamoto 2007	37	62.2	86.5
Koga 2007	42	50	66.7
Cheon 2008	22	50	63.6
Tiberio 2008	11	62.2	86.5
Makino 2010	16	25	63.6

Table 5. Recurrence after curative surgery.

3.3 Multimodal treatment

Multimodal treatments can further enhance survival rates, in particular if modern, state-of-art chemotherapy protocols are employed. For example we signal that Ueda and coll. reported in the cited work an outstanding 75% 5-year survival rate in a subgroup of 8 patients submitted to radical surgery followed by hepatic artery infusion chemotherapy.

Radio-frequency ablation is another front-line, state-of-art technique to be considered in designing the treatment strategy of hepatic metastases from gastric cancer. This ablative technique is employed either as alternative or in association to hepatectomy, following the guidelines for HCC or for metastases from colo-rectal cancer. It is a minimally invasive and low-cost procedure whose interest is particularly enhanced in case of poor general conditions contraindicating surgery, which is often the case in gastric cancer patients. Its exact role is yet to be defined, as the number of reported procedures is low, follow-up short, data can't always be effectively extrapolated from the context and reports are not unanimous as far as survival results are concerned. However, one paper by Hwang et coll., considered 72 patients with metachronous metastases submitted to different treatments but not to hepatectomy (table 5). They showed that 15 patients without extrahepatic disease treated by RFA ± chemotherapy displayed a median survival of 22 months, with 3- and 5-year survival rates of 50% and 40%, respectively, similar to those reported in the best surgical series. These data are coherent to those by Yamakado et al. which, however, suffer of short follow-up, and to those by Cheon et al.: in their experience a subgroup of 9 patients submitted to RFA compared favourably with 22 patients submitted to radical surgery, with a 4-year survival of 40% and 20%, respectively. Kim and collaborators appear less enthusiastic and report survival results superimposable to those of classic systemic chemotherapy alone. These data need further confirmation but highlight the interest of RFA in the management of these particular cases.

Author	No.	Timing	MST (months)	1-; 3-; 5- year survival rates
Yamakado (2005)	7	Methachronous	RFA + HAIC: 16.5	RFA + HAIC: 85%; n.a; n.a.
Cheon (2008)	9	Synch. + metach	n.a.	RFA: 57%; 40%; n.a.
Hwang (2009)	73	Metachronous	BST*: 3	BST*: 5%; 0%; 0%
			TACE*: 8	TACE*: 38%; 0%; 0%
			Chemoth.*: 15	Chemoth.*: 100%; 0%; 0%
			RFA*: 27	RFA*: 82%; 50%; 40%
Kim (2009)	7	Metachronous	RFA± Chemoth.: 10	RFA: 40%;14%; n.a.

n.a. = not available; HAIC = hepatic artery infusion chemotherapy; BST = best supportive treatment; TACE = trans arterial catheter embolization; * = patients without extrahepatic metastases.

Table 6. Radio-Frequency-Ablation (RFA) of hepatic metastases from gastric cancer.

3. Conclusion

Unexpected 5-year survival rates can be achieved in a subgroup of gastric cancer patients presenting hepatic metastases as sole metastatic site if an adequate treatment is selected. Simple clinical and biological characteristics of both the gastric primary and hepatic involvement display prognostic value which may be helpful in choosing therapeutic strategy, keeping in mind that the best results are achieved by aggressive treatments, which must be proposed whenever possible.

4. References

Adam R, Chiche L, Aloia T, Elias D, Salmon R, Rivoire M, Jaeck D, Saric J, Le Treut YP, Belghiti J, Mantion G and Mentha G for the Association Française de Chirurgie. Hepatic resection for noncolorectal nonendocrine liver metastases. Ann Surg 2006; 244: 524-535.

Ambiru S, Miyazaki M, Ito H, Nakagawa K, Shimizu H, Yoshidome H, Shimizu Y & Nakajima N. Benefits and limits of hepatic resection for gastric metastases. Am J Surg 2001;181:279-283.

Cao W, Yang W, Lou G, Jilang J, Geng M, Xi W, Li H, Ma T& Jin Y. Phase II trial of infusional fluorouracil, leucovorin, oxaliplatin and irinotecan (FOLFOXIRI) as first-line treatment for advanced gastric cancer. Anticancer Drugs 2009; 20: 287-293.

Cheon SH, Rha SY, Jeung H-C, Im C-K, Kim SH, Kim HR, Ahn JB, Roh JK, Noh SH & Chung HC. Survival benefit of combined curative resection of the stomach (D2 resection) and liver in gastric cancer patients with liver metastases. Ann Onc 2008; 19: 1146-1153.

Chiche L, Ducreux M, Lebreton G, Alkofer B & Rouleau V. Métastases hépatiques des cancers de l'estomac. In : Adam R, Chiche L, eds. Chirurgie des métastases hépatiques de cancers non colorectaux non endocrine. Monographies de l'association Française de Chirurgie. Paris: Arnette; 2005: 45-59.

Cocconi G, Carlini P, Gamboni A, Gasperoni S, Rodinò C, Zironi S, Bisagni G, Porrozzi S, Cognetti F, Di Costanzo F, Canaletti R, Ruggeri EM, Camisa R & Pucci F for the Italian Oncology Group for Clinical Research. Cisplatin, epirubicin, leucovorin and 5-fluorourail (PELF) is more active than 5-fluorouracil, doxorubicin and methotrexate (FAMTX) in advanced gastric carcinoma. Ann Oncol 2003; 14: 1258-1263.

D'Angelica M, Gonen M, Brennan MF, Turnbull AD, Bains M & Karpeh MS. Patterns of initial recurrence in completely resected gastric adenocarcinoma. Ann Surg 2004; 240: 808-816.

Dicken BJ, Bigam DL, Cass C, Mackey JR, Joy AA & Hamilton SM. Gastric adenocarcinoma. Review and considerations for future directions. Ann Surg 2005; 241: 27-39.

Faiçal J, Bessaguet C, Nousbaum JB, Cauvin JM, Cholet F, Bideau K, Robaszkiewicz M & Gouerou H. Epidemiology and long term survival of gastric carcinoma in the French district of Finistère between 1984 and 1995. Gastroenterol Clin Biol 2005; 29: 23-32

Fujii K, Fujioka S, Kato K, Machiki Y, Kutsuna Y, Ishikawa A, Takamizawa J, Ko K, Yoshida K, & Nimura Y. Resection of liver metastasis from gastric adenocarcinoma. Hepatogastroenterology 2001; 48: 368-371.

Hwang S-E, Yang D-H & Kim C-Y. Prognostic factors for survival in patients with hepatic recurrence after curative resection of gastric cancer. World J Surg 2009; 33: 1468-1472.

Imamura H, Matsuyama Y, Shimada R, Kubota M, Nakayama A, Kobayashi A, Kitamura H, Ikegami T, Miyagawa SI & Kawasaki S. A study of factors influencing prognosis after resection of hepatic metastases from colorectal and gastric carcinoma. Am J Gastroenterol 2001; 96: 3178-3184.

Japanese Gastric Cancer association. Japanese classification of gastric carcinoma. 2nd English edition. Gastric Cancer 1998; 1: 10-24.

Kerkar SP, Kemp CD & Avital I. Liver resections in metastatic gastric cancer. HPB 2010; 12: 589-596.

Kim HO, Hwang SI, Hong HP & Yoo CH: Radiofrequency ablation for metachronous hepatic metastases from gastric cancer. Surg Laparosc Endosc Percutan Tech 2009; 19 (3): 208-12

Koga R, Junji Y, Shigekazu O, Akio S, Makoto S, Yasunyuki S & Toshiharu Y. Liver resection for metastatic gastric cancer: experience with 42 patients including eight long-term survivors. JJCO 2007; 37: 836-842

Lee J, Kang WK, Kwon JM, Oh SY, Lee HR, Kim HJ Park BB, Lim HY, Han MJ, Park JO & Park YS. Phase II trial of irinotecan plus oxaliplatin and 5-fluorouracil/leucovorin in patients with untreated metastatic gastric adenocarcinoma. Ann Oncol 2007; 18: 88-92.

Makino H, Kunisaki C, Izumisawa Y, Tokuhisa M, Oshima T, Nagano Y, Fujii S, Kimura J, Takagawa R, Kosaka T, Ono HA, Akiyama H, Tanaka K & Endo I. Indication for hepatic resection in the treatment of liver metastasis from gastric cancer. Anticanc Res 2010; 30: 2367-2376.

Marrelli D, Roviello F, De Stefano A, Fotia G, Giliberto C, Garosi L & Pinto E. Risk factors for liver metastases after curative surgical procedures for gastric cancer: a prospective study of 208 patients treated with surgical resection. J Am Coll Surg 2004; 198: 51-58.

Miyazaki M, Itoh H, Nakagawa K, Ambiru S, Shimizu H, Togawa A, Shiobara M, Ohtsuka M, Sasada K, Shimizu Y, Yoshioka S, Nakajima N, Suwa T & Kimura F. Hepatic resection of liver metastases from gastric carcinoma. Am J Gastroenterol 1997; 92: 490-493.

Ochiai T, Sasako M, Mizuno S, Kinoshita T, Takayama T, Kosuge T, Yamazaki S & Maruyama K. Hepatic resection for metastatic tumours from gastric cancer: analysis of prognostic factors. Br J Surg 1994; 81: 1175-1178

Okano K, Maeba T, Ishimura K, Karasawa Y, Goda F, Wakabayashi H, Usuki H & Maeta H. Hepatic resection for metastatic tumors from gastric cancer. Ann Surg 2002; 235: 86-91.

Roh HR, Suh KS, Lee HJ, Yang HK, Choe KJ & Lee KU. Outcome of hepatic resection for metastatic gastric cancer. Am Surg 2005; 71: 95-99.

Saiura A, Umekita N, Inoue S, Maeshiro T, Miyamoto S, Matsui Y, Asakage M & Kitamura M. Clinicopathological features and outcome of hepatic resection for liver metastasis from gastric cancer. Hepatogastroenterology 2002; 49: 1062-1065.

Sakamoto Y, Sano T, Shimada K, Esaki M, Saka M, Fukagawa T, Katai H, Kosuge T & Sasako M. Favorable indications for hepatectomy in patients with liver metastasis from gastric cancer. J Surg Oncol 2007; 95: 534-539.

Shirabe K, Shimada M, Matsumata T, Higashi H, Yakeishi Y, Wakiyama S, Ikeda Y, Ezaki T, Fukuzawa S, Takenaka K, Kishikawa K, Ikeda T, Taguchi K, Maehara Y & Sugimachi K. Analysis of the prognostic factors for liver metastasis of gastric cancer after hepatic resection: a multi-institutional study of the indications for resection. Hepatogastroenterology 2003; 50: 1560-1563.

Tiberio GAM, Coniglio A, Marchet A, Marrelli D, Giacopuzzi S, Baiocchi L, Roviello F, de Manzoni G, Nitti D & Giulini SM. Metachronous hepatic metastases from gastric carcinoma: a multicentric survey. EJSO 2009; 35: 486-491.

Tsujimoto H, Ichikura T, Ono S, Sugasawa H, Hiraki S, Sakamoto N, Yaguchi Y, Hatsuse K, Yamamoto J & Hase K. Outcomes for patients following hepatic resection of metastatic tumors from gastric cancer. Hepatol Int 2010; 4: 406-413.

Ueda K, Iwahashi M, Nakamori M, Nakamura M, Naka T, Ishida K, Ojima T & Yamaue H. Analysis of the prognostic factors and evaluation of surgical treatment for synchronous liver metastases from gastric cancer. Langenbecks Arch Surg 2009; 394: 647-653.

Yamakado K, Nakatsuka A, Takaki H; Mori Y; Tonouchi H, Kusunoki M, Kida H & Takeda K: Prospective Study of Arterial Infusion Chemotherapy Followed by Radiofrequency Ablation for the Treatment of Liver Metastasis of Gastric Cancer. J Vasc Interv Radiol 2005; 16 (12): 1747-1751.

Yoshida M, Ohtsu A, Boku N, Miyata Y, Shirao K, Shimada Y, Hyodo I, Koizumi W, Kurihara M, Yoshida S & Yamamoto S. Longterm survival and prognostic factors in patients with metastatic gastric cancers treated with chemotherapy in the Japan Clinical Oncology Group (JCOG) study. JJCO 2004; 34: 654-659.

Zacherl J, Zacherl M, Scheuba C, Steininger R, Wenzl E, Muhlbacher F, Jakesz R & Längle F. Analysis of hepatic resection of metastasis originating from gastric adenocarcinoma. J Gastrointest Surg 2002; 6: 682-689.

17

Perspectives in the Treatment of Incurable Gastric Cancer

Yves Dittmar and Utz Settmacher
University Hospital Jena
Germany

1. Introduction

Gastric cancer is the second most frequent malignancy in the Western world [1]. The prognosis remains poor despite of advances in diagnostic techniques and therapeutic management: approximately 800.000 new cases und 620.000 cancer related deaths are reported worldwide per year [2]. More than 50% of gastric cancer patients and approximately 40% of esophageal cancer patients either die from a primary unresectable tumor or from tumor recurrence after radical treatment within five years [3]. The main reasons for this are the late onset of predominantly unspecific symptoms and the aggressive biological behavior [4]. Palliative chemotherapy, best supportive care and the interdisciplinary management of severe tumor-related complications (tumor bleeding, tumor perforation, complete obstruction, treatment-refractory pain) are well accepted treatment options whereas non-curative resections of the primary tumor as well as resection of secondary tumor lesions are controversially discussed [5]. However, there is growing evidence that non-curative tumor resections can prolong the remaining life time with acceptable perioperative morbidity [6-8]. Furthermore, the quality of life can be improved by reducing the incidence of severe tumor-related complications [9].

2. General aspects of incurable gastric cancer

Patients who do not undergo surgical or cytoreductive treatment die within three (stage 4) to six months (stage 3) [10,11].

The only option for cure is radical surgical treatment, recently more and more in combination with neoadjuvant and adjuvant chemotherapy [12,13]. With advanced tumor stage survival of resected patients dramatically declines: at UICC stage 1 the 5-year-survival rate of patients with R0 resection is 95%, whereas at stage 2 it ranges from 35% to 65%, depending on the presence of positive lymph nodes and the number of dissected lymph nodes [14,15]. In the rare cases where curative resection is achieved, the 10-year-survival rate ranges from 3% for stage 3b to 5% for stage 4 (according to UICC classification from 2002)[16]. Following the standardized treatment for locally confined gastric cancer the main determining factor for survival is the extent of lymph node involvement although the impact of extended surgical lymph node removal is still under discussion [17].

Unfortunately, the majority of patients with gastric cancer is diagnosed at an advanced stage of the disease and may not be suitable for treatment with curative intent [18]. But which alternatives can be offered to those patients? Especially patients with an incurable stage of the disease have to face the fact that they will die from their tumor within short time. Furthermore, 50% of those patients will develop severe tumor related complications necessitating invasive endoscopic, radiological or surgical treatment [19]. There are two important aspects of individuality in incurable gastric cancer patients: the individuality of the patients and the individuality of the tumor. The decision as to whether aggressive palliative treatment should be used rather than best supportive care or no treatment at all at patients' request depends on the personal expectation of the individual patient [20]. The reponse to that treatment on the other hand is crucially influenced by the molecular biology and the pathological behavior of the tumor [21,22]. Considering these circumstances, it becomes clear that the currently available tumor classification systems are limited with respect to the decision making process [3].

In fact, palliative strategies are much less standardized than curative treatment. A multitude of protocols has been introduced to improve and prolong the remaining life span of palliatively treated patients [23]. Recently first steps towards molecular-based target-specific therapy using trastuzumab and bevacizumab have been undertaken. The importance of surgery for palliative treatment is controversially discussed for more than 40 years [6,7,9,24-26]. Numerous authors reported about prolonged survival, improvement of quality of life and symptom relief and, therefore, supported palliative gastric resection [6,9,26]. Other investigators presented limited retrospective data and recommended gastric resection only in cases of otherwise not controllable complications, such as tumor bleeding or organ perforation [5,27].

Currently two basic palliative treatment strategies can be defined: a canonical palliative treatment strategy including palliative chemotherapy, best supportive care and invasive treatment for severe life-threatening tumor related complications versus cytoreductive (neoadjuvant) chemotherapy plus non-curative tumor resection.

3. Canonical palliative treatment strategy

The widely as beneficial accepted palliative chemotherapy and best supportive care is aimed to improve overall survival and to improve or at least to stabilize the quality of life [5]. Long term survival can be observed in few unusual cases but is not originally an aspired treatment outcome.

Overall, it is generally accepted that patients with incurable gastric cancer who are treated with chemotherapy live longer than those who receive best supportive care only. Several studies indicate that patients who underwent chemotherapy have longer overall survival (11 versus 4 months) and a longer time to progression (6-8 versus 2-3 months) as compared to those patients whose received best supportive care only [28].

The variety of available chemotherapy protocols that have been published during the last 30 years is very wide. Most chemotherapy protocols contain one or a combination of several of the following drugs: antimetabolites (5-Fluoruracil), platinum-containing analoga (cisplatin, oxaliplatin), topoisomerase-1-inhibitors (anthracyclins: epirubicin, doxorubicin), topoisomerase-2-inhibitors (irinothecan), tubulin depolymerisation inhibitors (taxans: paclitaxel, docetaxel) and mitomycin. All abovementioned agents are targeted to somehow disrupt the natural mechanisms of DNA synthesis or of the cell division process. Therefore, these agents manifest their effect not only on tumor cells but also on any other cells within the organism that undergo cell division to maintain the biological tissue and organ integrity.

The most frequently used agent is 5-fluoruracil and its oral analogon capecitabine. It has been described to elucidate an overall response of 20% when administered as a single agent treatment. Wagner and co-workers. compared 13 studies with a total of 1914 patients to evaluate the impact of a combination versus a single agent chemotherapy. Patients with a combination therapy had longer median survival (8.3 vs 6.7 months), longer progression free survival (5.6 vs 3.6 months) and a higher overall response rate (35% vs 18%). Based on these data, most oncologists in western countries do not treat their patients with a single-agent protocol, whereas in Japan the use of S-1 as a single-agent therapy is widely utilized. Furthermore, it was shown in this study that a three-drug combination is better than a two-drug combination in terms of survival as well as tumor response [10].

Clinical trials to study the effectiveness of the novel microtubule-dynamic-instability-inhibiting agent eribulin are currently underway.

But which patients are best siuted for palliative chemotherapy? Overall, the effectiveness of chemotherapy has to be weighed against chemotherapy-related toxicities and side effects. The most important factor to predict the benefit of palliative chemotherapy is to evaluate whether the patient is generally fit for this aggressive treatment. Hepatic, renal and carciopulmonary function should be taken into account. The toxicity increases with the number of chemotherapy agents which are administered in combination. To date, there is no evidence about preoperatively available clinical or pathohistological factors that could predict the response to chemotherapy.

A first step towards a target specific chemotherapy might be the administration of trastuzumab, an inhibitor of the Her2/Neu-receptor. Van Cutsem and co-workers published the data from the ToGA study in 2009 with the main result that patients who were positive for the Her2/Neu receptor chemotherapy plus trastuzumab had a median survival of 13.8 as compared to a median survival of 11.1 months in patients who underwent chemotherapy only. Furthermore, the study group who was treated with the combination chemotherapy showed a higher overall tumor response rate (47% versus 35%), a higher complete response (5% versus 2%) and a longer time to progression (7.1 versus 5.6 months). This treatment has been shown to be effective in patients who are at least double positive for the receptor measured by the FISH test [29]. Trastuzumab was the first molecular target agent showing a survival benefit in patients with advanced gastric cancer. The next step towards target-specific treatment might be the AVAGAST trial which investigates the benefit of the angiogenesis inhibitor bevacizumab plus chemotherapy versus chemotherapy alone [30]. Several studies investigating the survival benefit of further novel angiogenesis inhibitors, such as sorafinib, sunitinib, cediranib and axitinib are currently underway. The survival benefit of cetuximab - an inhibitor of the epidermal growth factor receptor - is currently investigated in a phase 3 trial. In summary, there is a growing selection of target specific agents that are thought to have an impact on the clinical course of advanced gastric cancer but to date only one agent (trastuzumab) has been approved for use in the clinical routine.

The second column of the canonical palliative treatment strategy is the management of severe tumor related complications. Many authors suggest that patients who develop such complications should be treated most preferably by interventional procedures, such as endoscopy or radiological intervention. Only in those cases where interventional approaches are not feasible or where interventional treatment fails and the complication either relapses or persists, patients are considered for surgical treatment. Furthermore, this surgical treatment should be limited to the most restricted possible procedure whereas larger tumor resections should be reserved for rare individual cases. In particular, palliative resections should be avoided [5,27].

The most frequently occurring complications are tumor bleeding, gastric obstruction and tumor perforation. Kang and co-workers analyzed data from 1856 patients with metastasized gastric cancer. Among these, there were 32 patients who had a tumor perforation during palliative chemotherapy. 17 patients underwent emergency surgery with a median survival of 5 months after the perforation whereas 15 patients received antibiotics only and had a median survival of 1 month after the perforation [31]. These data show that survival in patients treated by surgery was longer as than that with non-surgical treatment strategies. Other studies demonstrated that patients who were treated with palliative resection had a lower perioperative mortality as compared to those who underwent simple closure of the perforation only [32].

Tumor bleeding is a frequently observed event in patients with unresectable gastric cancer. Some authors regard substitution of up to 2 units of red blood cells per week as acceptable with respect to tumor bleeding which can be treated by blood transfusion alone [33,34]. However, palliative chemotherapy administration might be limited by persistent bleeding which finally may affect overall survival. Other authors suggest treatment of those patients with short-course radiotherapy up to 30 Gy. Recently, Asakura and co-workers reported a response rate to radiotherapy of 73% [35]. The endoscopic approach provides the opportunity for active and direct hemostasis by local injection of epinephrine, clip application, fibrin application, argon plasma coagulation or stent implantation. In cases of persistent uncontrolled tumor bleeding, surgical treatment has been suggested as an last resort [27]. However, emergency surgery for tumor bleeding usually requires palliative resection and is associated with a high rate of perioperative mortality [35].

The symptoms of progressive tumor-related gastrointestinal obstruction range from dysphagia and nausea to manifest ileus. The endoscopic approach provides a multitude of procedures, such as stent implantation (or even in due course stent-in-stent implantation), argon plasma beam, laser therapy and percutaneous endoscopic assisted gastrostomy. A considerable number of patients receiving endoscopic treatment relapse with obstructive symptoms. Selected patients may undergo surgical treatment, especially those who develop manifest ileus or in cases of endoscopic treatment failure. Whereas patients with lower gastric cancer benefit from a gastrointestinal bypass with low perioperative mortality rates, patients with gastric cancer at the gastroesophageal junction usually require palliative resection associated with higher perioperative mortality rates.

In summary, severe tumor-related complications frequently occur in patients with unresectable gastric cancer. They not only require invasive treatment in the majority of cases but also affect further palliative chemotherapy and, thus, affect overall survival and quality of life.

4. Neoadjuvant chemotherapy plus non-curative surgery for incurable gastric cancer

Whereas the canonical palliative treatment strategy can be regarded as the widely used standard, the combination of chemotherapy with cytoreductive non-curative resection is still under intensive debate.

4.1 Intentions of primary non-curative resection

One intention is to reduce the overall tumor mass by removing the primary tumor with a local R0 stage and by resecting secondary tumor mass. The reduction of secondary tumor growth includes liver metastases, positive lymph nodes and peritoneal carcinosis.

Several molecular considerations make this strategy sensible. Gross tumor formations are thought to be affected in a limited way by chemotherapy agents. Furthermore, it has been demonstrated that the primary tumor produces a local environment presumably via currently not fully understood molecular pathways that creates the precondition for the nidation of circulating tumor cells which subsequently can develop into distant metastases.
The second intention is to reduce the incidence of tumor related complications. In other words, the potentially complications-producing tumor is removed before these complications occur. In fact, the natural course of gastric cancer growth is associated with a considerable number of severe tumor related complications. At least 50% of all patients with non-resected advanced gastric cancer will develop such complications within the remaining life time. These complications frequently require invasive treatment by endoscopic or radiological interventions and emergency surgery in a considerable number of cases. However, emergency procedures are associated with high mortality rates. Based on a retrospective analysis, we found that by primary non-curative gastric resection the incidence of severe tumor related complications decreased as compared to that in patients who did not undergo resection (data not published).
Based on these intentions, primary non-curative resections are implemented to improve overall survival of palliative patients and to improve the quality of life within the remaining life time.

4.2 Study results on non-curative gastric resection

Gastric resections in patients with incurable gastric cancer have been reported for more than 50 years now. The intention to perform such procedures as well as the criteria dedicated to define suitable patients have changed over that relatively long period. Furthermore, the allocation of patients to curative and non-curative strategies becomes increasingly complex: a considerable number of patients with an initially unresectable stage of gastric cancer respond to neoadjuvant chemotherapy and eventually become resectable. To date and for the understanding of this chapter it is important to distinguish two different categories of gastric resections with a postoperative non-R0-result: first the so-called palliative resection, which encompassed initially a collective term for patients who were resected with curative intention but had R1- or R2-situations postoperatively, as well as for those who were primarily resected with palliative intention either due to tumor-related complications or for potential improvement of overall survival; and secondly the term "non-curative gastric resection" which includes patients who have at least one non-curative factor but nevertheless undergo primary gastric resection as a part of the multimodal concept.
Based on data of the last decades, the range of recommendations for palliative surgical treatment is wide. Some authors recommend to perform surgical treatment only in those cases where severe tumor related complications or symptoms are evident and interventional options have failed [27,36]. Other authors proposed that primary palliative resections should be performed whenever technically possible [9]. Palliative gastric resection is not a novel procedure. According to today´s benchmarks, the early beginnings of gastric surgery can be regarded as palliative procedures: the first documented gastric resections have been performed by Pean in 1879 and by Rygydier in 1880, both patients died within the perioperative period. The first successfully performed gastric resection traces back to Billroth (1881). The patient survived four months and died from local tumor recurrence.
The first publication on larger series of palliative gastric resections was in 1958 by Lawrence and McNeer. Data of 1.623 patients who underwent surgery for gastric carcinoma from 1931

to 1955 were analyzed. It was demonstrated that palliative resections (141 cases) achieved remarkable symptom relief as well as it increased the survival time. Perioperative morbidity and mortality, however, were high [24].
Another frequently quoted paper was published in 1979: ReMine et al. reported about 206 patients with non-curable gastric carcinoma who underwent surgical treatment. Palliative partial gastric resection was reported in 46 cases, while gastrectomy was performed in six cases. The other patients underwent gastroenteral bypass or no surgical treatment at all. The decision to extend the procedure from gastric resection to gastrectomy was due to additional proximal tumor infiltration. Although the perioperative mortality was 0% in the gastrectomy group, further survival was disappointing: five of the six patients died within nine months. Patients with palliative gastric resection showed significantly better survival: 20% of these patients lived more than two years. According to these findings, ReMine et al. judged resection to be the superior procedure compared with gastrectomy [25].

Author	Year of publi-cation	Number of patients	Median survival (months)	Peri-operative morbidity	Peri-operative mortality
Huang et al. [7]	2010	n=365	10.5	14-27%	0.5-6%
Kunisaki et al. [8]	2008	n=164	9	15%	4%
Lin et al. [6]	2008	n=183	20	No data	No data
Mizutani et al. [37]	2007	n=13	12	65%	0%
Onate-Ocana et al. [38]	2007	n=71	12.4	32%	8.5%
Lim et al. [39]	2007	n=63	13	No data	No data
Nazli et al.[40]	2007	n=29	10.4	35%	27%
Saidi et al. [41]	2006	n=24	16.3	33%	9%
Miner et al. [27]	2004	n=147	8.3	54%	6%
Medina-Fr. et al. [42]	2004	n=40	13	26%	2.6%
Hartgrink et al. [26]	2002	n=156	8.1	38%	12%
Monson et al. [43]	1991	n=53	19	12%	8%
Bozetti et al. [9]	1987	n=61	8	No data	11%
Meijer et al. [44]	1983	n=26	9.5	No data	8%

Table 1. Published data on palliative gastric resection from 1983 - 2010

Over the last 20 years, several published series of palliative gastric resections showed significant improvement in symptom control, survival and quality of life [6,9,26,37]. In addition, several cases of long term survival following combined palliative treatment have been described. However, in the majority of the published data the definition of "palliative intention" was not properly outlined. Frequently, curatively intended procedures with a postoperative R1-situation were included. In some publications, elective and emergency resections were not separated even though for emergency surgery there is a high rate of perioperative mortality. In several studies, the period of inclusion spans more than 20 years. An overview of the most important publications on palliative gastric resections is shown in Table 1. The median survival ranged from 8 to 20 months, whereas morbidity and mortality ranged from 12% to 65% and from 0% to 27%, respectively. In comparison, data from our hospital based on retrospectively analysed data from 48 patients with non-curable gastric cancer showed a median survival of 15 months with a morbidity of 32% and a mortality of 4% (emergency gastrectomies excluded). Furthermore, long term survival was observed in three cases.

Which patients are suitable for the non-curative gastric resection? The most pronounced benefit can be expected in cases with a limited number of tumor locations (2 tumor locations = primary tumor plus one more secondary tumor formation). Furthermore, younger patients seem to have a better survival following non-curative gastric resection. In a recently published study, Kunisaki and co-workers identified chemotherapy as an independent factor for longer survival in patients with no more than one "non-curative" factor. In our own study population, we found a significantly longer survival for younger patients (<50 years) and for those who had no more than two tumor locations, furthermore the highest benefit was achieved in those patients who underwent chemotherapy according to the ECF scheme.

Generally, at present, non-curative gastric resections should be performed preferentially in patients who can be included in a clinical trial investigating the clinical outcome of palliative surgery. Furthermore, non-curative resections should be part of a multimodal treatment strategy. The personal preferences of the individual patient should be taken into account in the decision-making process and every patient should be discussed in an interdisciplinary tumor conference.

4.3 Surgical treatment for peritoneal carcinosis

Peritoneal carcinosis from gastric cancer commonly indicates an advanced stage of the tumor disease and most frequently is associated with poor prognosis. The median survival time of patients with peritoneal carcinosis from gastric cancer is 3 months [45,46]. In comparison, for colorectal cancer it is 5 months and for ovarian cancer it is 12 - 23 months [47,48]. The degree of peritoneal involvement prior to cytoreductive resection is most frequently described by the peritoneal carcinosis index score (PCI) [49,50]. This index is a combination of peritoneal tumor size and the number and distribution of peritoneal tumors. There is a strong correlation between the PCI value and the prognosis. This has been demonstrated in patients with peritoneal carcinosis from colorectal cancer: patients with PCI up to 10 had 50% overall 5-year survival whereas for PCI 11-20, it was 20% and for PCI more than 20, there was no 5-year survival at all. The cytoreductive surgery in combination with intraperitoneal chemotherapy was first described by Sugarbaker in 1989. The surgical procedure may include parietal and visceral peritonectomy, resection of the liver capsule and the resection of adjacent organs located within the peritoneal cavity [51]. The surgical result is determined by the "completeness of cytoreduction score (CCR)" based on the macroscopic presentation to the surgeon at the end of the procedure [52]. Table 2 gives an overview on the details of PCI.

<table>
<tr><th>Number of the region</th><th>Region</th><th>Size of the largest regional lesion</th><th>Score</th></tr>
<tr><td>0</td><td>central</td><td>no lesion detectable</td><td>0</td></tr>
<tr><td>1</td><td>right cranial</td><td>lesion size smaller than 5mm</td><td>1</td></tr>
<tr><td>2</td><td>epigastric</td><td>lesion size from 5 to 50mm</td><td>2</td></tr>
<tr><td>3</td><td>left cranial</td><td>lesion size larger than 50mm</td><td>3</td></tr>
<tr><td>4</td><td>left side</td><td rowspan="9" colspan="2">Calculation of the PCI-score:

Every region is allocated to the score 0-3.
Then all scores are added up.

PCI can reach a maximum score of 36.</td></tr>
<tr><td>5</td><td>left caudal</td></tr>
<tr><td>6</td><td>pelvic</td></tr>
<tr><td>7</td><td>right caudal</td></tr>
<tr><td>8</td><td>right side</td></tr>
<tr><td>9</td><td>upper jejunum</td></tr>
<tr><td>10</td><td>lower jejunum</td></tr>
<tr><td>11</td><td>upper ileum</td></tr>
<tr><td>12</td><td>lower ileum</td></tr>
</table>

Table 2. Peritoneal carcinosis index

Table 3 shows the classification of the cytoreduction result according to the "completeness of cytoreduction score".

Size of residual tumor	**CCR value**
no residual tumor	0
largest residual tumor smaller than 2.5mm	1
largest residual tumor 2.5-25mm	2
largest residual tumor larger than 25mm	3

Table 3. Classification of the cytoreduction result according to the "completeness of the cytoreduction score"

It is generally accepted that cytoreductive peritoneal resection should be performed in combination with intraperitoneal chemotherapy. Surgery only or surgery in combination with intravenous chemotherapy are not sufficient because some chemotherapy agents, such as 5-FU do not reach an appropriate concentration within the peritoneal cavity to kill cancer cells whereas other agents, such as taxans do not even cross the blood-peritoenal barrier because of their high molecular weight. For that purpose, three procedures depending on the date of administration are available: preoperative intraperitoneal plus systemic chemotherapy (NIPS), hyperthermic intraperitoneal chemotherapy (HIPEC) and early postoperative intraperitoneal chemotherapy (EPIC) [52].

The best results from that combination therapy are achieved when the PCI is low, the CCR is 0 or 1 and there are no free intraperitoneal cancer cells. The Peritoneal Surface Malignancy Group (PSMG) defined several criteria that indicate a high probability for achieving a CCR 0 or 1 in patients with peritoneal carcinosis from colorectal cancer, these criteria are shown in Table 4.

For cytoreductive surgery for peritoneal carcinosis from gastric cancer, the PCI should be limited to a maximum score of 15.

Generally in cases of peritoneal carcinosis from gastric cancer, survival is worse than in other entities, such as ovarian cancer or colorectal cancer. For the combination of surgery with HIPEC, overall median survival from 10 to 16 months and 5-year-survival of 7%-8% have been reported. For colorectal cancer, it was demonstrated that HIPEC has a better clinical outcome in terms of survival than EPIC [53]. Cheong and co-workers observed a median survival of 11 months following cytoreductive surgery combined with EPIC in 154 patients with very advanced gastric cancer [52].

ECOG performance status 0-2*
no evidence of extraabdominal tumor lesions
up to 3 small, resectable parenchymal liver metastases
no evidence of bilary obstruction
no evidence of ureter obstruction
no evidence of intestinal obstruction at more than 1 location
small bowel involvement: no evidence of gross disease in the mesentery with several segmental locations of partial obstruction
small volume disease in gastro-hepatic ligament

*ECOG: Eastern Cooperative Oncology Group

Table 4. Several criteria that indicate a high probability for achieving a CCR 0 or 1 in patients with peritoneal carcinosis from colorectal cancer, defined by the Peritoneal Surface Malignancy Group

4.4 Surgical treatment of liver metastases from gastric cancer

Generally, liver metastases from gastric cancer develop less frequently as compared to other gastrointestinal tumor entities, but in most cases they are unresectable due to general as well as hepatic non-curative factors. Whereas liver metastases develop in approximately 50% of all patients with colorectal carcinoma, the incidence of liver metastases from primary gastric cancer ranges from 5% to 9%.

Liver resection for secondary tumor growth is performed mainly in cases of colorectal liver metastases with resection rates between 20% and 30% and a 5-year survival rate of 25% to 58% [54,55]. In contrast, liver resection for hepatic metastasized gastric carcinoma is a rarely performed procedure: resection rates of liver metastases from gastric cancer range from 11% to 21% [56,57].

The majority of patients remain incurable due to several frequently occurring factors even if extended or multivisceral surgery had been performed. Those incurable factors include bilobar multinodular tumor spread, gross peritoneal dissemination, diffuse affection of distant lymph nodes or unresectable local recurrence. Especially bilobar tumor spread within the liver is more frequent in gastric cancer as compared to other gastrointestinal malignancies in spite of the same venous drainage via the portal vein which rises the question if the pathway follows the portal venuous flow or if liver metastases from gastric cancer are caused by free circulating tumor cells and, thus, have to be regarded as a generalized stage of the tumor disease. This distinct biological behavior may also reflect that molecular signalling and gene expression pattern are different from other gastrointestinal tumors. Even in cases of potentially resectable gastric liver metastases, many medical professionals are reluctant to consider these patients for radical surgical treatment.

The first publication on the clinical outcome after liver resection for gastric cancer metastases was presented by Ochiai and co-workers: they described serosal perforation of the primary tumor (in cases of synchronous liver metastases) as well as lymphangiosis and venangiosis to be negative prognostic factors and reported a median survival time of 18 months and an overall 5-year survival rate of 19% [56]. One of the first western publications with focus on resection of gastric liver metastases was presented in 2001 by Zacherl and co-workers: the median survival of the 15 resected patients was 8.8 months while two of these patients survived more than three years [58]. In a recently published review, 19 studies were analysed to compare the survival following liver resection for hepatic metastasized gastric cancer. Median survival for all 436 patients was 17 months and 5 year survival was 26.5%. No prognostic factor was found to be statistically significant across all studies [59]. Table 5 shows further studies on the topic of radical surgery for gastric liver metastases that have been published since 1994. At present, there are no data available on results from a prospectively conducted trial. Although the currently available study results indicate a significant improvement in terms of disease free and overall survival, all conclusions drawn from these studies are based on retrospectively performed analyses on small patient populations. Therefore, a prospective study should be performed to evaluate the impact of liver resection in patients with isolated liver metastases from gastric cancer.

Author	Year of publication	Number of cases	Median survival in months	Overall 5-year survival
Ochiai et al. [56]	1994	n=21	18	19%
Miyazaki et al. [60]	1997	n=21	NA	9,5%
Fujii et al. [61]	2001	n=10	16,3	10%
Imamura et al. [62]	2001	n=17	12	0%
Ambiru et al. [63]	2001	n=40	12	18%
Zacherl et al. [58]	2002	n=15	8,8	NA
Saiura et al. [64]	2002	n=10	25	20%
Okano et al. [57]	2002	n=19	21	34%
Shirabe et al. [65]	2003	n=36	NA	36%
Sakamoto et al. [66]	2003	n=22	11	38%
Thelen et al. [67]	2006	n=26	9	10%
Tsujimoto et al. [68]	2010	n=17	34	31,5%

Table 5. Studies on radical surgery for gastric liver metastases from 1994-2010

5. The role of quality of life

Health-related quality of life has become a major criterion in the decision-making process in patients with gastric cancer as well as other malignancies. In most recently randomized trials it is an important endpoint parameter [20]. The ultimate challenge in this field, however, is to measure quality of life. In fact, health-related quality of life is a complex variable with a multi-dimensional structure [69]. Although a multitude of publications have been dedicated to this topic during the last two decades, a generally accepted and consistent definition does not exist. The essential tool for measurement of this variable are questionnaires. One of the major problems of interpretation of data related to quality of life is that uniform questionnaires are too unspecific and disease-related questionnaires are limited to small areas of clinical research. The questionnaires refer to four dimensions of patients' perception: physical functions, the emotional experience, the social interactions and symptoms related to the disease itself as well as adverse effects of treatment [69]. The QLQ-30 is one of the most frequently used site-specific questionnaires in the field of cancer research. It can be further particularized by entity-specific questionnaire modules, such as the STO-22 for gastric cancer. Moreover, it has been observed that the baseline physical scores as well as role function and the global quality of life correlate with overall survival which makes several paramaters measured by QLQ-30 valuable in predicting clinical outcome [70].

The impact of surgery on patients who underwent oesphagectomy for oesophageal cancer has been measured by using the QLQ-30 questionnaire. In the early postoperative course, all aspects of the quality of life except the emotional function decreased remarkably. Few scores, such as dysphagia were improved but were overshadowed by other symptoms, such as anorexia, nausea and diarrhoea. Overall, the deterioration of most key aspects resulted in reduced overall scores. Within the following nine months a gradual recovery of those symptoms was observed.

Svedlund and co-workers compared the quality of life of patients with gastric cancer at the time of diagnosis with that of the general population: lower mood, reduced sexual interest, insomnia and poor appetite have been observed in tumor patients as compared to the normal population. Several studies indicated that weight loss as a significant parameter not only for the quality of life but for survival and chemotherapy response. Furthermore, it has been shown by other authors that the preservation of a gastric remnant as well as construction of stomach-like reservoirs resulted in improved quality of life [71,72].

The course of quality of life in patients who undergo cytotoxic treatment mirrors the interplay of disease-related symptoms and treatment-associated toxicity. Glimelius and co-workers compared the clinical outcomes including quality of life of incurable gastric cancer patients who underwent palliative chemotherapy plus best supportive care in comparison to those who received best supportive care only. Both groups showed similar levels of quality of life [73]. Bamias and co-workers showed that patients who underwent palliative chemotherapy according to the ECF scheme had reduced physical and role functioning after 12 weeks whereas emotional functioning remained unaffected over that period. Within the posttreatment period, the global quality of life value improved in comparison to the baseline when the treatment had started. In addition to that, 6 years later it has been demonstrated that the ECF scheme is better tolerated than MCF (epirubicin exchanged with mitomycin) [74]. Furthermore, the comparison between irinothekan-based and docetaxel-based palliative chemotherapy resulted in similar effects on the quality of life: role function, emotional function, social function and sleep function improved 6 months after chemotherapy as compared to the baseline for both chemotherapy regimens but did not differ significantly from each other [75].

Currently, there is only little known about the impact of adjuvant and neoadjuvant chemotherapy in patients with advanced gastric cancer.

6. Perspectives for the strategy of non-curative resection

Due to the aggressive biological behavior of gastric cancer and the late onset of symptoms, 50% have to be regarded as non-curable cases. The well accepted treatment options of palliative chemotherapy as well as best supportive care including the management of severe tumor related complications can be summarized as the so-called canonical palliative treatment strategy.

Due to the lack of prospective randomized trials in this field, to date no recommendation for the value of palliative gastric resection can be given. Nevertheless, there are numerous references that indicate a survival benefit in selected cases. Therefore, the currently available study results show that the impact of non-curative gastric resection in combination with chemotherapy on survival as well as on the quality of life should be evaluated by conducting a prospective study.

Multimodal treatment of peritoneal carcinosis including cytoreductive surgery is effective in cases of PCI up to 15 and if CCR 0-1 can be achieved.

Liver resection or radiofrequency ablation can be performed in cases of limited liver involvement and if extrahepatic secondary tumor growth has been excluded.

7. References

[1] Jemal A, Tiwari RC, Murray T, et al.: Cancer statistics, 2004. CA Cancer J Clin 2004;54:8-29.
[2] Roukos DH, Kappas AM: Perspectives in the treatment of gastric cancer. Nat Clin Pract Oncol 2005;2:98-107.
[3] Dittmar Y, Posorski N, Rauchfuss F, et al.: Relationship between degree of chromosomal aberration and survival in intestinal-type gastric cancer - a preliminary report based on three cases of hepatic metastasized gastric cancer with long-time survival. Onkologie;33:591-596.
[4] Saif MW, Makrilia N, Zalonis A, et al.: Gastric cancer in the elderly: an overview. Eur J Surg Oncol;36:709-717.
[5] Moehler M, Lyros O, Gockel I, et al.: Multidisciplinary management of gastric and gastroesophageal cancers. World J Gastroenterol 2008;14:3773-3780.
[6] Lin SZ, Tong HF, You T, et al.: Palliative gastrectomy and chemotherapy for stage IV gastric cancer. J Cancer Res Clin Oncol 2008;134:187-192.
[7] Huang KH, Wu CW, Fang WL, et al.: Palliative resection in noncurative gastric cancer patients. World J Surg;34:1015-1021.
[8] Kunisaki C, Makino H, Takagawa R, et al.: Impact of palliative gastrectomy in patients with incurable advanced gastric cancer. Anticancer Res 2008;28:1309-1315.
[9] Bozzetti F, Bonfanti G, Audisio RA, et al.: Prognosis of patients after palliative surgical procedures for carcinoma of the stomach. Surg Gynecol Obstet 1987;164:151-154.
[10] Wagner AD, Unverzagt S, Grothe W, et al.: Chemotherapy for advanced gastric cancer. Cochrane Database Syst Rev:CD004064.
[11] Chu DZ, Lang NP, Thompson C, et al.: Peritoneal carcinomatosis in nongynecologic malignancy. A prospective study of prognostic factors. Cancer 1989;63:364-367.
[12] Cunningham D, Allum WH, Stenning SP, et al.: Perioperative chemotherapy versus surgery alone for resectable gastroesophageal cancer. N Engl J Med 2006;355:11-20.

[13] Jiang Y, Ajani JA: Multidisciplinary management of gastric cancer. Curr Opin Gastroenterol;26:640-646.
[14] Rajdev L: Treatment options for surgically resectable gastric cancer. Curr Treat Options Oncol;11:14-23.
[15] Feng XY, Chen YB, Chen S, et al.: [Relationship between the number of lymph node detection and prognosis in stage II gastric cancer after D(2) dissection]. Zhonghua Wei Chang Wai Ke Za Zhi;13:346-349.
[16] Hundahl SA, Phillips JL, Menck HR: The National Cancer Data Base Report on poor survival of U.S. gastric carcinoma patients treated with gastrectomy: Fifth Edition American Joint Committee on Cancer staging, proximal disease, and the "different disease" hypothesis. Cancer 2000;88:921-932.
[17] Coburn NG: Lymph nodes and gastric cancer. J Surg Oncol 2009;99:199-206.
[18] Shah MA, Kelsen DP: Gastric cancer: a primer on the epidemiology and biology of the disease and an overview of the medical management of advanced disease. J Natl Compr Canc Netw;8:437-447.
[19] Sarela AI, Miner TJ, Karpeh MS, et al.: Clinical outcomes with laparoscopic stage M1, unresected gastric adenocarcinoma. Ann Surg 2006;243:189-195.
[20] Conroy T, Marchal F, Blazeby JM: Quality of life in patients with oesophageal and gastric cancer: an overview. Oncology 2006;70:391-402.
[21] Carneiro F, Oliveira C, Leite M, Seruca R: Molecular targets and biological modifiers in gastric cancer. Semin Diagn Pathol 2008;25:274-287.
[22] Wu WK, Cho CH, Lee CW, et al.: Dysregulation of cellular signaling in gastric cancer. Cancer Lett;295:144-153.
[23] Menges M, Hoehler T: Current strategies in systemic treatment of gastric cancer and cancer of the gastroesophageal junction. J Cancer Res Clin Oncol 2009;135:29-38.
[24] Lawrence W, Jr., Mc NG: The effectiveness of surgery for palliation of incurable gastric cancer. Cancer 1958;11:28-32.
[25] ReMine WH: Palliative operations for incurable gastric cancer. World J Surg 1979;3:721-729.
[26] Hartgrink HH, Putter H, Klein Kranenbarg E, et al.: Value of palliative resection in gastric cancer. Br J Surg 2002;89:1438-1443.
[27] Miner TJ, Jaques DP, Karpeh MS, Brennan MF: Defining palliative surgery in patients receiving noncurative resections for gastric cancer. J Am Coll Surg 2004;198:1013-1021.
[28] Boku N: Perspectives for personalization in chemotherapy of advanced gastric cancer. Discov Med;9:84-89.
[29] Bang YJ, Van Cutsem E, Feyereislova A, et al.: Trastuzumab in combination with chemotherapy versus chemotherapy alone for treatment of HER2-positive advanced gastric or gastro-oesophageal junction cancer (ToGA): a phase 3, open-label, randomised controlled trial. Lancet;376:687-697.
[30] Shah MA, Jhawer M, Ilson DH, et al.: Phase II Study of Modified Docetaxel, Cisplatin, and Fluorouracil With Bevacizumab in Patients With Metastatic Gastroesophageal Adenocarcinoma. J Clin Oncol;29:868-874.
[31] Kang MH, Kim SN, Kim NK, et al.: Clinical outcomes and prognostic factors of metastatic gastric carcinoma patients who experience gastrointestinal perforation during palliative chemotherapy. Ann Surg Oncol;17:3163-3172.

[32] Shih CH, Yu MC, Chao TC, et al.: Outcome of perforated gastric cancer: twenty years experience of one institute. Hepatogastroenterology;57:1320-1324.
[33] Mackay S, Hayes T, Yeo A: Management of gastric cancer. Aust Fam Physician 2006;35:208-211.
[34] Kumagai K: [Oncologic emergencies in gastric cancer patients]. Nippon Geka Gakkai Zasshi 2004;105:281-285.
[35] Asakura H, Hashimoto T, Harada H, et al.: Palliative radiotherapy for bleeding from advanced gastric cancer: is a schedule of 30 Gy in 10 fractions adequate? J Cancer Res Clin Oncol;137:125-130.
[36] Moehler M, Galle PR, Gockel I, et al.: The multidisciplinary management of gastrointestinal cancer. Multimodal treatment of gastric cancer. Best Pract Res Clin Gastroenterol 2007;21:965-981.
[37] Mizutani S, Shioya T, Maejima K, et al.: Significance of gastrectomy as palliative surgery for gastric carcinoma with pyloric stenosis. J Nippon Med Sch 2007;74:241-245.
[38] Onate-Ocana LF, Mendez-Cruz G, Hernandez-Ramos R, et al.: Experience of surgical morbidity after palliative surgery in patients with gastric carcinoma. Gastric Cancer 2007;10:215-220.
[39] Lim S, Muhs BE, Marcus SG, et al.: Results following resection for stage IV gastric cancer; are better outcomes observed in selected patient subgroups? J Surg Oncol 2007;95:118-122.
[40] Nazli O, Yaman I, Tansug T, et al.: Palliative surgery for advanced stage (stage IV) gastric adenocarcinoma. Hepatogastroenterology 2007;54:298-303.
[41] Saidi RF, ReMine SG, Dudrick PS, Hanna NN: Is there a role for palliative gastrectomy in patients with stage IV gastric cancer? World J Surg 2006;30:21-27.
[42] Medina-Franco H, Contreras-Saldivar A, Ramos-De La Medina A, et al.: Surgery for stage IV gastric cancer. Am J Surg 2004;187:543-546.
[43] Monson JR, Donohue JH, McIlrath DC, et al.: Total gastrectomy for advanced cancer. A worthwhile palliative procedure. Cancer 1991;68:1863-1868.
[44] Meijer S, De Bakker OJ, Hoitsma HF: Palliative resection in gastric cancer. J Surg Oncol 1983;23:77-80.
[45] Sakata Y, Ohtsu A, Horikoshi N, et al.: Late phase II study of novel oral fluoropyrimidine anticancer drug S-1 (1 M tegafur-0.4 M gimestat-1 M otastat potassium) in advanced gastric cancer patients. Eur J Cancer 1998;34:1715-1720.
[46] Koizumi W, Narahara H, Hara T, et al.: S-1 plus cisplatin versus S-1 alone for first-line treatment of advanced gastric cancer (SPIRITS trial): a phase III trial. Lancet Oncol 2008;9:215-221.
[47] Hardy JR, Wiltshaw E, Blake PR, et al.: Cisplatin and carboplatin in combination for the treatment of stage IV ovarian carcinoma. Ann Oncol 1991;2:131-136.
[48] Curtin JP, Malik R, Venkatraman ES, et al.: Stage IV ovarian cancer: impact of surgical debulking. Gynecol Oncol 1997;64:9-12.
[49] Jacquet P, Sugarbaker PH: Clinical research methodologies in diagnosis and staging of patients with peritoneal carcinomatosis. Cancer Treat Res 1996;82:359-374.
[50] Glehen O, Gilly FN: Quantitative prognostic indicators of peritoneal surface malignancy: carcinomatosis, sarcomatosis, and peritoneal mesothelioma. Surg Oncol Clin N Am 2003;12:649-671.

[51] Esquivel J, Sticca R, Sugarbaker P, et al.: Cytoreductive surgery and hyperthermic intraperitoneal chemotherapy in the management of peritoneal surface malignancies of colonic origin: a consensus statement. Society of Surgical Oncology. Ann Surg Oncol 2007;14:128-133.
[52] Yonemura Y, Endou Y, Sasaki T, et al.: Surgical treatment for peritoneal carcinomatosis from gastric cancer. Eur J Surg Oncol;36:1131-1138.
[53] Elias D, Benizri E, Di Pietrantonio D, et al.: Comparison of two kinds of intraperitoneal chemotherapy following complete cytoreductive surgery of colorectal peritoneal carcinomatosis. Ann Surg Oncol 2007;14:509-514.
[54] Manfredi S, Lepage C, Hatem C, et al.: Epidemiology and management of liver metastases from colorectal cancer. Ann Surg 2006;244:254-259.
[55] Shimada H, Tanaka K, Endou I, Ichikawa Y: Treatment for colorectal liver metastases: a review. Langenbecks Arch Surg 2009;394:973-983.
[56] Ochiai T, Sasako M, Mizuno S, et al.: Hepatic resection for metastatic tumours from gastric cancer: analysis of prognostic factors. Br J Surg 1994;81:1175-1178.
[57] Okano K, Maeba T, Ishimura K, et al.: Hepatic resection for metastatic tumors from gastric cancer. Ann Surg 2002;235:86-91.
[58] Zacherl J, Zacherl M, Scheuba C, et al.: Analysis of hepatic resection of metastasis originating from gastric adenocarcinoma. J Gastrointest Surg 2002;6:682-689.
[59] Kerkar SP, Kemp CD, Avital I: Liver resections in metastatic gastric cancer. HPB (Oxford);12:589-596.
[60] Miyazaki M, Itoh H, Nakagawa K, et al.: Hepatic resection of liver metastases from gastric carcinoma. Am J Gastroenterol 1997;92:490-493.
[61] Fujii K, Fujioka S, Kato K, et al.: Resection of liver metastasis from gastric adenocarcinoma. Hepatogastroenterology 2001;48:368-371.
[62] Imamura H, Matsuyama Y, Shimada R, et al.: A study of factors influencing prognosis after resection of hepatic metastases from colorectal and gastric carcinoma. Am J Gastroenterol 2001;96:3178-3184.
[63] Ambiru S, Miyazaki M, Ito H, et al.: Benefits and limits of hepatic resection for gastric metastases. Am J Surg 2001;181:279-283.
[64] Saiura A, Umekita N, Inoue S, et al.: Clinicopathological features and outcome of hepatic resection for liver metastasis from gastric cancer. Hepatogastroenterology 2002;49:1062-1065.
[65] Shirabe K, Shimada M, Matsumata T, et al.: Analysis of the prognostic factors for liver metastasis of gastric cancer after hepatic resection: a multi-institutional study of the indications for resection. Hepatogastroenterology 2003;50:1560-1563.
[66] Sakamoto Y, Ohyama S, Yamamoto J, et al.: Surgical resection of liver metastases of gastric cancer: an analysis of a 17-year experience with 22 patients. Surgery 2003;133:507-511.
[67] Thelen A, Jonas S, Benckert C, et al.: Liver resection for metastatic gastric cancer. Eur J Surg Oncol 2008;34:1328-1334.
[68] Tsujimoto H, Ichikura T, Ono S, et al.: Outcomes for patients following hepatic resection of metastatic tumors from gastric cancer. Hepatol Int;4:406-413.
[69] Fayers PM: Quality-of-life measurement in clinical trials--the impact of causal variables. J Biopharm Stat 2004;14:155-176.

[70] Blazeby JM, Conroy T, Bottomley A, et al.: Clinical and psychometric validation of a questionnaire module, the EORTC QLQ-STO 22, to assess quality of life in patients with gastric cancer. Eur J Cancer 2004;40:2260-2268.
[71] Svedlund J, Sullivan M, Liedman B, Lundell L: Relationship of tumor burden and patients' minimization of distress in facing surgery for gastric cancer. Psychosomatics 2005;46:233-243.
[72] Gockel I, Pietzka S, Junginger T: [Quality of life after subtotal resection and gastrectomy for gastric cancer]. Chirurg 2005;76:250-257.
[73] Glimelius B, Ekstrom K, Hoffman K, et al.: Randomized comparison between chemotherapy plus best supportive care with best supportive care in advanced gastric cancer. Ann Oncol 1997;8:163-168.
[74] Bamias A, Hill ME, Cunningham D, et al.: Epirubicin, cisplatin, and protracted venous infusion of 5-fluorouracil for esophagogastric adenocarcinoma: response, toxicity, quality of life, and survival. Cancer 1996;77:1978-1985.
[75] Bouche O, Raoul JL, Bonnetain F, et al.: Randomized multicenter phase II trial of a biweekly regimen of fluorouracil and leucovorin (LV5FU2), LV5FU2 plus cisplatin, or LV5FU2 plus irinotecan in patients with previously untreated metastatic gastric cancer: a Federation Francophone de Cancerologie Digestive Group Study--FFCD 9803. J Clin Oncol 2004;22:4319-4328.[